SIXTH EDITION

INTRODUCTION TO COMPUTERS for Healthcare Professionals

Irene Joos, PhD, RN
Associate Professor
La Roche College
Pittsburgh, Pennsylvania

Ramona Nelson, PhD, RN-BC, ANEF, FAAN
Professor Emerita, Slippery Rock University
President, Ramona Nelson Consulting
Allison Park, Pennsylvania

Marjorie J. Smith, PhD, RN, CNM
Emerita Professor of Nursing
Winona State University
Winona and Rochester, Minnesota

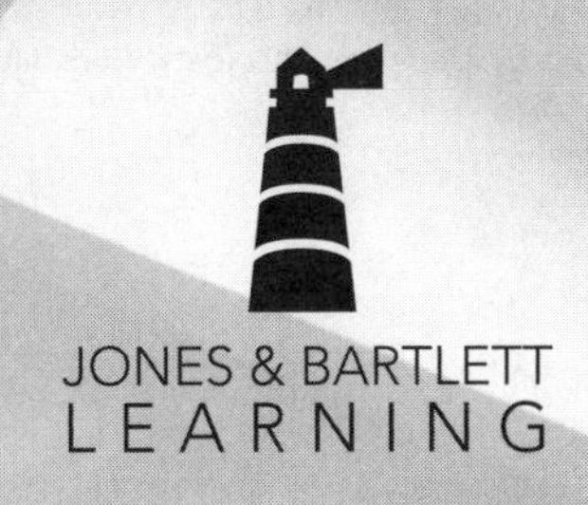

JONES & BARTLETT
LEARNING

World Headquarters
Jones & Bartlett Learning
5 Wall Street
Burlington, MA 01803
978-443-5000
info@jblearning.com
www.jblearning.com

Jones & Bartlett Learning books and products are available through most bookstores and online booksellers. To contact Jones & Bartlett Learning directly, call 800-832-0034, fax 978-443-8000, or visit our website, www.jblearning.com.

Substantial discounts on bulk quantities of Jones & Bartlett Learning publications are available to corporations, professional associations, and other qualified organizations. For details and specific discount information, contact the special sales department at Jones & Bartlett Learning via the above contact information or send an email to specialsales@jblearning.com.

Production Credits

Executive Publisher: William Brottmiller
Senior Editor: Amanda Harvey
Associate Managing Editor: Sara Bempkins
Production Editor: Keith Henry
Senior Marketing Manager: Jennifer Stiles
V.P., Manufacturing and Inventory Control: Therese Connell
Composition: Laserwords Private Limited, Chennai, India
Photo Research and Permissions Coordinator: Joseph Veiga
Cover Design: Scott Moden
Cover Image: © Inga Ivanova/ShutterStock, Inc.
Printing and Binding: Edwards Brothers Malloy
Cover Printing: Edwards Brothers Malloy

To order this product, use ISBN: 978-1-284-03026-6

Library of Congress Cataloging-in-Publication Data

Joos, Irene Makar, author.
Introduction to computers for healthcare professionals / Irene Joos, Ramona Nelson, Marjorie J. Smith.—6e.
p. ; cm.
Includes bibliographical references and index.
ISBN 978-1-4496-9724-2 (pbk.)
I. Nelson, Ramona, author. II. Smith, Marjorie J., 1936- author. III. Title.
[DNLM: 1. Computer Systems. 2. Medical Informatics. 3. Computer Literacy. 4. Computer User Training—methods. W 26.55.C7]
R858
610.285—dc23

2013025624

6048

Printed in the United States of America
17 16 15 14 13 10 9 8 7 6 5 4 3 2 1

Dedication

The sixth edition of this book is dedicated to our families, including our children and our grandchildren. These are the people who continue to provide us with new meaning and joy during the mad rush of our busy lives.

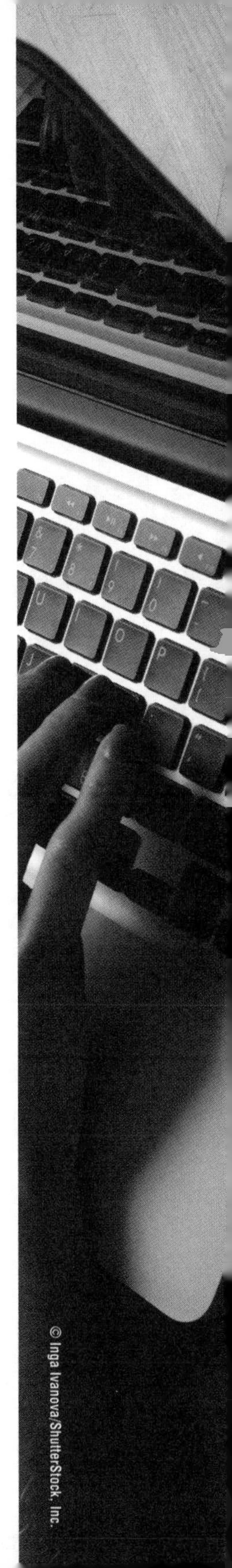

Contents

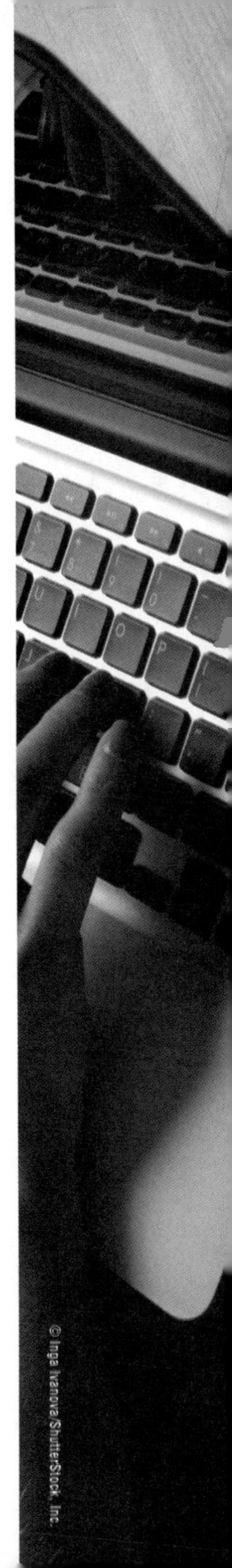

About the Authors

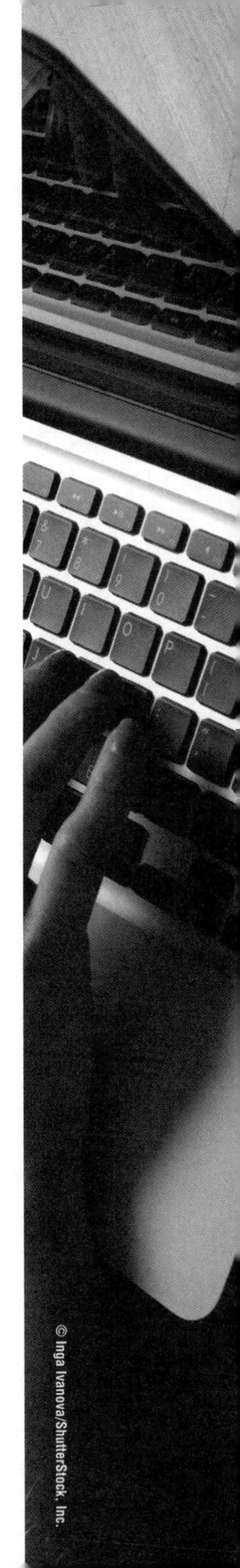

Irene Joos

Irene Joos is an associate professor in the Information Systems Technology (IST) Department at La Roche. Dr. Joos has also served as the Director of Online Learning, and the Director of Library and Instructional Technologies at La Roche College. Dr. Joos received her baccalaureate degree in nursing from Pennsylvania State University. She holds a master's degree in both medical-surgical nursing and information science and a doctorate in education from the University of Pittsburgh.

Dr. Joos has taught medical-surgical nursing, foundations, basic nursing concepts and theories, professional nursing role, and nursing informatics courses at diploma, baccalaureate, and graduate programs. With two grants, she was instrumental in the installation of interactive video units in the skills laboratory and she managed both the microcomputer and skills laboratory at the University of Pittsburgh School of Nursing, Learning Resources Center. She teaches office automation, management of information systems, cyberspace, computer based training, senior seminar, virtual communities and social media, and nursing informatics courses to both undergraduate and graduate students in on-campus and online formats. As the Director of Online Learning she was instrumental in planning and implementing the online initiative at La Roche College. This included supporting online students and faculty as well as conducting training sessions for faculty in online teaching and use of Blackboard. She serves as the faculty advisor for the website of the student's literary journal, *Nuances*.

Dr. Joos's area of interest is the use of technology to help us do our work in an efficient and effective manner. This includes using technology in whatever arena you might find yourself—education, research, or practice. This has been the focus of her publications and presentations, the most recent being *Social Media for Nurses* (2013) published by Springer Publishing and a chapter on distance education in *Health Informatics: An Interprofessional Approach* (2014) published by Elsevier (Mosby).

Ramona Nelson

Ramona Nelson holds a baccalaureate degree in nursing from Duquesne University and a master's degree in both nursing and information science, as well as a PhD in education, from the University of Pittsburgh. She has also completed a postdoctoral fellowship at the University of Utah with Dr. Judy Graves. Currently president of her own consulting company, Dr. Nelson was previously a Professor of Nursing and chair of the Department of Nursing at Slippery Rock University, which led to her appointment as Professor Emerita. Her teaching at the University included courses related to healthcare informatics, community health, nursing research, and school nurse courses. All of these courses were offered via Web-based distance education. Her primary area of research is nursing informatics with a focus on theoretical concepts in health informatics, consumer informatics, and distance education. Dr. Nelson's consulting services are focused on the development of informatics courses and the integration of informatics concepts/skills in the curriculum of healthcare professionals as well as on the delivery of learning via distance education.

Dr. Nelson has been an active member of several professional organizations including NLN, ANA, AMIA, and HIMSS. She is a fellow in the American Academy of Nursing and the NLN Academy of Nursing Education. She has written textbooks, monographs, book chapters, journal articles, Internet publications, abstracts, and newsletters. Her most recent publications include *Social Media for Nurses* (2013) published by Springer Publishing and *Health Informatics: An Interprofessional Approach* (2014) published by Elsevier (Mosby).

Marjorie J. Smith

Marjorie J. Smith is an Emerita Professor of Nursing at Winona State University, Winona and Rochester, Minnesota, where she was the first Director of the Master's Program in Nursing. Dr. Smith received her baccalaureate degree in nursing from the University of Wisconsin, Madison. Her master's degree in childbearing/childrearing family nursing and doctorate in adult education are from the University of Minnesota. She is a certified nurse–midwife.

Dr. Smith taught medical-surgical nursing, pediatric nursing, and obstetrical nursing at the undergraduate level in diploma, associate degree, and baccalaureate programs. She also taught graduate courses in nursing theory, research, women's health care, instruction and evaluation, nursing informatics, and healthcare technology and computers. She was chief editor of the textbook *Child and Family: Concepts of Nursing Practice*, published by McGraw-Hill. She has also written a computer assisted learning program, *The Client Using the Birth Control Pill*, published by Medi-Sim.

Dr. Smith received the Outstanding Educator Award from the Mayo School of Health Related Sciences in 1998. In 2000 she received the Outstanding Nurse Educator award from the Minnesota Association of Colleges of Nursing. In 2009 Dr. Smith was selected as one of the 100 distinguished alumni of the University of Minnesota's School of Nursing in celebration of its centennial. Outstanding individuals were selected from some 8500 living alumni who were deemed to have made great achievements to advance health care or who were doing significant work in the nursing profession that has had a profound impact on families, communities, the school, or the nursing profession. Dr. Smith continues her work related to CenteringPregnancy, a model of group prenatal care that is part of the Centering HealthCare Institute. She also continues her work with computers and enjoys an active travel and family life.

Preface

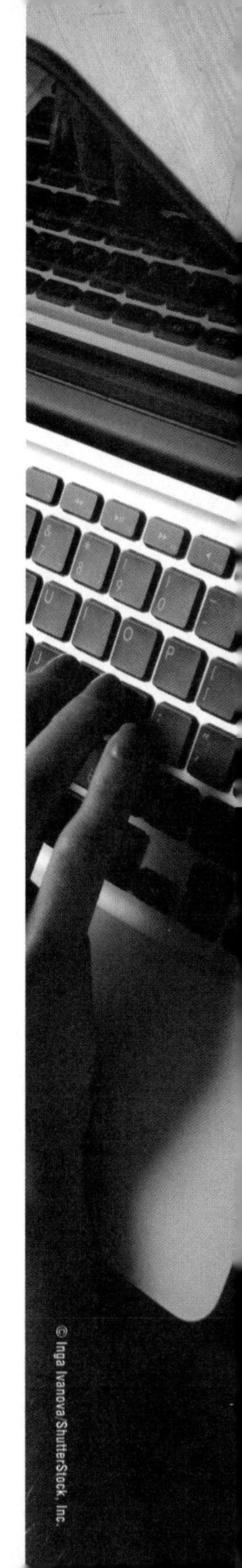

The need for computer- and information-literate healthcare professionals has been well documented in the professional literature of the healthcare disciplines. On November 29, 1999, the Institute of Medicine (IOM) released a report called *To Err Is Human: Building a Safer Health System* (Kohn, Corrigan, & Donaldson, 2000). This report estimated that medical errors kill between 45,000 and 98,000 hospitalized Americans each year. Additional fatal errors also occur in nonhospitalized patients. Automated healthcare information systems and electronic health records have been identified as a critical element in improving the safety of all patients; the development and use of such systems require that health professionals are computer and information literate.

As a follow-up to this report, more than 150 experts attended a Health Professions Education Summit in 2002, the goal of which was to assist the IOM Committee on Health Profession Education Summit, develop strategies to ensure that educational systems for health professionals are consistent with the principles of the 21st century healthcare system. Based on this summit, the IOM issued a seminal report titled *Health Professions Education: A Bridge to Quality* (Greiner & Knebel, 2003).

The report stated that doctors, nurses, pharmacists, and other health professionals are not adequately prepared to provide the highest quality and safest medical care possible. To meet this challenge the report called on educators, as well as accreditation, licensing, and certification organizations, to ensure that students and working professionals develop and maintain proficiency in five core competencies: patient-centered care, interdisciplinary teams, evidence-based practice, quality improvement, and informatics. To obtain competency in informatics, healthcare professionals must be computer and information literate. The IOM publication called upon the healthcare professions to make this a reality, and several healthcare professional organizations have taken up this call. The Joint Task Force of the American Health Information Management Association (AHIMA) and American Medical Informatics Association (AMIA) have focused on the education of healthcare workforce as shown in the follow example:

> *There are several important cross-cutting issues, including the wide variety of health professionals—from physicians and nurses to therapists and admissions staff—who are or will be using EHRs as part of their day-to-day activities. This, in turn, has an impact on the broad range of training needed, from basic computer literacy to more sophisticated computer applications and health information technology.* (AHIMA & AMIA, 2008, p. 5)

In nursing, this call was answered by the American Nurses Association (ANA), the National League for Nursing (NLN), and the American Association of Colleges of Nursing (AACN). The American Nurses Association's *Nursing Informatics: Scope and Standards of Nursing Informatics Practice* (2008) identified informatics competencies that are required of all nurses. "These competencies are categorized in three overall areas: computer literacy, information literacy and professional development/leadership" (ANA, 2008, p. 36).

In 2008 both the NLN and the AACN documented the need for computer, information, and informatics literacy within nursing. The AACN stated in the revised *Essentials of Baccalaureate Education for Professional Nursing Practice* that "graduates must have basic competence in technical skills, which includes the use of computers, as well as the application of patient care technologies such as monitors, data gathering devices, and other technological supports for patient care interventions. . . . Computer and information literacy are crucial to the future of nursing" (2008, p. 17). The NLN's focus is on preparing nursing faculty and administrators to provide the education needed in schools of nursing. Its recommendations for faculty and administration preparation are outlined in its position paper, *Preparing the Next Generation of Nurses to Practice in a Technology-Rich Environment: An Informatics Agenda* (2008). In addition, the NLN posted an Informatics Toolkit as a resource for faculty. (This toolkit, which can be seen at http://www.nln.org/facultyprograms/facultyresources/index.htm, builds from computer literacy to information literacy to informatics literacy.) This text is listed as a resource within this toolkit at http://www.nln.org/facultyprograms/facultyresources/computer.htm.

At the same time that these professional associations were encouraging educational institutions to prepare healthcare professionals who are computer and information literate, the TIGER Initiative was established by a group of informatics specialists in 2004. The acronym TIGER stands for **T**echnology **I**nformatics **G**uiding **E**ducation **R**eform. This initiative brought together nursing stakeholders "to develop a shared vision, strategies, and specific actions for improving nursing practice, education, and the delivery of patient care through the use of health information technology (IT)" (TIGER Initiative, n.d., p. 2).

The TIGER Nursing Informatics Competencies Model consists of three units:

1. Basic Computer Competencies
2. Information Literacy
3. Information Management (including use of an electronic health record)

These competencies are detailed in the TIGER Collaborative Summary Report, which can be found at http://www.tigersummit.com/9_Collaboratives.html. The TIGER initiative has now been established as a tax-exempt formation, and continues to develop resources supporting competencies in informatics, including computer and information literacy. Additional information on these current initiatives can be seen at http://www.thetigerinitiative.org/default.aspx

The topic of computer and information literacy has also been the focus of research studies. For example, in 2009 B. L. Elder and M. L. Koehn reported on their research comparing nursing students' self-rated computer skills with their ability to perform those skills. Most faculty who teach these skills would not be surprised to learn that the Elder and Koehn research demonstrates that students rate themselves higher on their computer skills than their actual performance warrants. They went on to conclude that "many students still need assistance with basic computer skills, especially those related to college course expectations. Therefore, faculty in higher education will be faced with this ongoing problem for several years" (2009, p. 152).

The failure to provide students with effective computer and information literacy skills has a negative impact on healthcare delivery. Campbell and McDowell (2011) assessed the computer and information literacy needs of RNs who face increasing pressure to quickly implement the Meaningful Use requirements for electronic health records. They found that 47% of the nursing staff surveyed had little or no self-perceived competency with most of the hardware/software items in the study. As this study demonstrates, healthcare institutions are rushing to implement electronic health records but are forced to provide remediation for healthcare professionals who lack the necessary computer and information literacy skills needed in today's healthcare environment.

The sixth edition of *Introduction to Computers for Healthcare Professionals* reflects the ever-changing world of computers, their applications, and the "real world" of today. It features updated lesson material, exercises, and activities that provide additional experience with the Internet, social media, Windows 7, and Microsoft Office 2010.

The first chapter incorporates information about computer and digital literacy and its importance in the workforce; it also includes basic steps in computer use and provides an introduction to email and OneNote. Chapter 2, "Information Systems: Hardware, Software, and Connectivity," which presents basic information necessary to understand current technology, has been updated to reflect changing technology. Chapter 3, "The Computer and Its Operating System Environment," now includes more desktop and Windows management concepts and exercises, while still providing foundational concepts on managing files and folders. Chapter 4, "Software Applications: Common Tasks," provides information and activities common to Microsoft Office software programs. These include, for example, the common Microsoft interface; using online help; creating, opening, and saving files; printing; and the cut/copy/paste functions.

Chapters 4–8, the software application chapters, have been updated to reflect the skill set needed to use the Office 2010 suite effectively. Chapter 8 was revised to reflect current database concepts and functions, including database functions within Excel.

Chapters 9 and 10, the Internet and communications chapters, have been updated to reflect the evolving world of the Internet and related communication activities including Web 2.0 tools and the growing influence of the mobile technology workforce on communication. Chapter 11 has been updated to reflect the evolving use of the Internet in delivering distance education. This chapter is written from the perspective of a student with the goal of maximizing student learning in the online environment.

Chapters 12–14 move on to concepts in automation in health care. Chapter 12 "Information: Access, Evaluation, and Use," discusses specific information literacy skills that are imperative to the implementation of evidence-based practice in today's healthcare setting. It includes concepts and exercises about search strategies and the subsequent evaluation and use of the retrieved health-related information, including information from social media sites. These concepts can be used to educate patients as well as to search the professional literature, including gray literature. Chapter 13 focuses on privacy and security. It addresses threats to and procedures for protecting privacy, confidentiality, integrity, and security of personal data including health-related data. The book concludes with the chapter "Introduction to Healthcare Informatics and Health Information Technology," which provides the learner with an introduction to the discipline and specialty of health informatics, as well as information systems used in healthcare delivery.

It is our sincere hope that this book will serve as a sound foundation for developing computer and information literacy skills for healthcare professionals and, in turn, improve the quality of patient care delivered by these professionals.

References

American Health Information Management Association & American Medical Informatics Association. (2008). *Health information management and informatics core competencies for individuals working with electronic health records.* Retrieved from http://www.ahima.org/schools/FacResources/RESOURCEworkforce_2008.pdf

American Association of Colleges of Nursing. (2008). *The essentials of baccalaureate education for professional nursing practice.* Retrieved from http://www.aacn.nche.edu/Education/pdf/BaccEssentials08.pdf

American Nurses Association. (2008). *Scope and standards of nursing informatics practice.* Silver Spring, MD: Author.

Campbell, C. J., & McDowell, D. E. (2011). Computer literacy of nurses in a community hospital: Where are we today? *Journal of Continuing Education in Nursing, 42*(8), 365–370.

Elder, B. L., & Koehn, M. L. (2009). Assessment tool for nursing student computer competencies. *Nursing Education Perspective, 30*(3), 148–152.

Greiner, A., & Knebel, E. (Eds.). (2003). Institute of Medicine: Committee on the Health Professions Education Summit: *Health Professions Education: A Bridge to Quality.* Washington, DC: The National Academies Press.

Kohn, L. T., Corrigan, J. M., & Donaldson, M. S. (Eds.). (2000). *To err is human: Building a safer health system.* Washington, DC: National Academy Press.

National League for Nursing. (2008). *Preparing the next generation of nurses to practice in a technology-rich environment: An informatics agenda.* Retrieved from http://www.nln.org/aboutnln/PositionStatements/informatics_052808.pdf

The TIGER Initiative. (n.d.). *Collaborating to integrate evidence and informatics into nursing practice and education: An executive summary.* Retrieved from http://www.tigersummit.com/uploads/TIGER_Collaborative_Exec_Summary_040509.pdf

Acknowledgements

First, we would like to acknowledge the personnel at Jones & Bartlett Learning who made this book possible, beginning with Amanda Harvey, Senior Editor, Nursing. Amanda provided much-needed support, information, and guidance as we decided when to write the sixth edition of this book, especially in regard to which versions of the different technologies and software would most likely meet the needs of the readers and the faculty who use this book. Second, we would like to acknowledge Sara Bempkins, Associate Managing Editor, Nursing, who was our "go to" person, handling scheduling, manuscript preparation, ancillary development, and any other questions or problems that are inherent in writing a book of this size. Sara's quick responses and problem-solving ideas greatly helped to keep the project on schedule. Next, we would like to acknowledge Keith Henry, Production Editor, Nursing, who handled the copyediting and page proof management and who guided the manuscript preparation through to publication. Finally, we would like to acknowledge Jennifer Stiles, Senior Marketing Manager, who provided all of the marketing and promotional efforts and materials to support the distribution of this book.

In addition to these Jones & Bartlett Learning personnel, we would also like to acknowledge friends, family, and colleagues who provided specific assistance, beginning with Chris Meyer, PhD, RN, Sr. Consultant–Accelerated Services at McKesson Corporation, who worked carefully with Fairfield Medical Center (http://www.fmchealth.org) to ensure that the book includes actual and current screen shots of an electronic health record while ensuring that the information within the EHR screenshots do not divulge actual patient data.

Special thanks also go to Carolyn Ryno, Administrative Assistant, Master's Program in Nursing, Winona State University; and Jane Timm, MS, RN-BC, Supervisor, Nursing Informatics, and Linda Griebenow, MS, RN-BC, Informatics Nurse Specialist from the Mayo Clinic Rochester, for their reviews and suggestions.

And last, we would like to thank LaVerne Collins and Jackie Bolte, librarians at La Roche College, for their ability to quickly locate and provide reference materials, and Brian Joos for his research and reviews.

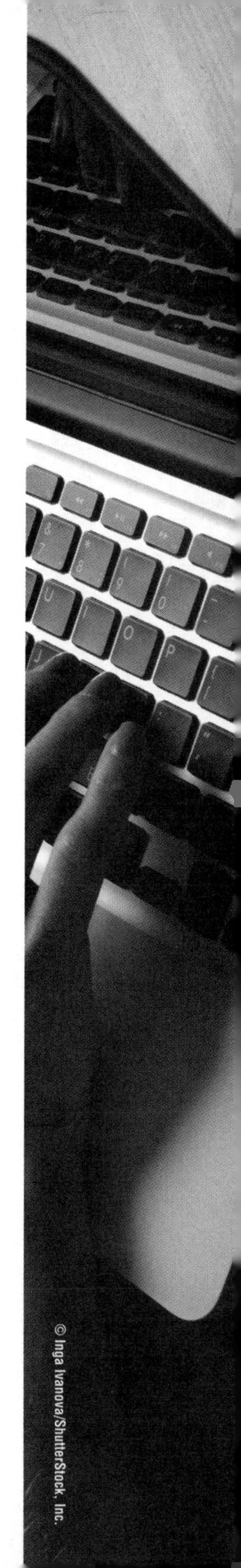

chapter 1

On The Way to Computer and Information Literacy

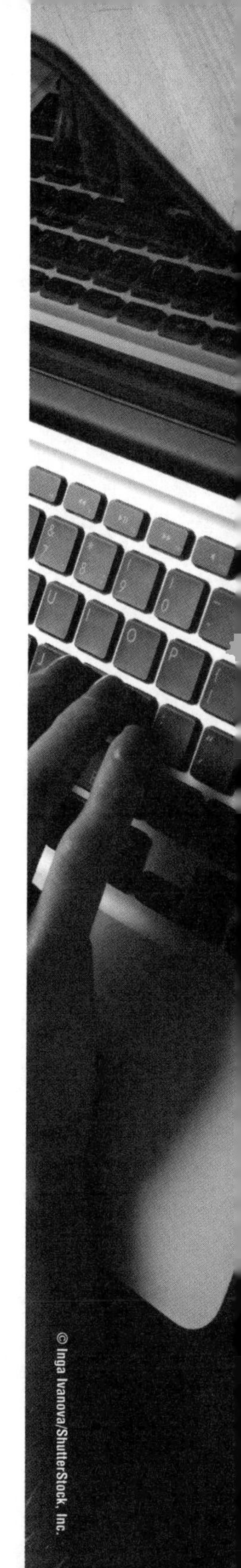

Objectives 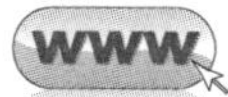

1. Define the concepts of information and computer literacy.
2. Review the organization of this text.
3. Identify elements of a computer lab system.
4. Identify the hardware and software components needed for email communication.
5. Log in to a computer system.
6. Send email messages.
7. Download and upload an email attachment.
8. Identify and prevent security threats when using email.
9. Create a PDF file.
10. Compress and unzip a file.
11. Use selected features in OneNote.

Introduction

Healthcare professionals increasingly rely on information systems to assist them in providing quality care. They realize that a large percentage of their practice involves the management of information. Computers are often required to perform information-related functions such as identifying patient needs; documenting care; providing remote patient care through telemedicine facilities; organizing, calculating, and managing financial data; and accessing healthcare literature. To use the tools of automation in meeting their responsibilities and to take advantage of evolving computer technologies, healthcare professionals must be computer and information literate.

The purpose of this text is to help you develop the essential computer and information literacy skills that all healthcare professionals need. Its focus is the introduction of concepts that cross specific applications, the development of practical computer skills, the access and use of information to provide quality patient care, and the development of electronic communication skills. Each chapter provides exercises from the healthcare arena that demonstrate the concepts and skills and provide practice in applying those concepts and skills.

Literacy

Healthcare providers learn to use the tools necessary to provide patient care, such as a stethoscope to assess patients and a pulse oximeter to measure a patient's pulse and oxygen saturation. This practice involves understanding the function and purpose of the stethoscope and pulse oximeter as well as developing skill in using them. Just as healthcare providers learn to use the right tools, so they must learn the function and purpose of computers and software in health care as well as develop skill in their use. In other words, healthcare providers must become "computer and information literate."

Literacy

Literacy means the ability to locate and use information to make decisions and to function in society, both personally and professionally.

Computer Literacy

Add "computer" to the term "literacy," and it refers to the ability to use the computer to do practical tasks. A variety of viewpoints exist that identify computer skills required for computer literacy, but there is general agreement that **computer literacy** includes the ability to use basic computer applications to complete tasks.

Information Literacy

This term describes a set of skills that enables a person to identify an information need, locate and access the required information, evaluate the information found, and communicate and use that information effectively. With the explosion of information, both good and bad, **information literacy** has taken on a major role in all educational settings.

Digital Literacy

Digital literacy is the ability to effectively and critically use digital technology to navigate, evaluate, and create information. It includes the ability to understand and use information that is presented in multiple formats.

People who are computer, information, and digital literate have the following characteristics. They:

- Use the computer, appropriate digital technologies, and associated software as tools to complete their work in a more effective and efficient manner.
- Recognize the need for accurate and complete information as the basis for intelligent decision making.
- Find appropriate sources of information using successful search strategies.
- Evaluate and manage information to facilitate their work.
- Communicate information in various formats.
- Integrate technology and information strategies into their daily professional lives.

Many professional organizations and accrediting agencies now include information and computer literacy requirements as part of their criteria. For example, the Association of College and Research Libraries (ACRL) produced a document defining and outlining specific criteria and standards for demonstrating information literacy in higher education (ACRL, 2000). To support the development of information literacy, they developed a Web site with links and citations to information literacy standards and curricula developed by accrediting agencies, professional associations, and institutions of higher education. You can view the ACRL Web site at http://www.ala.org/acrl/standards/informationliteracycompetency. Chapter 12 provides additional information on the concept of literacy.

Organization of the Text

This text consists of 14 chapters and an index that features highlighted terms. Most chapters begin with information that introduces the content, describes key concepts and terms, and, in application chapters, provides descriptions of common application functions and keystrokes. Each chapter also includes one or more exercises for use in the classroom or computer laboratory to practice application of lesson concepts and one or more assignments to demonstrate your knowledge and acquired skills. Additional materials for exercises and assignments are available to download from the text's Web site.

The first chapter provides material that is useful to understanding and using this text as well as an introduction to email and OneNote. Chapters 2, 3, and 4 contain content about hardware and software. Computer hardware and software terms are introduced in Chapter 2. Chapter 3 focuses on managing the computer environment. Chapter 4 covers tasks that are common to most application programs. As a consequence of this consistency, many applications in a graphic environment have common looks and functions. The next four chapters present word processing (Word), presentation graphics (PowerPoint), spreadsheet (Excel) and database applications (Excel database features), including database functionality within the spreadsheet application. We use Microsoft Office applications to illustrate the basic concepts of each of these chapters. The text then introduces basic Internet concepts for connecting and browsing, and related software such as Internet Explorer and Chrome. Chapters 9, 10, and 11 share tips for successful communication over the Internet and in distance education endeavors. Chapters 12 and 13 review means of accessing information resources and issues of security, integrity, and ethical use of electronic data. Chapter 14 provides an introduction to the field of healthcare informatics.

The authors have made every attempt to select current quality Internet sites that demonstrate the presented concepts. Remember, however, that Internet sites can and do change, so some of the links may not work. You may have to practice your searching skills to find the current location of the page or a similar site.

Before Beginning: Some Helpful Information

Every computer system and every computer laboratory have subtle differences that can cause problems for the beginner; therefore, learning something about the computer environment in use is essential. Professors or computer laboratory personnel as well as university documentation can help to answer questions about the following topics.

Accounts

Is an **account** necessary to use the computer laboratory or university's resources? If so, what is the process for getting one? Some schools have at least a 24-hour wait time before you can use the laboratories. By comparison, other schools automatically create an account when a student registers or provide facilities and directions to create an instant account. Some schools require students to own laptops or mobile devices, but you will still need an account to sign in to the school's network. A separate account may also be necessary to access course materials made available through the Internet or that reside on course management software servers. Other schools use a one login option that provides access to all the resources to which a student may be entitled.

Cost

Is there a user charge for accessing and using the university's computer equipment and software? Do the rates vary (less at night or during off-peak times)? Is a computer fee included in tuition charges? What does the fee cover? For example, there may be an additional fee for computer equipment and/or applications with selected courses or for activities like printing.

Documentation

Most universities provide user **documentation**. This includes user documentation that provides helpful information for starting and learning specific software programs. Where is the documentation? Are handouts available in the computer laboratory and/or are the documents available online to read and/or print? Which documentation is necessary to begin? For example, the university might have a document called "Getting Started with Outlook" or "Accessing the Network from Home," or "Accessing the University Resources with a Mobile Device."

Computer Laboratories

Are there computer laboratories and who has access to them? Is an identification card required to use the equipment and software? Are some laboratories reserved for specific student populations—for example, health professional students or engineering students—or are all laboratories general-purpose facilities that are available to all students, staff, and faculty?

Equipment/Mobile Devices/Storage

Which type of hardware is available? Are the computers always left on? If not, how do you turn them on? Can you bring your own laptop or mobile device to the computer labs and connect to the network? Is it wireless or wired? What are the requirements for connecting your laptop or mobile device to the network while on campus? Where can students store data files? Do you automatically have storage space on the network? If so, how much? Which types of storage devices can you use and where can you purchase them? Does the bookstore sell removable storage devices?

Laboratory Hours

What are the laboratory hours? Do they change during the term? Is the laboratory open over the weekend? Some laboratories expand their hours of operation toward the end of the term when many papers and projects are due. Does a laboratory assistant need to be present for the laboratory to be open, or is the laboratory left unattended? If so, do you need an ID to enter a closed lab?

Lease or Buy

Does the university have a program whereby students lease or buy a laptop computer or mobile device for use at home, in the dormitory, or in the classroom? If so, how long does it take to get a computer? How does the university support this program in terms of repair, software, and other technical issues? Is there a protection plan offered? Can you buy the computer or mobile device at the end of the lease? Is a certain operating system (i.e., Windows or Mac OS) required?

Logging In

Most resources that you will need as a student and as a professional will require you to **log in** to the system. Some institutions have a universal login that provides a customized home page (referred to as a portal) with all your resources a click away; other institutions require separate accounts for each resource like the network, email, library online databases, student records, course management software, and so forth. Is there a log-in procedure (a series of steps to access the computer software)? If so, how do you log into the system? Is there a help sheet to follow?

Policies/Rules

What are the policies that govern use of the university resources? Policies can include anything from how often to change a password to how many pages one can print each term to respecting the rights of other users. What are the penalties for not adhering to the policies? Penalties might range from a warning for a minor offense to dismissal or expulsion for a major offense. Most universities as well as other organizations and businesses provide policies to each account holder. For example, most institutions will address confidentiality of data and protection of a password in the policies. Individuals who hold dual roles, such as a student employee, may need to follow policies for both roles.

In addition there may be rules or policies that apply to certain areas or applications. For example, what are the rules that govern use of the computer laboratories? Many laboratories prohibit eating and drinking, chatting, and game playing. Laboratories can restrict the lab to academic use only. Some laboratories also check all removable storage devices that one brings into the laboratory for viruses. What are the rules for mobile devices?

Printing

Which printing capabilities are available at the university? Can you print to college printers with your mobile device? Is there access to color printing? Is there a charge for printing? Some schools use a prepaid print card, keep an electronic record of printing that allows individual billing, or use a software program such as PaperCut to keep track of printing costs. When the printing credits go to zero, the student must add more print credits to continue printing. Other schools permit unlimited printing.

Support/Help

What kind of support is available when one needs help? Many universities provide a help desk to assist students, faculty, and staff who have questions or are experiencing problems. In addition there are often online help services and quick reference guides. Are there orientation classes for the laboratories and/or training classes on specific software? Key questions in accessing these resources include (1) What is the telephone number for the help desk? (2) What is its email address? (3) What are the hours for live support? (4) What automated services are available for support and (5) Who can use the services?

Getting Started with Your Computer

It is wise to review the material in this section before beginning work on a computer.

Enter	Throughout this text, **Enter** refers to the Enter or return key. When the word "Enter" appears in this text, do not type it. Instead, press the Enter or return key with a left-pointing (↵) arrow.
Bold	Instructions in bold indicate what to click on, which keys to press, or what to type. Computers are very exacting. A misspelled word or failure to place a blank where a blank is required may result in an error message. When instructions indicate to type, make sure you type exactly what is in bold.
Ctrl+X	When Ctrl (or Alt or Shift) appears with a plus sign (+) and function key number or letter, press the first key and then, while holding it down, press the correct function or letter key. Release both keys together. On a Mac computer the Command key, next to the space bar, works like the Ctrl key on a Windows computer.
Version	The specific sequence and location of commands vary with different **versions** of software. In this text, we use Microsoft Office 2010 for the word processing, presentation graphics, spreadsheet, and database content, and Internet Explorer (version 9) and Chrome (version 25.0.1364.97) for the two browsers. If you are using different versions or a Mac, some of the specific commands will be different.
Windows/Mac OS	Although the exercises for Word, Excel, PowerPoint, Internet Explorer, and Chrome are intended for Windows 7 users, you can just as easily use Mac-based programs for these exercises. Most of the keystrokes are exactly the same. A few menu items and a few keys on the keyboard are different. Although we made every attempt to replicate the windows in true form, your system may display some variations in terms of how the window "looks." Despite these minor differences, you should be able to follow along in the exercises.

Developing a Few Basic Skills

This section covers concepts and skills of logging in, working with PDF files, and compressing/extracting zip files/folders.

Logging In

To log in:

1. From off campus, you may be required to type an **address** in a browser, such as intranet.laroche.edu, to access the main internal Web page, press **Ctrl+Alt+Delete** to access the log-in screen, or open an **icon** on the desktop for a specific system. **Figure 1-1** provides two examples.
2. Type your **UserID** or **user name** in the appropriate textbox.
3. Type your **password** in the appropriate text box. NOTE: The password will not show but will have asterisks or black dots in place of the typed letters and numbers. Some system passwords are case sensitive.

NOTE: Some systems you access may require specific settings to function properly. For example, Blackboard requires you to enable JavaScript and cookies while Microsoft's Web-based access to Outlook requires you to enable pop-ups. Your institution should provide you with instructions to enable these should they be required.

Working with PDF Files

Working in the computer environment requires some knowledge of working with files that you might need for a class or that you might need to send to your professor. Many professors use PDF (portable document format) files as they are files

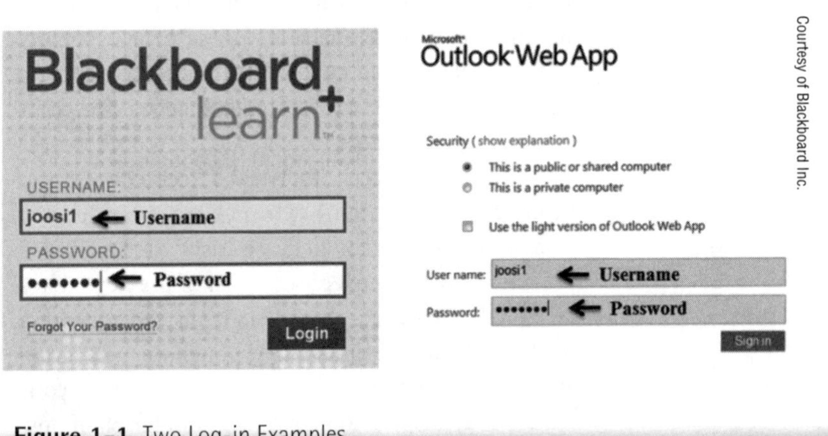

Figure 1-1 Two Log-in Examples

with a fixed-layout, neutral format for file exchange and publishing. Two popular fixed-layout, neutral formats are Adobe PDF and Microsoft PDF or XPS (XML Paper Specification).

To open a PDF file you must have a PDF reader on your computer such as Acrobat Reader, which is available for download from Adobe Systems.

To save a file as PDF:

1. Click the **File** tab File in Word.
2. Click **Save As**. The Save As Dialog Window opens (See Chapter 4).
3. In the File Name Box, type a **name** for the file if it has not been saved before.
4. In the Save as type list, click **PDF**. See **Figure 1-2a**.
5. After choosing PDF other choices become available. See **Figure 1-2b**.
    a. If the document requires high-quality print, click **Standard** (publishing online and printing).
    b. If file size is more important than print quality, click **Minimum size** (publishing online).
    c. If you want the file to open in the selected format after saving, select the **Open file after publishing** check box.
6. Click **Option** button to set the page to be printed, to choose whether markup should be printed, and to select output options. Click **OK** when finished.
7. Click **Save**.

NOTE: The procedure for saving a file in PDF format may vary depending on the program you are using. Some require you to select **Publish to** or **Print, Print**, and to change the printer to Adobe PDF. For more information, search Microsoft Office Help online for "Save as PDF or XPS format."

Compressing Files and Folders

Windows 7 comes with a compression utility that allows you to send or receive large or multiple files. Other programs that zip and unzip files include WinZip and StuffIt. Faculty may send textbook files in zip or compressed format to you as email attachments, place them on a file server, or post them to a CMS (Course Management System).

To compress a file:

1. Select the **file** or **folder** from your storage device or space.
2. Right-click the **file** or **folder**.
3. Choose **Send To** and then **Compressed** (Zipped) Folder. See **Figure 1-3**. A compressed folder appears in the same place as the original folder.

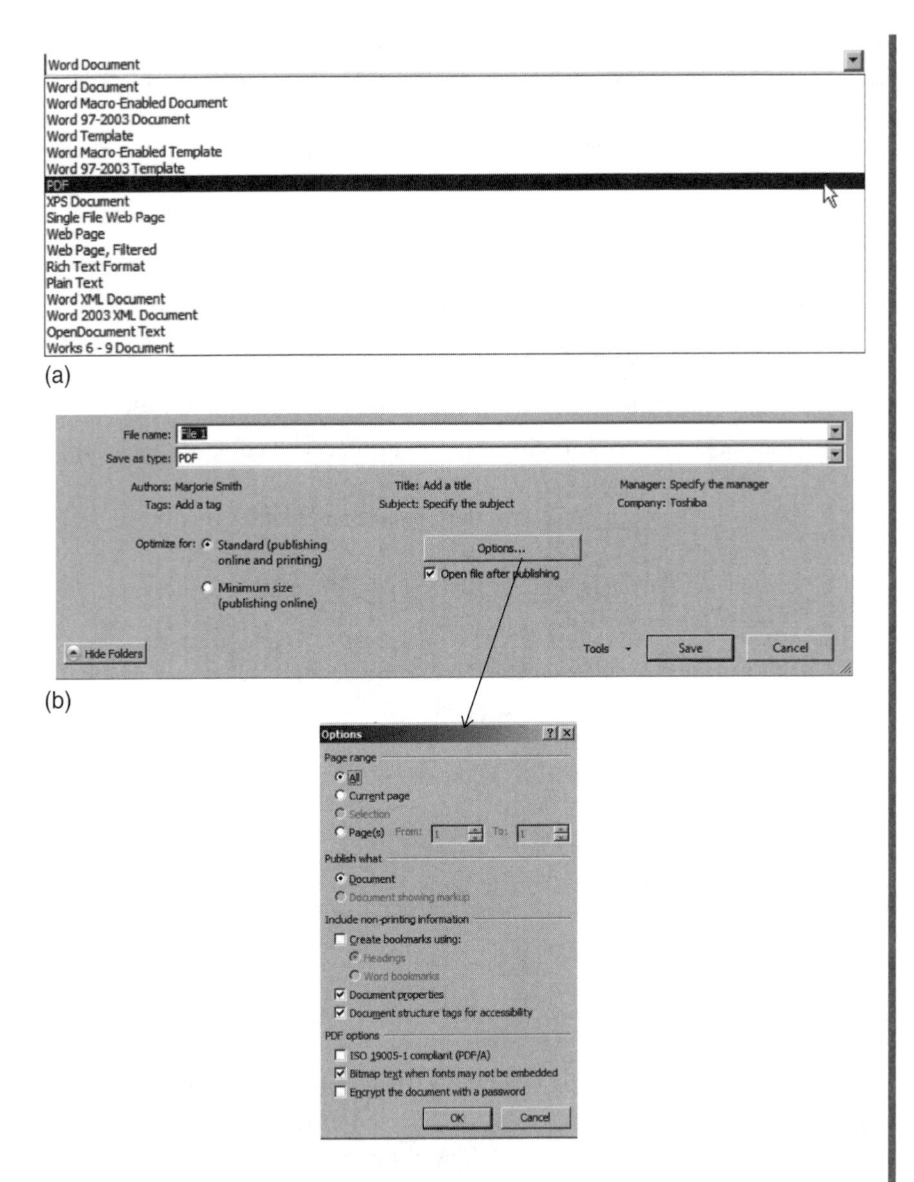

Figure 1-2 (a) "Save As Type" List for Saving a File as a PDF (b) Choices When Saving a File as a PDF

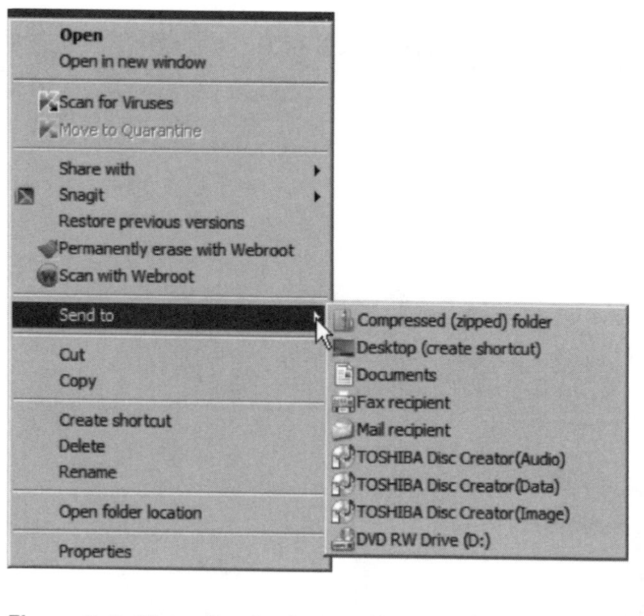

Figure 1-3 Dialog Box for Compressing a File/Folder

To unzip a file:

1. Double-click the **compressed file** or **folder**. (See **Figure 1-4a**.) You may also **right-click** the compressed file or folder. Choose **Open with**, and then **Compressed** (Zipped) Folder or WinZip. (See **Figure 1-4b**.) Note that your window might look slightly different but will function similarly.
2. Select the **appropriate file** or **folder** to extract and then click the **extract all files** text. Again, a button may be available on a toolbar that you can use to extract files, depending on the program.

NOTE: Although you can view compressed files, they will *not* work properly until you extract them.

Communicating by Email

The basics of technology-assisted communication such as email require a sender, channel, medium, and receiver, as illustrated in **Figure 1-5**. Both the sender and the receiver of an email message must have the appropriate hardware and software, and

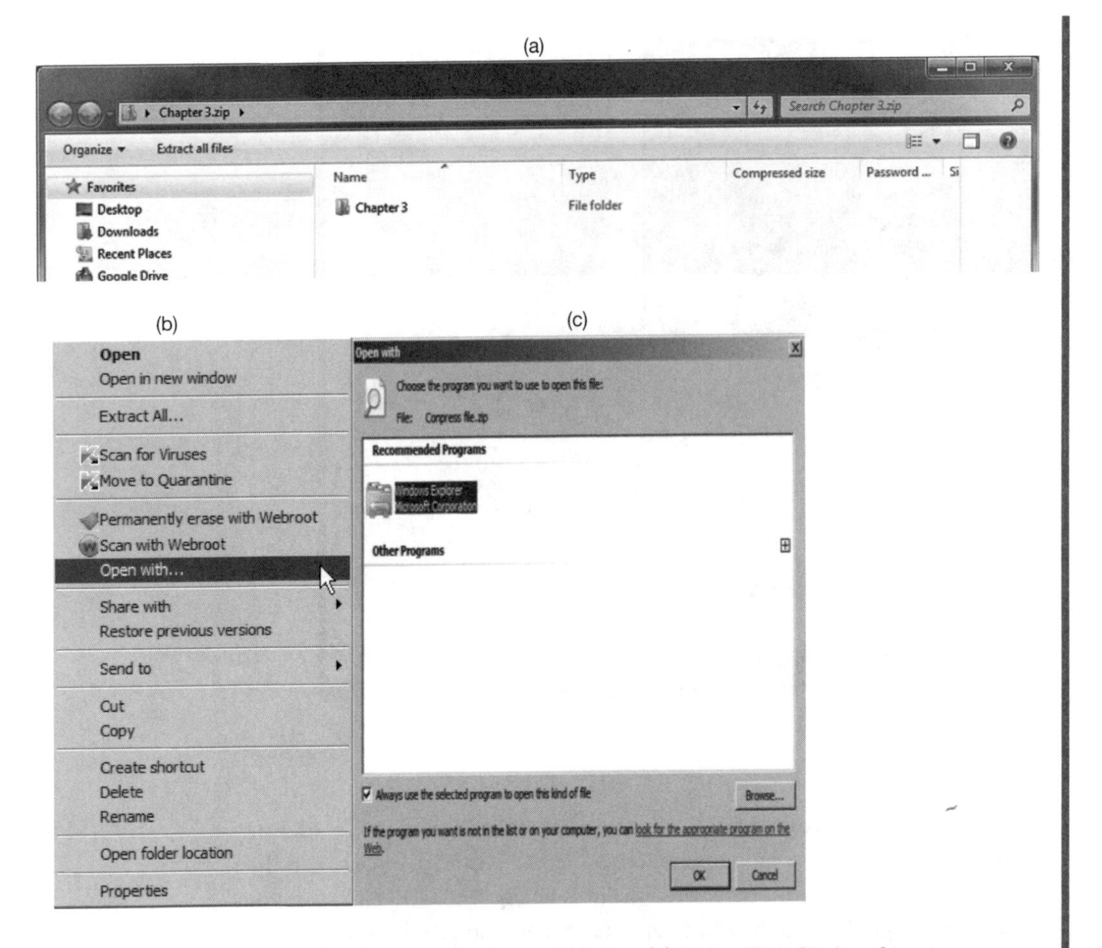

Figure 1-4 (a) Double-Click Compressed File/Folder Window (b) Right-Click Choices for Compressed File/Folder (c) Open With Dialog Box for File/Folder

a connection to the network if they are to communicate successfully. The sender creates the message and, using a specific application on a device, codes the message for transmission across a channel. The channel includes equipment such as telephone wires, twisted-pair, fiber-optic cables, radio waves, or satellites as well as the software that actually transmits the message to the decoder. You must connect the technology device to the communications channel by a modem, a router, a network card, or a wireless card in the computer. The computer that receives the message must then decode or translate the message back into a format that the receiver can

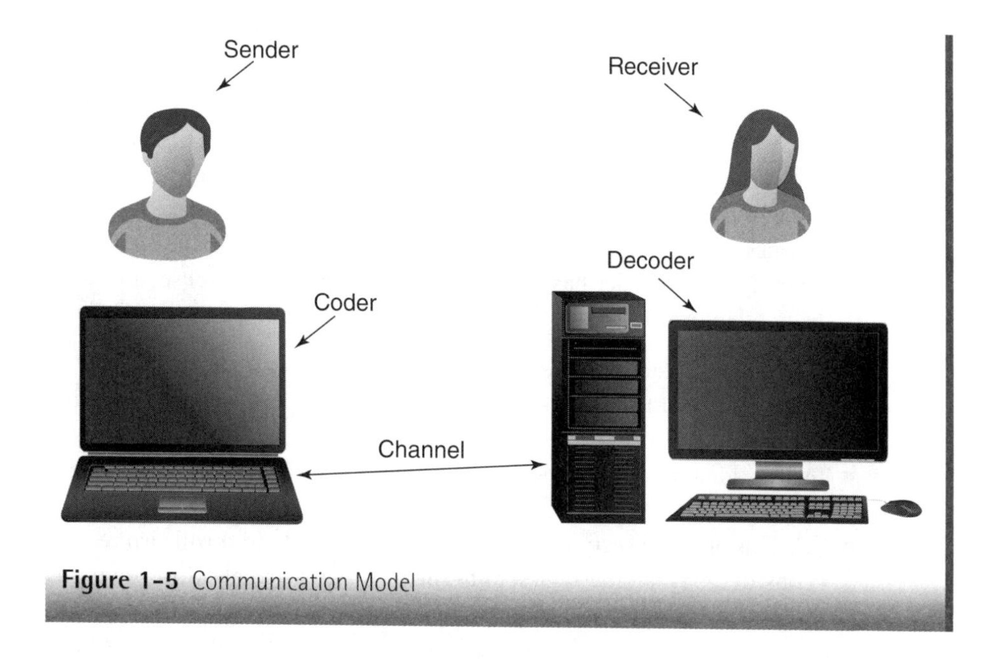

Figure 1-5 Communication Model

understand. It is essential that both computers, as well as the channel, support the same communications protocol and standards if they are to "talk" to each other. For cell phones you use the same wireless connection for making and receiving calls but instead the phone connects to a cell tower and then the Internet.

Obviously, most computers do not have a direct channel as seen in **Figure 1-5**, but rather send messages through a network. Most universities and hospitals are networked. A network consists of all computers and related devices connected together for the purpose of sharing devices, programs, and data. Refer to Chapter 2 for additional information on networks and to Chapter 9 for additional information on the Internet. Chapter 10 discusses other forms of technology assisted communication.

Electronic Mail

Electronic mail (email) is a way to send messages to others in electronic form. Users write an email just like they would write a letter with word processing software. However, instead of printing the message and sending it via the postal system, email users typically click a Send button in the email program. The email message arrives at its destination within a matter of seconds or minutes, depending on where it is going and the traffic on the network. Just as there are many different word processing, graphics, and spreadsheet programs, so there are many different email programs.

Many search sites and Internet service providers offer free email services. **Table 1-1** outlines common functions shared by almost all email programs. Although this chapter provides general information about using email, it does not provide step-by-step procedures for using a specific program. For assistance in using your specific email system, check the help information online or the documentation for the system at your institution.

Email messages consist of two parts: the header and the body. The body is the actual message. The header has at least four (and sometimes five) sections that provide useful information:

- **Date:** This includes the date and time that the message was sent.
- **From:** This identifies the sender's email address and, in many cases, the sender's name.
- **To:** This identifies the receiver's email address and can include the receiver's name.
- **CC:** This optional section identifies the other people who will also receive a copy of the email message sent to the primary recipient. Most programs also provide an optional blind carbon copy (BCC). When you use the BCC function, a copy of the email is sent to one or more additional receivers; their names will not appear in the header and are not visible to the other receivers. Only the sender will know who has been sent a blind copy of the message. Using the BCC option also avoids sending an email with a large distribution list in the header.
- **Subject:** Use the subject line to convey the essence of the body of the email. This field will be blank if the sender omitted this information. Some university email systems will not accept email if the subject field is blank. Always include one to three words in this section.

Email users are given a certain amount of space to store email messages on the server of their email provider. If you never delete email messages, eventually the allotted space will become full and the system will return all new messages. Thus people with email accounts should read their email often and delete messages that are no longer needed. By moving previously read messages to folders, the inbox of the email system remains uncluttered and new messages are more readily visible when you start the email program. In addition, some organizations have policies where they will automatically delete email sitting in the inbox, sent folder, or delete folder after a set time. Therefore, moving important email to folders will save it from deletion. It is possible, however, to occupy all of your allocated space with email messages that you have moved to folders. Most programs allow users to systematically store the messages that they wish to keep in folders off the mail server, either on the local drive or on another network server. Note that storing on the local drive means you won't have access to those messages if you are not using that particular computer.

TABLE 1-1 COMMON EMAIL FUNCTIONS

Function	Description
Configure your email settings	When you set up your email program you will make several decisions such as how you want your name displayed, your incoming and outgoing mail server name, and your password. Some of this information you will need to obtain from your Internet service provider.
Compose and send an email message	There are significant variations in the type of formatting available when composing an email message. Some will permit all of the same text formatting available in your word processing package while others only accept plain text with no formatting.
Reply to an email	When replying to an email check to see if you are replying to everyone who received the original email or only the author of that email message.
Forward an email	Never send an email you are not willing to have published. All emails can be forwarded to another person or even several people whom you may not intend to read your words.
Maintain an address book	This is a list of your contacts and their email addresses. It is also possible to maintain distribution lists in your address book.
Attach files to your message	Any type of file can be attached to an email message including word files, graphics, spreadsheets, audio, and even video. Remember the receiver will need the appropriate software to open these files.
Create and attach a signature to your email	Your signature file includes your name and contact information that you want to share in your emails. This can be attached automatically to all of your emails.
Organize and save your email	Most email programs make it possible for you to create folders where you can categorize and save emails. For example, you may want to save all of the emails related to a course in a folder with the name of the course.

Email Addresses

All email systems provide users with individual addresses. On a **local area network (LAN)**, an email address operates much like an interoffice mail address; that is, the user's local email address usually consists of the user's ID only. In contrast, email sent over a wide area network (WAN) is like mail sent via the postal service, in that a full Internet address is needed. An "at" symbol (@) in an email address always separates the user ID from the rest of the address. There are three parts to an Internet email address. Suppose the address is janesmith@gmail.com.

- The **user ID** is the name of the individual on the computer system where one receives email. No one else on that system has the same user ID. The user's ID in the previous example is janesmith.
- The "at" (@) symbol is always typed between the user's ID and the user's email system address.
- The **user's domain** is the location address for everyone who uses that email system. This part of the address functions like the home address of a person in postal service mail delivery; that is, everyone in the same family uses the same apartment or house address. In this example, the location address is gmail.com.

One of the email application's functions that is especially useful when sending a message to a group of people is the ability to create a **distribution list** (also called an **alias** or **mailing list**). The distribution ID is the name assigned to the list. Each time the sender addresses an email message using the distribution ID, each person on that list receives the message. For example, a list called ClassN402 might contain the addresses of all students in a healthcare informatics class. When you send a message to the ClassN402 distribution address, the message arrives in the inbox of everyone on that list.

Email-Related Terms

Attachment — An **attachment** is a file that accompanies an email message but is not in the body of the message itself.

Bounce — **Bounce** is a message that failed to be delivered promptly. Emails can bounce for many reasons. For example, you typed the wrong email address, the recipient's mailbox is full, or the account no longer exists (Email Experience Council, n.d.).

Emoticon — This is a way to show an emotion via text on the computer. **Emoticons** are symbols or combinations of symbols substitute for facial expressions, body language, and voice inflections.

Filter	**Filter** is a tool that automatically moves incoming emails into separate folders according to criteria that either you or your Internet provider specify. Virus checkers or a software programs that you use may include filters. An example is the Junk Mail folder in Microsoft Outlook or the Spam folder on AOL.
Phishing	**Phishing** is fraudulent email that solicits private information such as passwords or credit card numbers. It can result in **identity theft**.
RSS (Really Simple Syndication)	This scheme makes it possible for you to subscribe to and receive information about a specific topic that blogs, podcasts, and other social networking applications publish. **RSS (Really Simple Syndication)** feeds deliver this aggregated information, and you may read this content through a feed reader or email message.
Spam	**Spam** is electronic junk mail. It is unsolicited and may or may not be from an identifiable source. It may be deceptive in addition to being irritating and wasting time. Spam can lead to identity theft, disrupt your personal computer with malware, and turn your system into a zombie for distributing spam (FCC, 2011).
Spim	**Spim** is the spam of instant messaging. It is part spam and part instant message. An increasing number of advertisers are using spim.

Email Etiquette (Netiquette)

Just as there are rules governing what is acceptable to say and do during social interactions, guidelines exist for acceptable ways of communicating using email. Many of these rules also apply to other forms of online communication. **Netiquette** is the name given to electronic communication conventions. Some of the main rules of netiquette include the following:

1. Start the message with a greeting, just like with any communication, and make it specific to the recipient(s): "Hi, Kurt," "Mary," or "Greetings, Colleagues." With email, there is a tendency to be less formal than is common in a face-to-face communication. However, when dealing with faculty and medical personnel, it is better to use formal titles. It is also important to use the recipient's correct title. For example, do not refer to a PhD-prepared professor or a physician as Mr. or Mrs.; use Dr. instead.
2. Include in the message only what is appropriate for others to read. Never assume the message is private.

3. Be clear and concise. Email messages include only words. When people communicate face to face, they use intonation and body language as well as words to send the message. With email, no observation of the recipient is possible, so no immediate feedback or the ability to adjust the message midway is available. As a general rule, if a message can be misinterpreted, it will be. "Emoticons," like the smiley face, are available to signify feelings. Standard emoticons include the following:

   :-) Basic smiley
   ;-) Winking smiley—means "just kidding"
   :-(Sad face
   8-) Smiley with sunglasses
   -o : Surprised

   There are several other emoticons, and several Web sites that list these symbols. As with all communication tools, the sender and recipient must understand the symbol for the symbol to be effective in supporting communication. Consider text messaging abbreviations unacceptable in most email messages. For example, do not use the letter "U" to stand in for "you."
4. Keep it short. Do not quote huge amounts of material. When replying, put the reply early in the message body so that readers do not have to wade through material to get to the response. If a longer message is necessary, attach a file with the message.
5. Always specify the content of the message in the subject line so that readers know what to expect. This information can also help readers discriminate between what might be a legitimate message from an acquaintance and what might be a message containing a virus.
6. Never type in all capital letters. THIS IS CONSIDERED SHOUTING.
7. Ensure that the message is well written. Check the spelling and grammar.
8. Respect copyright. Always give credit to others for their work, and follow copyright rules for using material (see Chapter 12 for guidelines as to copyright).
9. Avoid flaming, which is voicing very strong antagonistic opinions or verbally attacking someone. Never respond when you are angry. It is hard to look professional or explain your thinking if you are in the middle of a "flaming war."
10. Sign the message. The signature should include at least the sender's name and email address. It can also include the sender's postal mail address, telephone number, title, and professional affiliation. It is possible to create a "signature" file ahead of time and use it as a standard addition to all email.
11. Do not send chain letters. A chain letter is an email that ends with the suggestion that the recipient forward the message to several other people.

One of the best ways to stop this type of junk email is not to forward it. If there is a specific email with a message you do want to share with a specific person, delete the part of the email suggesting you forward the email to others before you send it forward. Keep in mind that when you receive an email that has been forwarded the email message may also have been edited or modified by anyone who had forwarded that email message.

Email Attachments

An **attachment** is a file sent along with an email message. You can send any type of file via email, including text files (Word files), graphics (PowerPoint files), spreadsheets (Excel files), audio (.wav files), and even video. Be certain that the recipient of the file has the appropriate software to open and run the file being sent. For example, if you send an Excel spreadsheet, the recipient will need to have the Excel software or a plug-in to access that document. Some email systems limit attachment sizes. If the receiver's email system does not accept your attachment because it is too large, the system will bounce it back to you. Some email systems also do not accept files with certain extensions, such as .exe or .accdb.

To attach a file to an email:

1. Open the **email program** and look for words like compose mail, new message, or a symbol . Click the **words** or **symbol** to start and **compose** a message.
2. Once you have composed the message, look for a paper clip or attachment words. Click the **words** or **paper clip**.
3. Make appropriate choices in the window that appears asking for the location and file to attach. Click **Open** on the appropriate file/document. Make sure the attachment (such as this: Exercise 1.docx (30 KB) ×) appears in the mail message window before you send the message.

Most email programs provide the ability to attach multiple attachments at once; however, most of these email applications also will limit the number of attachments that you can include with one email message. Others like Microsoft Web Mail permit you to upload one file at a time requiring you to repeat the process to attach more than one file.

To download an email attachment:

1. Open the **email** program and display the **mail message**.
2. Look for words or a paper clip that indicates an attachment. The attacment should look similar to this: Document1.docx (212 KB).
3. Double-click the **file** and click **Save** or click **Open** with … (or something similar to those words).
4. Select a **place** to download the file.

Each mail program is slightly different in terms of the location and display of the attached file. Nevertheless, all programs should give you the ability to right-click and save the file to a specific location. Typically, clicking the attachment indicator either opens the file or opens a dialog box that allows the viewer to save the attachment to a file or to open the attachment. Sometimes you will need to right-click to see these options.

Safe Email Practices

To protect the computer, it is wise not to open attachments without checking them for a virus. Most virus-checking software will give you the option for configuring your virus checker so that it scans all attachments automatically as they come into your email program. However, no virus checker will catch every virus. Malicious computer hackers have developed systems that enable them to access a user's address file and send messages to everyone in the list, making it appear as if the message is from that user. Thus it is prudent not to open attachments unless you expect them. It is also wise to configure your virus software to scan email attachments before you open them if you do not configure your virus-checker to do so automatically. While all attachments can include malicious applications, executable (.exe) attachments are highly suspect. Once you open an infected file, these attachments may create a variety of problems on the computer.

While most university systems routinely check all attachments before delivering the email to the individual user, new viruses can slip through this safety net. Therefore, the safest course of action is to save the attachment to a folder—just be sure to note in which folder you are saving the file—and then explicitly check it with an antivirus program such as BitDefender, Norton Utilities, or Webroot SecureAnywhere Antivirus software before opening the file. If the antivirus program finds a file with a virus, delete the file from both your email list and the computer's delete folder without opening it.

Today, at least 77% of the U.S. population has Internet access in the home, and email has become a primary tool for communication, rivaling even the telephone (ITU, 2012). The percentage goes up when you talk about other Internet access through schools, libraries, and work. Along with its advantages, however, has come the irritating problem of unsolicited messages—that is, spam. Many Internet providers offer spam-blocking products for their customers, and some email programs have filters that you may set to block spam related to specified subjects or from specified addresses. It is wise to never open messages from anyone or any company that you do not know. Never respond to spam because this reply can confirm that your email address is active and you are reading these emails. Always report spam to your Internet service provider. Most ISPs that provide email functionality make sending such reports easy, through an option on the email menu. In an attempt to prevent advertising spam from coming into email accounts, some individuals set up a separate account for electronic discussion groups, ordering online, and registering warranties to control the number of advertisements coming to their personal email account.

No matter what address appears on an email or which trademarks appear on the email, you should never provide personal information such as your password, account number, or Social Security number in response to an email message. Some emails fraudulently represent commercial companies by including the company's headers or logos on the email message and then request personal information. Your bank and any other company that you do business with will never request this type of information by email.

These so-called phishing scams can lead to identity theft. A common phishing scam on campus is to send emails offering part-time work. The email will look like it is coming from a campus email address. However, when students apply for the job by providing their personal information, including their Social Security number, they have just been caught in a phishing scam. If you receive such an email job offer, call the university's human resources department by phone and ask if the message is legitimate.

While email is a frequently used Internet tool, another tool that comes with Microsoft Office and that is less frequently used is OneNote. This tool has many capabilities that you need to exploit and that can assist you in gathering information as you use the Internet.

Using OneNote

Microsoft Office OneNote 2010 provides you with an electronic tool for creating, gathering, organizing, storing, and sharing information such as notes from class, reference materials, and Internet sources. You gather information in digital notebooks that are equivalent to traditional three-ring binders, where each notebook has sections and pages. You can store almost any kind of electronic information in OneNote, such as photos, text, graphics, audio, Web clippings, and video clips. You can write a note with the keyboard, write a note with a "pen," or copy something from the screen and paste it into OneNote or even into another Office document. When you copy something from the Internet, the OneNote page will automatically display the URL from the source site. Collaborative tools help you work with others in shared notebooks both offline and online. The program highlights unread notes and indicates the author in shared notebooks. You can link notes to Word or PowerPoint documents. OneNote also supports touch-enabled operating systems. If you sync your notebooks to SkyDrive they are available anywhere from any computer. We captured some of the small figures or icons in this text using OneNote. OneNote in Office 2010 now uses tabbed ribbons like other Office applications.

OneNote Basics

OneNote in Office 2010 comes with one preset notebook called Personal. **Figure 1-6** shows the window that appears when you open OneNote for the first time. Under the General Section the first page provides a summary of OneNote. On the right, under New Page New Page, is a list of all pages in this section. These pages describe what's new in OneNote, what it does, its top uses, and the basics of use. To explore this guide, click each page tab and read its contents to get an idea of how OneNote works. You can expand or collapse Page tabs by clicking the chevron > to the right of New Page. There are also up and down chevrons

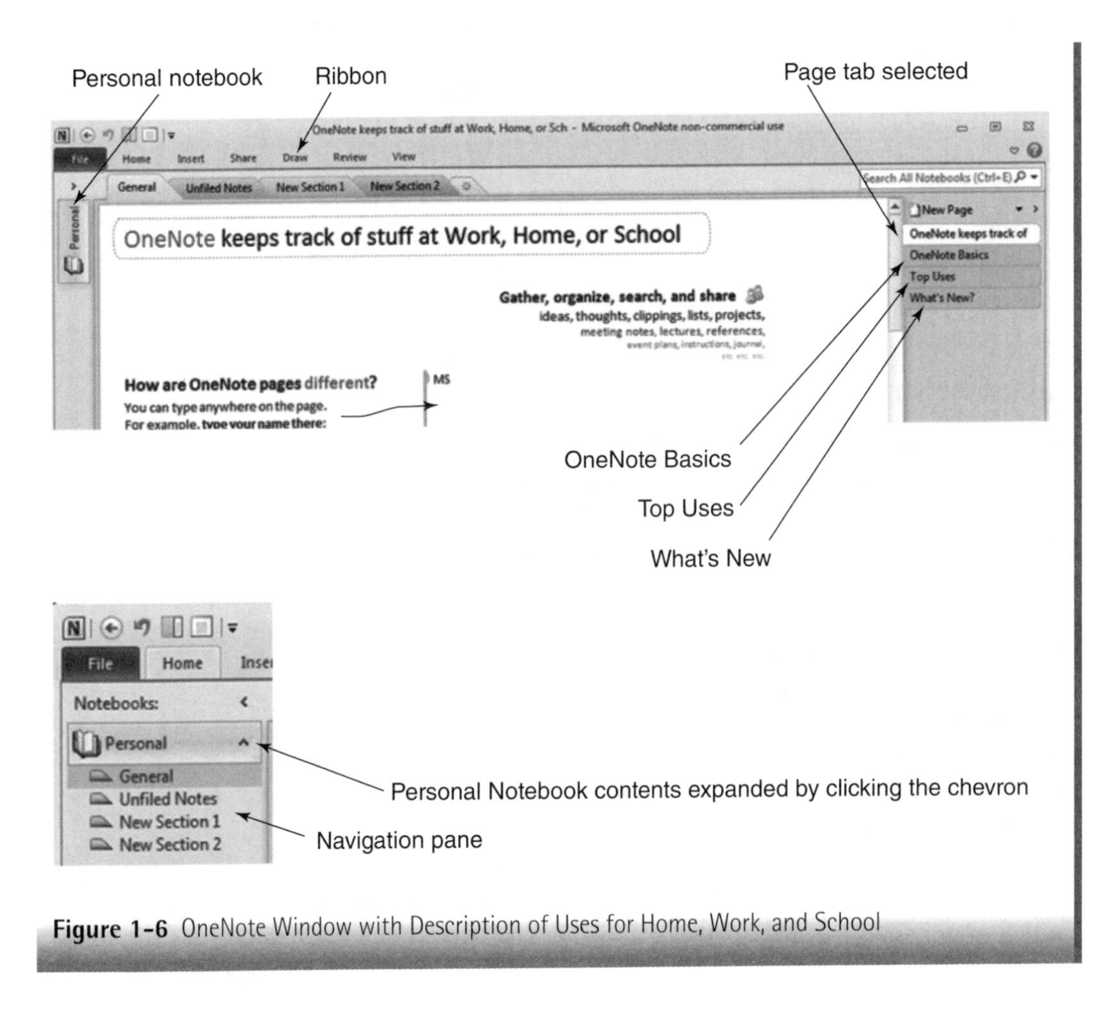

Figure 1-6 OneNote Window with Description of Uses for Home, Work, and School

on the Navigation pane that expand and collapse the view of each notebook as Figure 1-6 shows. **Figures 1-7a** and **b** show the material provided in *OneNote Basics*. **Figures 1-8a, b,** and **c** provide a partial list of what is in the *Top Uses* page. You will also find it worthwhile to review the online training available from Microsoft for OneNote. Click Help in the menu bar and choose Microsoft Office Online to discover the options available. You can also choose Help under the File tab.

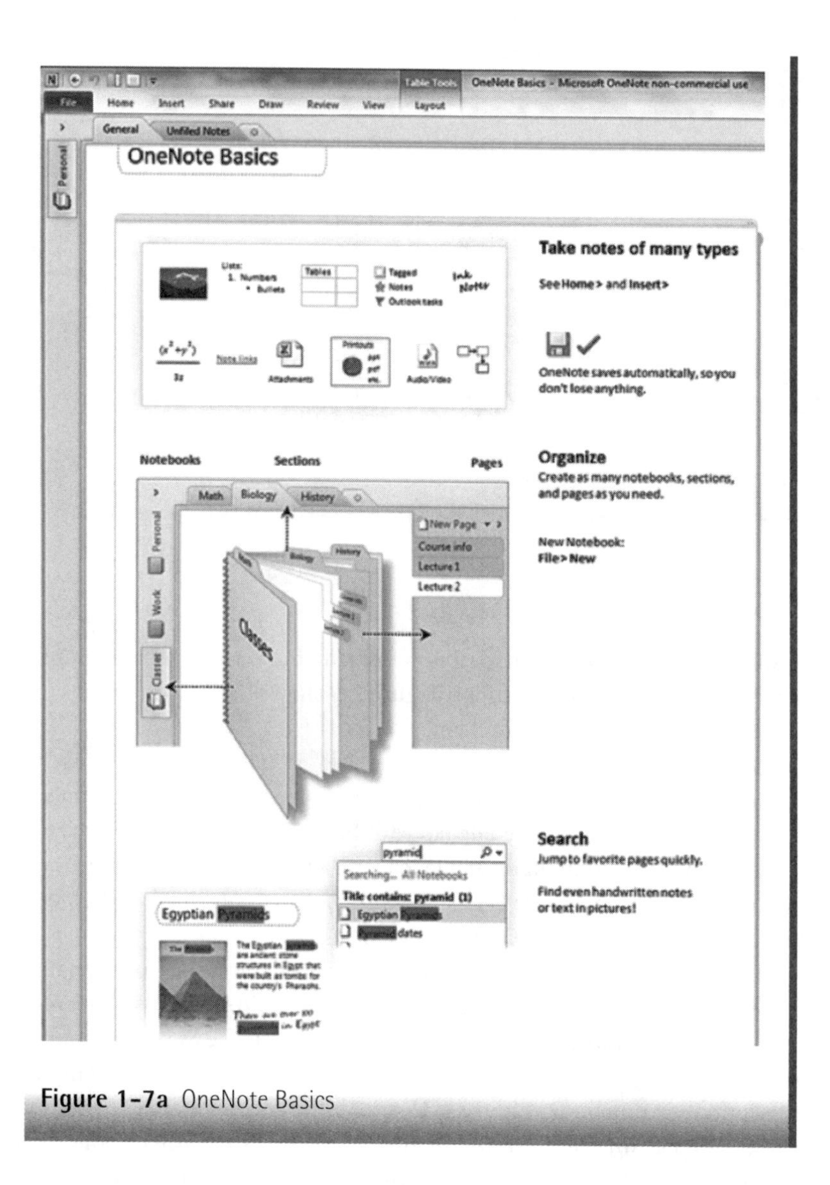

Figure 1-7a OneNote Basics

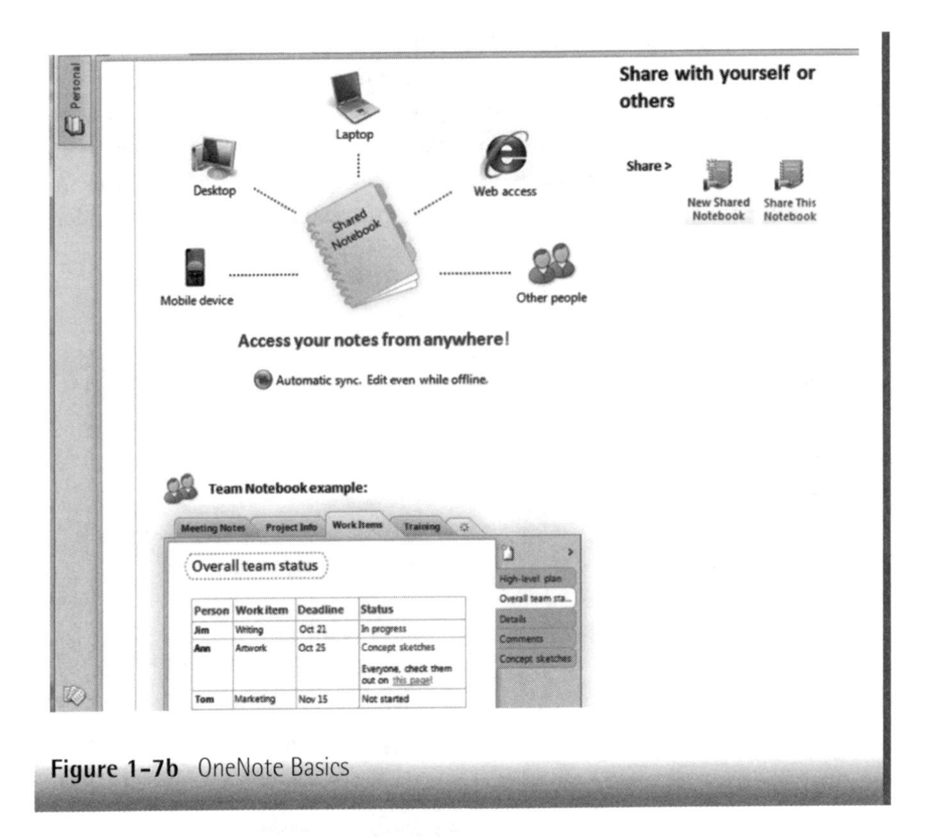

Figure 1-7b OneNote Basics

Working with OneNote's Tabbed Ribbon

OneNote 2010 now uses a tabbed ribbon instead of toolbars to hold commands, just like other Microsoft applications. **Figure 1-9** shows the individual tabs in the OneNote ribbon when you select them.

As with other Office applications, the File [File] tab offers a backstage view of all the things you do with a document such as opening, saving, printing, and so forth. **Figure 1-10** shows the File tab with **Info** selected. This shows the list of notebooks in OneNote (in this example Personal and Research) as well as ways to access other notebooks. **Figure 1-11** shows the choices available of where to find a notebook when you select the **Open** command.

Figure 1-12 shows the **New** command that offers choices for storing, naming, and creating a notebook. The **Share** command provides choices for posting a notebook to the Web or network. (See **Figure 1-13**.) The **Save As** command, shown in **Figure 1-14**, lets you select a format (Word, PDF, etc.) for saving your page, section, or notebook. **Figure 1-15** shows the choices available when you choose **Send** or **Print**. **Figure 1-16** lists the **Help** options you can explore as well the choices available under **Options** for customizing your display, mini-toolbar,

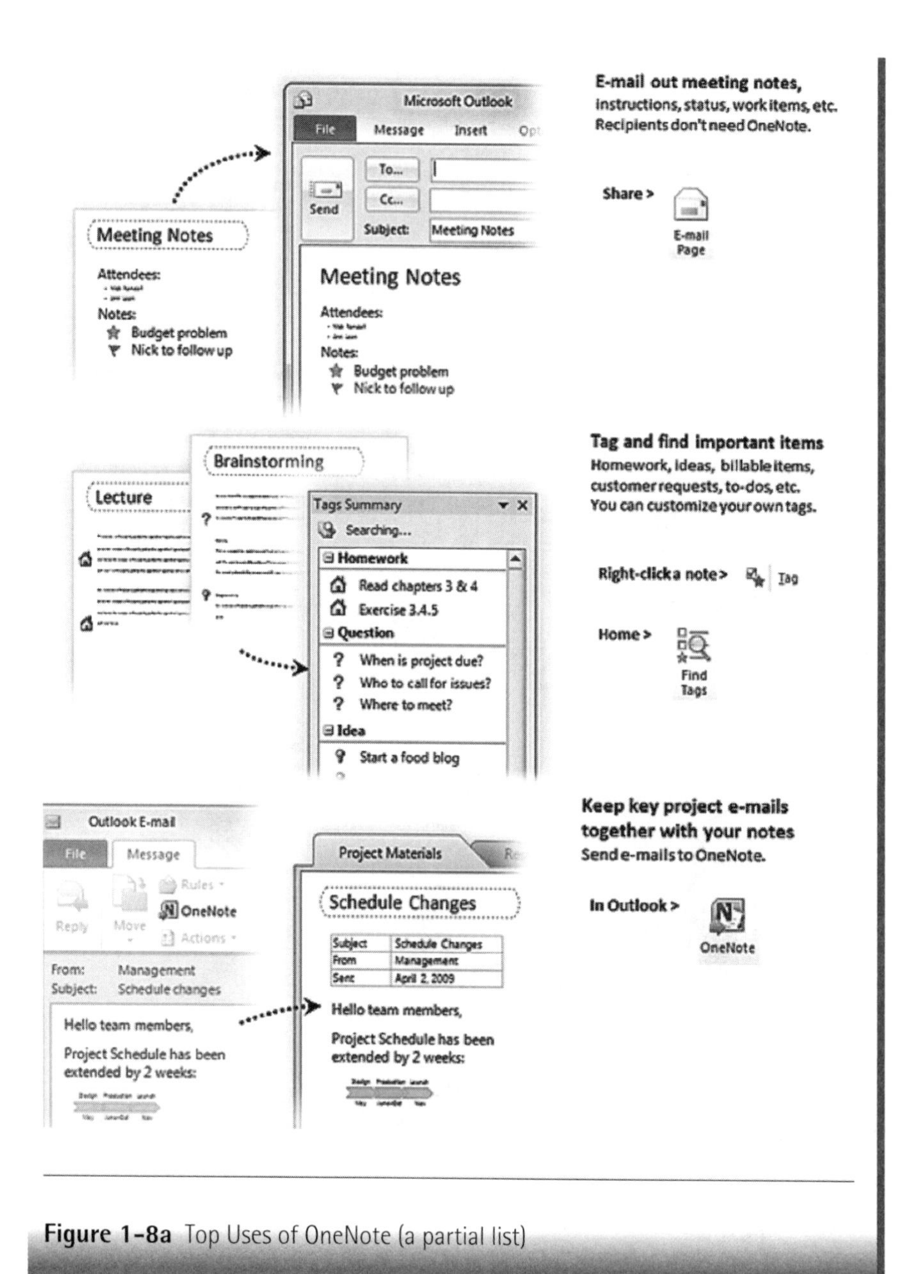

Figure 1-8a Top Uses of OneNote (a partial list)

ribbon, audio, and video among others. Figure 1-16 also shows the General option choices. On the right side of the OneNote window is an arrow. If the arrow looks like this ⌄ the ribbon is not expanded and you won't see the contents of each tab as they appear in Figure 1-9. Click the arrow and it turns into this ⌃; the ribbons expand so that when you click a tab the ribbons look like they do in Figure 1-9.

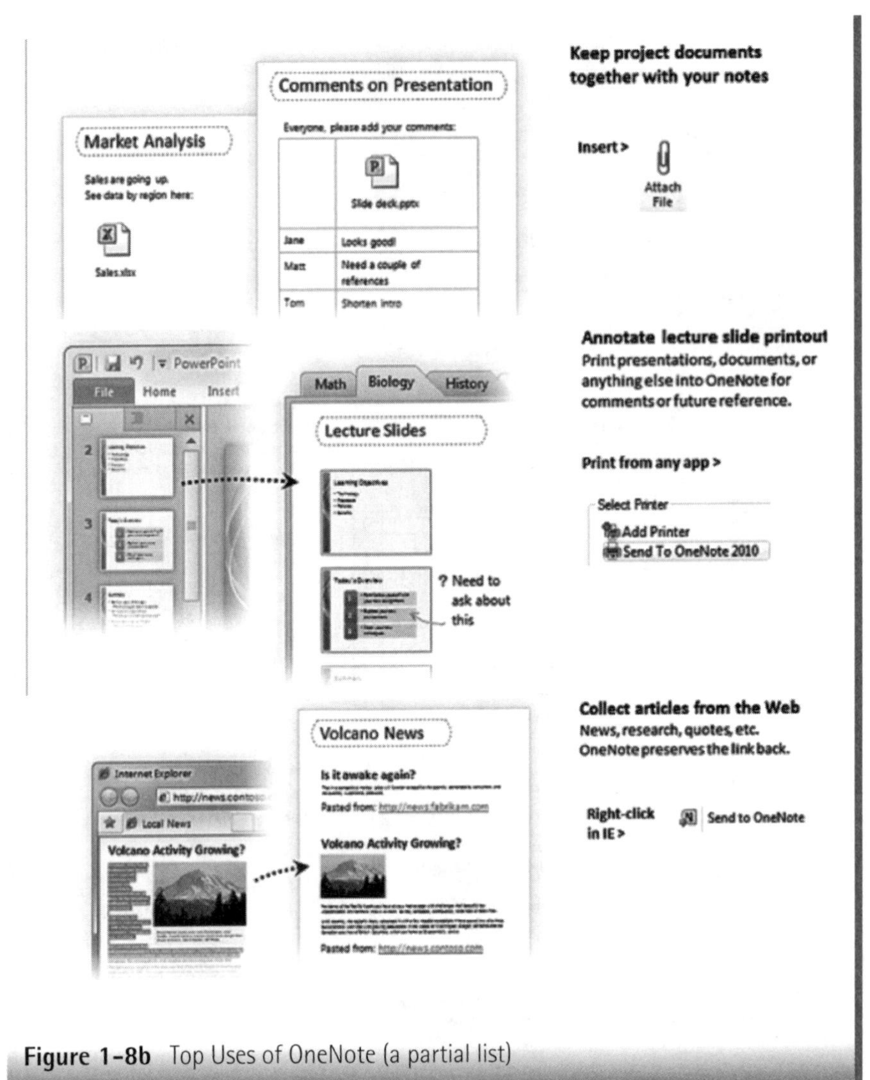

Figure 1-8b Top Uses of OneNote (a partial list)

Using OneNote

When you open OneNote for the first time, you will see a window like that shown in **Figure 1-17**—an untitled new page. You can click anywhere inside the page and write a note, draw something, or paste text or a picture. The note will appear in a "container" or text box like this: with the cursor inside. You can modify the container using traditional Microsoft protocols. If you don't see the Untitled Note Page, click the New Page button N. (See Figure 1-17.)

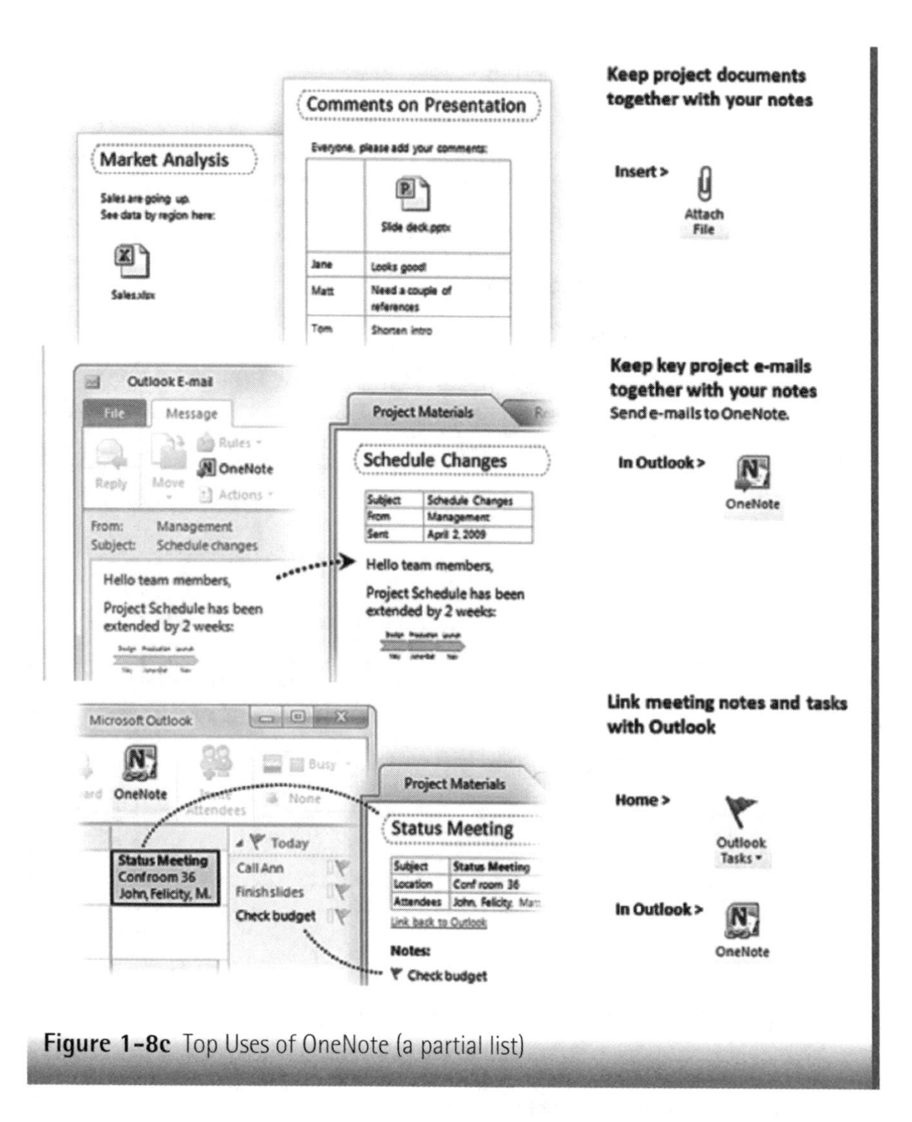

Figure 1-8c Top Uses of OneNote (a partial list)

To move the container:

- Click the **container** and the cursor changes to a four headed arrow.
- Drag the **container** anywhere on the page.

To size the container:

- Click the **container edge** and the cursor changes to a two-headed arrow.
- Drag the **edge** to change the width of the container.

Home Tab

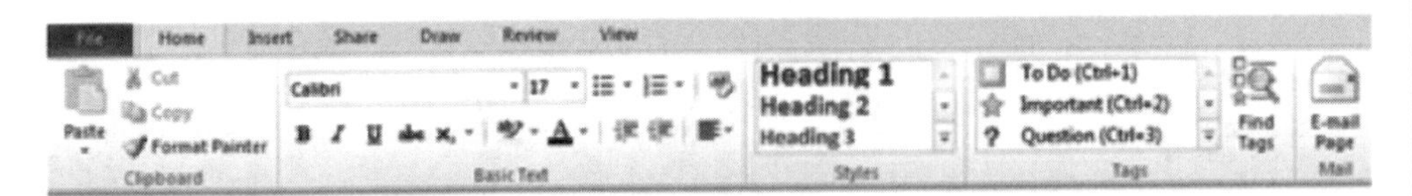

Insert Tab

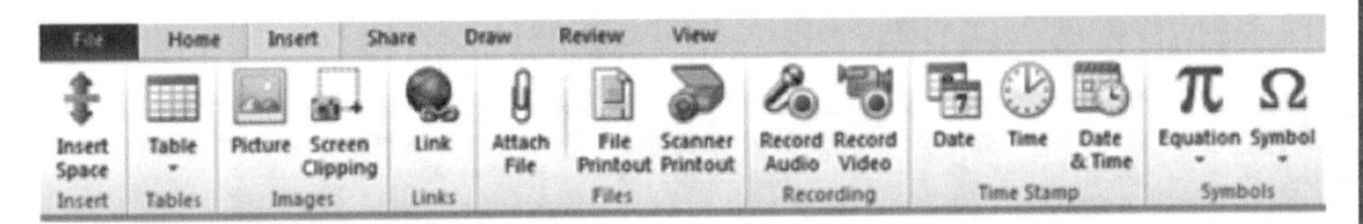

Share Tab

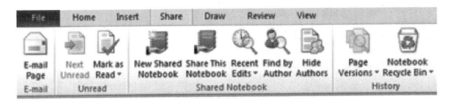

Draw Tab

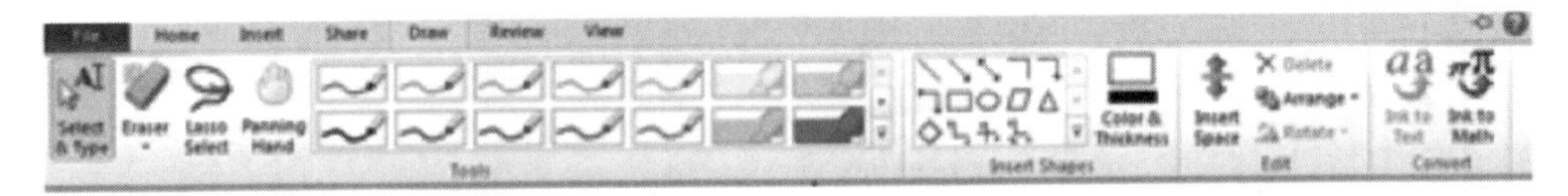

Review Tab

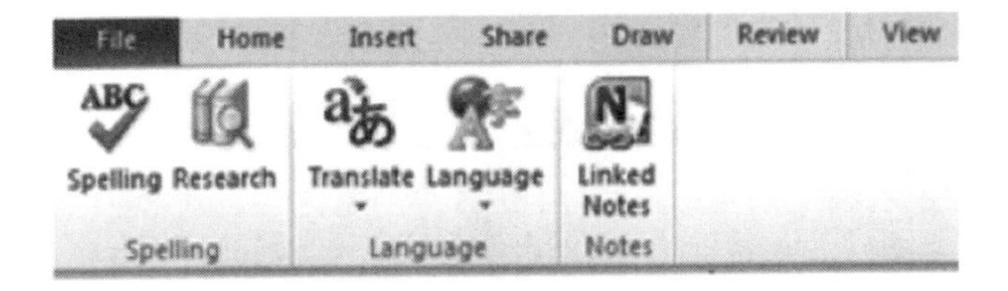

View Tab

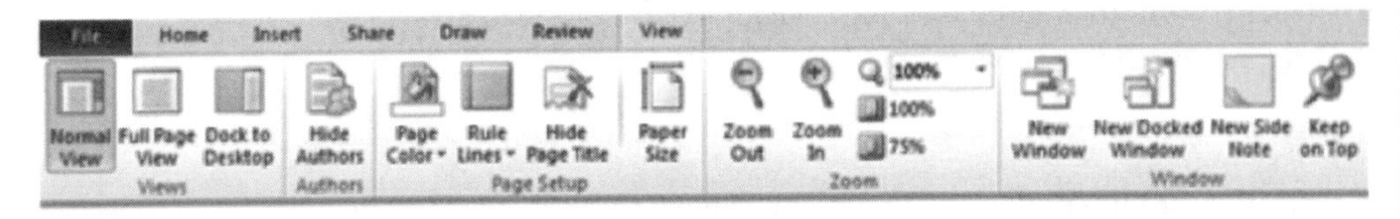

Figure 1-9 Tabs in OneNote

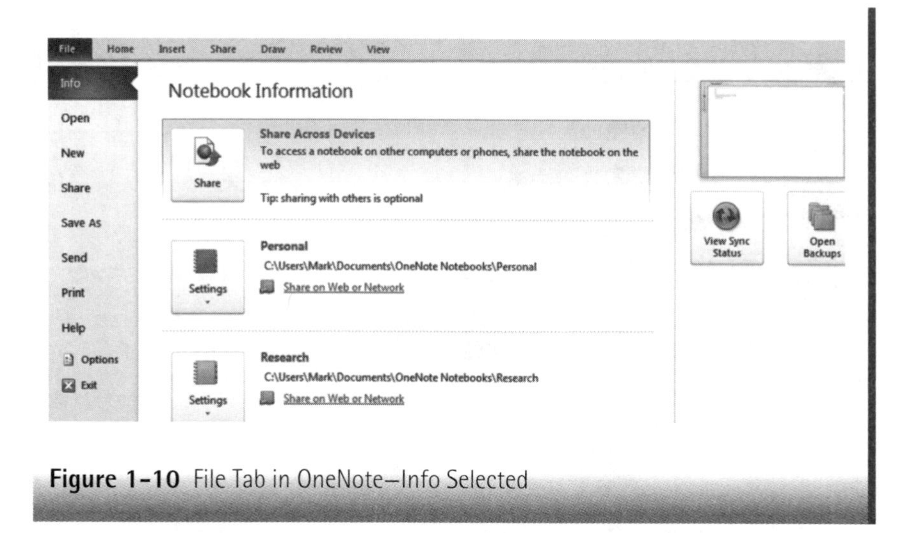

Figure 1-10 File Tab in OneNote—Info Selected

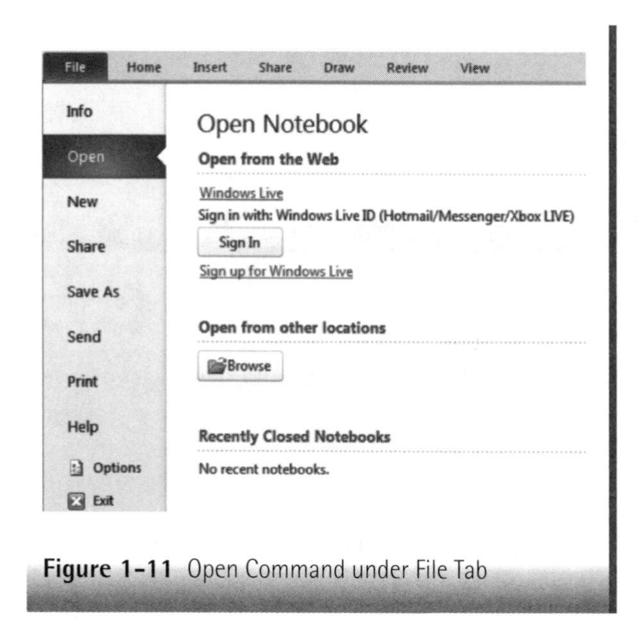

Figure 1-11 Open Command under File Tab

To remove what you typed:

- Select the **text**.
- Press the **Backspace** or **Delete** key. Alternatively, you can right-click and choose Cut from the menu that appears.

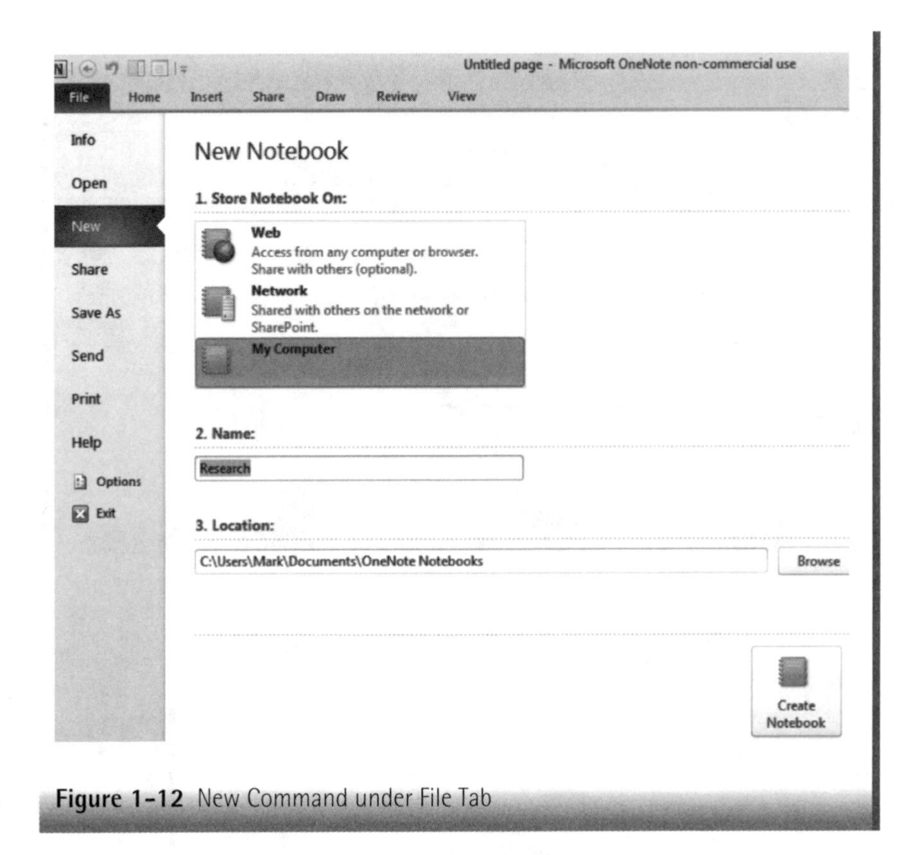

Figure 1-12 New Command under File Tab

Creating a New Notebook, Section, or Page

You can create a new Notebook and then add new pages and sections to the notebook.

To create a new notebook:

- Click **File** [File].
- Click **New** [New]; a menu will appear as shown in Figure 1-12.
- Select a **storage space**—Web, Network, or My Computer.
- Type a **name** for the notebook.
- Select a **location** (type it in or click browse button) and click **create notebook**.
- In addition to the 2010 templates, templates from OneNote 2007 are available online that deal with house hunting, research, job applications, school, and work, for example. Each notebook can have several sections. You can add new notebooks at any time.

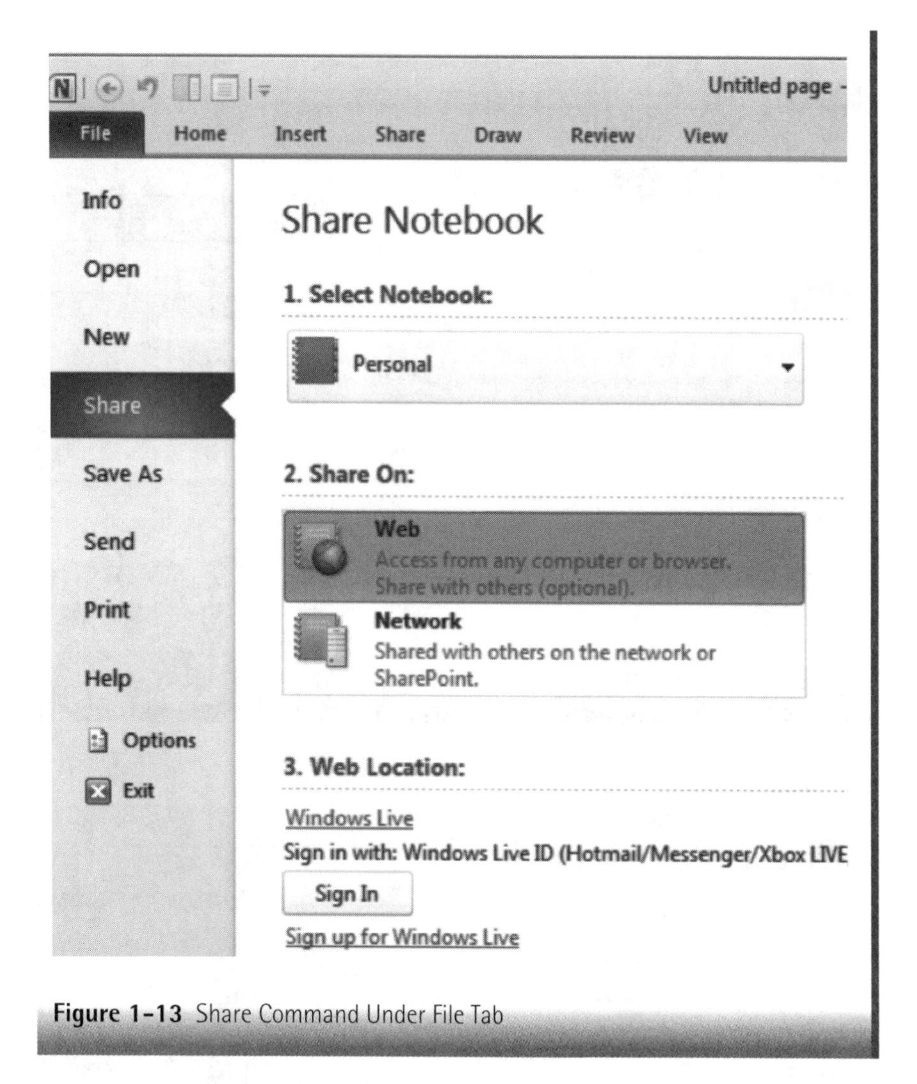

Figure 1-13 Share Command Under File Tab

To add a new section to a notebook:

- Click the **starburst icon** in the far right mini-tab.
- Select the **text** on the new section tab.
- Type a **name** for the section.

To add a new page:

- Open the **Notebook** or **section** where you want to insert the page.
- Click **New Page** in the page tabs list on the far right. The Page task pane lists any untitled or named note pages. You can also click the arrow next to

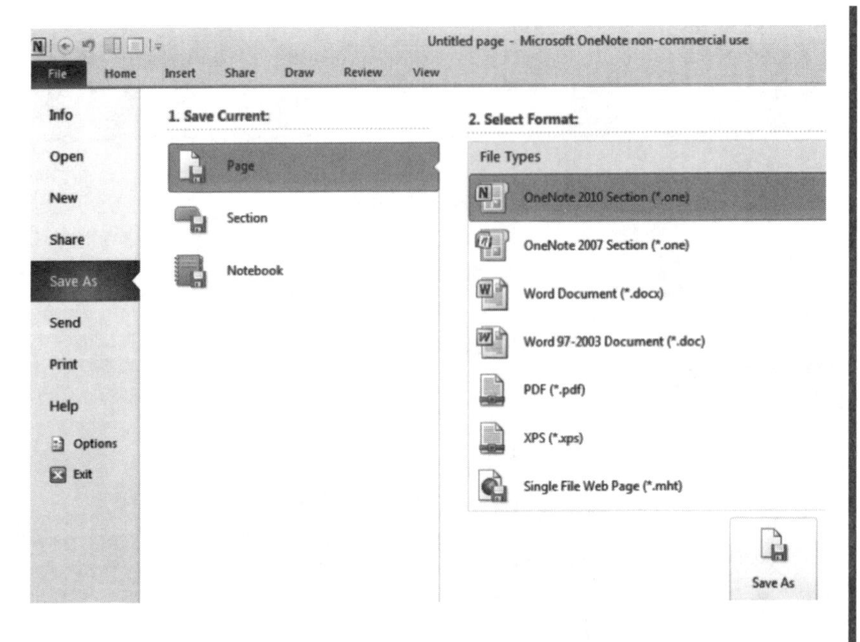

Figure 1-14 Save As Command Under File Tab

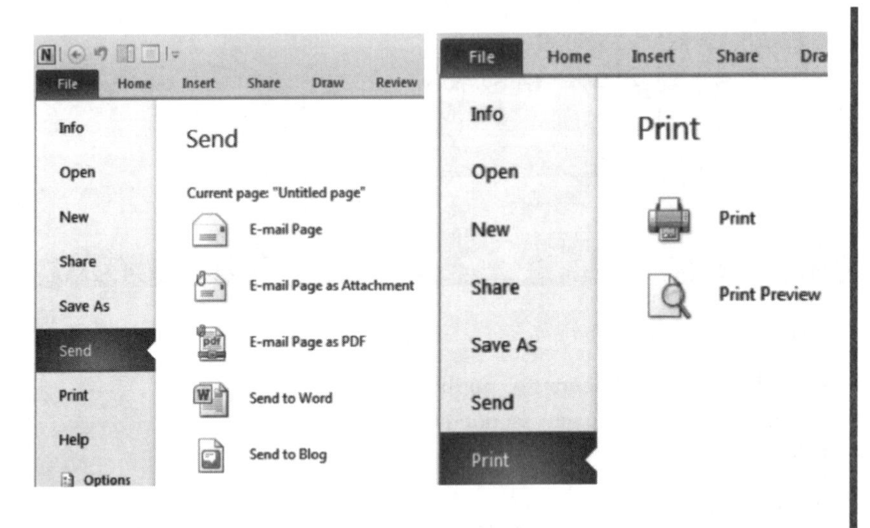

Figure 1-15 Send and Print Commands Under File Tab

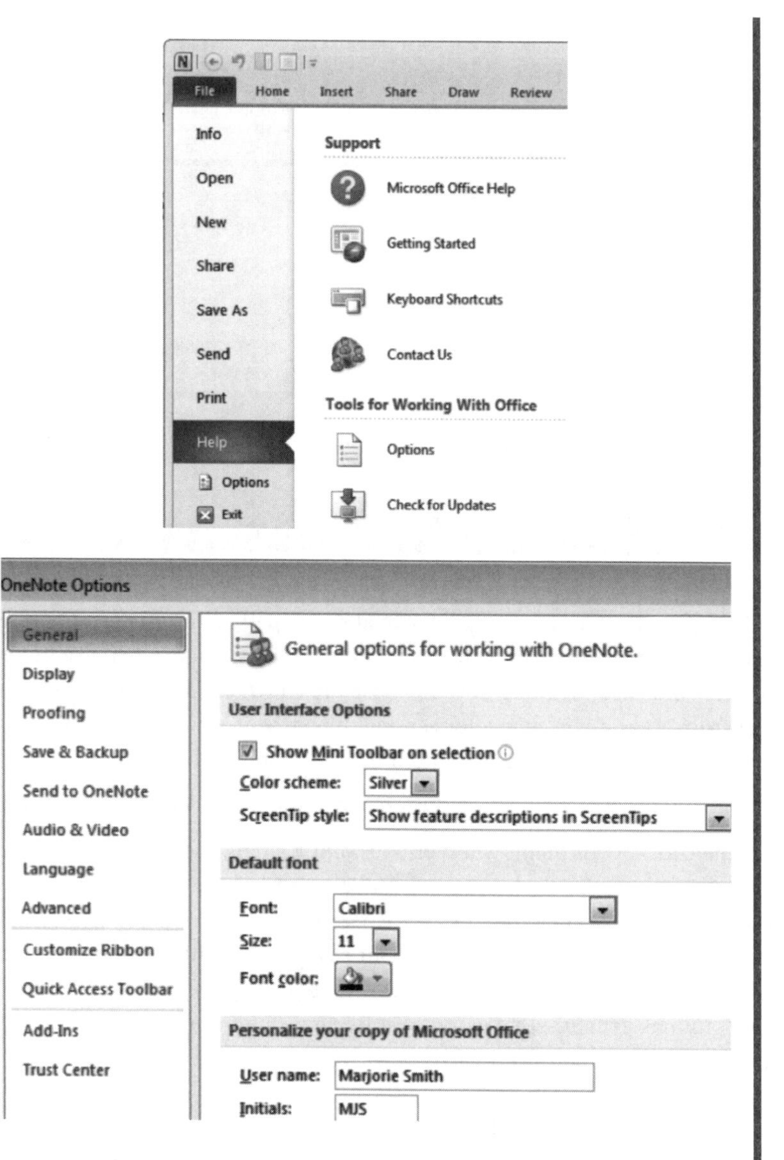

Figure 1-16 Help and Options Commands Under File Tab

New Page and a popup menu appears (see **Figure 1-18** for options). You can also choose a template.

- Click the **placeholder** and type a **name** for the page Summary .
- You are now ready to add Notes to the **page**. Click on the page and add the **note** to the container that appears.

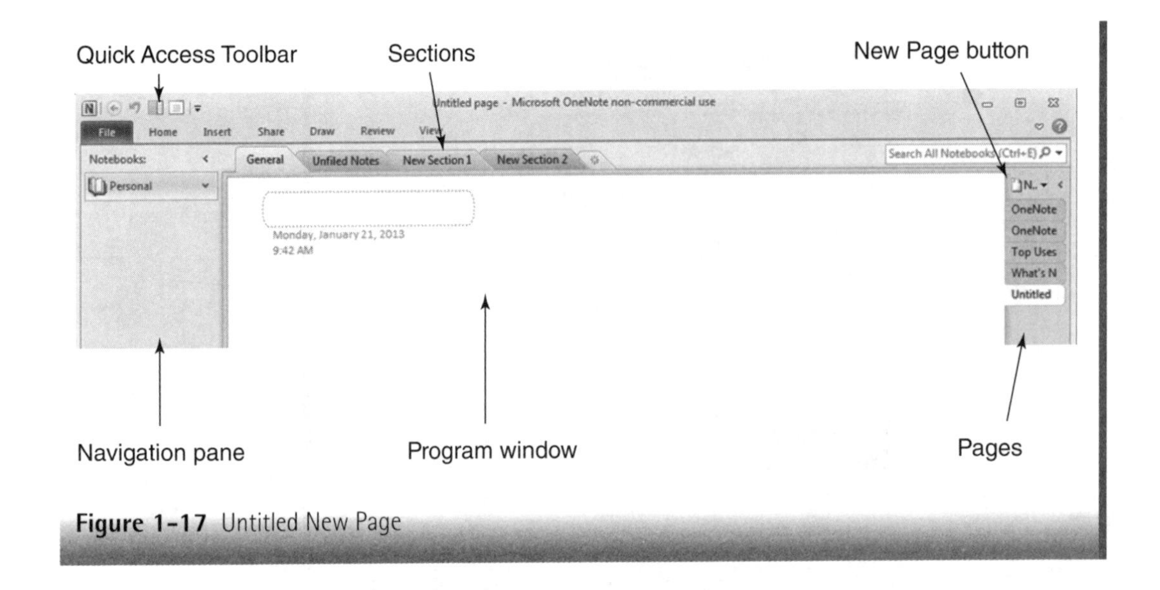

Figure 1-17 Untitled New Page

Once you select a new page, you can alter the page setup to meet your needs. For example, you can change the font, add rule lines, make a list, use bullets or numbers, and check spelling. If you choose the Draw tab (see Figure 1-9) you can select from a variety of pen colors and widths. If you have a pen or stylus tablet PC you can just draw. Otherwise hold down the mouse button after selecting a pen tool and draw. If you make a mistake, click the Eraser button and choose from the drop-down menu whether you want a small, medium, large, or stroke eraser. You can resize each image or move it around the page in the same way that you can move other containers. Remember that you can add notes and sections to a notebook at any time. You can easily move unfiled notes to sections or notebooks. However, it is wise to consider the type of tasks and the type of organizational structure that works best for the content. Also note that OneNote automatically saves notes and notebooks.

Capturing Screen Clippings

You can use the OneNote Screen Clipper to copy an image of anything you see on your computer screen.

To capture a picture, icon, or piece of text on your screen:

- Press the **Windows** **logo key** + **S**. The screen changes to a filmy white and the cursor changes to a plus sign.
- Place the plus sign over a corner of the object/picture you wish to copy; click and drag until you have selected the image you desire. Release the mouse button.

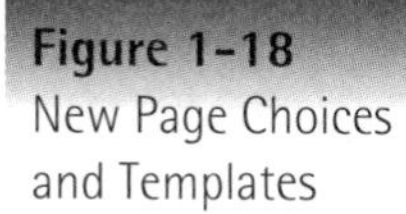

Figure 1-18
New Page Choices and Templates

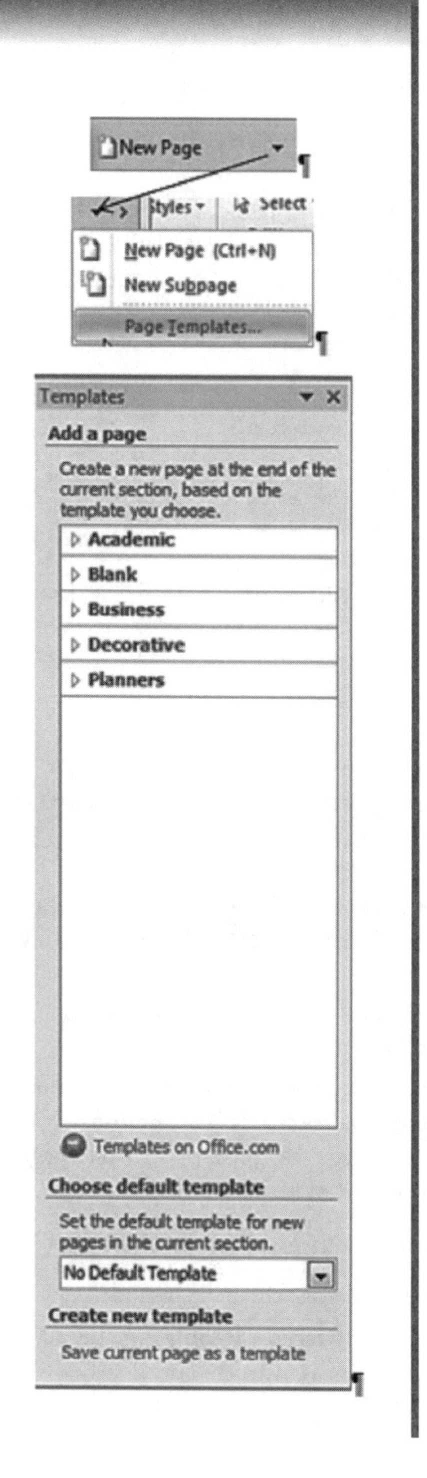

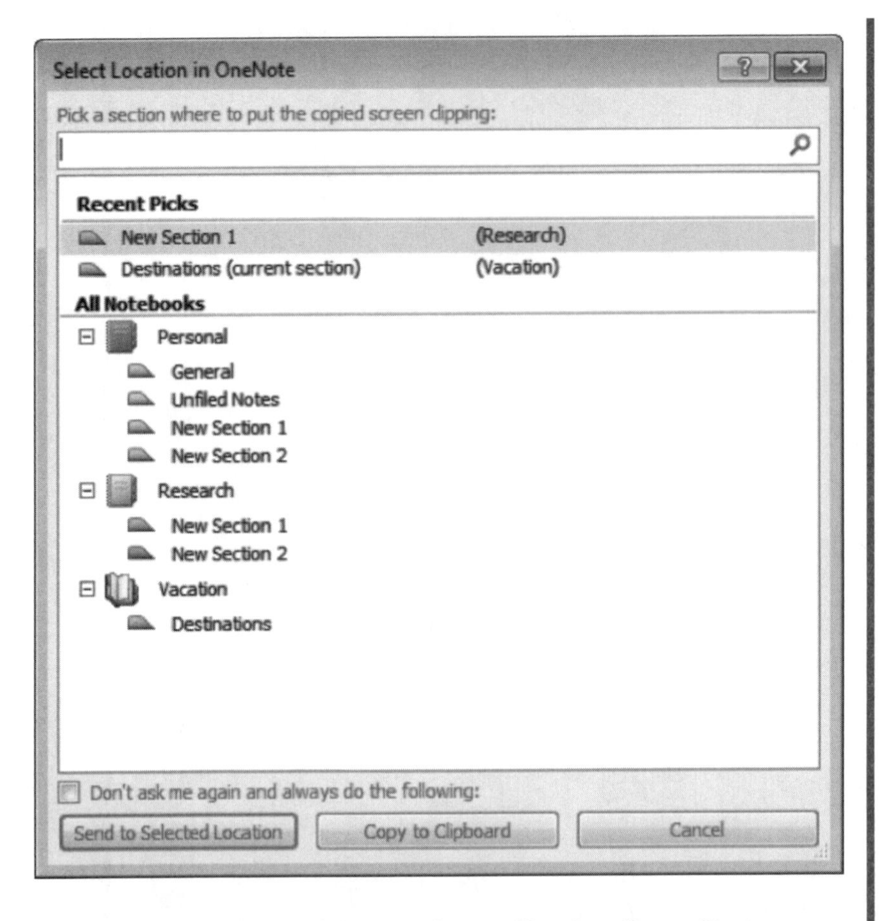

Figure 1-19 Menu Box for Selecting a Storage Place for a Screen Clipping

- A menu box appears asking you where you want to store the image. (See **Figure 1-19**.)
- Select a destination from the list and click the **Send to Selected Location** Send to Selected Location **button**.
- The image will appear on a Notes page along with the date and time when you clipped it.

Here is another way to prepare to take a screen clipping:

- Click the **Insert** tab in OneNote.
- Choose **Screen Clipping** Screen Clipping; the screen turns white and you proceed the same way as instructed previously.

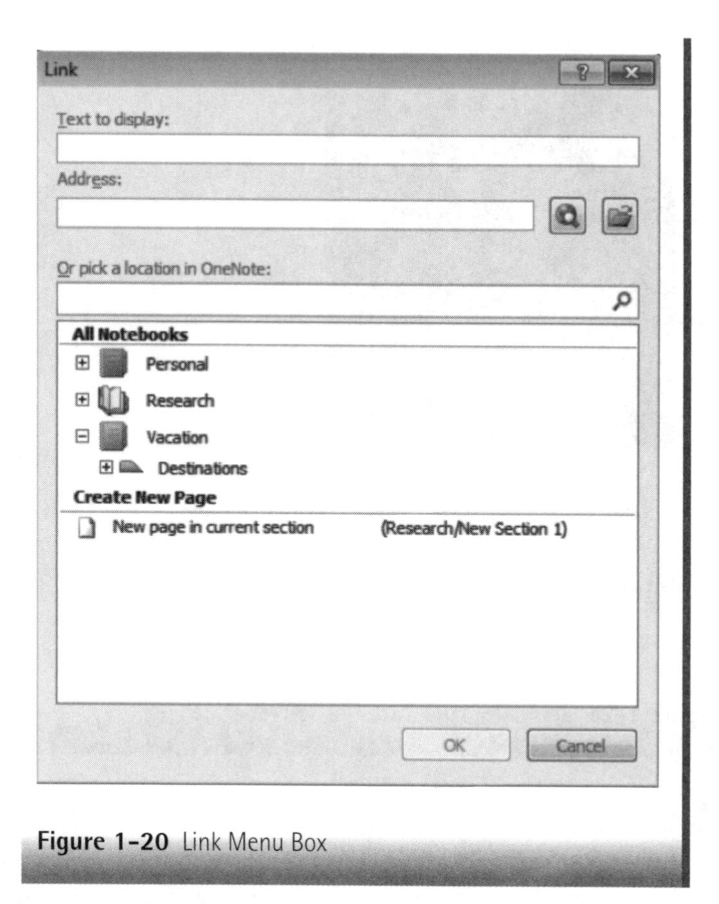

Figure 1-20 Link Menu Box

To capture an image from a Web page:

- Go to the **Web page** and locate the **image** to capture.
- Switch to **OneNote**, select the **page** to place the image, and click **where you want the image** to go in OneNote.
- Click the **Insert** tab, **Screen Clipping** in the images group. OneNote minimizes and you see a dimmed Web page.
- Click and **drag to select the image**. When you release the mouse button, OneNote captures the image and inserts the image in the location you selected.

When you capture an image from the Internet, you can also display the Internet address. Choose **Link** from the Insert tab, type a title for the image, and copy the Internet address to the provided box. See **Figure 1-20**. When you

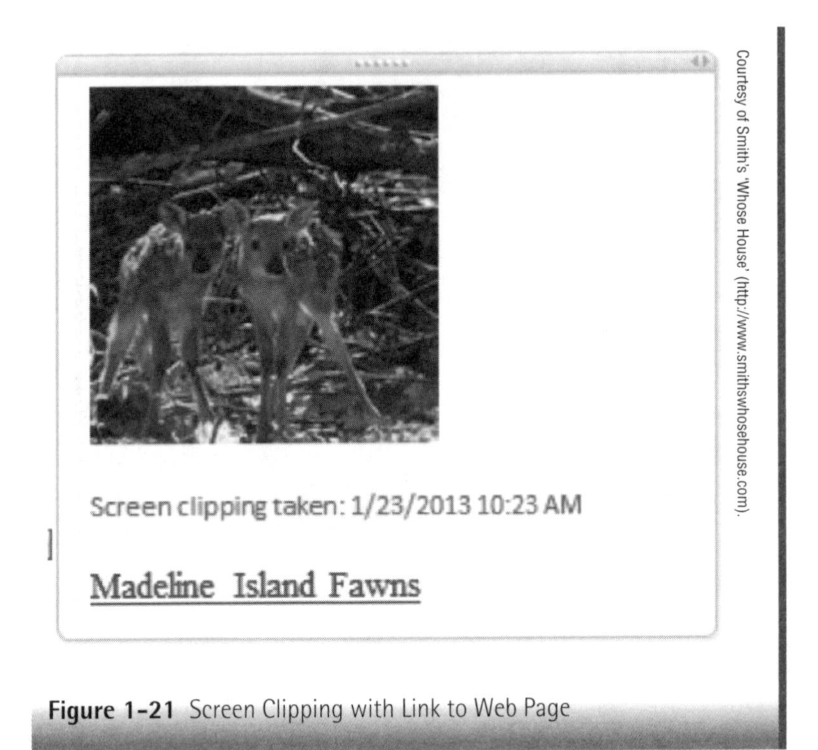

Courtesy of Smith's 'Whose House' (http://www.smithswhosehouse.com).

Figure 1-21 Screen Clipping with Link to Web Page

return to that page you can hold the cursor over the title of the image and the Internet address where the image came from will appear as shown in **Figure 1-21**.

Copying Text or Images to Other Documents

Once you capture an image, OneNote also places it on the Windows Clipboard. This provides you with the ability to paste the image into other documents such as Word or PowerPoint. If you are now reviewing your notes in OneNote and decide to copy several images captured previously, follow these directions:

To copy an image or text from OneNote and paste it into another document:

1. When you place your mouse arrow over the **image/text**, it turns into a four-headed arrow. Click to select the text.
2. You have several ways to copy it:
   a. Under the Home tab, choose **Copy**, or
   b. Right-click the **image** and select **Copy** Copy on the short cut menu, or
   c. Click the **Copy** icon in the Quick Access toolbar if it is present, or
   d. Press **Ctrl+C**.

3. Go to the document where you want to place the image:
   a. Choose **Paste** under the Home tab, or
   b. Right-click the **image** and select **Paste** Paste Options: on the short cut menu, or
   c. Click the **Paste** icon on the Quick Access Toolbar if it is present, or
   d. Press **Ctrl+V**.

NOTE: If you don't have the Copy and Paste icons on the Quick Access Toolbar, go to the down arrow in it and click it to bring up the menu for customizing the Toolbar.

Working with Side Note

Side Note is a small version of OneNote and functions much like a sticky note. It appears in its own small window. It will stay open on your desktop when you click the **Dock to Desktop** icon as shown in **Figure 1-22**. Use Side Note to make notes when you are working in other programs. The ribbon is a smaller version of the one on OneNote with tabs containing many of the same choices. OneNote automatically saves Side Note in the Side Notes section of your notebook.

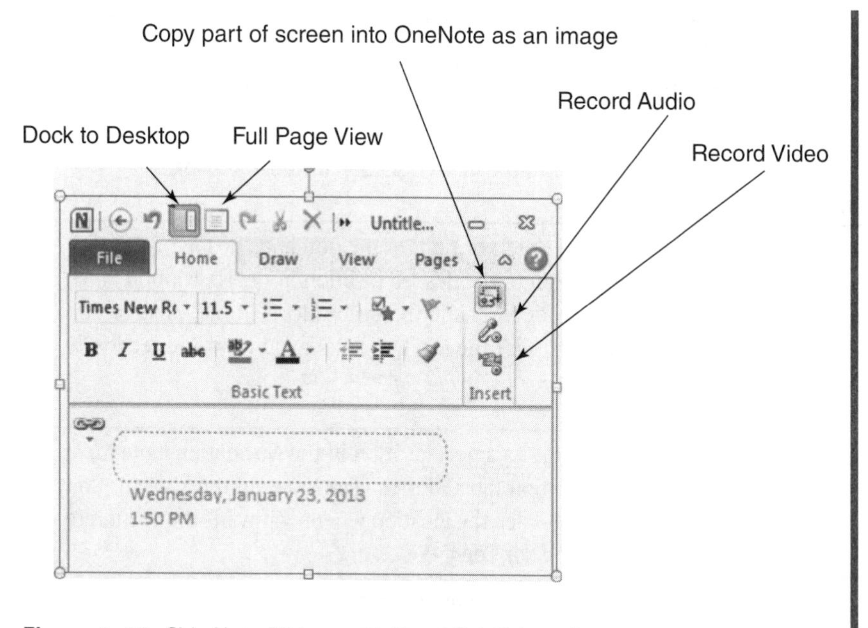

Figure 1-22 Side Note Ribbon with Home Tab Selected

To open a Side Note window and add notes:

1. Press the **Windows logo** key + N or right-click the **OneNote icon** in the notification area of the taskbar and click **Open New Side Note.**
2. Click in the **blank area** of the OneNote and type your **message**. OneNote saves this Side Note in the open notebook.

To create a Linked Note:

1. If you are using Word or PowerPoint and want to make quick notes about something to remember later, select **Linked Notes** under the Review tab in Word or PowerPoint.
2. Select the **location** for the Side Note and click **OK**. This will associate the notes with the application.
3. Type the **Side Note**.

Moving Pages, Sections, and Notebooks

Moving large pieces of information is easy in OneNote. The following are some ways you can do this. Be aware that the target notebook must be open in order to move content into it.

To Move This	Do This
A page or subpage within a section	Drag the page tab up or down on the page task pane.
A page to another notebook	Drag the page tab to the desired section in the notebook.
A section within a notebook	Drag the section tab left or right in the notebook header; or Drag the section tab to the desired location in the Navigation Pane; or Right-click the section tab and then click Move. In the Move or Copy Section dialog box, click the location where you want the section to go, and then click Move or Copy Move or Copy....
A section to another notebook	Drag the section tab to a new location in the Navigation Pane; or Right-click the section tab and then click Move. In the Move or Copy Section dialog box, click the location where you want the section to go, and then click Move or Copy.
A notebook on the Navigation Pane	Drag the notebook title up or down the notebook list.

Other Features

A few other important features include sending information to other Office programs, tagging notes, sending an image or text from a browser, and search OneNote. Tags mark notes for easier return to that reminder, for follow-up, and to send to others. Tags also let you set priorities and categorize your notes.

Sending a piece of information, a table, or picture to another Office Program:

1. Select the **pages** or **section** you want to send.
2. Go to **File** and click **Send**. Choose one of the listed options as shown in Figure 1-15.

Tagging notes:

1. Select a **note** to tag.
2. Find the **Tag Box** Tags on the Home ribbon.
3. Click the **Important Tag**. A star will appear in the note's container.

If you click the down arrow, a menu appears as shown in **Figure 1-23.** Many more choices become available on this menu.

Sending a note or image from a browser to OneNote:

If you are working in Internet Explorer or Firefox, you can send an image or text to OneNote. Chrome requires the installation of an extension.

1. Find an **image** or **portion of text** or even a whole Web page.
2. Press the **Windows logo** key + S.
3. Drag the mouse over the **section/picture** you wish to capture.
4. Double click the **section/page** in the OneNote menu where you want to send the image. (See **Figure 1-24.**)

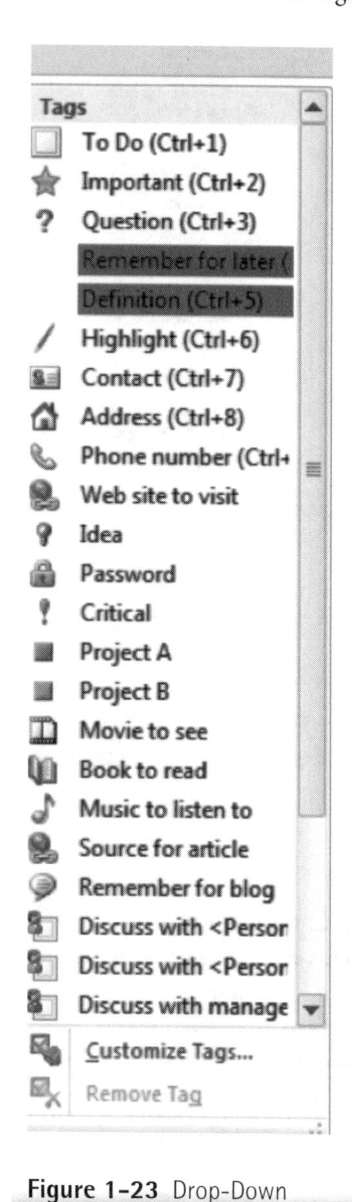

Figure 1-23 Drop-Down Menu for Tags in OneNote

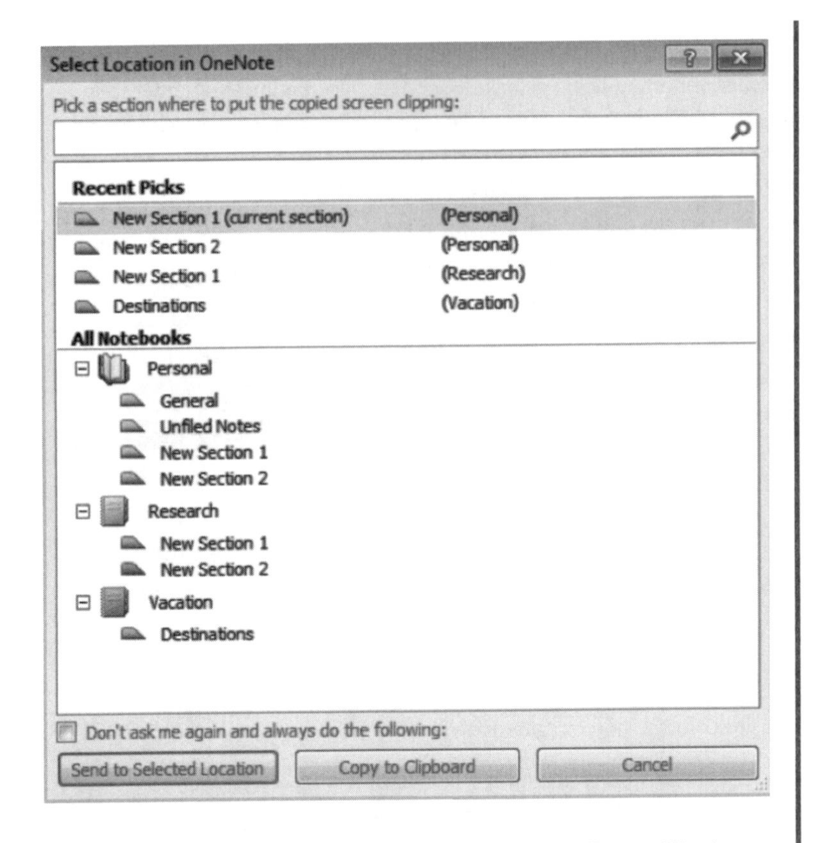

Figure 1-24 Location Selection Menu in OneNote for Screen Clipping

Searching OneNote

This section has highlighted just a few of the many things you can do with One-Note. If you use this program properly, you will end up with a large collection of information. Even if you use all the tools possible to organize your information, you may need to search for some information.

1. Go to the Search text box Search All Notebooks (Ctrl+E) and **click in it**.
2. Type the **word(s)** that represent the information for which you are searching.
3. Click the **magnifying glass**.
4. A list of the matches appears, highlighted in yellow. Click **View List**, and a partial description of each match appears on the right side of the window.

Additional Tips

Some additional tips described here will prove helpful as you work through this text to develop your technology literacy skills.

1. Do not try to complete all of the text exercises at once. Sometimes it is helpful to come back later, especially when the exercises are not going well or when fatigue sets in.
2. Pay attention to messages on the screen. They are the computer's way of trying to provide help.
3. Use the software sequences at the end of each lesson on an application program to complete the exercises or assignments for that software program. It is not necessary to memorize the commands, mouse clicks, or sequences of events. Use the screen clues, prompts, and online help to guide you through the sequence.
4. Explore additional functions by referring to other reference sources such as online help, manuals, or reference books. We've chosen the functions highlighted in this book to help you complete the exercises and learn some basics of how the programs work. Many more functions are available within each of the software programs presented here.
5. Always back up your files. This point is especially important for the beginner so that you will not lose hours of work. Open a document and then save it immediately; don't wait until you have finished it or finished your session on the computer.
6. Practice doing assignments from all courses using your computer. It takes practice to develop computer literacy. The more you use the computer, the easier and faster tasks will become.
7. Be patient. Learning a new vocabulary and developing new skills take time and energy.
8. Start collecting information for your e-portfolio using OneNote.

Summary

This chapter provided an introduction to computer and information literacy. It described how this book is organized and the conventions used to denote user actions. The chapter presented helpful information about getting started using the school or laboratory facilities. Instructions related to creating a PDF file and compressing files are included. The chapter addressed the essentials of email communication. Also described were the basics of using OneNote—getting started, opening new notebooks, adding pages or sections, using the drawing tools, and taking screen clippings. Finally, it described resources for learning more about OneNote.

References

Association of College and Research Libraries (ACRL) (2000). *Information literacy competency standards for higher education*. Chicago: ACRL. Retrieved from http://www.ala.org/ala/mgrps/divs/acrl/standards/informationliteracycompetency.cfm

Email Experience Council (EEC) (n.d.). Email Glossary. New York: EEC. Retrieved from http://www.emailexperience.org/email-resources/email-glossary/

Federal Communications Commission (FCC) (2011). *How to proctect yourself online*. Columbia, MD: FCC. Retrieved from http://www.fcc.gov/guides/how-protect-yourself-online

International Telecommunications Union (ITU) (2012). *Internet Usage and Broadband Usage Report*. Geneva: ITU. Retrieved from http://www.internetworldstats.com/am/us.htm

Exercises 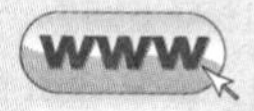

EXERCISE 1 Using an Email System

Objectives

1. Access an email system.
2. Change the password for an email account.
3. Read, save, and delete email.

Activity

1. If you do not already have an email account, obtain an account from the university computer center. An account gives you permission to use the system. This permission comes in the form of a user ID and a unique password. If you were not provided with an account, you need to set up a computer account before doing this exercise. If you have a user ID and password, you are ready to begin this exercise. If your university does not provide email accounts, use an Internet search engine to find one of the free online services that provide email accounts.
2. Find the documentation. Most institutions have documentation for computer programs available to users. Short handouts are usually available for free either in print or at the institution's Web site. Find out where and how you can obtain documentation at your institution. Obtain a copy of or view the documentation for signing on to the system and for using email. With an account, you may also be able to access online help.
3. Sign in to the network. Follow the directions for signing on to the computer system. Typically, you will type the **user ID**, and press the **Tab** key to go to the next text field. Type the **password**, and then either press **Enter** or click **OK**.

   Remember that the password will not appear on the screen. In most email programs, it appears as a series of asterisks (******) or black dots in the Password text box.

   If a message appears on the screen saying Invalid password, Login incorrect, or something similar, try typing the user ID and password again. Some systems are case sensitive; thus you need to note whether you should or should not use capitals in either the user ID or the password. Most systems give you at least three tries to get in before the account is locked out; you will then need to see the account administrator or call the Help Desk to have it unlocked.

4. Change the password. When signing in for the first time, most email systems require you to change the password before proceeding. If the system does not require you to change the password, this should be your first action after signing in. Check the documentation for the specific process for changing a password.

In email programs:

a. Click the **Password icon**, *or* select an option on a **menu**, *or* click a **hypertext** link.
b. When prompted for the current password, type the **current password**, and then either press **Enter** or click **OK**.
c. When prompted, type the **new password**, and either press **Enter** or click **OK**.
d. When prompted, type the **new password** a second time and either press **Enter** or click **OK**.

When you are typing passwords throughout this procedure, the passwords will not appear on the screen. The change is usually processed immediately, although on some systems there may be a time lag before the new password takes effect. Check the system documentation. Also note that many universities have a one log-in system. Once you change the network password, your email password also changes; other places require you to log-in to the network and then the email program.

5. Access the email system. This may be as simple as selecting **MS Outlook** from the programs list on the Start menu of the desktop or clicking an **email** link to another email program such as gmail. You may also be able to type the URL for the email program directly into your browser. For example, mail.yahoo.com/. For personal emails, you may need to use a browser to access an email program such as gmail or yahoo.
6. Once you log in to your email, open and read each message.
   a. Double-click or highlight the email **message** and press **Enter**.
   b. If this approach does not work, look at the screen for directions and read the documentation for the system. After you read each email message, look at how the email directory changed.
7. Send a message. Find the **email address** of a friend. Asking your friend for his or her address is the easiest way to do this. In college settings, there may be a faculty, staff, and student online address book that contains listings of addresses. One way to test your understanding of the correct procedure at the location is to practice by sending yourself a message. Once you master the procedure, practice sending messages to a friend.
   a. Start the **email** program.
   b. Type the **email address** of the friend in the **To** text box. Many programs permit you to select the address from the email address book by double-clicking it.

c. Press the **Tab** key or click in the **Subject** text box.
d. Type in the **subject**, and press the **Tab** key or click in the **Message** text box. Most likely you do not need to CC yourself. Most email programs automatically place a copy of all email sent out in your Sent folder.
e. Type and format the **message**.
f. Click the **Send** icon.

The procedure for composing an email message varies greatly from one system to another. The previous information outlines the general process used by many of today's email programs. If this procedure does not work, read the local documentation for the following information:

How do you initiate the function to compose a message?
How do you enter the address of the person who will receive this message?
How do you enter the email message?
When the email message is ready, how do you give the send command?

8. Reply to a message.
   a. Open an email **message** (double-click it).
   b. Click the **Reply to Sender** icon. This symbol may look different for different programs. The program inserts the sender's address and subject in the appropriate text boxes. The Subject text box uses the same subject and adds the prefix "RE:" to it. Note the difference in the option Reply to All versus simply Reply.
   c. If you receive a message as part of a distribution list, find out how to reply to the author and how to reply to everyone on the list.
   d. Compose the **response**, and click the **Send** button.
9. Save or delete each message.
   a. Highlight the **message**.
   b. Press the **Delete** key or click the **Delete** button. In some Web-based email programs, you delete messages by clicking in the square box next to the message, and then clicking the Delete button.

Read the local documentation for the delete procedure. In many email applications, you must "empty the trash" or "purge the Delete folder" to remove a message. Once you complete this step, you will not be able to recover deleted messages. If you do not delete messages, the mailbox will become full and eventually new messages will bounce back to the sender. Most email programs automatically save a copy of all sent messages in a Sent folder. If these sent messages accumulate, this folder will eventually take up too much space and new email sent to your mailbox will bounce. The system administrator may also automatically empty the sent message folder after a set time period. Some email programs leave the undeleted messages in the inbox, whereas others move them to an older message folder. You will know if an unread message is in your inbox because it will be listed in the message list each time you start the email program.

c. Read the documentation for the save procedure. Most systems also permit you to move messages into online folders. Read the documentation for a procedure for saving messages in folders.

10. Exit the email program.

    In Windows-based email programs, follow one of these procedures:

    a. Click the **Close** button in the upper-right corner of the screen, or
    b. Select **File**, **Exit** from the menu bar.

    It is important to exit the email system with the computer still running. If you turn the computer off or just walk away without exiting email, someone else may be able to access your account without signing on. Once you exit the email program, complete the computer sequence for shutting down the computer as specified by the laboratory, library, or other locale.

EXERCISE 2 Log In, Download, and Send an Email Attachment

Objectives

1. Log in to the email program.
2. Download and send an email attachment.

Activity

1. **Log in** to the mail program you will be using for this course. You will receive an email with an attachment from your professor.
2. **Open** the email and follow the instructions contained in it. It will contain a compressed file. Download the compressed file using the directions provided in this chapter. Extract the contents of the file. What was in the compressed file?
3. Send an email to your classmates and professor that contains the following information:
   a. A brief introduction about you, your interests, and so on.
   b. A picture of yourself as an attachment.
4. Read and respond to your classmates' emails. Open their attachments.

EXERCISE 3 Information Literacy Competency Standards for Higher Education

Objectives

1. Develop a personal definition of information literacy.
2. Add the definition to OneNote.

■ **Activity**

1. Go to the Web site of the Association of College and Research Libraries.
   a. Type **http://www.ala.org/ala/mgrps/divs/acrl/index.cfm.**
   b. Click **Guidelines and Standards** on the left side of the screen.
   c. Move down the list and click **Information Literacy Competency Standards for Higher Education (Jan. 2000).**
   d. Review the standards by selecting **Standards, Performance Indicators, and Outcomes.**
   e. Review the material on information literacy and information technology at this site.
2. From this material, develop your own definition of information literacy.
3. Place this definition in OneNote for later addition to your e-portfolio. Keep a weekly journal of the skills you are developing in this course.

EXERCISE 4 Electronic Reference Formats

■ **Objectives**

1. Find sources for styling electronic references.
2. Recognize the appropriate format for electronic references used by the American Psychological Association (APA).

■ **Activity**

Use OneNote to keep a notebook of your findings regarding how to format electronic references. If necessary, review the processes described earlier in this chapter. In the Word chapter, you will learn how to use templates and the References tab to automatically format your papers and references in the correct style.

1. Go to the Dartmouth Institute for Writing and Rhetoric.
   a. Type **http://www.dartmouth.edu/~writing/.**
   b. Click **Sources & Citation at Dartmouth.**
   c. Download a copy and review it. (Note: You will need the **PDF add-in utility** on your computer. If necessary, review the process for adding the PDF utility that was described earlier in this chapter.)
2. Go to APA Style.org.
   a. Type **http://www.apastyle.org/.**
   b. Click **Websites.**
   c. Review the page.
3. Review the following sources:
   a. Type **http://www.dianahacker.com/resdoc/.**
      i. Hold the mouse pointer over Finding Sources in the **Sciences Section** and click **Nursing and health**.
      ii. Review the sections on **Databases & Indexes** and **Web resources**.

b. Go to "The Owl at Purdue" and review its APA Formatting and Style Guide.
   i. Type **http://owl.english.purdue.edu/owl/resource/560/01/**.
   ii. Under General Format, scroll down and choose **Reference List: Electronic Sources**.
   iii. Review the materials.

EXERCISE 5 Compare Three Information Literacy Tutorials

■ Objectives

1. Review three different information literacy tutorial series.
2. Compare and evaluate them.
3. Use OneNote to write your comparison.

■ Activity

1. Compare the following three information literacy tutorial series in terms of their ease of use, ease of navigation (i.e., ability to move around them), content, and value to you.
   a. Information Literacy Tutorial: University of Wisconsin-Parkside Library
      i. Type **http://www.uwp.edu/departments/library/**.
      ii. Under Quick Links, click **Information Literacy**.
      iii. Click **Start the Tutorial** under Quick Links.
      iv. Select **Module 5**. Review any other modules that are of interest to you.
   b. Information Literacy Tutorial: University of Wisconsin-Milwaukee
      i. Type **http://guides.library.uwm.edu/infolit**.
      ii. Review the six modules—especially **Module 6**.
   c. Information Literacy Video Tutorials: University of Pittsburgh
      i. Type **http://www.library.pitt.edu/services/classes/infoliteracy/teaching.html**.
      ii. View **Avoiding Plagiarism** and **Surfing the Cyber Library**. View any other videos of interest to you.
2. Add a new notebook to OneNote named **Chap1-Exercise5-LastName**. Create a new page in the notebook named **InfLitComparison**. Add your comparison to the new page.

EXERCISE 6 Explore the Uses of e-Portfolios

■ Objectives

1. Describe the essentials of an e-portfolio.
2. Describe the relationship between information literacy and e-portfolios.

■ Activity

1. Go to the e-portfolio site at Penn State.
   a. Type **http://portfolio.psu.edu/**.
   b. Click the **Featured Portfolio** and view the video.
2. What is an e-portfolio?
3. How does it relate to information literacy?
4. Next click **Featured Resource**. Review the page and check out other links such as **Information Literacy**, **Copyright**, and **Plagiarism Prevention Resources**.
5. If you are interested in learning more about e-portfolios, you will find an **Overview of E-Portfolios** by the *Educause Learning Initiative* at this site: **http://net.educause.edu/ir/library/pdf/eli3001.pdf**.

Assignments

ASSIGNMENT 1 Learning about Your School's Computer Policies

■ Directions

Use your school's intranet site to answer the following questions:

1. Find your school's Web site. What is its Uniform Resource Locator (URL)?
2. Is there a technical support center? Is it known by another name?
3. What are the policies and procedures of the academic computing center?
4. Can you download these policies?
5. How does a student set up network and email accounts?
6. Which operating systems and software does the center support?
7. Is there a laptop or mobile device lease/buy program at your school?
8. Does your school have an e-portfolio system for students?
9. Is there an e-learning center? If so, which classes are available?
10. What are the hours for technical support?
11. What was the most valuable thing you learned from this assignment?
12. Write a summary of your learning from answering these questions. Save the file as **Chap1-Assign1-LastName**. Submit the file as directed by your professor.

ASSIGNMENT 2 Setting Up an Online Email Account

■ Directions

1. Use an Internet search engine to find a free email application.
2. Select a free email application from one found.

3. Click the new **user sign-in link** and follow the instructions given. Read all of the privacy information. When given the choice, be sure that you select the free email service. How much storage space does this email system provide?
4. Once you register, read the welcome message. How often do you need to use this system for your account to remain active?
5. Print this message to hand in, and answer the previous questions on the printout.

chapter

2

Information Systems: Hardware, Software, and Connectivity

Objectives 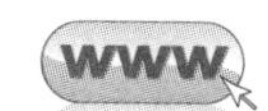

1. Define information systems.
2. Describe the major components of computer systems and their related functions.
3. Define basic terminology related to hardware, software, and connectivity.
4. Describe the main categories of computer software.
5. Appropriately utilize the language of information systems.

Introduction to Information Systems

A recent announcement in *InformationWeek* entitled "Pittsburgh Healthcare System Invests $100M in Big Data" (Lewis, 2012) states that the money will be spent to "create a comprehensive data warehouse that brings together clinical, financial, administrative, genomic, and other information from more than 200 sources across UPMC, UPMC Health Plan and other affiliate entities" (para 1). We are truly in an "information age" where technology is being increasingly used to manage the exponential growth of data to produce information necessary for healthcare professionals to provide safe, efficient client care that results in quality outcomes. To do this requires information- and computer-literate healthcare professionals who can identify needed data and who can communicate with technical experts to produce systems that can transform data into useful information.

A system is a set of interrelated parts; an **information system** is a system that produces information using an input/process/output cycle. A basic information system consists of four elements: people, policies and

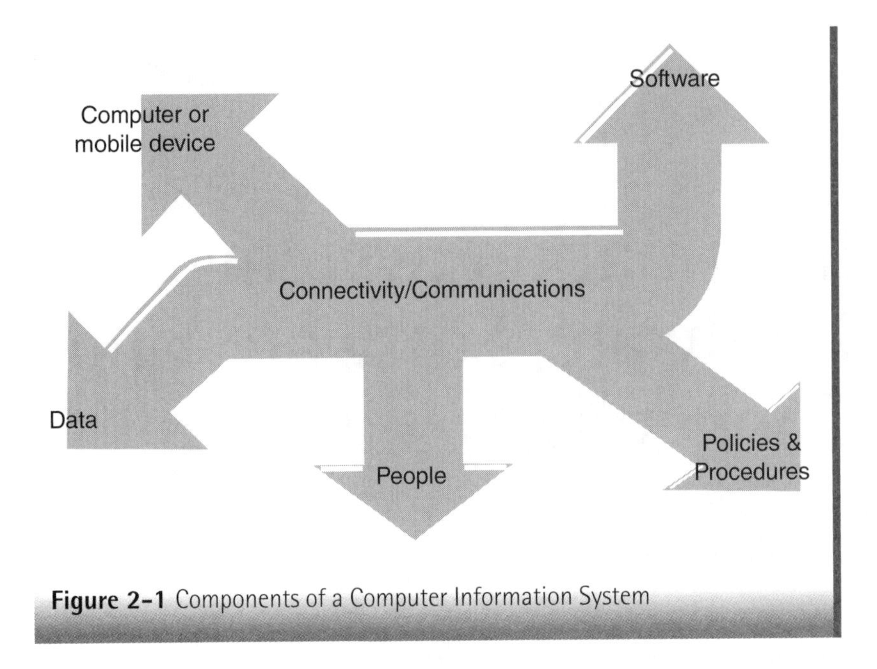

Figure 2-1 Components of a Computer Information System

procedures, communication (connectivity), and data. A computer information system then adds two more elements: hardware and software. (See **Figure 2-1**.) Types of information systems include transaction systems, such as payroll and order entry systems; management information systems, which facilitate running an organization; decision support systems, which support user in making decisions; and expert systems, which attempt to mimic a human expert in providing advice or recommendations regarding diagnosis or treatment.

The purpose of an information system is to provide information to the users to facilitate the work of the organization. A brief description of each of its elements follows.

People

People are the most important part of the system as they are the ones who need to use the information generated in order to provide quality patient care and improve patient outcomes; they—and ultimately their organizations—benefit from the information provided by these systems. Information systems typically identify three basic types of users: end users, technical professionals, and informatics specialists. In health care, end users are the healthcare providers who use computers as tools to assist them in delivering care and the consumers who access healthcare information on the Internet and/or store their personal health records (PHR) on Internet-accessible servers.

Technical professionals are the information technology professionals who develop, maintain, and evaluate the technical aspects of information systems. They are generally responsible for the network, databases, software and hardware updates, security, communications, and so forth. These are the people who respond to end-user problems and questions. They do not have the healthcare knowledge to determine what healthcare professional need to provide quality care.

Informatics specialists are professionals who bridge the gap between the healthcare provider as end user and the technical expert. Their education and professional experience include both health care and computer/information science. Chapter 14 provides examples of types of Information Technology personnel found in health care

Critical to bridging the gap in communications between technical experts and end users is the basic computer and information literacy of the end users. Both parties must speak the same language for quality healthcare information systems to move forward. Achieving the goal of computer and information literate healthcare providers is the mission of this text.

Policies and Procedures

Policies and procedures outline the guiding principles as to information and technology use and give step-by-step directions for how the system works and how you do things to accomplish the end results. Most systems have a manual or documentation—mostly online but some in print form—that includes the necessary directions and/or instructions, rules or policies, and special guidelines for using the system. Later chapters dealing with communications in healthcare systems (Chapter 10) as well as data integrity and security (Chapter 13) provide examples of specific policies and procedures for healthcare technology.

Data

Data are the basic units used in the creation of information. Topics relating to data use and access are provided throughout the text. The chapter on healthcare informatics and information systems (Chapter 14) describes data and information, along with knowledge and wisdom. The chapter on databases (Chapter 8) presents basic database concepts and the chapters on using the Internet and information access, evaluation, and use (Chapters 9 and 12) cover information access.

Hardware

Hardware consists of the devices that personnel use to input and access information in the system. The trend is for more mobile devices to be used at the point-of-care delivery such as in the home, a clinic, a hospital, or remotely as in telehealth.

Software

Software programs and apps (software applications for mobile devices) provide directions to the hardware to tell it what to do. Without software or apps, the devices would not be able to process data or create information.

Connectivity/Communication

Connectivity (also known as communication) refers to the electronic transfer of data from one place to another. This is an area of rapid development that is changing how work is done. We are living in a mobile technological society with 24/7 connectivity via smartphones and tablets.

Communication also refers to how people use the technology to enhance their communications with each other and with healthcare consumers. Basic communication concepts covered in this text include appropriate and professional communications within the healthcare setting. The use of social media has expanded the communication options (1) among patients, (2) between patients and healthcare providers, and (3) among healthcare providers.

Hardware, software, and connectivity are the focus of this chapter. Other chapters in this text contain more information about specific software applications and communications.

Introduction to Information Systems: Hardware

The hardware for a computer system consists of input devices, the system unit (processing unit, memory, boards, and power supply), output devices, and secondary storage devices. The basic function of the computer is to accept data and instructions from a user, process the data to produce information, store the data for later retrieval, and display the information. More advanced functions involve the creation, communication, and storage of knowledge used in the provision of health care. Supporting the implementation of evidence-based care at the point of delivery is an example of this advanced function.

A Few Definitions

Computer

A **computer** is a programmable machine capable of performing a series of logical and arithmetic operations. One of the most frequent uses of a computer in health care is the conversion of data into information. As an electronic device, the computer uses a series of 0s and 1s to describe data and to represent information. It does not understand the spoken word as we do, but must convert words to a sequence of 0s and 1s.

Bit	A **bit** is the smallest unit of data, the lowest level; the term "bit" is an abbreviation for "binary digit." A bit represents one of two states for the computer, 0 or 1; these two states are equivalent to off or on (like the two states possible for a light switch). Everything the computer understands uses combinations of 0s and 1s.
Byte	A **byte** is a string of bits used to represent a character, digit, or symbol. It usually contains 8 bits.
Default	**Default** means the setting the computer will use unless told otherwise. For example, users will have difficulty printing to a color printer if the default printer is a black-and-white laser printer. This would require the user to select the color printer before sending the job to the printer. Another example relates to the default folder where files are saved unless otherwise instructed.
Toggle	**Toggle** means to switch from one mode of operation to another. For example, by default the Show/Hide mode in Word is turned off. If you want to see the paragraph marks, tab marks, and so forth you must click the Show/Hide icon to toggle it on.
Update	**Update** means to install the latest patches for an application or device driver. Updating is critical to maintain a secure computer. This is especially true for an antivirus program to be able to recognize the latest viruses.
Upgrade	**Upgrade** means to enhance a piece of hardware or to obtain the latest version of a software program.

Types of Computers and Mobile Devices

Computers come in various sizes and configurations. Over the years, the power, speed, storage capacity, and capabilities of computers have increased, while their size and cost have decreased. **Figure 2-2** illustrates two types of larger computers and **Figure 2-3** illustrates some mobile and personal devices. Some common types of computers are described next.

Supercomputer

Supercomputers are the fastest, most expensive, and most powerful type of computers available. While some are single computers, most supercomputers consist of multiple high performance computers that work in parallel as if they were a single computer. They tend to focus on running a few programs requiring a lot of computations; by comparison, other types of computers typically run many

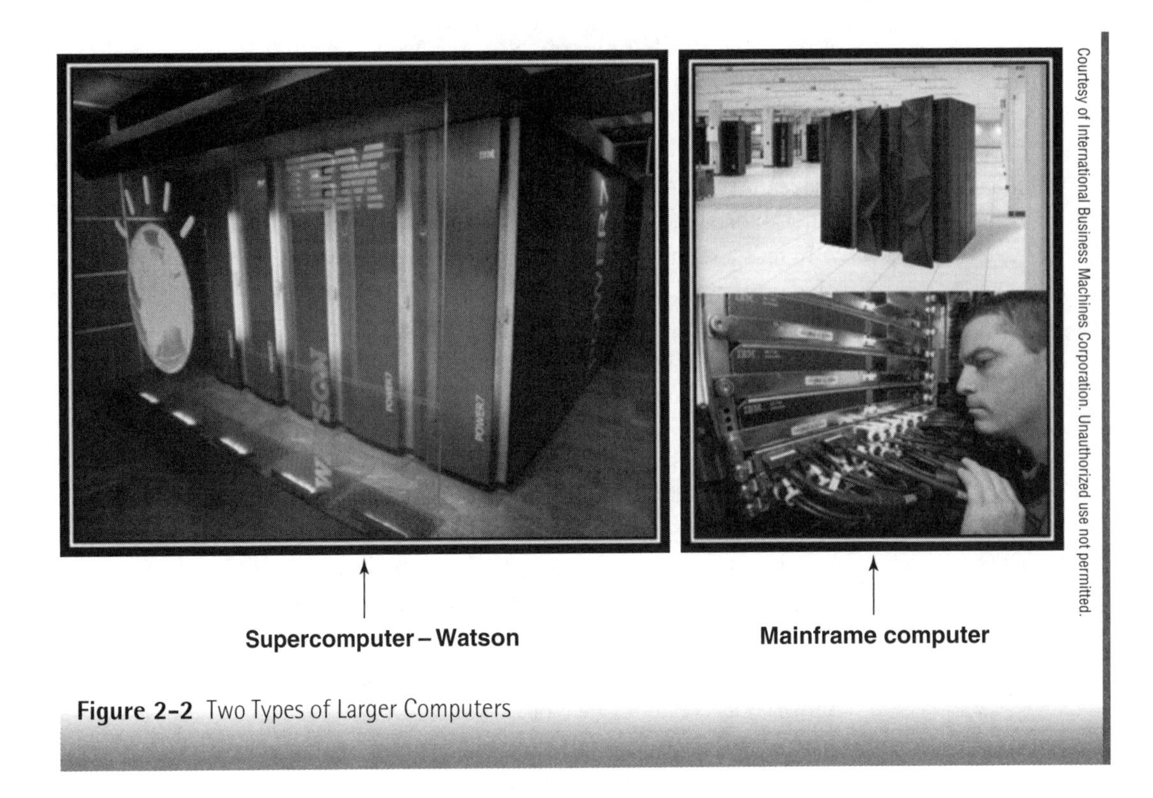

Figure 2-2 Two Types of Larger Computers

programs concurrently. Uses of supercomputers include development of animation graphics, weather forecasting, and research applications. Some medical-related examples include recreating the internal architecture of bone structures to guide bone replacement in reconstructive surgery, designing new molecular compounds for drug-related therapies, genetic mapping in understanding Parkinson's disease, analysis of tumor cells, and aiding in unlocking information buried in large amounts of data. The newest supercomputer on the scene is IBM's Watson. This supercomputer has teamed up with Cleveland Clinic to work together on improving health care (Magaw, 2012).

Mainframe (Enterprise Server)

A **mainframe** is a large computer that accommodates hundreds of users simultaneously. It has a large data storage capacity, a large amount of memory, multiple input/output (I/O) devices, and a speedy processor(s). Many universities and hospitals run their computer systems on mainframe computers, as do larger big box stores.

With more powerful smaller computers, enterprise servers are replacing mainframes in many smaller businesses such as local health centers. The enterprise

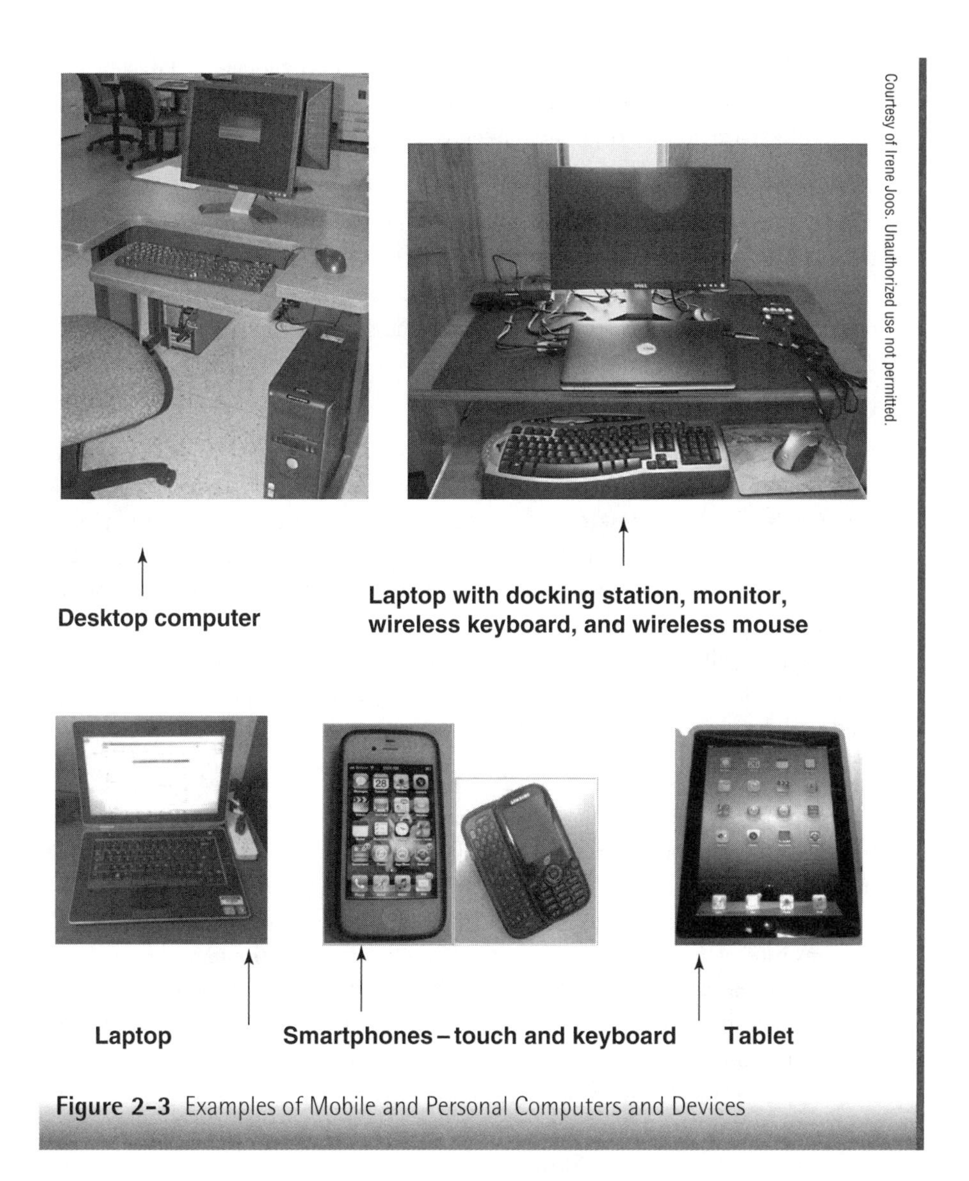

Figure 2-3 Examples of Mobile and Personal Computers and Devices

server contains programs that the whole company or enterprise uses. Two examples are Sun Microsystems' computers running Unix or Linux operating systems and IBM's Power Series.

Servers

A **server** is a computer that controls access to the software, hardware (like printers on the network), and such specialized services as the Web server, the firewall server, the database server and so forth. Users utilize their personal computers to access the resources on the network and to store data on specialized servers or file servers. Many facilities do not permit storing files on the local hard drive where only the person using that computer can access the work. Companies provide users with space on the corporate file server to save their work.

Workstations

A **workstation** is basically a desktop computer with more power, memory, and enhanced capabilities for performing specialized tasks. Some public relations (PR) departments in hospitals use them for 3D graphics development and to support Web sites and publications. Users may employ them to produce patient educational videos and simulations/games.

Microcomputer/PC/Desktop

A **microcomputer** is a small, one-user computer system with its own central processing unit (CPU), memory, and storage devices. Also referred to as personal computers (PCs) and desktops, these models are growing in processing power, speed, and storage capacity. They are designed to be used in one location and are less expensive than some of the portable devices. In clinics and hospitals you see them in patient/examining rooms and nurses stations/offices. Some people predict they will go the way of the dinosaur as mobile devices grow in use and capabilities or we will redefine them as personal devices and include what we currently call laptops, tablets, and smart phones (Aamoth, 2013).

Laptops/Notebooks/Netbooks

Laptops, sometimes called **notebooks,** are generally more expensive than PCs, but can have the same power and capabilities. Their small size and portability make them a good choice for use in airplanes, libraries, and homes, or in small spaces such as a nurse's station. Batteries or AC outlets provide power to laptops. Laptops integrate the monitor, keyboard, and mouse into the laptop case. Users can convert laptops into a PC by using a docking station, ports, or a laptop interface that accepts a larger monitor, full-size keyboard, mouse, or printer. **Netbooks** are ultraportable laptops that are smaller and cheaper than traditional laptops, but also less powerful. Many students use them as they can do most of what a traditional student needs to do, i.e., papers and presentations, perform research on the Internet, send email, and so forth.

Personal Digital Assistants

Personal Digital Assistants (PDA) are being replaced by smartphones. They perform many of the same functions as PCs, but are meant to supplement PCs, not replace them. PDAs have a processor, an operating system (OS), memory, a power source (batteries), a display, an input device (newer ones use color touchscreens), audio capability, I/O ports, and software, but no hard drive. Basic information such as a calendar, address book, or contacts, is stored on a read-only memory (ROM) chip; programs added later, such as drug reference material, are stored on a **random access memory (RAM)** chip. Most PDAs can access the Internet via wireless connections, and some models have **Global Positioning System (GPS)** capabilities. Their ability to store information such as contacts, drug references, laboratory tests, and other diagnostic reference material as well as their small size make them favorites in the healthcare field. An increasing number of nursing programs have chosen to provide their students with PDAs as quick reference sources to use in clinical rotations.

Smartphones

Smartphones such as the iPhone and Android phones provide access to the Internet, email, texting, references, GPS, books, and games, as well as the ability to make phone calls. Increasing numbers of healthcare professionals are using these devices to provide quick access to references during patient care. The distinction between PDAs and smartphones is also blurring as their functions increasingly overlap.

Tablets

Tablets are smaller than laptops but bigger than smartphones. If you look on the inside of a tablet it looks much like a computer but with a snug, more efficient fit (think smaller processor). Tablets generally run on a rechargeable battery that lasts on average 10 hours. The bestselling tablet is the iPad but there are now others on the market like the Android tablets, Kindle Fire, and the new Windows tablet, Surface. Tablets are being used in health care because they are mobile, convenient, and contain a larger screen than a smartphone. They are used in hospital operating rooms, to provide patient education, to look up resources, to access the Internet, to access an EMR, and the list goes on. The latest trend in this area are **convertibles**, which are laptops that turn into tablets when the top part (screen and tablet) is removed from the bottom part (keyboard).

Computer Components: Input Devices

Input devices are hardware components that convert data from an external source into electronic signals understood by the computer. The user interacts with the computer through an interface and an input device.

While there are other input devices, the three most common are the **keyboard**, **mouse**, and **touchscreen**. For the keyboard and mouse interaction, the term "**cursor**" or "**pointer**" is used to describe the "visible indicator" on the screen that marks the current location and the point at which the work begins. The cursor can appear as a pointer (generally an arrow ( )), a vertical line ( ), a horizontal line (__), or an I-beam ( ). The cursor also changes to reflect processes and functions. For example, in Windows, it changes to a spinning circle ( ) or a circle and left slanted arrow ( )when the program is processing a command. In Internet Explorer (a Web browser), it changes to a hand ( ) when placed over linked text or objects (text or objects that can lead to more information either at this site or at another site). There are also other symbols that look like double-headed arrows (⟷, ⤡, etc) used for resizing windows and graphics. For each of the Office applications you will see additional pointer shapes like the size column shape in Excel.

Keyboard

The **keyboard** is an input device for typing data into the computer. The most common layout includes the typical alphanumeric keys with the function keys at the top and the cursor movement keys and the numeric keypad (calculator layout) on the right. In contrast, laptop computers have a slightly different layout because of their size limitations. Mobile devices such as smartphones and PDAs have fewer keys, each key representing multiple characters that the user cycles through. For example, the number 2 also represents the letters A, B, and C. Newer keyboards may also include additional keys for Internet access and media controls. Mac keyboards have many of the same keys, but they may be called by another name. Some have fingerprint and card readers. **Figure 2-4a** shows a wired keyboard, a wireless, ergonomic keyboard, and a laptop keyboard.

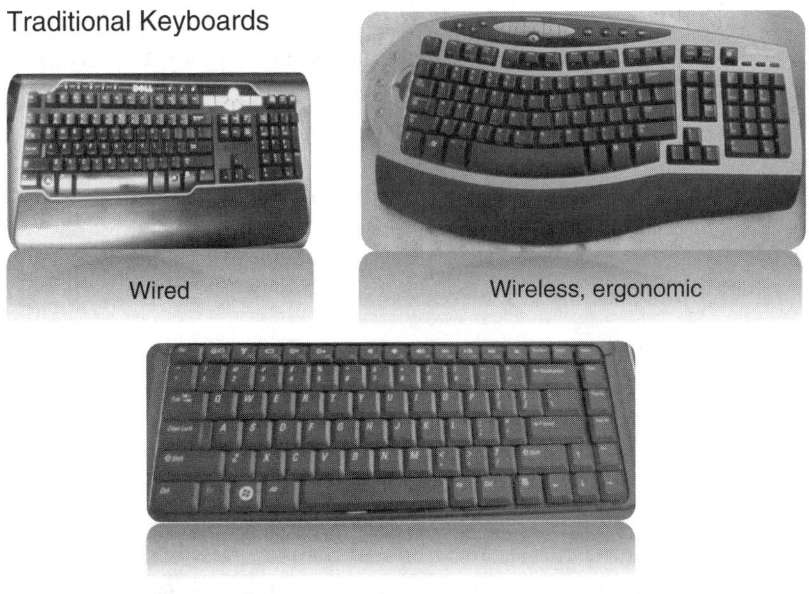

Traditional Keyboards

Wired

Wireless, ergonomic

Laptop

Figure 2-4a Traditional Input Devices

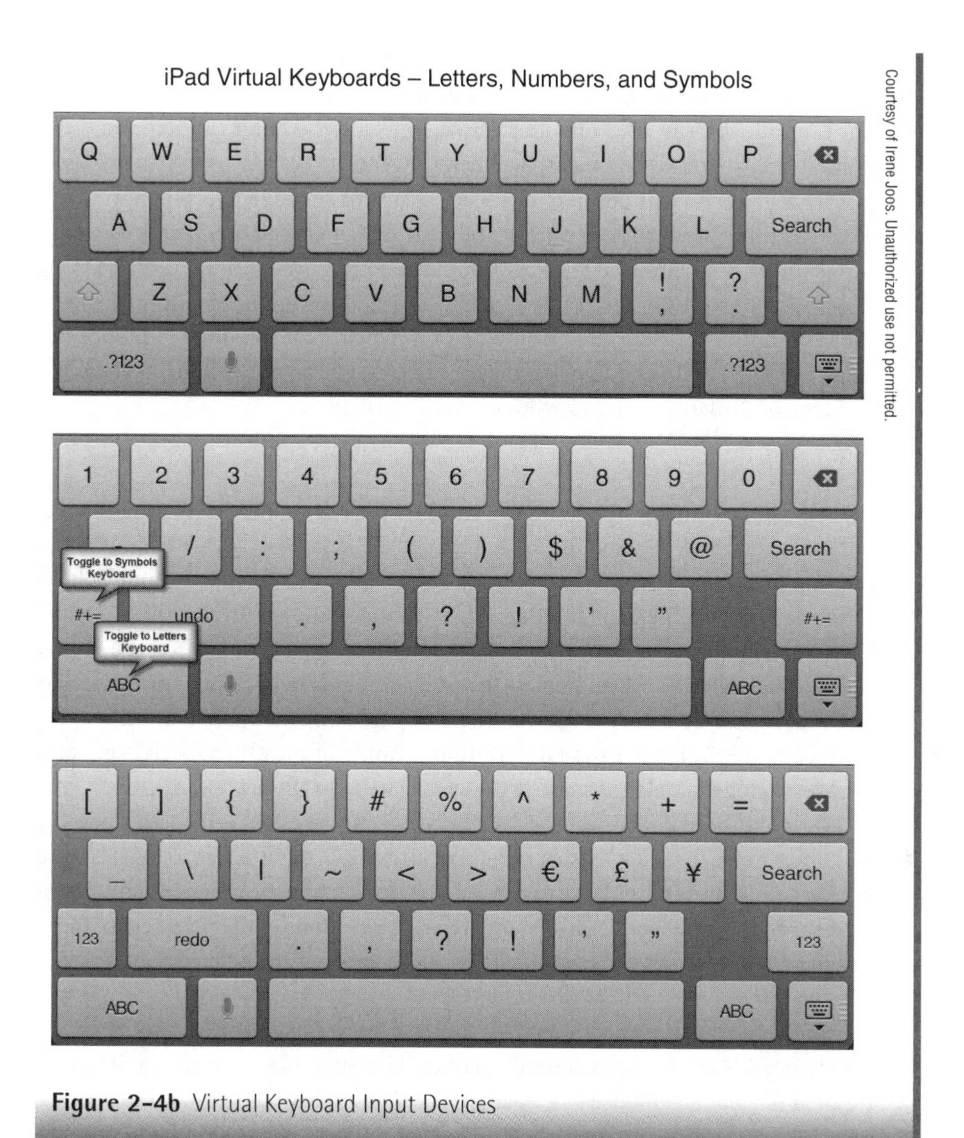

Figure 2-4b Virtual Keyboard Input Devices

Virtual keyboards, as shown in **Figure 2-4b**, are growing in popularity with the advent of touch phones, tablets, and touch computer monitors. Virtual keyboards are software components that permit the user to type on an optical-detectable surface instead of pressing physical keys. There are two flavors of virtual keyboards—projection keyboards in which the image of the keyboard is projected on a flat surface as is the case with white or smart boards. and soft keyboards in which the image of the keyboard is displayed on the device screen. Virtual keyboards for mobile devices generally limit the type of characters available and may require switching back and forth between two or three types of keyboards. For example, on the iPad one must move between the letter keyboard and the numeric keyboard, which may slow down the typing.

Physical keyboards connect to the system unit through the keyboard port, although some use the **serial port** or the **USB port.** Cordless keyboards use radio waves or infrared light waves to communicate to the system unit via an **IrDA** or **Bluetooth** port in the system unit. Laptop keyboards are integral to the top of the system unit. The design of some newer keyboards is intended to reduce the chance of wrist and hand injuries; they are referred to as "ergonomic" keyboards.

Some of the keys used on keyboards are described next.

Keyboard Keys

Most keyboards today still maintain the QWERTY layout for arranging the letters, numbers, and punctuation keys. Some of the keys have dual functions when they are pressed in conjunction with the Shift, Ctrl, or Alt key. For example, lowercase letters become capital letters when pressed along with the Shift or Caps Lock key; numbers become symbols such as $, %, and * when pressed along with the Shift key. Use the Caps Lock key to switch or toggle between all uppercase and lowercase letters. This key is helpful when a significant amount of text needs to be in all caps. See **Table 2-1** for a description of some of the other special keys and **Figure 2-5** for examples of some of the special keys on the keyboard.

For touchscreens, the alphabet is present; sometimes with one letter per key and other times three letters share a key requiring 1, 2, or 3 presses to toggle to the correct letter. Most of the time one has to toggle to make the number and symbol keyboards appear. Figure 2-4(b) shows the three versions of the iPad keyboard.

Mouse

Currently, most computers (not tablets or smartphones) come with another input device in addition to the keyboard—namely, a mouse. (See **Figure 2-6)** The traditional mechanical mouse has a ball on the underside of the unit. To use such a device, the user slides it over a mouse pad or desktop. Most of today's mice are "optical" models that do not use such a a ball but rather sense changes in light reflection to detect mouse movement. An optical mouse has no moving mechanical parts. It can be used on almost all surfaces, thereby decreasing the need for a mouse pad. The optical mouse also requires no cleaning and is more precise than a traditional mechanical mouse.

Some laptops have a **trackball,** pointing stick, or touchpad that serves as the mouse or pointing device. A trackball is a stationary mouse with the ball on the top part of it; the user moves the ball instead of the mouse. A **pointing stick** looks like a pencil eraser and uses pressure to detect mouse movement. A **touchpad** is another

TABLE 2-1 ADDITIONAL KEYBOARD KEYS

Key	Function
Special Keys	
Delete (Del)	Used to delete characters to the right of the cursor.
Backspace	Used to delete characters to the left of the cursor.
Insert	Used to insert characters at the insertion point, moving all characters to the right.
Space bar	Used to separate words on a line; do not use to spread items out on a line.
Tab	Moves the cursor along the screen at defined intervals or to the next field in a dialog box; use it instead of the space bar to arrange items on a line.
Alt and Ctrl	Used in combination with another key to initiate a command or complete a task.
Esc	Used to back out of a program or menu one screen at a time.
Fn	Used in conjunction with other keys to initiate special actions that vary with applications; commonly seen on laptops.
Function: F1, F2, etc.	Used by applications to perform special tasks; used many times in conjunction with the Alt, Ctrl, and Shift keys. Use is decreasing in favor of mouse clicks and shortcuts like Ctrl+P for print.
Print screen	Used to capture the screen and place it on the clipboard; can be used in conjunction with the Alt key to capture the active window.
Lock	Used to lock part of the keyboard to change how the keys' functions; for example, the Num Lock key to toggle the shared keys of numbers and cursor movement or cap lock to switch to all caps.
Cursor or Navigation	
Up/down/left/right arrows	Moves the cursor one space or line in the direction of the arrow; not always present on abbreviated keyboards found on laptops.
PgUp/PgDn Home/End	Quickly moves the cursor from one place to another, for example to the top or bottom of a page or to the beginning or end of a document; present on some laptop keyboards.
Numeric Keypad	
Used to quickly enter numbers; found on full keyboards and on a few laptops. In most cases it shares keys with the cursor movement keys; must have Num Lock light on to use numeric keypad.	

(continues)

TABLE 2-1 ADDITIONAL KEYBOARD KEYS (continued)

Key	Function
Special Windows Keys[1]	
Menu or application	Used to display the shortcut menu for selected items; for example, when pressed and working in this text, it will display the shortcut menu.
Windows logo	Used to display or hide the Start menu; also used in combination with other keys to execute commands. For example, Windows logo key + F opens the Search for a file or folder dialog window.
Special Applications and Media	
Application buttons	Special keys to access email, a computer application for seeing files saved on storage devices, and the calculator.
Media control buttons	Special buttons on the keyboard to access volume, forward, backward, pause, etc., for use with multimedia programs.

[1] Mac keyboards have many of the same keys, but they may be called by another name. Mac keyboards do not have Windows keys.

stationary pointing device for which the user moves a finger around on the pad to move the cursor. These devices were designed for mobile computers in recognition of the fact that there may not be a desktop upon which to move the mouse.

The mouse connects to the computer via a cord plugged into the mouse port. Alternatively, radio waves and infrared light waves may be used as a mode of communication between the system unit and a wireless mouse. Touchpads, trackballs, and pointing sticks on laptops are integral to the system and require no separate form of connection.

The mouse is used to access menus or functions, open application programs, and create graphic elements without using the function or cursor keys. A button is a place on the mouse that the user presses to invoke a command or activity; it clicks when pressed. A mouse generally has two buttons, denoted as left and right. Some models also have programmable thumb or side buttons that enable the user to perform additional functions. For example, on the Microsoft wireless mouse, the left thumb button activates the magnifier. In addition, a mouse may have a scroll wheel in the center for scrolling in windows or on Web sites. **Table 2-2** lists common mouse operations.

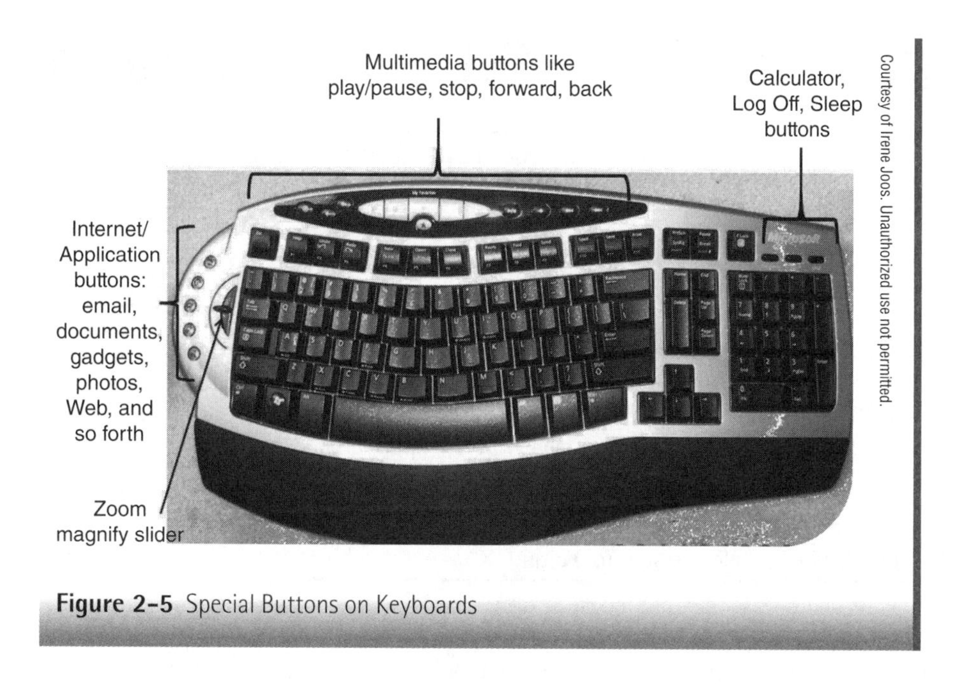

Figure 2-5 Special Buttons on Keyboards

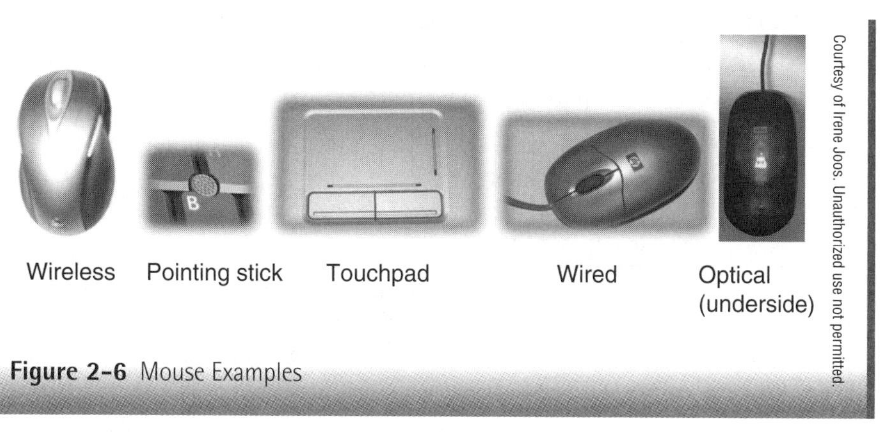

Figure 2-6 Mouse Examples

Touchscreen

A **touchscreen** allows the user to enter commands or actions by pressing specific places on a special screen with a finger. Most smartphones and tablets use touchscreens as the main input device. When it is necessary to type text, a virtual keyboard appears on the screen. Newer computers now offer touchscreen options for PCs and laptops. **Table 2-3** describes a few common touchscreen operations.

TABLE 2-2 COMMON WINDOWS MOUSE OPERATIONS[1]

Action	Description
Point	Move the mouse so that the cursor is on or over a particular command or icon on the screen.
Click (press)	Press and hold the mouse button down, as on a menu item to see the commands, or to scroll through a window until the desired command is selected. Often this term is inappropriately used to mean single-click. Click requires the user to hold down the mouse button.
Single-click	Press and release the left mouse button once to activate a command or to select an icon or menu option. Use a single-click to insert the I-beam (cursor in the shape of a capital I) at the point in the document where typing is to occur.
Double-click	With the cursor on an icon or option, press and release the left mouse button twice in quick succession. Use a double-click to start an application program, to open a file or folder, or to select a word for editing.
Right-click	Press and release the right mouse button once. This operation is used to activate the shortcut menu. Make sure to right-click in the appropriate place because different shortcut menus appear depending on what object or place is clicked. Use this operation only when instructed to right-click; otherwise, use the left mouse button.
Triple-click	Press and release the left mouse button three times. In word processing programs, this operation selects an entire paragraph.
Drag	Left-click an icon, menu option, or window border; then, without lifting the finger off the mouse, roll the mouse to move the object to another place on the screen. This operation can change a window's size, copy a file or document, select text, or take something to the trash.
Right-drag	Hold down the right mouse button, move the mouse to a different location, and then release the mouse button. This operation generally results in the appearance of a shortcut menu from which to select a command. The commands vary depending on the object that is right-clicked by the user.
Rotate wheel	Move the wheel forward and backward. Use this action to scroll up and down in a document or at a Web site.
Press wheel button	Click the wheel once and move the mouse on the desktop. This action causes the mouse pointer to scroll along the document automatically until the user presses the wheel button again.

[1] Note the Mac mouse has a different configuration (one button), but you should be able to complete most of these functions.

TABLE 2-3 TOUCHSCREEN OPERATIONS

Operation	Action
Touch/Tap	Touch a place on the screen to select an icon or option.
Double-tap	Touch the screen twice in the same location, much like double-click. On many touchscreens this results in zooming in or out on images or other items.
Tap and hold	Touch a place on the screen and hold your finger down. This may place you in edit mode or may open an options menu depending on the device.
Scroll/Drag	Place your finger on the screen and drag it up or down, left or right to show more apps. It also scrolls through pages as when reading a book.
Swipe	Touch a spot on the screen and drag your finger left, right, up, or down.
Flick	Swipe a spot on the screen except do it faster. This makes the screen scroll quickly.
Pinch	Use two fingers to touch the screen and bring both fingers together as you continue to touch the screen. This makes the item smaller.
Spread	Use two fingers close together and then spread them apart, touching the screen as you spread them. This enlarges the item.

Other Input Devices

A variety of other devices are used to input data to the system. See **Figure 2-7** for some examples of these input devices.

Gaming input devices such as light guns, joysticks, dance pads, and motion sensing controllers are not covered here. Nevertheless, a number of these devices have become increasingly important tools in the rehabilitation and maintenance of patients with limitations or disabilities. For example, gaming systems such as the Nintendo Wii, along with the newest addition, the Wii U, with its bowling and tennis games, are a big hit in nursing homes as a means of having fun while participating in some exercise.

Cradles or **docking stations** are input devices that laptops, iPods, and cameras use to input data from the mobile device to the desktop computer, and vice versa. Connecting them to the computer facilitates the movement of data from one device to the other. To use this input strategy, the user places the mobile device in the cradle or on the docking station. Some cradles require the user to press a button to perform the data transfer between the mobile device and the desktop computer. In addition, some users use docking stations to expand the capabilities of their mobile device such as using a widescreen monitor, full keyboard, and/or regular mouse.

A **digital camera** is used to take photographs and then to upload them to the computer or a special picture printer. Digital cameras eliminate the need for both

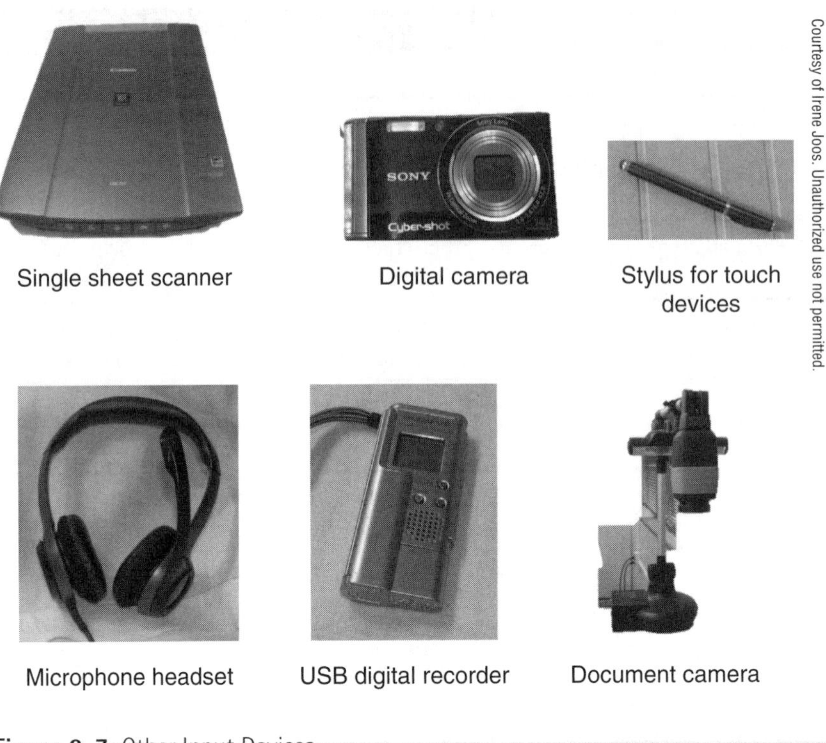

Figure 2-7 Other Input Devices

film and film development. Some cameras are stand-alone units that look much like traditional film-based cameras; others are built into smartphones or other mobile devices like tablets. Increasingly, digital and video cameras are being used to monitor people from remote places.

A **light pen** is a light-sensitive, pen-like device used in some older hospital clinical information systems. Some models require a special monitor to enter data. Light pens and **electronic pens** are not the same thing, however; electronic pens permit the construction of electronic signatures and require the user to hold the pen and write on a special pad. In contrast, light pens enable the user to enter data only with special screens. Touchscreens are replacing these special screens.

A **microphone** (voice input device) permits the user to speak into the computer to enter data or give instructions. A quadriplegic might use this device to give commands to computer-controlled robots that help the person complete activities of daily living or do work. Healthcare providers use these applications in settings such as the operating room where they are using their hands to provide patient care.

A **video camera** is an input device that the operator uses to capture video. It may be used to send video images as email attachments, to make video telephone calls (**video conferencing**), and to post live, real-time images to a Web server. A video camera that captures and displays images on a Web server is called a webcam. Many smartphones and tablets also have this capability.

RFID (radio-frequency identification) uses radio signals to communicate information on a tag first to an RFID reader and then to the computer. In health care, RFID technology is useful for tracking confused patients, inventory control, and monitoring staff movements. New passports contain RFID technology to aid in going through customs. Smart cards may also use this technology to input data.

A **scanner** is an input device that converts character or graphic patterns into digital data (discrete coded units of data). Such a device can scan a picture and then display the image on the computer screen. Software programs can then import this converted data. Two main types of scanners are image readers (for text and graphics) and barcode readers (for database work). Growing in popularity are data collection devices that collect data at remote places and then upload these data to the main computer. In high-security areas, some scanners now collect biometric (body-specific) data such as a fingerprint, voiceprint, or retinal scan to verify the user. Many hospitals use barcode scanners to input data as to supplies or medications used by patients.

Tablets may use a **stylus** or **digital pen** to create an image on the tablet surface. The tablet then converts the marks or images to digital data that the computer can use.

Computer Components: System Unit

The **system unit** is in a case, which varies in size and shape depending on which device you are using. It may be a separate unit found inside the display screen, or inside a mobile device. In any event, the system unit contains the control center or "brains" of the computer; it is not visible to the eye on most computers unless someone removes the cover of the computer. For most computers, the input and output devices reside outside the system unit; for most mobile devices, the input and output devices and the system unit are contained within one unit.

Motherboard

The **motherboard** (also referred to as the system board) is the main circuit board of the system unit. It provides the connections and sockets for other components to communicate with each other. The processor and memory chips reside on the motherboard.

Chip

A **chip** is a tiny piece of semiconducting material (usually silicon) that packs many millions of electronic elements onto an area the size of a fingernail. The circuit boards found in computers consist of many chips. The specialized chip called a processor or CPU contains an entire processing unit; in contrast, memory chips hold only programs and data.

Processor

The **processor** is the central unit in a computer that contains the circuitry for manipulating the data and carrying out the program instructions. An older term for the processor is "central processing unit" (CPU); both terms are sometimes used interchangeably. A **microprocessor** is a processor that fits on one integrated circuit chip. A dual-core processor refers to two complete execution cores per physical processor on a single chip. These processors are well suited for multi-tasking because each core can function independently of the other, providing more resources to complete the tasks.

The processor has two parts: the control unit and the arithmetic/logic unit. The control unit coordinates the computer's activities. It receives, interprets, and implements instructions. The arithmetic unit performs math functions such as addition, subtraction, multiplication, and division. The logic unit compares two values of data to determine whether they are equal or whether one is greater than or less than the other. The arithmetic/logic unit temporarily uses registers and memory locations to hold data being processed.

Microprocessors have specific names dependent upon the manufacturer (such as Intel or AMD [Advanced Micro Devices]). Examples are the AMD Athlon X2 and Phenom II and Intel Core 2 Duo L7400/7500 and Core i7. Specially designed processors are also available for smaller mobile devices such as portable media players, smartphones, and so forth that use the system on a chip (SoC) processor called a microchip. As **nanotechnology** development moves forward, smaller and smaller devices may be used for a variety of healthcare-related applications. Potential examples include nanobots performing as programmable antibodies to fight infections or to deliver medications to treat chronic conditions. Tiny devices may even be implanted in the brains of blind clients so they can see.

The important point to remember is that processor names, speed, size, and uses will inevitably change over time, but the basic functions of processors will remain the same.

Memory

Memory is a form of semiconductor storage that resides inside the computer, generally on a motherboard, and takes the form of one or more chips. It stores operating system commands, programs, and data. Primary memory storage is fast but has low density (amount of data stored per square inch) and costs more per unit of storage than does secondary storage (discussed later). Other terms used to describe memory include main storage, internal storage, main memory, and primary storage. Most forms of memory are intended to be temporary storage and include RAM, virtual memory, cache, and the CPU register. Permanent memory (generally called storage) includes ROM/BIOS, removable devices, network/cloud file servers, and the hard drive. These components will be discussed in the section on storage.

Random access memory (RAM) stores data that the computer needs to use temporarily. It is faster than secondary storage devices like the hard drive. This type of memory is volatile—the data disappear from RAM when the power is off. The most common unit of measurement for RAM is the byte, which is the amount of storage space it takes to hold a character. The more RAM a computer has, the greater its computing capabilities. When a software program starts, the computer loads the necessary program and user data files into RAM. As additional functions are requested, the computer loads the required software files. If the memory is not large enough to hold all of these files simultaneously, software files are swapped in and out of the system as needed, slowing down the work.

Several variations of RAM are available. For example, dynamic RAM (DRAM) must be reenergized constantly or else will lose its contents. By contrast, static RAM (SRAM) does not need to be reenergized, so it is much faster—and more expensive—than DRAM. Generally, the size requirements for RAM increase with new software releases.

Flash memory is a type of nonvolatile memory that the user can erase and rewrite, making it easier to update the memory contents. Some computers hold their startup instructions in this type of memory so that the user can upgrade the instructions. This type of memory is common with mobile devices, digital cameras, and digital voice recorders.

Cache memory stores frequently used instructions and data. The computer accesses cache memory before RAM memory, thereby speeding up processing.

Ports

Ports are the highways that lead into, out of, and around the computer. They take the form of plugs, sockets, or hot spots that are found on the back, front, and sides of most system units and on some monitors. Ports allow the computer to communicate with peripheral devices, carrying information to and from these devices. For example, many computers have built-in game, mouse, keyboard, card reader, and monitor ports that allow the computer to "talk" with these devices. The ports described here are also considered external data buses, where a bus comprises a series of connections or pathways over which data travels. Computers today generally come with multiple USB (universal serial bus) ports. Some computers can be configured with **FireWire**, IrDA, and/or Bluetooth ports that connect to peripheral technologies such as digital cameras, PDAs, and MP3 players. **Figure 2-8** shows some examples of ports. Many manufacturers configure their computers with multiple ports on the front to facilitate access . Some monitors also contain ports. The term "jack" is sometimes used to refer to connections for audio and video ports. On some multimedia computers, audio and video ports are color coded to match the cable tip so that there is no confusion about which device plugs into which port.

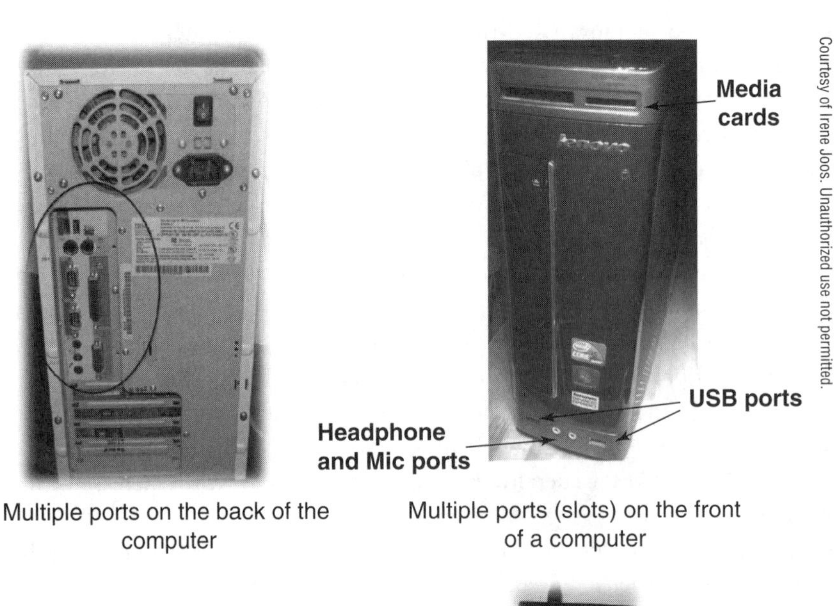

Multiple ports on the back of the computer

Multiple ports (slots) on the front of a computer

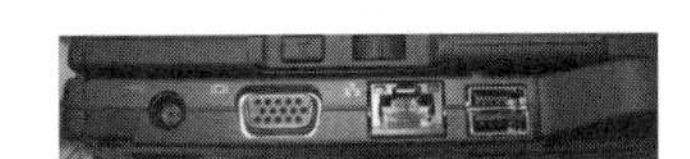

Multiple ports on a laptop

USB hub for multiple USB storage devices

Figure 2-8 Ports

Serial ports, also known as "com" ports, arrange data in serial form, sending it to the destination one bit at a time. This strategy allows data to move from the internal, parallel form in the computer to external devices. Because serial ports allow two-way communication, the reverse data flow also occurs, from the external devices back to the computer. These ports were common in devices that did not require much speed such as a keyboard or mouse, but serial ports are almost obsolete and wireless keyboards, wireless mouse, and USB ports have all but replaced them.

USB (universal serial bus) is a port standard that supports fast data transfer rates (480 million bits per second for 2.0 and 4.8 billions of bits per second for 3.0). It can support as many as 127 peripheral devices simultaneously as well as plug-and-play technologies. Devices that can connect to a USB port include the mouse, printers, cameras, microphones, PDAs, USB removable storage devices, and game consoles. In recent years, the USB port has virtually replaced audio, mouse, keyboard, serial, and parallel ports.

FireWire is a special-purpose port that is similar to a USB port in that the user can attach multiple devices to it. A variety of devices that require faster data transmission than is possible with normal ports, such as cameras and camcorders, connect to FireWire ports. A FireWire port can support a maximum of 63 devices simultaneously. In recent years, this type of port has largely replaced audio, parallel, and SCSI ports.

There are also special purpose ports that the computer does not generally include unless the user specifically orders or installs them. These include ports such as IrDA infrared light beam ports to connect wireless devices to the computer using light waves and Bluetooth ports that compete with IrDA ports, although Bluetooth uses radio waves to communicate between the devices instead of infrared light waves. The Bluetooth advantage over the IrDA port is that it eliminates the line-of-sight requirement. Many electronic devices today, such as cell phones, baby monitors, and garage doors, are Bluetooth enabled.

Power Supply

A **power supply box** converts the power available at the wall socket (120-volt, 60-MHz, AC current) to the power necessary to run the computer (+5 and +12 volt, DC current). The power supply must ensure a high-quality, steady supply of both 5- and 12-volt DC power for the computer to operate effectively. It includes a built-in fan that cools the system (computer processing generates lots of heat). Laptops and many external peripherals, such as wireless routers and modems, have their own AC adapters. Many laptop power adapters can use both 110 and 220 volts, which is most advantageous in other countries such as Europe where 220-volt power is common.

For mobile devices, one must consider the battery and its life. These batteries are rechargeable but vary in how long they last before recharging is necessary. While there are three basic types of batteries—lead acid, nickel-based, and lithium-ion—most mobile devices today run on lithium batteries (Wallen, 2012; Odegard, 2011). **Table 2-4** provides some tips about how to care for these batteries.

Additional Terms

In addition to the processor in the computer, other factors in the system unit affect how fast the computer works. They include the computer's registers, the RAM, the clock speed, the internal data bus, and the cache.

Registers are temporary, high-speed storage spaces that the processor uses when it processes data. They are part of the processing unit, not the memory. The size of the registers affects processing speed: Simply put, the larger the register, the faster the processing. For example, a 64-bit register is faster than a 32-bit register.

TABLE 2-4 CARE OF THE MOBILE DEVICE BATTERY—LITHIUM

Care Tip	Reason
Avoid temperature extremes both hot and cold	Overheating causes battery corrosion; batteries last longer in cooler temperatures. Heat above 140 degrees or subzero cold can reduce the battery life. Avoid leaving in a car or direct sunlight.
Charge often	Lithium batteries can take partial and random charging with partial charge being better. Charge the battery to 50% of capacity every 6 months when not using regularly.
Keep discharge above 50%+	Don't try to fully discharge the battery. This only adds strain to the battery. Try to keep the battery around 50% capacity.
Use the right charger	Different kinds of batteries have their own technology and rate of charge. Using the right charger is one way to extend the life of the battery and avoid damage to the battery.
Check local, national, and international regulations before transporting your battery—it can't be placed in checked luggage; you may pack spare batteries in carry-on luggage and so forth	There are some restrictions on what you can and can't do with lithium batteries when flying for safety reasons as these batteries can overheat or be overcharged and lead to combustion. These batteries are found in cell phones, hearing aids, laptops, and AA/AAA batteries.

Sources: Odegard, A. (2011). *Treat your tablet battery correctly.* Retrieved from www.pocketables.com/2011/02/treat-your-tablet-battery-the-right-way.html.

SafeTravel.dot.gov (n.d.). *DOT rule for passengers traveling with lithium batteries.* Washington, DC: US Department of Transportation Pipeline and Hazardous Materials Safety Administration. Retrieved from http://safetravel.dot.gov.

Wallen, J. (2012). *How and when to charge your tablet battery.* San Francisco: TechRepublic. Retrieved from www.techrepublic.com/blog/tablets/how-and-when-to-charge-your-tablet-battery/814.

The amount of RAM available (discussed earlier) also has implications for the processing speed. A program runs faster when more of it fits into RAM simultaneously. Cache memory (described earlier) also affects how fast the computer works. It is time-consuming to move data back and forth between the processor registers and the memory. Data stored in a cache can be accessed much more quickly than other data, so more cache memory means faster processing.

The **clock speed** is a function of the quartz crystal circuit that controls the timing of computer work. The faster the internal clock (which is used to time processing operations) runs, the faster the computer works. The unit of measurement for the clock speed is gigahertz (GHz; 4 GHz = 4 billion cycles per second). Theoretically, the higher the clock speed, the faster the computer works.

Data buses, which comprise a collection of wires, move data around the computer system. The two types of buses are internal (also called internal data bus, memory bus, system bus, or front-side-bus) or external (also called expansion bus). The internal bus connects the CPU and memory to the motherboard while the external bus connects external devices like the printer or scanner. The wider the bus (determined by the number of wires or pins), the faster it can move data. All buses consist of two parts: an address bus (where the data is going) and a data bus (the actual data), but high-end computers also add a control bus. The most important factors for the bus are its width (16, 32, or 64 bits) and its speed. The width determines how much data the bus can move at a time, and the speed determines how fast it moves the data.

Computer Components: Output Devices

Output devices take the processed data, which is called *information*, and present it to the user in display (text, graphics, or video), print, or sound form. **Figure 2-9** shows some of the most popular output devices.

Monitor

Monitors display graphic images from the video output of a computer. Other terms used for this device include display screen and flat panel. In recent years,

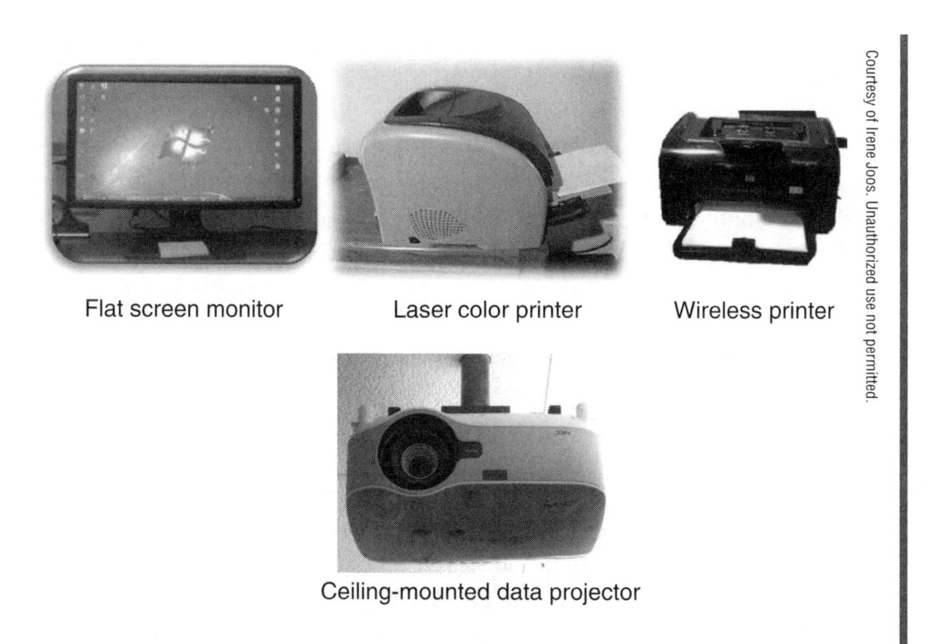

Figure 2-9 Output Devices

flat panel **LCD (liquid crystal display)** monitors have replaced cathode ray tube (CRT) monitors. Flat panels have a smaller footprint, smaller power requirement, and no flicker effect. As a consequence, most computers now use LCD technology for the display device. Computers in many industries, including health care, are rapidly moving to adopt touchscreen technologies. Gas plasma monitors provide an option for display screens in larger spaces like those seen in convention centers and large lecture halls.

Monitors vary in terms of their size, footprint, color, resolution, inputs, and adjustability. The ability of a monitor to project an image that can be used for diagnostic purposes is of key importance in health care. One should consider the following factors when selecting a monitor.

Size refers to the diagonal measurement from corner to corner of the display unit. The active viewing area refers to the actual measurement from left to right and top to bottom of the screen. The appropriate monitor size depends on the proposed usage and application. Commonly encountered computer display sizes are 17, 19, and 21 inches; larger sizes are appropriate for desktop and Internet publishing as well as for diagnostic imaging in healthcare facilities. Mobile devices typically have smaller viewing areas, ranging from a few inches for some smartphones, 7 to 9 inches for some tablets, and up to 17 and 20 inches for larger laptops.

Footprint refers to how much space the monitor takes up on the desktop. Flat screen monitors require far less space than older traditional monitors and have all but replaced them. LCD monitors generally come with a stand and may also be adjustable in height and rotation.

Color refers to whether the monitor is monochrome (one color, usually green or amber, on a black background) or colored. The number of displayed colors ranges from 256 to much higher numbers. Most monitors today are colored monitors, but there are still some monochrome in use. Contrast ratio is the ratio of the brightest color (white) to the darkest color (black) on the screen. Today's monitors produce contrast ratios of 20,000:1. Higher ratios provide better representation of colors.

Resolution describes the number of horizontal and vertical pixels (dots) found on the screen. Monitors display images by projecting tiny dots of light on the screen and they vary widely in terms of the number of pixels per screen (resolution). The more pixels on the screen, the sharper the image will be. A common resolution for 21- to 24-inch displays is 1920 × 1200. Higher resolutions stress the graphics card and warrant investment in a better graphics card. Smaller monitors use the highest resolution, so the objects on the screen will be very tiny.

Other features for consideration are sound, ports, webcam, and video options. Some monitors come with sound, ports, and **webcams** in the monitor; others do not. Some monitors also have video options for picture-in-picture displays. All of these features depend on the primary use of the system. For example, cell phones may not have the best displays for reading large documents but work well for email checking and texting. Remember though, this is an ever-changing environment.

The last key point to consider when it comes to monitors relates to their conformance to two standards. First, a monitor should be energy efficient and should conform to the U.S. Environmental Protection Agency (EPA) Energy Star guidelines. To meet the EPA standard, the monitor must meet certain energy requirements when it is on, in standby mode, in suspended mode, and off. In July 2007, the EPA adopted new energy-efficiency standards that many older monitors do not meet. Second, consider the amount of electromagnetic emissions produced by the monitor. Specifically, the monitor should comply with the Swedish MPR-II or TCO emissions standard.

Printers

Printers come in an array of types, configurations, sizes, and costs. This section examines the concepts of venue, technology, function, output, and purpose (Westover, 2011).

Venue refers to the location of the printer—home or office. Most home printers tend to be on the low-end of cost, speed, and size and are not designed for high-volume printing. They may come with Wi-Fi capabilities and adjustable trays for various types of paper, and they are generally inkjet-type printers, although there are some lower-end black-and-white and color laser printers for use at home. Office printers are generally high-volume, multifunction machines that are larger, faster, and more costly than home printers.

Technology refers to the underlying operation of the printer.

- **Laser printers** are the most expensive of the common types of printers. They produce high-quality print, are fast, and generate little noise. They come in black-and-white and color versions relying on toner cartridges instead of inkjets.
- **Inkjet printers** are usually reasonably priced and less expensive to purchase than laser printers, making them the most common type of consumer printer. They work by firing droplets of ink onto the paper and may require multiple ink cartridges. They generally produce quality photos.
- **Thermal printers** press heated pins against special paper to produce the printed image; the quality of this output is low, so such printers are generally used in sites such as retail sales and gas station pumps.

Depending on the printing requirements, laser printers can be cheaper than inkjet printers. For example, if one is printing a large volume of black and white text, a laser printer might be cheaper because of lower toner costs. Growing in popularity are photo printers, which use inkjet technology to produce color pictures in varying sizes. Some **plotters** also use inkjet technology to produce large banners and architectural drawings.

Function refers to single-purpose printers or multifunction printers (MFPs). Single-function printers only print. Multifunction printers may also act as scanners, copiers, and fax machines. Usually they are cheaper than purchasing each device separately and take up less space. However, if the device breaks down, all functions are gone. In addition, stand-alone devices may offer more advanced features.

Output refers to the nature of the output—black-and-white or color. If one prints only documents, a black-and-white printer will do; if, however, there is a need to print marketing materials, photos, or full-color graphics, a color printer will be necessary.

Purpose refers to general-purpose printers or specialty printers. For example, a healthcare provider making home visits may need a portable printer that can attach to a mobile device or may need a wireless connection to use the device. There are also plotters, label printers, and photo printers that can print banners.

When purchasing or requesting a printer, consider some of these specifications: speed referred to as pages per minute (ppm), internal memory on the printer, duty cycle, paper handling, and network or wireless capabilities. If printing multiple copies of large documents, a slow printer will not do. If printing documents with lots of graphics or pictures, will the printer's memory be able to handle it? How many pages can this printer print in a month without failing? That is the duty cycle. Make sure the printer exceeds the volume per month of anticipated printing. Next, do you want duplex printing capabilities, multipurpose trays, and/or a manual feed slot? Do you want this printer to print from any device that you might use or only from one computer? Make sure the printer has the capabilities to meet the printing requirements.

Other Output Devices

As end users have become more adept at using technology, the demand for other output devices has increased.

Speakers come with most computers and many mobile devices today and usually reproduce high-quality sound. Speakers can be integral to the monitor, be attached to the monitor, stand separately on the desktop, or be integral to the computer. Some high-level multimedia computers also come with a subwoofer to handle bass sounds. Most computer laboratories now require users to wear **headphones** so that computer-generated sounds do not disturb other users; if users do not use headphones in the labs, they may need to turn off the sound capability.

Data projectors display graphic presentations to an audience. Such a device takes the image on the computer screen and projects it onto a larger screen. Data projectors may be either portable or ceiling-mounted. As with all electronic devices, the price and quality of these output devices vary dramatically, ranging from low-end to high-end models.

Interactive whiteboards are display devices that connect to a computer and permit the user to interact with the computer as well as the Internet using remote controls, special pens, a writing tablet, or a finger.

SmartTVs, also called connectedTVs, are televisions that integrate Internet and Web 2.0 tools. These TVs permit browsing the Internet, using Web 2.0 tools like Facebook, and the sharing of information from laptops, tablets, smartphones and so forth.

Computer Components: Secondary Storage

Storage comprises a place or space for holding data and application programs. The computer has both primary (memory storage—covered earlier in this chapter) and secondary storage (e.g., hard drives, optical drives, USB storage devices, and the cloud) storage spaces.

Secondary storage media hold programs such as Word and Excel and user data when these are not in use. It takes longer to access data held in secondary storage. Secondary storage has a higher density (amount of data per square inch) and is less expensive than primary storage. Data storage is measured in the same units as memory—bytes, kilobytes, megabytes, gigabytes, and terabytes. A byte is equal to one character. One kilobyte is 1024 bytes; one megabyte (MB) is 1 million+ bytes; one gigabyte (GB) is 1 billion+ bytes; and one terabyte is 1 trillion+ bytes. **Figure 2-10** shows examples of storage devices.

Storage Devices

Storage devices refer to media that holds the data used by devices, from computers to smartphones. They come in a variety of types and storage sizes as outlined below.

Read-only memory (ROM) is memory as well as storage. The contents of the chip (ROM) were burned onto the chip during manufacturing; the computer can read instructions from it but cannot alter them. This memory is permanent, not volatile, which is why some consider it storage — it holds data until the system needs it. Computer start-up instructions reside in ROM; these instructions tell the computer what to do when it is turned on (see Chapter 3 for more on the start-up process). Other types of ROM include programmable read-only memory (PROM), which permits instructions to be programmed on the chip only once, and erasable programmable read-only memory (EPROM), which permits a user to program the instructions many times.

Hard disks (also known as **hard drives**) are fixed data storage devices in sealed cases that read stored data on platters in the drive. These magnetic storage devices store data in sizes ranging from gigabytes to terabytes. Hard drives are generally slower than primary memory (RAM). They are either external to the system unit

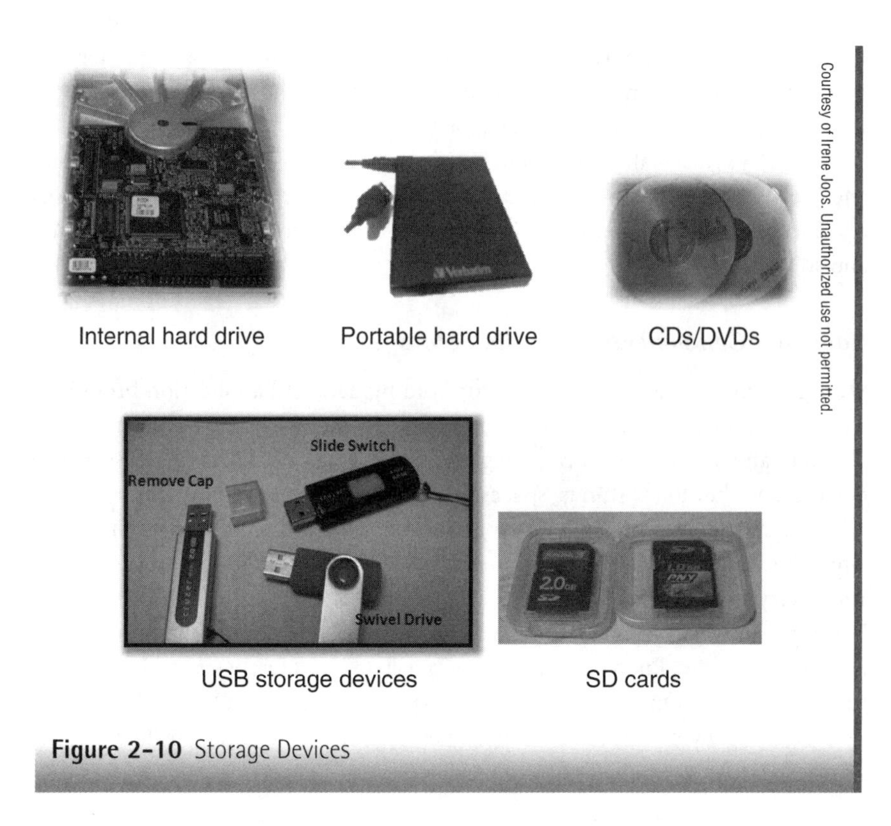

Figure 2-10 Storage Devices

(portable) or internal to the system unit (fixed). Hard cards are hard disks that are inserted in an expansion slot; portable drives are generally connected to a USB or FireWire port. Both PCs and laptops generally come with one hard disk drive and most last at least three to five years. Proper maintenance of the hard disk drive requires periodic defragmentation and periodic disk scans.

Optical drives are an alternative to magnetic storage. They hold large amounts of data, which are usually written (pressed) once and accessed many times. Almost all computers come with at least one internal optical drive while mobile devices have none by default. The most common example is the **DVD** drive. The design of earlier DVDs accommodated video—hence the name "digital video discs." As use of these discs increased as data storage media, DVD has come to mean "digital versatile disc." These discs can hold more data, such as a full-length movie, than can CDs. Variations of DVDs include DVD-ROM with a storage capacity of 4.7 GB; BD-ROM (Blu-Ray disc) with a storage capacity of 100 GB; and HD DVD-ROM (high-definition) with a storage capacity of 60 GB. RW DVDs are rewritable. DVDs can last anywhere from 5 to 100 years with proper care, which includes storing the disc in a case and holding the disc only by its edges. One should not stack discs but rather they should be stored on their edge; it is best not to touch the underside, expose the disc to excess temperatures, or eat or smoke around a DVD.

CDs were earlier optical storage devices and typically hold 650 MB of data, although the capacity of some models goes as high as 1 GB. Other variations of optical drives include CD-R (compact disc–recordable) drives, which permit users to write data only once (but not erase data), and CD-RW (compact disc–rewritable) drives, which permit users to write and erase data many times.

Solid-state media such as **flash memory** cards and USB storage devices consist of electronic components and have no moving parts. The life expectancy of solid-state media is in the range of 10 to 100 years, depending on the manufacturer. The maximum storage capacity of these devices changes regularly. Today, 32 GB USB storages devices are commonplace. Sony's Memory Stick XC has a theoretical capacity of 2 TB but is not in common use at this point in time. Flash memory cards are commonly found in digital cameras, smartphones, and PDAs; they are more expensive than other storage media. USB storage devices are popular for portable storage because of their capacity and size. **Figure 2-11** illustrates the appropriate care instructions for a USB storage device.

Cloud storage has gained in popularity with the growth of mobile devices. End users may use hosted cloud computer services, specifically Infrastructure-as-a-Service (IaaS), to provide storage. The service provider owns the equipment and is responsible for housing, running, and maintaining it, and for setting the policies for its use. Many of these services provide a certain amount of free storage with associated costs for amounts above the free range. Chapter 9 discusses cloud computing services in more detail.

Secure digital (SD) cards are nonvolatile cards used in portable devices such as smartphones, PDAs, digital cameras, and tablet computers. Most of us are familiar with their use in cameras because you can easily remove and replace them, though in most phones the cards are inside the phone and not accessible to the user. These cards vary in size (mini, micro, and standard) and storage capacity (from 2 GB to 128 GB with 2 to 4 GBs being most common).

Smart cards (also called chip cards and integrated circuit cards) store data on a credit card–sized card that contains a microprocessor, input and output functions, and storage. Increasingly, various industries are using smart cards to store personal information such as a person's medical record and credit card information. Smart cards are already in extensive use in Europe and China for storing healthcare information.

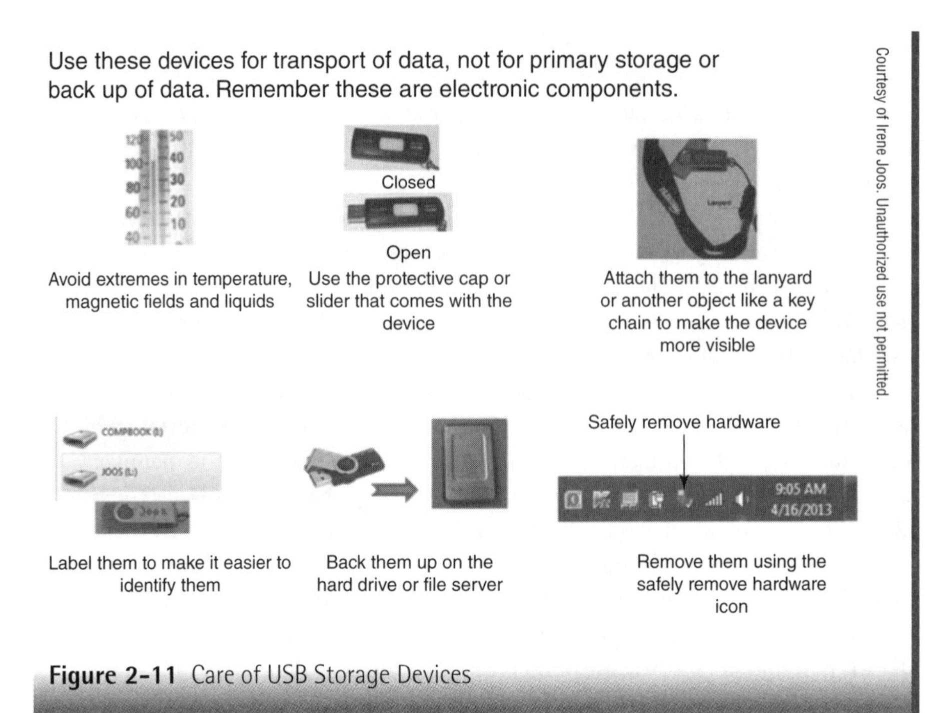

Figure 2-11 Care of USB Storage Devices

Labeling Devices

Operating systems assign letters to storage drives. The use of drive letters and drive icons with letters allows users to access stored information on a specific drive. The letters "C" and "D" usually refer to hard disk(s); the default hard drive is C. Other drives and devices use the letters "D," "E," "F," or "G." The letters "A" and/or "B" were reserved for floppy drives and are rarely seen today. In the Windows environment, words appear next to the letters describing the nature of that storage device as well as the assigned letter. As an example, **Figure 2-12a** shows disk drive labeling on a networked computer using Windows 7 versus disk drive labeling on a stand-alone computer using Windows 7. Because many variations for drive labeling exist, consult the laboratory assistant or instructor for the applications of conventions in your laboratory.

When using smart devices like phones or tablets, one often sees the name of the storage app like Dropbox or Skydrive. There is generally no drive letter associated with storage on these devices. One accesses the service by selecting the app. **Figure 2-12b** shows the CloudStorage apps on an iPad and folders on a cloud service.

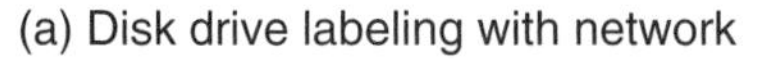

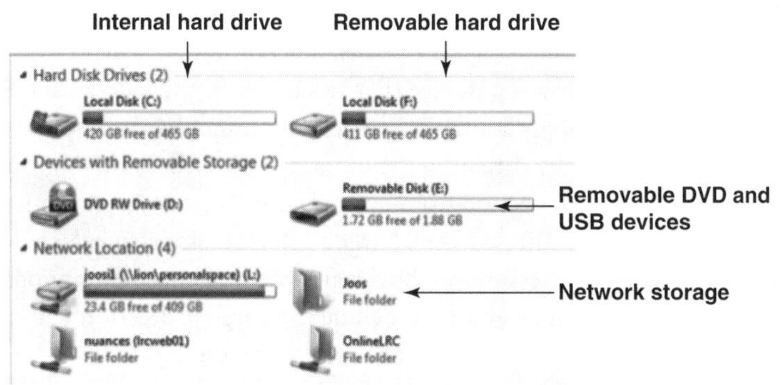

Disk drive labeling without network

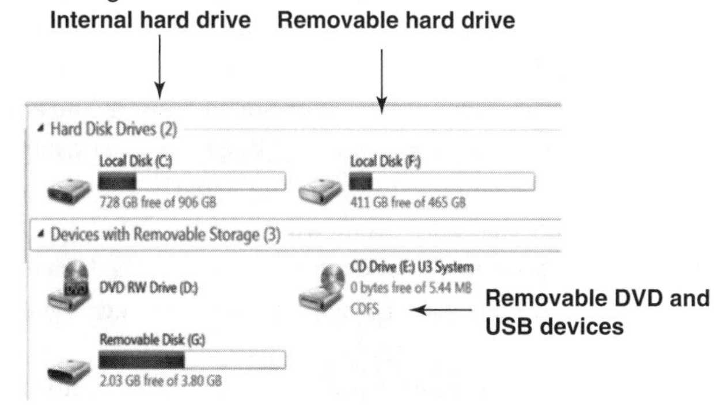

(b) Cloud storage services and folders

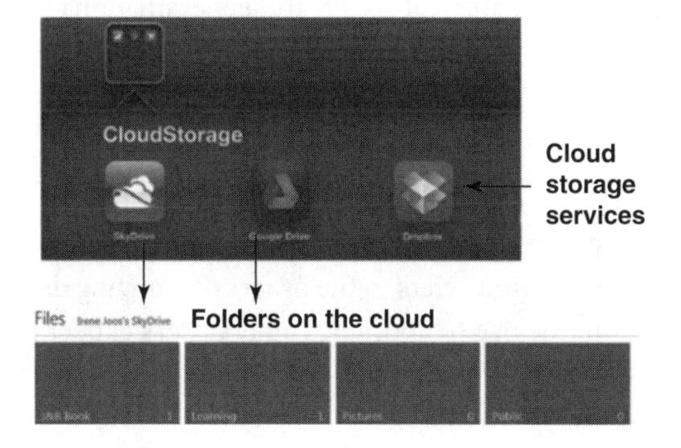

Figure 2-12 (a) Disk Drive Labeling and (b) Storage on the Cloud

Other Peripherals

Two other peripheral devices to consider when selecting hardware are the surge protector and the uninterruptible power supply.

A **surge protector** is a device that sits between the electrical outlet and the computer power supply source. It protects the computer from low-voltage surges in electrical power by directing the extra power to the outlet's grounding wire. Although it offers protection from normal surges in voltage, it cannot protect the computer from lightning strikes. Surge protectors are also referred to as power strips and surge suppressors, but be careful when making assumptions about their capabilities. Not all power strips include the surge protection feature. This also applies to laptops when plugged into an electrical outlet.

An **uninterruptible power supply (UPS)** provides electrical power generated by a battery in the event of a power outage. The battery keeps the computer going for several minutes after the outage occurs. During this time, the user can save data and properly shut down the computer. Two types of UPS systems are available: standby and online. Standby devices monitor the power line and switch to battery power when they detect a problem. Online devices constantly provide power even when the power line is functioning properly, thereby avoiding the momentary lack of power that may occur when the UPS switches from power to battery. Online devices are more expensive. Think of UPS devices as standby generators, much like hospitals use in case of a power outage, albeit on a much smaller scale.

Generally one should plug printers, speakers, and scanners into surge protectors, and plug computers, monitors, and storage devices into the UPS. Printers can cause a large drain on the battery of a UPS and generally don't require uninterruptible power. Many UPS units also bundle surge protection in one device. (See **Figure 2-13**.)

Introduction to Computer Systems: Connectivity

Most people now assume that a computer has the ability to communicate with other computers. **Communication** refers to the process of moving data and information from one computer device to another. Today's users expect to be able to easily communicate from a PC to a laptop to a handheld device to a Web server with very little effort on their part.

The basic communication process includes a sender and receiver, a channel, and a communication device. Chapter 9, The Internet, and Chapter 10, Technology-Assisted Communication and Collaboration, discuss some of the services people use when communicating using the Internet. Relevant terms for understanding basic computer communications or connectivity are discussed in this section.

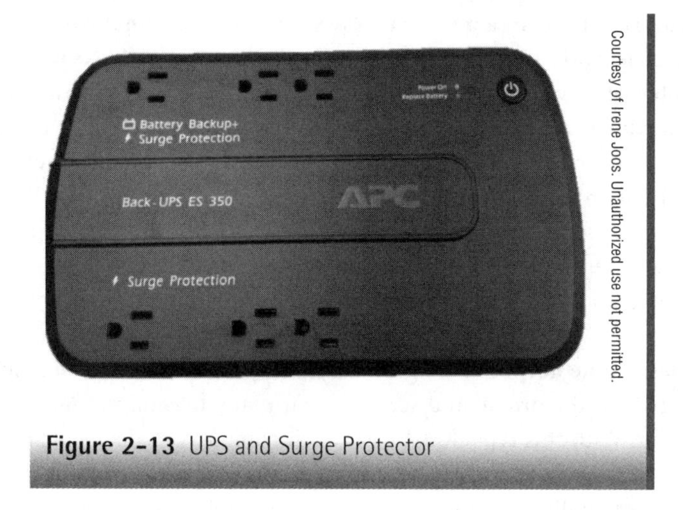

Figure 2-13 UPS and Surge Protector

Networks

A **network** is a collection of computers and other hardware devices, such as a printer, scanner, or file server, that are connected together using communication devices and transmission media.

A **local area network (LAN)** is a type of network with distance limitations. A building or small campus environment might use a LAN. Some departments within healthcare institutions use LANs to connect various types of equipment for the purpose of communicating and sharing information. LANs typically use a communications standard called **Ethernet**.

A **wireless local area network (WLAN)** does not use wires for communication between the server and the client computer or mobile device. Most WLANs physically connect to a LAN for the purpose of accessing resources on the LAN. Many campuses now have a WLAN for use with mobile devices such as laptops, tablets, and smartphones. Access points are scattered around the building or facility that provides the local computer with access to the LAN. Communication standards or protocols in the wireless world include **Wi-Fi (wireless fidelity)**, Bluetooth, IrDA, and **RFID (radio-frequency identification)**. Wi-Fi permits two Wi-Fi devices to communicate with each other or with a Wi-Fi–enabled network. Bluetooth enables communication with laptops, tablets, microphones, and similar devices. IrDA provides line-of-sight communication between two devices. RFID allows the reading of tags on objects as varied as supplies and passports. One of the key problems with wireless connections in hospitals are dead spaces that are the result of interference to the signal by such things as lead-lined rooms or doors or not enough access points.

The **metropolitan area network (MAN)** and **wide area network (WAN)** are high-speed networks that cover larger geographic distances. MANs may include a city or Internet service provider (ISP) that provides the connection for city agencies or individual users with access to the Internet. The best example of a WAN is the Internet, which uses the **Transmission Control Protocol/Internet Protocol (TCP/IP)** communications standard. These networks may also use Worldwide Interoperability for **Microwave Access (WiMAX)** when the network includes use of wireless towers. **Wireless Application Protocol (WAP)** is a standard used by mobile devices such as smartphones when they are communicating with Internet services.

Wireless home networks are growing in both popularity and simplicity, and are now part of the broadband services that many telecommunications companies offer. With this type of network, each computer or device that connects to the wireless network must have a wireless network card or built-in wireless networking capabilities (found on many laptops, tablets, and smartphones). The network also must have a wireless access point or a combination **router/wireless device** that connects to one of the desktop computers in the home. **Figure 2-14** shows an example of a wireless router for a home network connected to a Verizon FiOS connection and wireless access points in a library.

Communication Devices

A **communication device** is any type of hardware capable of transmitting data and information from one computer to another. This section discusses some types of modems and cards commonly used to communicate with a network. Computers and mobile devices must have a communication device to communicate with a network. Dial-up modems are rapidly disappearing and will not be discussed here.

A **cable modem** is a device that connects to the network using television cable services. The cable company that provides the connection service also supplies the cable modem. A **DSL (digital subscriber line) modem** is a device that connects to the network over a DSL connection. The telecommunications company that provides the connection service generally provides or rents the modem or the

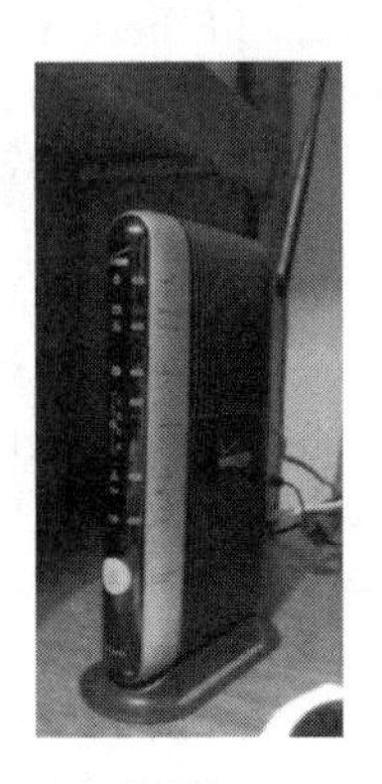
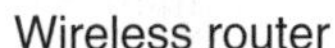

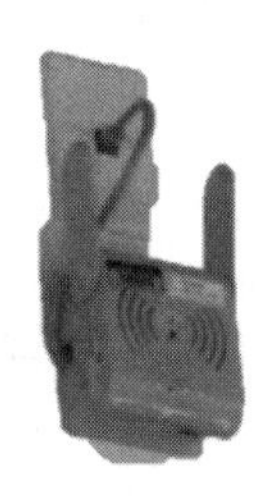

Figure 2-14 Wireless Router and Access Point

subscriber can purchase one from another source. The telecommunication company assumes no responsibility for setup or maintenance of a modem purchased elsewhere. A **wireless router** performs the functions of a router (a network device that forwards packets from one network to another) as well as providing a wireless access point for devices with wireless cards, such as a laptop. Generally, FiOS connections use a router to provide wireless access to other devices used in the home. The router is generally provided by an ISP such as Verizon which then will support and resolve router issues.

An **Ethernet card** fits into a computer slot and provides connectivity to an internal network. Schools, offices, and businesses often use Ethernet cards to connect computers and peripheral devices to their network.

A **wireless card** fits into a computer slot or is built into the devices to permit access to a wireless network via radio-based connection. The device must be in range of the wireless access point to access the network. See Figure 2-14 for an example of an access point.

A **wireless modem** (also known as mobile broadband modem, connect card, or data card) is a device with an external or built-in antenna for use with mobile devices such as laptops and cell phones. Some mobile phones can function as data modems serving as a hotspot for other devices. These modems use the cell phone network to connect to the Internet. Most of these connect through the USB port at 3G and 4G speed connections.

Communications Channels

A **communications channel** is the transmission pathway that data take to arrive at the other end of a connection.

Bandwidth describes the amount of data that can travel over a communications channel at one time. The larger the number, the more data the channel transmits at one time. Remember that music, video, and graphic files take up more bandwidth than plain text. Healthcare systems typically need a larger bandwidth because they often transmit data-intensive images such as CAT scans and MRIs along with text.

Broadband refers to the ability to transmit multiple signals at the same time in a faster mode than traditional dial-up and the connection is always on. DSL, cable, fiber, wireless, satellite, and BPL (Broadband over Powerline) are examples of broadband connections (FCC, n.d.).

Transmission media refers to the materials or substances capable of transmitting a signal. They are of two types: physical media and wireless media. Physical media include twisted-pair cable, which is widely used but slow; coaxial cables, which are common in cable TV connections and offer faster data transmission than twisted-pair; and fiber-optic cables, which connect large networks as well as private homes through some telecommunication company media. Fiber-optic cable is the fastest of these media and is replacing the other physical media. Wireless transmission media include infrared, broadcast radio, cellular radio, microwave, and satellite. Wireless media is more convenient in that the user does not have to install cables to make a connection and it provides more flexibility in moving equipment around; however, it may experience service interruptions during bad weather.

Connection Options

A **DSL connection** makes a faster connection than dial-up service, usually through the phone system over copper lines. DSL connections have severe distance limitations. The device must be within 18,000 feet of a phone switching station; as the device moves farther away from the switching station, the data transmission rate declines. Data transmission rates via DSL range from 128 Kbps to 9 Mbps. These connections provide both voice and data signals simultaneously.

The **cable** lines coming into most homes provide another option for a communications channel. This type of communications channel is faster than either dial-up or DSL, but degrades in speed as more people access the cable lines at the same time.

Fiber-optic cables, such as those used in Verizon's FiOS service, are a broadband option for connecting to a network using fiber-optic cable run to homes and businesses by some phone companies. **T1** and **T3** are communication connections that some large businesses use. They are commonly leased lines with reserved circuits that operate over either copper or fiber optics. These are very expensive and out of the reach of most individuals. Larger healthcare facilities and some colleges and universities may connect using this connection service.

Wireless connections use a radio signal to access the Internet. These connections can be mobile or fixed. Most mobile devices also use wireless connections at 3G and 4G speeds while a router provides a fixed wireless access point.

Satellite Internet connection employs a microwave dish generally located outside the building. This is another form of wireless connection. This data transmission option is subject to noise interference during rain and snowstorms, but may be the only option for people located in rural areas, on an ocean liner, or for those who travel widely.

Broadband over Powerline (**BPL**) connections go through the existing electric power distribution network. This is an emerging technology with limited availability but with great potential because power lines are everywhere.

The important point to remember here is that for a computer to communicate with other computers, it needs a communication device, a communications channel, media, and network service. Most ISPs provide these tools and services to enable their customers to connect to the Internet. Most large organizations provide these tools and services through their Information Technology (IT) department. The IT department typically provides the hardware specifications for connecting individual devices to the organization's network (either wired or wireless). Many organizations are working on policies and procedures for dealing with issues related to BYOD (bring your own device).

Introduction to Computer Systems: Software

Computers and mobile devices are unable to complete any task without directions from software programs. **Software programs** consist of step-by-step instructions that direct a device to perform specific tasks such as multiplying, dividing, fetching, or delivering data. All computers require software to function. When the computer is using a specific program, users say they are *running* or *executing* the program. The three major categories of software are operating systems (OSs), languages, and applications (or apps).

Operating Systems

The **operating system (OS)** is the most important program that runs on a computer or mobile device: It tells the computer how to use its own components or hardware. No general-purpose computer or mobile device can work without an OS.

Operating systems perform some functions necessary to all users of the computer system. These basic functions include keeping track of files and folders, communicating to peripheral devices such as printers, receiving and interpreting input from the mouse or keyboard, displaying output on a screen, and managing how data move around inside the computer. In other words, operating systems coordinate the computer hardware components and supervise all basic operations. The most common operating system for PCs is the Windows family (Windows XP, VISTA, Windows 7, and now Windows 8). Apple computers use the Macintosh operating system (OS 10). Some computers also use variations of UNIX called Linux and Xenix. Larger computer systems or networks and workstations may use Windows Server 2010 and UNIX or a UNIX variation such as Solaris.

A mobile operating system is the software that runs smartphones, tablets, PDAs, and other digital mobile devices. These include some of the same features that PCs use plus a variety of connectivity options (cellular, Bluetooth, Wi-Fi), cameras, recorders (both video and speech), players (music and video), and so forth. Examples of mobile device operating systems are Google's Android, Apple's iOS, Research in Motion's BlackBerry OS, Nokia's Symbian, Hewlett-Packard's webOS (formerly Palm OS), and Microsoft's Windows Phone OS. Some, such as Microsoft's Windows 8, function as both a traditional desktop and mobile OS. Critical to selection of the mobile device and its related OS are the apps that will run on it. Remember that most mobile operating system software is developed for a specific piece of hardware and may not be portable to other mobile devices. See Chapter 3 for more on operating systems.

Languages

Language software presents a simplified means to execute a series of instructions. Specifically, a language consists of a vocabulary and an accompanying set of rules that tell the computer how to work. Languages permit the user to develop programs to perform specific tasks. Popular languages include C, C++, C#, Java, and Visual Basic. Users do not need to be programmers to use the computer; however, understanding programming concepts and developing programming skills are helpful when trying to do more advanced work on the computer.

Several types of programming languages exist. Machine-level languages are the lowest level and consist of numbers only; this type of language is the only one that the computer recognizes directly. Assembly languages are the next generation of languages, and they give the programmer the ability to use names instead of numbers when telling the computer what to do. Procedural or 3GL (third-generation level) languages are what users normally think of when they say "programming language." They include the previously mentioned languages such as Visual Basic and C. Object-oriented programming languages include the ever-popular Java, C++, and Visual Basic. The 4GL (fourth-generation level) languages include SQL (Structured Query Language), which is used when working with large relational databases.

Although many people include HTML (Hypertext Markup Language), SGML (Standard Generalized Markup Language), and scripts such as PERL (Practical Extraction and Report Language) and PHP as programming languages, in reality they are not. These standard protocols are considered organizing and tagging languages that are designed to manage the layout and formatting of documents between different computer systems or scripting languages.

Applications

Application programs meet the specific task needs of the user; running these programs to complete your work in an efficient and effective manner is the primary use of any computer system. Programmers use language software to write application programs. Major types of applications or programs include the following:

- General-purpose software such as word processors, spreadsheets, database managers, presentation graphics, communications programs, and Web page authoring programs.
- Educational programs such as simulations or computer-assisted learning.

- Utility programs such as virus scanners, personal firewalls, screen savers, spyware and adware removers, hard disk managers, media players, and Internet filters such as antispam programs, pop-up blockers, and phishing filters.
- Personal programs such as calculators, calendars, and money managers.
- Entertainment programs such as games and simulations.

This term has taken on a new meaning with mobile devices and is commonly referred to as apps. **Apps** are software that can run on a mobile device and allow the users to perform certain tasks. Many apps are stripped down versions of more powerful software while other apps are unique to mobile devices. Apps are downloaded from an app store that is generally affiliated with the company that produces the mobile device, such as Apple iTunes or Amazon Kindle Store, or open app stores such as Handango.com. Apps are generally cheaper than full function applications like Word, Excel, and so forth.

This text covers the more commonly used general-purpose application software.

General-Purpose Software

Electronic mail (email) software permits the sending and receiving of messages from one person to one or many other people. The computers send and receive these messages by using standard communication protocols (rules and procedures that govern the communication between the computers). While the majority of the United States population uses email, a significant portion of electronic communication is now moving to text messages.

Database software helps organize, store, retrieve, and manipulate data for the purpose of later retrieval and report generation. These types of programs are the foundation for many specialty applications. For example, there are programs for organizing photos, bibliographical references, recipes, and electronic health records.

Desktop publishing software permits the user to create high-quality specialty publications such as newspapers, bulletins, and brochures. It handles page layouts better than word processors and can import a variety of text and graphic files from other application programs.

Document management and exchange software allows individuals and teams to share ideas and information in a common format that is seamless as to the platform (OS), original file integrity, accessibility, and readability. This software may be stand-alone or an add-in application. Adobe Reader is an example that permits the exchange of files regardless of system used.

Graphics and related design software facilitates the creation of a variety of graphics and design documents. There are three types of graphics/design programs:

Presentation graphics permit the user to create or alter symbols, display a variety of chart styles, make transparencies and slides, and produce slide shows. Paint programs permit users to create symbols or images from scratch. Computer-aided drafting and design (CADD) programs meet the drawing needs of architects and engineers.

Integrated software includes multiple capabilities in one program, such as word processing, database, spreadsheet, graphics, and communication programs.

Spreadsheet software permits the manipulation of numbers in a format of rows and columns. Spreadsheet programs contain special functions for adding and computing statistical and financial information. They are used for financial functions and number crunching. The functionality provided by a spreadsheet program often overlaps with the functionality provided by a database program.

Analytical software includes software programs for analyzing both qualitative and quantitative data. Quantitative data refers to numeric data while qualitative data refers to text, audio, and video types of data. An example of this software is SAS Analytics.

Suites are value packages that include several programs in one package. These usually include a word processor, a spreadsheet, a database, a presentation graphics program, and sometimes a personal information manager along with other applications. The main advantage of these suites is their cost (lower than buying each program individually) and the ability to share data easily between each program. They are different from the integrated software listed previously which is one program with multiple functions.

Web browsers permit the displaying of Web pages from the Internet. a Web browser may come with the operating system or be a stand-alone program.

Word processing software permits the creating, editing, formatting, storing, and printing of text. Most have spelling and grammar checkers along with a number of other functions that can assist writers in editing their materials.

Education

Computer-assisted instruction software comprises a set of programs that help users learn concepts or specific content related to their discipline or area of study. In some circles, developers refer to this type of program as training software. CD-ROMs and DVDs hold educational programs that provide integrated sound and motion to provide a lesson. The Internet is a natural means for delivering computer-assisted instruction.

Increasingly, we are seeing software designed to take advantage of mobile devices and other related technologies. For example, Second Life (simulated environment), Blackboard, and other course management software for delivering instruction and promoting interactive learning using a variety of technology tools.

Utilities

Utilities are a group of software programs that help with the management or maintenance of the computer and protection of the computer from unwanted intrusion. Examples include hard disk managers, virus detectors, compression/decompression programs, spyware removers, firewalls, spam blockers, viewers, and so forth.

Personal

Personal software programs help people manage their personal lives. Examples include appointment calendars, checkbook balancing applications, money management applications, password managers, and calculators. Increasingly, these also include health-related applications for tracking and managing a range of healthcare needs.

Entertainment

The class of software programs that the industry has designed for fun is called **entertainment software.** Many games exist to provide diversion, including golf and football. Others challenge the user's problem-solving abilities. Some programs are like arcade-type games. Still others are strategy-based programs in which players takes turns and the game unfolds in real time.

When discussing software developments, the trend is toward easier-to-use, graphic interactive programs with certain built-in intelligence that anticipate the preferences of the end user.

Summary

This chapter presented the terminology and concepts necessary to become an intelligent computer user. To that end, it described the tenets underlying an information system, the major components of computers and connectivity/networking, and software basics broken down into three major classes: operating systems, languages, and applications. Although the specifics of computer systems will undoubtedly change as technology evolves, the basic concepts will remain the same. Users will always need to follow the input–process–output cycle and use some form of software and storage.

References

Aamoth, D. (2013). What is a PC? TimeTech, Feb 7, 2013. Retrieved from http://techland.time.com/2013/02/07/what-is-a-pc/

Federal Communications Commission (FCC) (nd). *Types of Broadband Connections.* Washington, DC: FCC. Retrieved from www.broadband.gov/broadband_types.html

Lewis, N. (2012). Pittsburgh healthcare system invests $100M in big data. *Information-Week*, October 15, 2012. Retrieved from www.informationweek.com/healthcare/clinical-systems/pittsburgh-healthcare-system-invests-100/240008989

Magaw, T. (2012). *IBM supercomputer Watson, Cleveland Clinic to work together.* Modern Healthcare, October 30, 2012. Retrieved from www.modernhealthcare.com/article/20121030/INFO/310309993

Odegard, A. (2011). *Treat your tablet battery correctly.* Retrieved from www.pocketables.com/2011/02/treat-your-tablet-battery-the-right-way.html

SafeTravel.dot.gov (n.d.). *DOT rule for passengers traveling with lithium batteries.* Washington, DC: US Department of Transportation Pipeline and Hazardous Materials Safety Administration. Retrieved from http://safetravel.dot.gov

Wallen, J. (2012). *How and when to charge your tablet battery.* San Francisco: TechRepublic. Retrieved from www.techrepublic.com/blog/tablets/how-and-when-to-charge-your-tablet-battery/814

Westover, B. (2011). Types of printers: a primer. *PC Magazine*, October 4, 2011. Retrieved from www.pcmag.com/article2/0,2817,2393904,00.asp

Online Resources

How Stuff Works (www.howstuffworks.com) is an excellent site for learning about computer hardware and connectivity.

Webopedia: Online Computer Directory for Computer and Internet Terms and Definitions (http://pcwebopedia.com/) is a great site for finding definitions and understanding basic concepts. It has a wonderful interface and is simple and easy to use. Another site of this type is WhatIs.com by Tech Target (http://whatis.techtarget.com/).

PC Magazine (www.pcmag.com) is an excellent site for reviews and the latest happenings regarding hardware and connectivity.

PC Tech Guide (www.pctechguide.com) covers a lot more detail and technical issues regarding technology.

Exercises 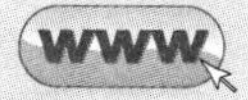

EXERCISE 1 What Do I Know about My Computer?

Objectives

1. Identify the specific computer hardware on your computer using the control panel.
2. Explore the information available to learn about the computer configuration using the control panel and computer.
3. Use the correct terms to describe computer components and functions.

> NOTE: Depending on the operating system edition you have (home, professional) the icons and organization on your screen may differ from the examples shown here, but you should still be able to obtain this information by looking around.

Activity

1. Start your computer and click **Start**, **Control Panel**.
2. Click the **System and Security** icon System and Security Review your computer's status Back up your computer. Now click the **System** icon System.
3. Who is the manufacturer and what is the model of this computer?
4. Identify the following: operating system and service pack, processor, memory, system type, and pen/touch availability.
5. Go to the control panel and click the **Appearance and Personalization** option Appearance and Personalization Change the theme Change desktop background. Click the **Display** icon Display located in the Appearance and Personalization section of the control panel. What can you do from this window? Why might you want to adjust the monitor settings?
6. Go to the control panel and click **Hardware and Sound** Hardware and Sound View devices and printers Add a device. Click the **Devices and Printers Manager** icon Devices and Printers Add a device | Add a printer | Add a Bluetooth device | Mouse | Device Manager. What is the model number of the monitor ? ________ Does the monitor automatically turn on and off when the computer is shut down? What other devices are attached to this computer? For example, wireless router, printer, scanner, and so forth.
7. Click the word **Mouse** in the Devices and Printers option Devices and Printers Add a device | Add a printer | Mouse. How do you change the mouse buttons if you are left handed? Can you change the speed of the clicks? Look at each tab and describe what is available for you to alter the settings.
8. Click the **Programs** icon Programs Uninstall a program in the control panel. Click the **Programs and Features** icon Programs and Features. What can you do from this window? List a few of the software programs available to you.
9. Click **Start, Computer**. What is the size of the hard drive (generally C:)? How much space is taken by your programs, utilities, and data?

10. How would you determine if you have any USB ports? How many do you have? How many are used by devices? How many are open?
11. Do you have a DVD storage device? Why would this be important to know?
12. How does this computer connect to the Internet or internal network? Why would you want to know this?

EXERCISE 2 Which One – Laptop, Tablet, or Smartphone?

Objectives

1. Distinguish features among laptops, tablets, and smartphones.
2. Evaluate the devices against a set of criteria.
3. Determine which is best for each intended use.

Activity

1. Based on your understanding of each device rate each on a 1 to 5 scale with 1 being poor and 5 excellent.

Statement/Feature	Laptop	Tablet	Smartphone
Supports creation of content such as documents, spreadsheets, presentations, school or corporate databases, and participation in discussion forums, taking tests, and so forth			
Provides a good reading experience in terms of viewing size and resolution			
Easily fits in a shirt or pant pocket			
Provides portability in terms of size and weight			
Provides for an easy and complete Web browsing experience			
Provides an email option			
Supports a wide range of apps or applications			
Provides excellent photo and video displays			
Provides excellent photo and video capture, both front and back			
Has a good battery life			
How good are the network options, e.g., Wi-Fi, 3G, and 4G?			
Provides reasonable storage options, e.g., RAM size, USB option, built-in storage			
Is the cost reasonable for the intended use?			
Communicates well with the other devices you use. equipment you own, e.g., syncing			

2. Before you make a decision about which device to purchase or which combination of the three types to purchase, you need to determine what features this/these device(s) must have in order to meet your needs. Select the appropriate device or devices that will meet the computing needs for computing based on the scenarios listed here. Explain your choice.
   a. Person A is an author who writes healthcare textbooks and travels doing research for those textbooks. This author is a producer of information and needs to type information into the software programs. This author believes a keyboard is mandatory for ease in producing the material.
   b. Student A is a consumer of information who needs access to diagnostic tests, drugs, and evidence-based data, and who communicates with the faculty through email. In the community, this student must capture images for entry into the patient's electronic medical record. Power and mobility are important when doing this job.
   c. Student B needs mobility with a voice option, access to the Internet, and some computing capabilities in all the patient rooms. In addition, Student B wants to check Facebook and Twitter to keep in contact with family and friends, send comments to the discussion board in the Course Management Software, and view communications from the faculty. Student B believes small and mobile is the key to meeting these needs.
   d. Student C needs to be able to connect the device to a printer and/or scanner, and to store confidential information on a portal hard drive. Student C also needs to create papers to submit for various courses. And, of course, Internet access is a must.

EXERCISE 3 How Do I Care for My USB Storage Device?

Objectives

1. Identify the rationale for each safety tip when caring for a USB storage device or external hard drive.
2. Insert a USB storage device or external hard drive into the computer properly.
3. Save a file to the device.
4. View the contents of the device.
5. Remove the device safely.

Activity

1. Match the safety tip in column A with its explanation from column B.

Column A – Safety Tip	Column B – Rationale
___ Avoid extremes in temperatures	A. Files might become corrupt if the safely remove feature is not used
___ Use the cap or slider when finished with the device	B. This makes it easier to see and not leave the device in the computer unintentionally
___ Attach the lanyard (strap) or key chain to the device	C. This protects the metal part of the device that is inserted into the USB port
___ Label the device	D. Electronic devices can be damaged when exposed to extremes
___ Back up the device	E. USB devices are storages devices for transport; they should not be considered reliable permanent copies. They can become corrupt during transport or exposure to the elements
___ Safely remove the device	F. This makes it easier to identify if lost or left in the computer

2. Insert a USB storage device into the computer. (Note: This also applies to inserting a portable hard drive.)
   a. Locate the USB port on the computer. It has the USB symbol above or below it.
   b. Depending on the USB device, **remove** the cap, **push** the slider button, or **swivel** the device to expose the metal tip.
   c. **Line up** the metal tip with the USB port and **push it** gently into the port. The ends should match, as shown in **Figure 2-15**. USB ports can be found on the front of many computers, on the left and/or right side of laptops, on the left side of some monitors (see **Figure 2-16**), and on the back of other computers.

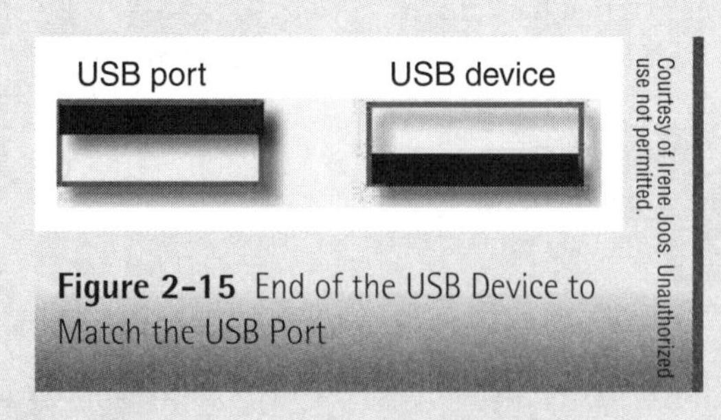

Figure 2-15 End of the USB Device to Match the USB Port

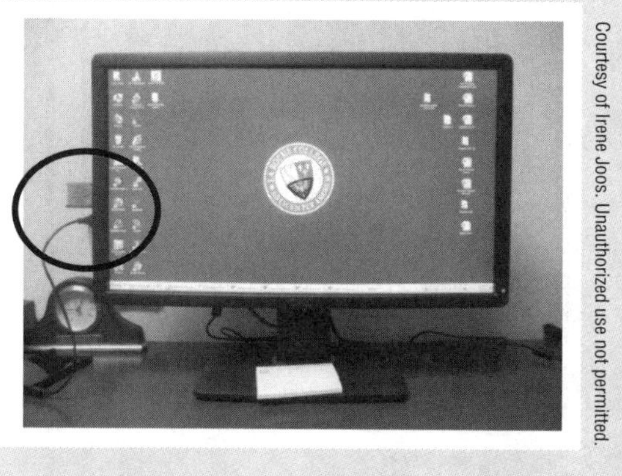

Figure 2-16 USB Port on Side of Monitor

NOTE: Some devices may require the installation of a device driver, as indicated by a message that appears at the lower-right side of the screen. The message will go away once the device driver is installed.

d. Once the USB storage device is engaged, the AutoPlay dialog box will appear unless this feature has been disabled. (See **Figure 2-17**.)

NOTE: Depending on the computer, the user may see a message such as "This device can perform faster ..."; click **X** to close the message balloon on the lower-right side of the screen. The user may also see another balloon on the upper-right side of the screen. If so, click **Cancel.**

NOTE: Some users disable the AutoPlay feature as a security feature. In this case, to access the storage device, click **Computer** and click the **device**. (See **Figure 2-18**.)

e. Click **Open Folder to view files** and click **OK**. You will now see a list of files or folders, if there are any, and the device letter in the computer window. The device is now ready to be used.

f. If a folder or file is present, double-click the **file** or **folder** to open it.

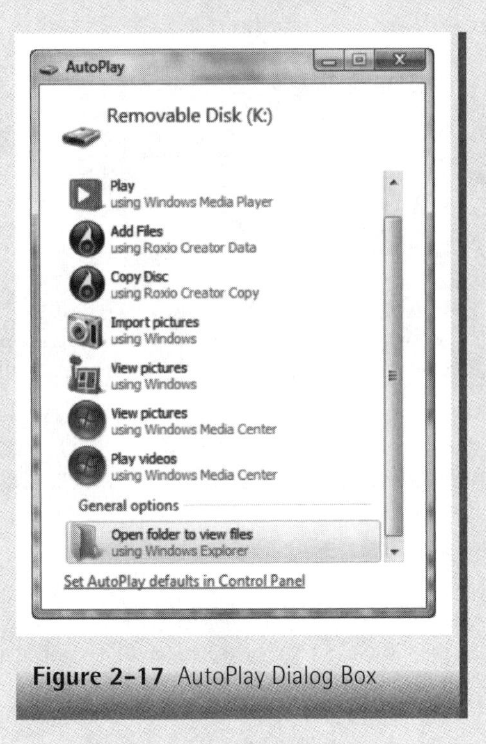

Figure 2-17 AutoPlay Dialog Box

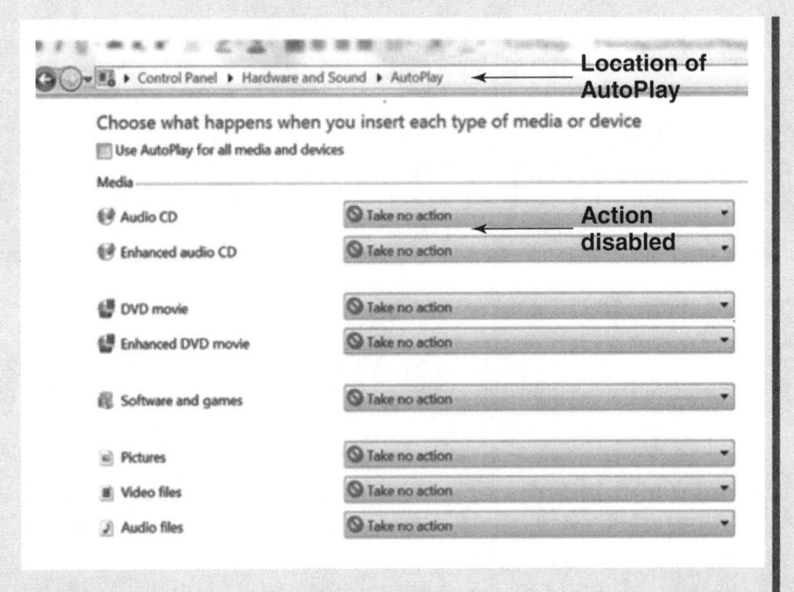

Figure 2-18 AutoPlay Dialog Screen Showing Diasabled Autoplay

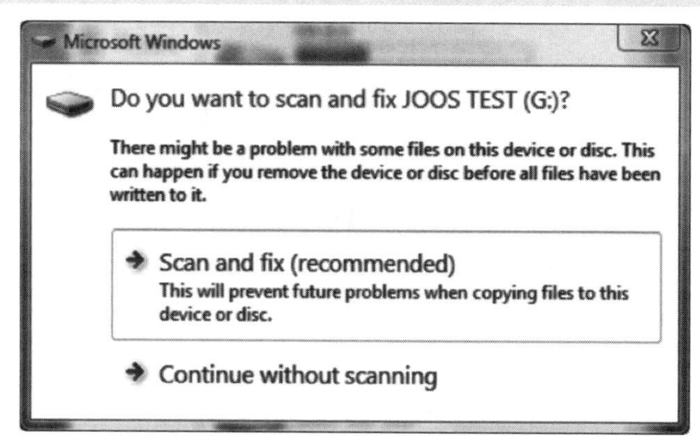

*This screen may or may not appear depending on your operating system settings.

Figure 2-19 Improper Removal of a USB Device

g. If the screen in **Figure 2-19** appears, it means the device was *not* removed properly the last time it was used. Choose **Scan and Fix (recommended)** and click **Close**. You are now ready to work with the USB storage device.

3. Save a file to the USB device.
   a. Open Word (**Start**, **All Programs**, **Microsoft Office**, **Microsoft Office Word 2010**). There are other ways to open the program, which you will learn later.
   b. Type **This is a test document for learning how to save a document to the removable USB storage device.**
   c. Click the **File tab** and then the **Save as** option. The screen shown in **Figure 2-20** appears.
   d. Click the **Computer** option on the left. Note that the default is Library/ Documents and may require scrolling down to see Computer on the left side.
   e. Click the correct **USB storage device.**
   f. Type **TestDocument** for the file name.
   g. Click the **Save** button. The file is now saved to the USB device. You can repeat the process to see that it was saved. Chapter 3 describes the process of saving files in more detail.
4. View the contents of the USB device.
   a. Click the **Start** button on the taskbar.
   b. Click **Computer** in the user identification area on the right side.
   c. Double-click the **USB storage device.** The file should now appear in the window.

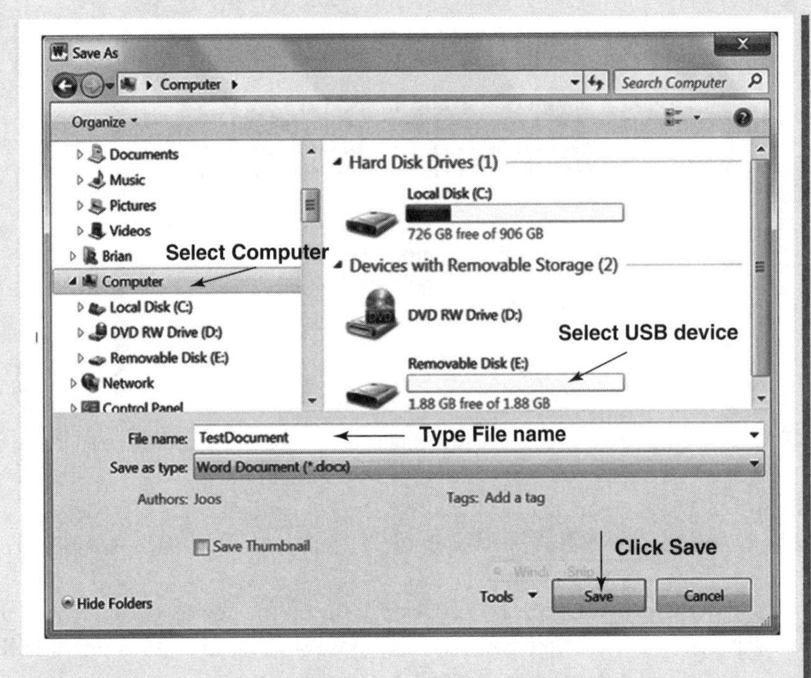

Figure 2-20 Saving to a USB Device

d. Click the **Close** button on the USB storage device window. The window closes.

5. Remove the USB device safely.

a. When finished using the USB device but *before removing* it, click the **icon** in the lower-right taskbar that reads "Safely Remove Hardware and Eject Media." For some computers, you must first click to see a menu of options and then to bring up the Safely Remove Hardware menu.

b. When the menu appears, click the **USB device**. A message appears stating that it is either safe to remove the USB storage device or that the device is currently in use and to close all programs and repeat the ejection process.

c. Click **OK** and **remove** the device. Replace the **cap**, retract the **metal tip** on the slider, or swivel the **metal tip** closed.

EXERCISE 4 Setting Up a Cloud Storage Service

(Using MS SkyDrive although any other service will also do.)

Objectives

1. Create an account on the storage services Web site.
2. Download the appropriate app to your device.
3. Create a folder on the cloud.
4. Upload a file and a picture to the cloud.
5. Examine the site for help and features.

Activity

Create an Account

(This assumes that you do not have Hotmail, SkyDrive, Xbox Live, or a Windows phone. If you have any of these you already have an account and can skip this part).

1. Open your **browser** and type **skydrive.com** in the URL text box.
2. Click **Sign Up Now** on the opening screen. (See **Figure 2-21**.)
3. Complete the **form** that appears requesting your name, birthdate, gender, userID (account sign in), password, phone number, and zip code, type in the nonsense characters to prove you aren't a robot, and click **Accept**.

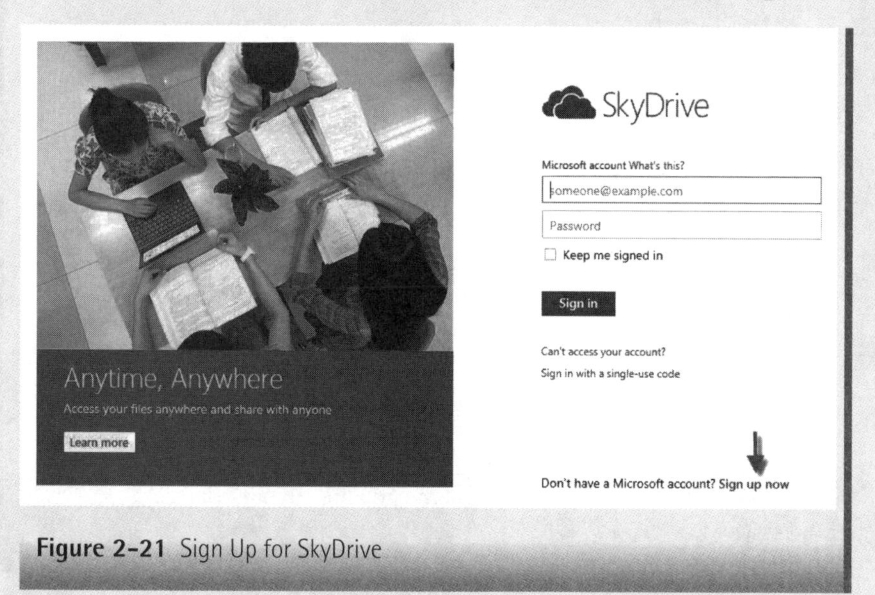
SkyDrive
Microsoft account What's this?
someone@example.com
Password
Keep me signed in
Sign in
Can't access your account?
Sign in with a single-use code
Anytime, Anywhere
Access your files anywhere and share with anyone
Learn more
Don't have a Microsoft account? Sign up now

Figure 2-21 Sign Up for SkyDrive

NOTE: You may remove the check mark in the box next to Send me email with promotional offers from Microsoft but do read the agreement before accepting it. (See **Figures 2-22, 2-23**, and **2-24**.)

Access SkyDrive

1. Open your **browser** and type **skydrive.com** in the URL text box.
2. Type your Microsoft **user account name** and **password**. Click **sign in**. *You should see three default folders.*

Upload a File to SkyDrive

1. Create a **simple Word document** and save it as **Practice-SkyDrive**.
2. Access your **SkyDrive account.**
3. Click the **Upload** button Upload.

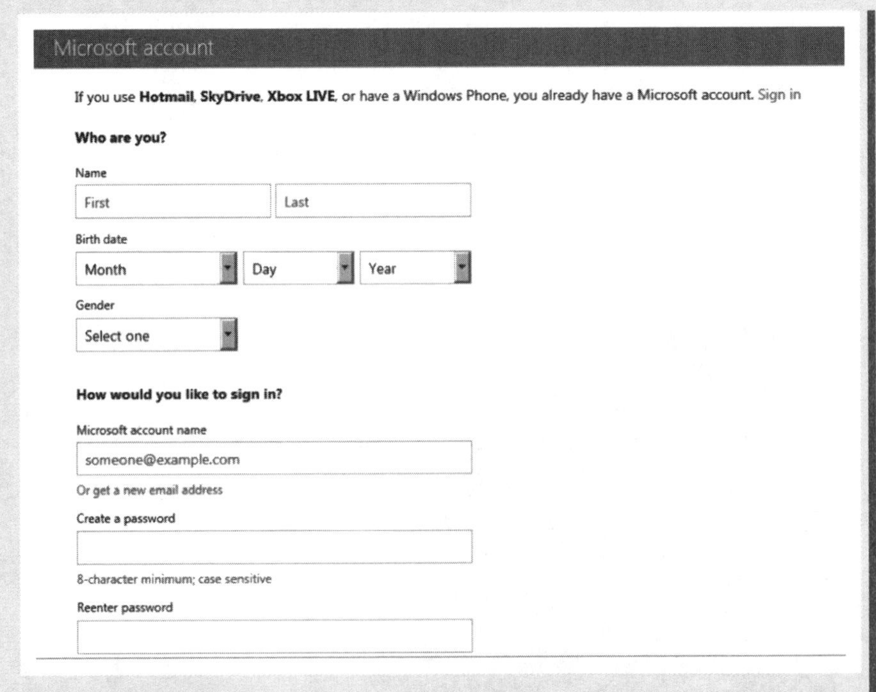

Figure 2-22 Additional Information—Who You Are, Account Name, and Password

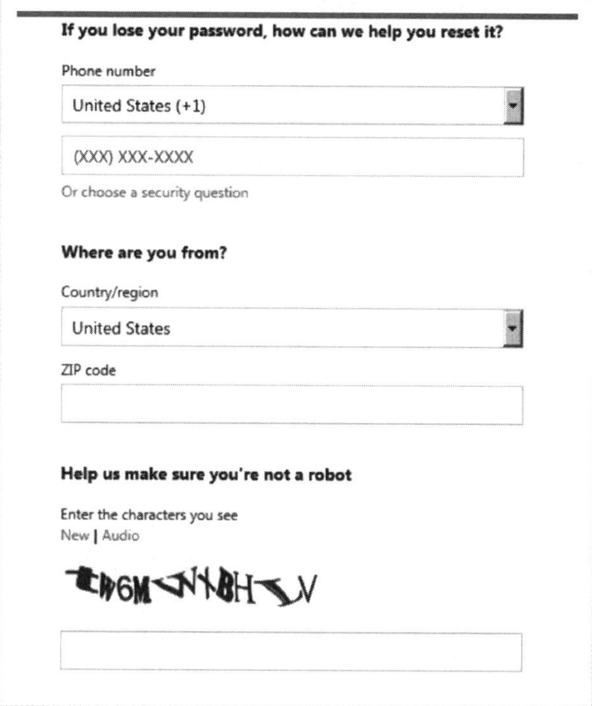

If you lose your password, how can we help you reset it?

Phone number

United States (+1)

(XXX) XXX-XXXX

Or choose a security question

Where are you from?

Country/region

United States

ZIP code

Help us make sure you're not a robot

Enter the characters you see

New | Audio

Figure 2-23 Additional Information—Phone Number, Location, Zip Code, and Proof You Are Not a Robot

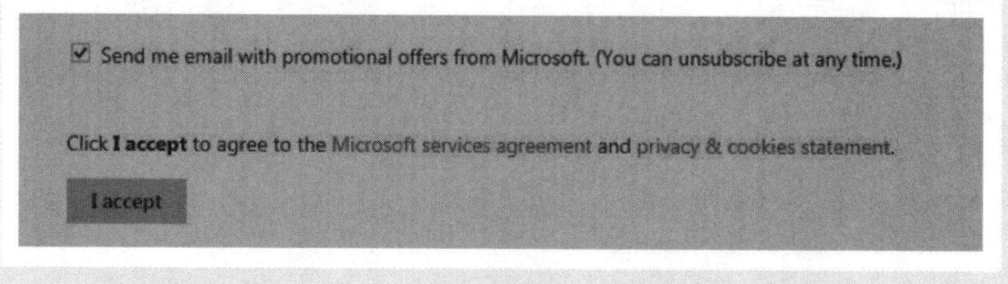

☑ Send me email with promotional offers from Microsoft. (You can unsubscribe at any time.)

Click **I accept** to agree to the Microsoft services agreement and privacy & cookies statement.

I accept

Figure 2-24 Additional Information—Email Promotions and Acceptance Agreement

4. Select the file **Practice-SkyDrive** and click **Open**. *The file is now on the cloud.*

NOTE: You may also upload to the main screen showing the folders and then drag and drop the file into the correct folder. Or you can use the Manage button and mouse right button click to manage the files, i.e., rename, delete, copy, and so forth.

Learning One New Feature

1. Look around SkyDrive and teach yourself one new feature. For example, how do you upload multiple files, share a file with others, open and save a document in SkyDrive, create groups, use the iPad SkyDrive app to email files, and so forth.
2. Find and share with your classmates one good reference that provides directions on SkyDrive features.

Access SkyDrive from the Desktop

You may decide you want to make sure you can upload and download files from mobile devices as well as from your desktop. By downloading the SkyDrive app you can synchronize the files on your local computer with SkyDrive. Any file or folder you place in the SkyDrive folder will automatically synchronize to your other devices that have the SkyDrive app installed.

1. Open your browser and type **http://windows.microsoft.com/en-US/skydrive/download**
2. Click the **Download SkyDrive** button Download SkyDrive. This will place the program on your computer.

NOTE: Download the free SkyDrive app on your Windows Phone, Android, iPhone, or iPad. On other phones just use the Web browser to sign in to SkyDrive.com.

NOTE: This will require downloading a file to your computer or mobile device; this probably will not be permitted in a public computer lab. Also note that ALL FILES placed in the SkyDrive folder you have created will automatically synchronize with your SkyDrive folder.

3. To access SkyDrive, click **Computer** and select **SkyDrive** located under the favorites areas. Favorites Desktop Downloads Recent Places SkyDrive You will see all your SkyDrive files. Now, when working on your desktop, you can place the file in this SkyDrive folder and it will automatically synchronize with the cloud SkyDrive.

EXERCISE 5 Computer Specifications

Objectives

1. Specify minimum hardware requirements for different scenarios.
2. Identify software needs.
3. Justify the recommendations for the requirements for both hardware and software.
4. Demonstrate knowledge of appropriate concepts and terms related to hardware and software.

Directions

1. You are serving on a school committee that is deciding what technology incoming students must purchase. You are one of several students representing the student point of view. Think about what tasks you will be required to complete as a student—papers, research, PowerPoint presentations, podcasts, group projects, and so forth.
2. Make a list of tasks students perform where technology would be a great asset.
3. Identify the technology specifications you believe will meet those requirements. Make sure you address hardware, software, data access, and connectivity.
4. Support your work with at least two articles identifying what schools in your area and across the country are doing related to technology requirements for students and how they anticipate using the technology.
5. Provide a two-page synopsis outlining the results of your thinking and research. Name it **Chap2-Exercise5-LastName**
6. Submit it as directed by your professor.

EXERCISE 6 Accessing Application Software

Objectives

1. Start application programs using a variety of techniques.
2. Identify the software programs or apps on your computer or mobile device.
3. Shut down the computer or mobile device.

Activity (for laptops or desktops running Windows operating system)

1. Start an application using the double-click method.
   a. Turn the **computer system on** if necessary. (Some computer labs leave the systems on all the time.) Text appears on the screen as the computer

goes through startup routines. If necessary, press **Ctrl+Alt+Del** to obtain the login screen. (In other words, hold down the Ctrl key, hold down the Alt key, and then press Del.) Release all three keys. If necessary, type **your login** (**user ID**) and **password** and press **Enter**. Use the **Tab key** to move between the user ID text field and the password text field.

b. Double-click the **Internet Explorer** icon on the desktop. The browser program opens. Alternatively, you can press the **Start** button and select **Internet Explorer** from the menu where it might be pinned or under all programs. You may also have the icon on the quick launch area of the Taskbar.

c. Click the **Close button** on the browser window to close the application.

2. Start an application using the Start button on the taskbar.
   a. Click the **Start button** on the taskbar. A menu appears.
   b. Select **All Programs**, **Accessories**, and **WordPad**. WordPad, a word processing program that comes with Windows, now starts.
   c. Click the **Close button** on the WordPad window to close the application.
3. Start an application using Computer.
   a. Double-click the **Computer** icon. Alternatively, you can click the **Start** button and then the **Computer** option. The Computer window opens.
   b. Double-click the **local (OS) drive** icon (usually C:), the **Windows** folder, and then the **System32** folder. Scroll through the window to find the calculator icon calc.
   c. Double-click the **Calc** icon. The calculator program opens.
   d. Click the **Close button** on the calculator window to close the application.
4. Identify application programs on the system.
   a. Click the **Start** button on the taskbar.
   b. Select **All Programs**.
   c. List the application programs that are accessible on this computer.
   d. Close all **open windows**.
5. Shut down the computer.
   a. Click the **Start** button.
   b. Click the **Closes all programs, shuts down Windows and then turns off your computer** button Shut down.

   At work and in some laboratories, users do *not* turn off the computer. In that case, select the option for log off Log off. At home, you might want to choose the option to save the session and turn off the computer. When you return, Windows will restore your session. Some computers automatically turn themselves off when shutting down; others require the user to turn them off physically. The same applies to the monitor.

■ **Activity (for a mobile device like a smartphone or tablet)**

1. Start an app (this example is from iPad but it should work similarly for others).
   a. Swipe to **find the app** on the screen (many mobile devices have multiple app screens).
   b. Tap the **app icon** on the screen; in this case, the **settings app**.
   c. Look at the various settings you can alter so the device functions as you prefer.
   d. To return to the main screen, while leaving the app running in the background, press the **Home** button or **pinch four or five fingers** together on the screen.
2. View open and recently used apps.
   a. Open the **settings** app and the **camera** app.
   b. Double-click the **Home** button. You now see your most recently used apps in the multitasking bar at the bottom of the screen.
   c. To close an app, hold and tap the **app in the multitasking bar**. They will now jiggle and a red circle with a minus sign will appear on the top left of each app. Tap and hold the icon to delete. It will now be closed.
3. Use your favorite search site and find the online manual for your mobile device. Download it to your device and search for one new function to learn about operating your device. Share that information with your classmates as directed by your professor.

Assignments

ASSIGNMENT 1 How Do I Compare Two Tablets?

■ **Objectives**

1. Justify the need for the tablet.
2. Select at least five criteria to use in making this comparison.
3. Explain why those criteria are important.
4. Compare two tablets using the criteria selected.
5. Recommend one of the tablets.

■ **Directions**

1. Write a short description about why you need a tablet and what you intend to do with it. Explain why a laptop or cell phone isn't the solution for your needs.
2. Decide on the criteria that are important when selecting a tablet. Ask yourself how important the apps are. How important is the operating system (there are several different ones on the market). How important are the hardware specifications listed in the following form.

3. Find the specifications for two tablets to make a comparison.
4. Complete the following form, making a recommendation and explaining why your selection will be best.
5. Submit the assignment to your professor in either print or electronic form.

Description:
Comparison:

Features/Specifications	Tablet 1	Tablet 2
Hardware Specifications		
Physical dimensions; viewing size		
Weight		
Battery life		
Resolution		
Internal flash memory		
Processor, core, and speed		
Cameras		
External ports		
Audio-mic and speakers		
Connectivity		
Bluetooth		
Cellular options		
Wi-Fi		
GPS		
Secondary Storage Options		
Storage size	_ GB	_ GB
Usability/Help		
Available apps for the task needed to be done		
Attachable keyboard		
Ease of use		
Warranty		
Cost	$	$

Recommendation:
Rationale/Comments:

ASSIGNMENT 2 How Do I Select a Cloud Storage Service?

Objectives

1. Identify specific criteria important to you when selecting cloud storage.
2. Compare two cloud storage services using those criteria.
3. Make a recommendation and justify that recommendation.

Directions

1. Select five of the criteria below that are important for your use of cloud storage.
   - Amount of storage
   - Accessible by all my devices (Windows, Mac, smartphone, tablet)
   - Works with Microsoft Office
   - Organize and showcase photos
   - Share files with anyone
   - Individual file size limitations
   - Cost
   - Additional storage options for additional price
   - Security of files
   - Post files/photos to Facebook, Twitter, etc.
   - Ease of backup or sync with local files
   - Optional (select any other criteria that might be important to you)
2. Select two online storage services (e.g., Microsoft SkyDrive, Apple iCloud, Google Drive, Dropbox, Amazon Cloud Drive, MediaFire.
3. Create a table—list the criteria in column 1 and the two devices in columns 2 and 3.
4. Make a statement about how the storage service meets those criteria.
5. Make a recommendation about which service you would select and why you chose that one over the service not selected.
6. Create an account on the selected service and upload a few documents.
7. Create a screen capture showing the documents you uploaded and paste that file to the end of your comparison document.
8. Submit the assignment as directed by the professor.

ASSIGNMENT 3 How Is Mobile Technology Changing Health Care?

Objectives:

1. Download a file to a storage device or to a cloud service.
2. Select two scenarios from the article to discuss.

3. Identify what the issue was, what technology was used as the solution, and what implications that may have for your practice and health care.

■ **Directions:**

1. Go to www.brookings.edu/research/papers/2012/05/22-mobile-health-west and on the right side download the paper to your mobile storage device or cloud service.
2. Read the article by Darrell West entitled *How Mobile Devices are Transforming Healthcare*.
3. Select two scenarios from the article. Identify the issue for which a particular technology was a solution. Argue for or against the technology selected and justify your answer. Discuss what implications this may have for your practice and health care.
4. Go to the Endnotes section of the document and review one of the related articles cited to support information provided. Would you agree or disagree with how that information was summarized in this article and why.
5. Write your results in a Word document and submit to your professor. Alternatively, this may be an assignment for discussion in a discussion forum.

chapter

3

The Computer and Its Operating System Environment

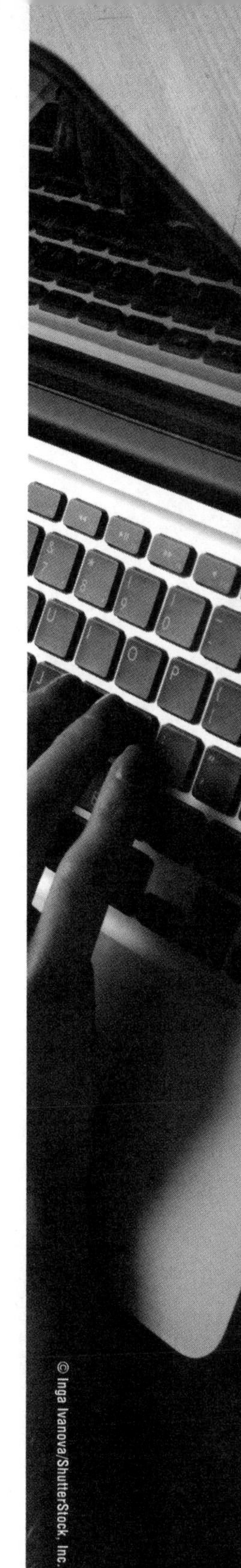

Objectives 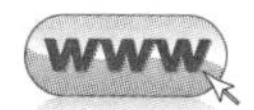

1. Describe the Windows operating system environment.
2. Perform the boot process.
3. Explain graphical user interfaces.
4. Describe operating system trends in end-user design and functions.
5. Start Windows and log off from Windows.
6. Manipulate windows and manage the desktop.
7. Identify the basic concepts underlying file and disk management, including file naming conventions.

Introduction

Every computer and mobile device relies on an operating system to function. Computers without a functioning **operating system (OS)** are just pieces of hardware (with the exception of simple, single-purpose computers like those that control microwave ovens). Many operating systems are available for different types of computers. Here are just a few examples:

- Microsoft Windows for personal computers.
- Mac OS for Apple computers.
- UNIX/Linux for workstations and larger computers.
- iOS for Apple's iPads and iPhones.
- Android OS from Google running on multiple mobile devices like the Kindle Fire, Nook, and Nexus tablets.
- Windows RT and 8 Pro for Microsoft's Surface tablet.

This chapter describes the operating system environment that many personal computers (PCs and laptops) use in the educational and healthcare arena: Microsoft Windows.

Every three to four years, Microsoft and Apple issue a new operating system or updated version thereof, making modifications to that OS as per users' needs, changes in technologies, and changes in the computer world. For example, the current focus is on increasing the functionality of mobile devices and the next wave may be ubiquitous computing. All operating systems give users the ability to manage the operating system environment and the user's own files and folders. With each version of the operating system, Microsoft and Apple add more functionality, but learning the basic concepts will help you adjust to the new look and functionality of each new version.

The Microsoft operating system after XP was Vista, which had a short life span. Following Vista was Windows 7. This version included a redesigned taskbar that closely resembles Apple's Dock, a new version of Internet Explorer, a new Windows Media Center and Windows Media Player, revised interfaces in Paint and WordPad, improved wireless support, pervasive touch screen support, and the removal of the side bar. Microsoft released its newest operating system version Windows 8 in late 2012 and only time will tell if it is a success or will go the way of Vista. Note that most operating system versions are not supported or updated after about 10 years.

The Windows 7 design provides a friendly interface between the user and the hardware. The intent of this **graphical user interface (GUI)** is to take advantage of the computer's graphic and mouse capabilities and make it easier to use the commands and applications. The user employs the mouse in a point-and-click approach to issue commands and manage the interface.

Critical to working in any operating system environment is the ability to manage files and folders. Files contain data and information, whereas folders are storage places for files. This chapter includes information on managing files and folders using Computer (My Computer in earlier versions of Windows). Computer provides quick access to Windows Explorer, which is used to create and manage folders.

The Operating System Environment

Operating systems are responsible for many of the computer's "housekeeping" tasks. The operating system "wakes" the computer through a set of commands and routines that make the computer recognize the central processing unit, memory, keyboard, disk drives, and printers. The purposes of the operating system are to supervise the operation of the computer's hardware components and to coordinate the flow and control of data. Without the operating system, the user cannot run language or application software.

There are several types of operating systems:

- Real-time operating systems (RTOS) that control machinery, scientific instruments, and industrial systems. There is very little user interface or interaction with the end user.
- Single-user, single-task OS to manage one user and one task at a time. One example is the OS on Palm devices, which are rarely seen today.
- Single-user, multitasking OS that permits multiple tasks and applications to run at the same time. This type of OS is the focus of this chapter.
- Multiuser, multitask operating systems on large computers like one might see in a hospital or educational system. An example of this type of OS is Unix (Franklin and Doustan, n.d. para 1).

Today, most operating systems (platforms) come preinstalled on the computer or mobile device. Several versions of the Windows operating system are in use: XP, VISTA, Windows 7, and Windows 8. For mobile devices, the operating system resides on a chip. General trends with these versions include the integration of Internet capabilities, the ability to perform multiple tasks at the same time, the ability to work in network environments, and increased inclusion of security and multimedia capabilities.

To become proficient in using the computer, the user needs a basic understanding of how the system works and how to manage the desktop environment. This means learning how to customize the desktop, manipulate the windows, switch between applications, and manage files and folders. One needs many of these same skills for using the mobile operating system environment that relies more on apps and touch screens.

Starting the Computer: The Boot Process

The boot process refers to turning on the computer or using the restart button if the computer has one and initiating a series of actions. A cold boot refers to turning on a computer that one has turned or powered off. A warm boot refers to the process of restarting a computer that is already on in one of two ways:

1. Press the **Ctrl+Alt+Del** keys together and then select the **Shut down** options button down arrow on the lower-right side of the screen.
2. Click the Start button, **Shut down** arrow Shut down, and click the Restart option on the menu.

See **Figure 3-1** for these two examples. Some computers may have other options for a warm boot depending on the edition and settings of that OS. Use a warm boot when you are installing new software or when the computer stops responding. Some school computers use the **Ctrl+Alt+Del** option to wake up the computer for you to login. When you click the **Start** button, you may see Log off Log off or Shut down Shut down depending on the configuration of the OS.

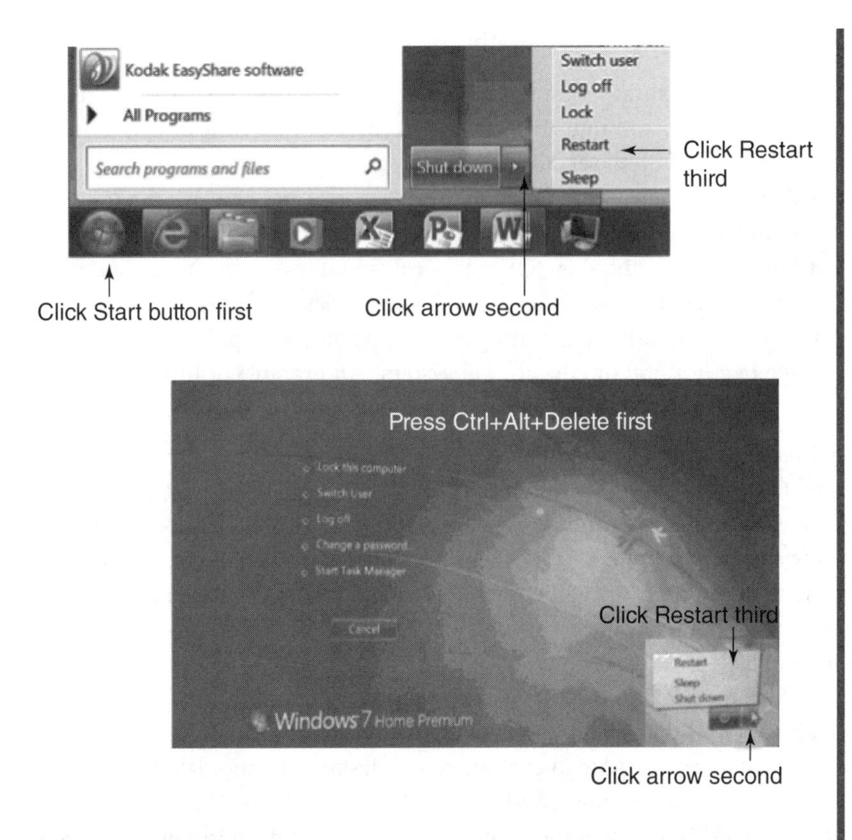

Figure 3-1 Warm Reboot

Power-On Self Test (POST)

When you boot the computer, the power supply sends an electrical signal to the processor, causing it to reset itself and find the basic input and output system (BIOS) instructions on the read-only memory (ROM) chip. The BIOS performs a **power-on self-test (POST)**, which analyzes the buses, clock, memory, drives, and ports to make sure that all of the hardware is working properly. The system compares the results of this test with data stored in the complementary metal-oxide semiconductor (CMOS) chip.

System Files and Kernel

Upon completion of the POST test, the software loaded in ROM activates the computer's disk drives and looks for a bootable sector of a disk—the part of the disk containing a program that loads the system files into memory (bootstrap loader). Generally, this activity involves checking the hard drive. Once found, the system files are loaded into memory. This central module of the operating system, called the **kernel**, is the part of the operating system that loads first and remains in memory as long as the computer is on. The operating system in memory is now in control of monitoring system resources.

This startup procedure runs very quickly on most computers. If the computer finds problems, the computer makes beeping sounds and then stops running. If all goes well, the user logs in to his or her account. On personal computers, the user may or may not need to log in depending on the configuration of the operating system. The desktop now appears.

Understanding the **boot** process makes problem solving easier when something goes wrong during this process. If you press the **On** button and nothing happens, the computer may have been unplugged or the battery may be dead. Without a power source to initiate the startup process, the computer can do nothing. Note that many tablets go to "sleep" but stay on, thus making it quicker to start using the device. However, you will need to know the specific steps to wake the computer. Information on how to do this is provided later in this chapter.

Graphical User Interface (GUI)

Windows, Macintosh OS, and mobile devices use GUIs as the means for the user to interact with the operating system. **Figure 3-2** shows a typical Windows desktop with its graphical interface. Your desktop may have all or few of the items shown in Figure 3-2, as individuals and companies often customize the GUI. Your mobile device may have many or a few icons visible and generally you must swipe to reveal more options.

The focus of this chapter is the Windows operating system and some features that are common to both the Windows and Mac operating systems. This chapter does not cover mobile device operating systems.

Desktop

The **desktop** is the area on the screen that displays the icons, folders, files, and taskbar. In the Windows environment, the desktop is the primary workspace that fills the screen. The monitor displays the desktop when you boot the computer or log in. The user may customize the desktop to suit his or her work style—that is, the user can change the colors and the location of objects, add images to the background of the desktop, add gadgets, and install screen savers.

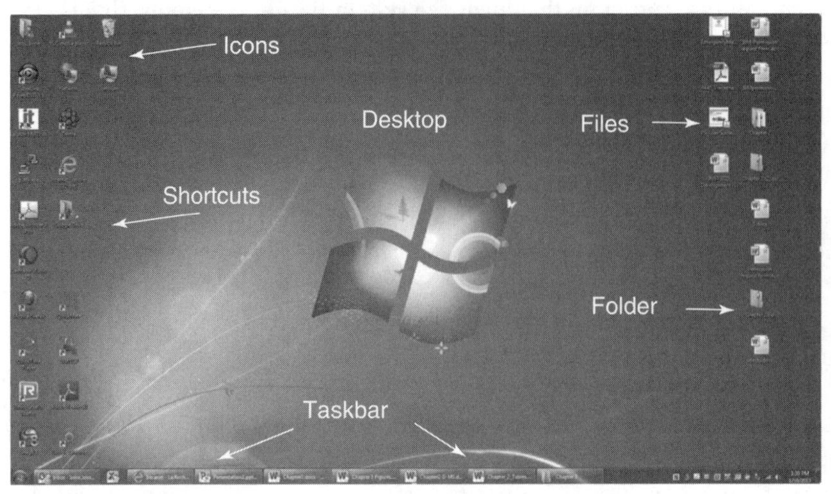

Windows 7 desktop

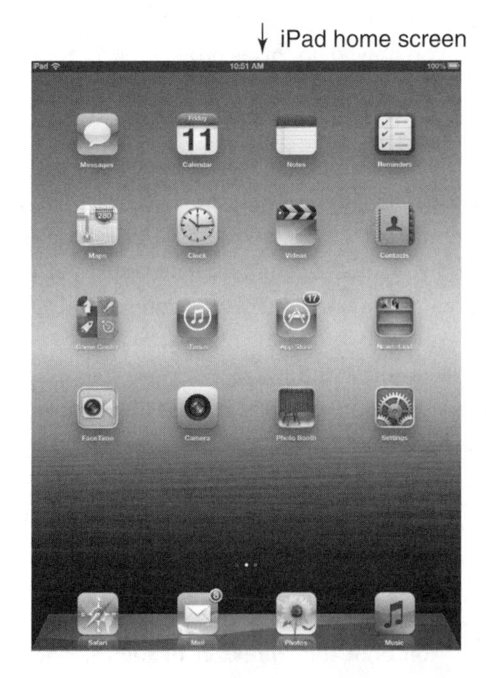

Figure 3-2 Windows 7 Desktop and Apple iPad Home Screen

Dialog Box

The **dialog box** is a special, secondary window that requires the user to make selections from options to implement the commands. Making a selection may require:

- Selecting from a list box,
- Clicking a square or circle to make a selection,
- Clicking a tab for another option, or
- Clicking a commit button. (See **Figure 3-3**.)

Gadgets

Gadgets are a Windows option for the desktop. Gadgets permit easy access to frequently used tools such as slideshows of pictures, newsfeeds, or the weather. **Figure 3-4** shows the gallery of gadget options that come with the operating system. More gadgets are available from independent developers but you need to make sure they come from a trusted source. Use a search site to find them.

Menus

Menus are lists of commands or tasks that become available when the user selects a command category from the menu bar. See **Figure 3-5** for an example of a menu and its drop-down menu. While many applications use the menu bar, Office 2010 uses the **ribbon** concept covered in Chapter 4.

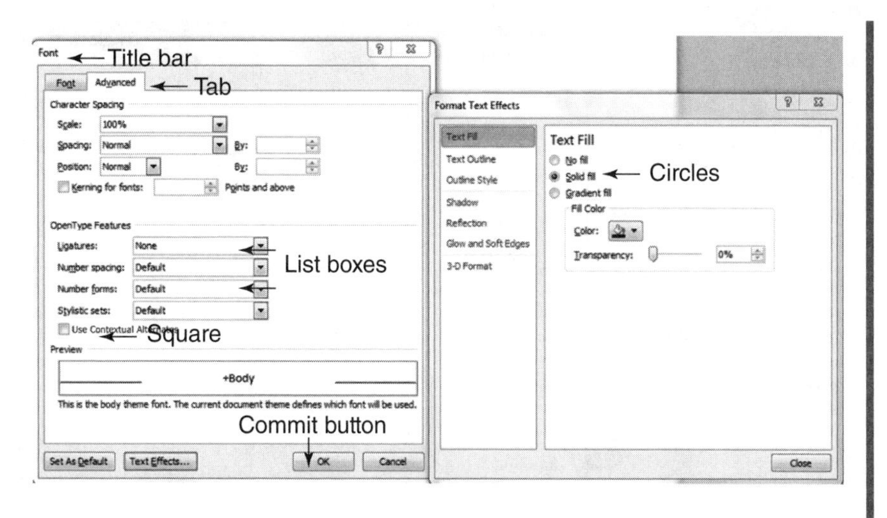

Figure 3-3 Example of a Dialog Box

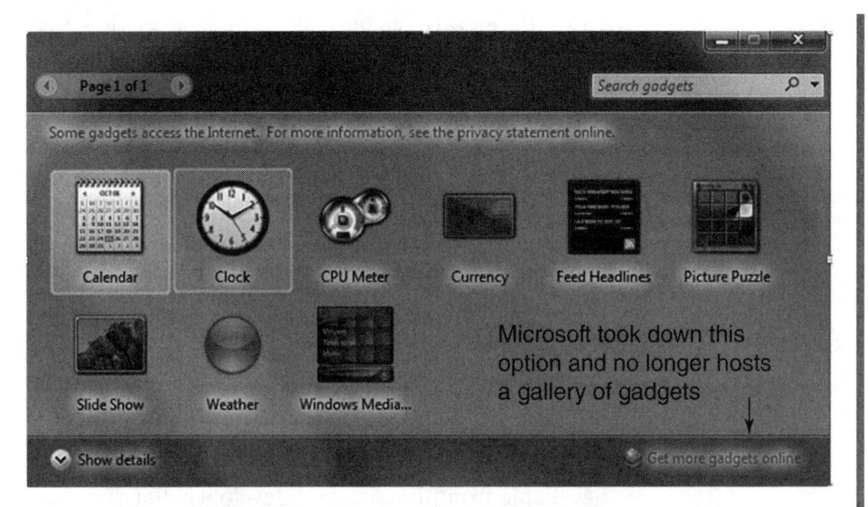

Figure 3-4 Add Gadgets to the Desktop

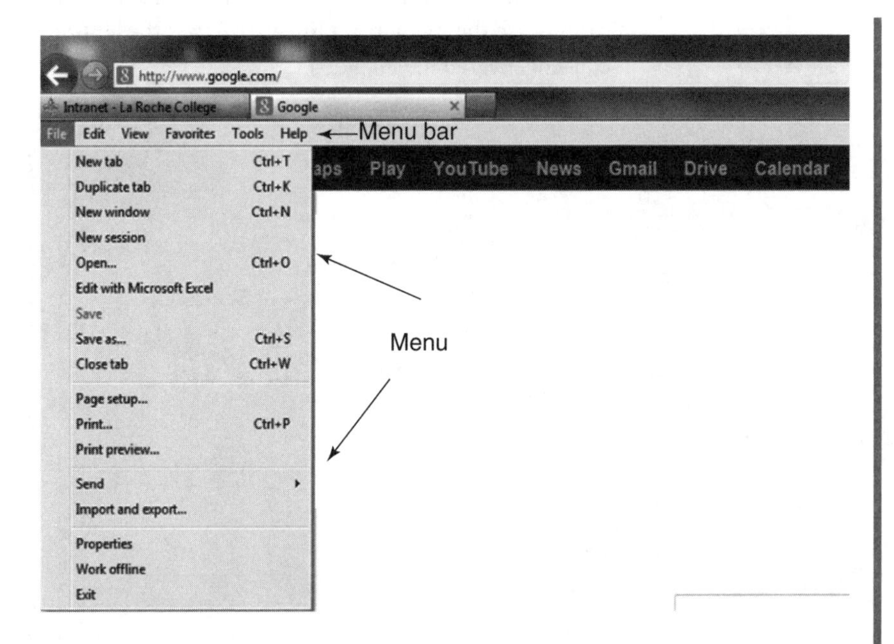

Figure 3-5 Menu Bar and Menu in a Typical Window

Mouse/Touchpad and Touchscreen

Devices that enable you to select objects and issue commands include the **mouse**, **touchpad**, and **touchscreen**. The idea behind the use of these devices is to make issuing commands faster, especially for the nontypist. GUIs depend on these devices to select objects or commands from menus, ribbons, and toolbars. Most of the commands that you access in this manner also have an equivalent keyboard stroke. Refer to Chapter 2 for a description of mouse actions.

Objects

Objects on the desktop are small pictures or graphic representations of icons, files, folders, and shortcuts. To select an object place the pointer on it and click. Double-clicking the object opens it. Right-clicking an object opens a shortcut menu, sometimes called a context-sensitive menu. See Figure 3-2 for examples of objects on the desktop.

Pointer

A **pointer** is the symbol that represents the mouse location on the screen. Many applications change the look of the pointer to reflect the process the system is expecting. For example, the pointer changes to a double-headed arrow (⟷) when you hover over a window border, indicating readiness for resizing the window. Use the pointer to select commands from menus and toolbars. This text presents different pointer shapes as they occur in discussions about application programs.

Taskbar

The **taskbar** is generally the long horizontal bar at the bottom of the desktop. It combines window management and program launching functions. Use it to switch between applications and files. All open windows become items on the taskbar. Windows 7 permits you to pin an application to the taskbar for quick access. A border appears around the icon of an open application. In the Windows Aero view, you can also see a **thumbnail** of the document. **Figure 3-6** shows the parts of the taskbar.

Window

A **window** on the desktop displays the contents of application programs, files, or folders. Each program

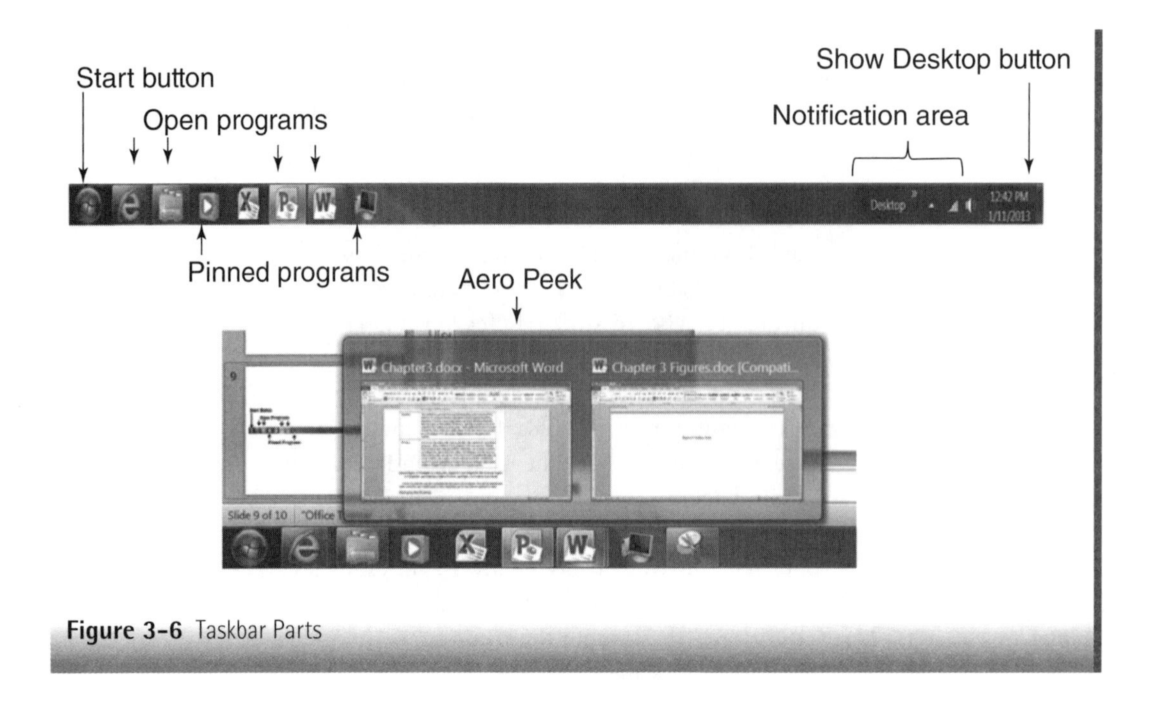

Figure 3-6 Taskbar Parts

or file has its own window. Each window may contain a title bar, menu bar, one or more toolbars, an address bar, tabs, and a status bar. Office 2010 displays the title bar and ribbon along with a status bar. If the window is too small to display all of the contents, the window will also contain scroll bars. Additional window controls include those that close, maximize, minimize, and restore windows. More information on this is found in the application chapters.

Even though applications have their own look, the GUI provides the user with a consistent feel and easy-to-use commands. The common features and looks enable the user to adjust quickly to other applications and to move between applications easily.

Managing the Desktop

NOTE: You may not have permission to alter the desktop or taskbar in the clinical environment or school labs.

This section discusses the layout of the desktop and explains how to manage the desktop in Windows 7. The desktop is the main window visible after logging on to the computer. Just as most workers enjoy arranging their desks in a specific way to make them more comfortable and productive in their work environment, a computer desktop can be customized in any number of ways.

When programs open, they run on top of the desktop. To display the desktop without closing any of the opened programs, click the Show Desktop button on the far right of the taskbar.

Objects on the Desktop

The desktop displays several objects by **default** unless the user changes the default. *Default* means that the computer uses a certain setting or configuration. Figure 3-2 shows some of these default objects: icons, folders, shortcuts, files, and the taskbar.

Icons

Icons or small pictures, represent applications, folders, and files. By default, the recycle bin is on the desktop. Other icons present on the desktop depend on the unique configuration of the computer. For example, the school computer may include the recycle bin, computer, and network icon. When you install a new program, the computer may ask you if you want an icon for the program placed on the desktop.

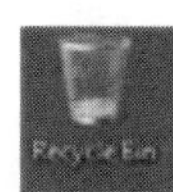

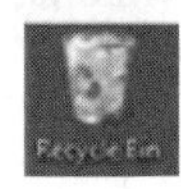

The Recycle Bin temporarily stores deleted files until you empty it. The system deletes files that you delete from external storage devices (such as USB storage devices) *immediately*. This icon is present by default. The top view is an empty Recycle Bin and the bottom view is one with files in it. You should empty the Recycle Bin periodically depending on how frequently you send items to the recycle bin.

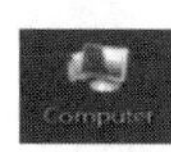

This icon may or may not be present on the desktop. This gives you access to your storage devices and files. To add it to the desktop, click **Start**, right-click **Computer**, and click **Show on Desktop**.

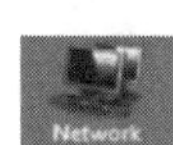

If the computer is connected to a network, the user has access to the Network icon. It may or may not be placed on the desktop. Use it for viewing and accessing network resources.

You may add other icons to the desktop or Quick Launch area of the taskbar as well as create shortcuts on the desktop.

Shortcuts

Shortcuts are pointers to an actual application, folder, or file. They contain the path to the executable file for the application, to the folder, or to the file, respectively. Deleting one simply deletes the shortcut, not the application, folder, or file. Shortcuts have a right curved arrow on the bottom left of the icon. Use shortcuts to provide quick access to commonly used applications, folders, or files. Later in this chapter the process of creating shortcuts is described. Here are a few examples of shortcuts:

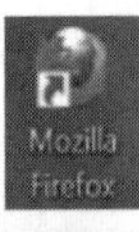

This is a shortcut to the Firefox browser.

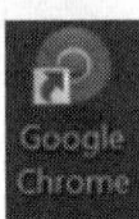

This is the shortcut to Google Chrome.

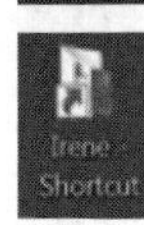

This is a shortcut to a folder called Irene-Shortcut located down a path on the hard drive.

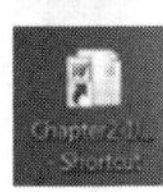

This last example is a shortcut to a file called Chapter2-IJ-Shortcut located on the hard drive in a folder.

Folders

Folders are holding places for files and may be on the desktop or other places on the hard drive or removable storage devices. They are represented by icons that look like manila file folders. By storing similar programs and files together in folders, your work is more organized. Subfolders are folders within folders that impose a hierarchical structure to the system. See Managing Files and Folders later in this chapter for more about creating and using folders.

Files

Files contain data that users create in applications such as Word, Excel, and PowerPoint. Files hold or store the work we do. Icons representing each file type assume the look that one associates with the application that creates them. For example, a Word file looks like a piece of paper with a W symbol on the icon representing the file. You create files when you save work in an application or when you select the **Create**, **New File** command from the shortcut menu.

This image shows a Word document file titled Chapter 2-Figures.

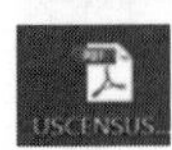

This image shows a pdf file titled USCENSUS… The dots indicate that the file name is longer than what you see.

Taskbar

The **taskbar**, by default, is at the bottom of the screen. The user may move it to any screen edge. It is actually three separate components, although it looks like one object. **Figure 3-6** shows the parts of the taskbar.

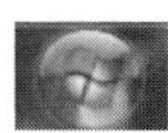

Use the **Start button** to open the Start menu. This will allow you to access programs, documents, settings (Control Panel), help, and shut down features. The Start menu contains the user name at the top right with an icon above it that you can change. On the left side are the recently accessed programs, pinned items, and a link to All Programs. To the right are the System Folders, Control Panel, Help and Support, and the Log off/Shutdown button. (See **Figure 3-7**.)

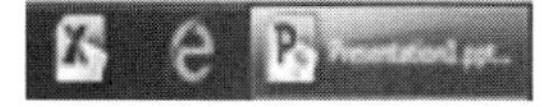

This setup represents Microsoft's approach to unclutter the desktop. A practice exercise at the end of this chapter demonstrates how to customize the Start menu. Between the Start button and notification area are the open and pinned programs/windows. Frequently used applications are pinned to this area to provide quick

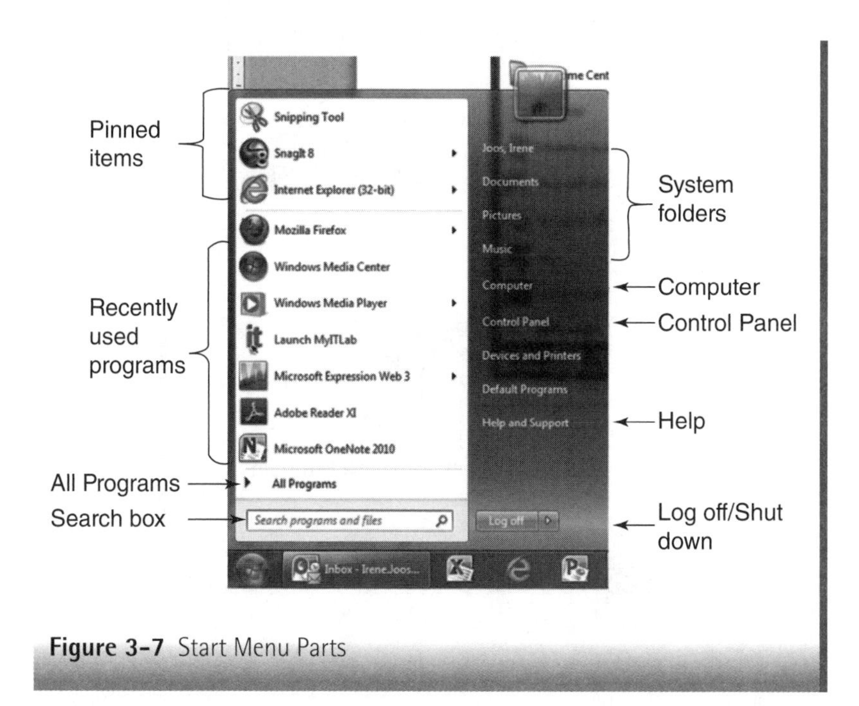

Figure 3-7 Start Menu Parts

access to them and to keep an uncluttered desktop. Open windows are also indicated in this area of the taskbar. **Figure 3-8** shows Excel and Internet Explorer as pinned programs and PowerPoint Presentation1 document as an open window.

To the far right of the Start button is the **notification area.** It contains programs that usually run in the background and need only occasional user input, such as antivirus programs, the battery charge indicator, the Safely Remove Hardware utility, the Internet access signal strength, and the volume control. If the mouse-controlled pointer pauses over one of these icons, the function or name of that icon appears. Periodically a small pop-up window will notify you of an action you should take or consider, such as "Your virus protection software needs to be updated." (See **Figure 3-9**.)

The date and time along with the Show Desktop button are to the far right on the taskbar.

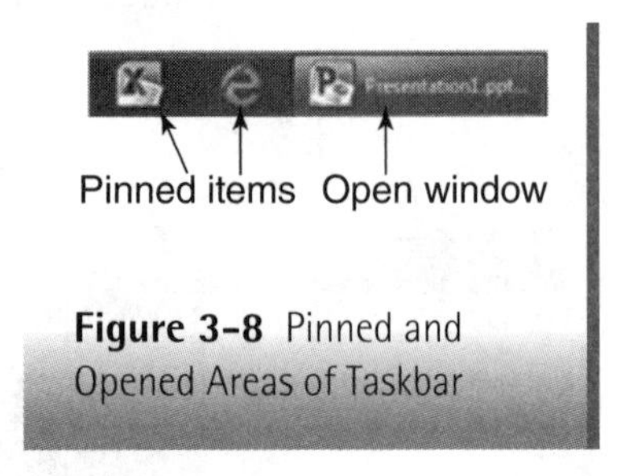

Figure 3-8 Pinned and Opened Areas of Taskbar

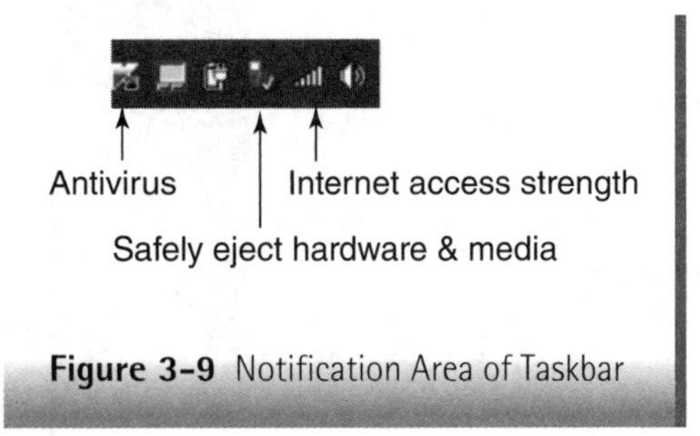

Figure 3-9 Notification Area of Taskbar

Pointer Shapes

As mentioned earlier, pointer or cursor shapes may change while the user is working in the Windows environment. When the pointer changes shape, the computer expects to complete certain operations and responds accordingly.

The ready arrow means that the computer is waiting for commands. Use it to select objects, double-click objects, right-click objects, drag objects, or choose menu or icon commands.

Use the I-beam to insert text. It appears when the user pauses over a text field, along with the insertion point (blinking vertical bar). Any text entered will be inserted at the location of the vertical bar or insertion point, not the I-beam location (which could be over any text field).

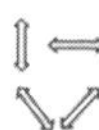

Window-sizing pointers appear when the cursor is over a window border. There are four versions: left–right, up–down, left slanted, and right slanted. Left–right arrows widen the window. Up–down arrows lengthen the window. Slanted arrows can widen and lengthen the window simultaneously.

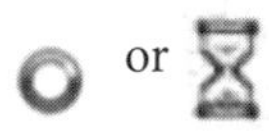

The moving circle or hourglass indicate that the computer is processing and cannot execute any further commands until it finishes processing. Wait. Do not type or click the mouse button until the hourglass disappears. If you click anything before the ready arrow appears, the computer may freeze, stop working, or crash.

The hand means that the mouse pointer is over a linked object or linked text. Clicking the text or object will bring more information from this site or take you to another site. Use the hand pointer to obtain additional information.

When the mouse pointer looks like this, the attempted action is not available. This is the forbidden cursor shape.

Additional pointer shapes will be discussed in appropriate application sections elsewhere.

Changing the Appearance of the Desktop

By default, Windows 7 will install the Windows 7 Basic theme on the computer. Each person with an account on the computer can set up the computer to display his or her own theme. In addition, users may customize or personalize the background (also called wallpaper) or color scheme. Some users never change the theme, color, or background; others find change in the workday world stimulating, so they change them regularly. Windows provides for both types of users by letting the user choose the theme, desktop background, and color. If the user changes the default settings, the new settings are in effect until the user changes them again. A variety of digital pictures are available as desktop backgrounds. Some users prefer to use their own personal digital pictures as background wallpaper. Some computer labs and companies may restrict the ability to adjust the desktop.

HINT: To see additional themes, you must first install them from Microsoft's Web site or from the Internet.

To change the default theme:

1. Right-click a **blank area** of the desktop. A shortcut menu appears.
2. From the shortcut menu, select **Personalize**. The screen shown in **Figure 3-10** appears.
3. Click one of the **themes** and the new theme appears.

To change the desktop background or color scheme:

1. Right-click a **blank area** of the desktop. A shortcut menu appears.
2. From the shortcut menu, select **Personalize**. The screen shown in Figure 3-10 appears.
3. Click the **Desktop Background** or **Window Color** options.
4. Select a **background** or **window color** from the presented options.
5. When satisfied with your choice, click **Save changes** and close the **Personalize** window.

A user can also change the desktop from the Control Panel. To access the Control Panel, select the **Start button** on the taskbar, the **Control Panel** option, and **Personalization** Personalization. Again, Figure 3-10 shows the available choices.

NOTE: The Control Panel is the same place to alter the appearance of the mouse pointer, to add sounds, and to add screen savers.

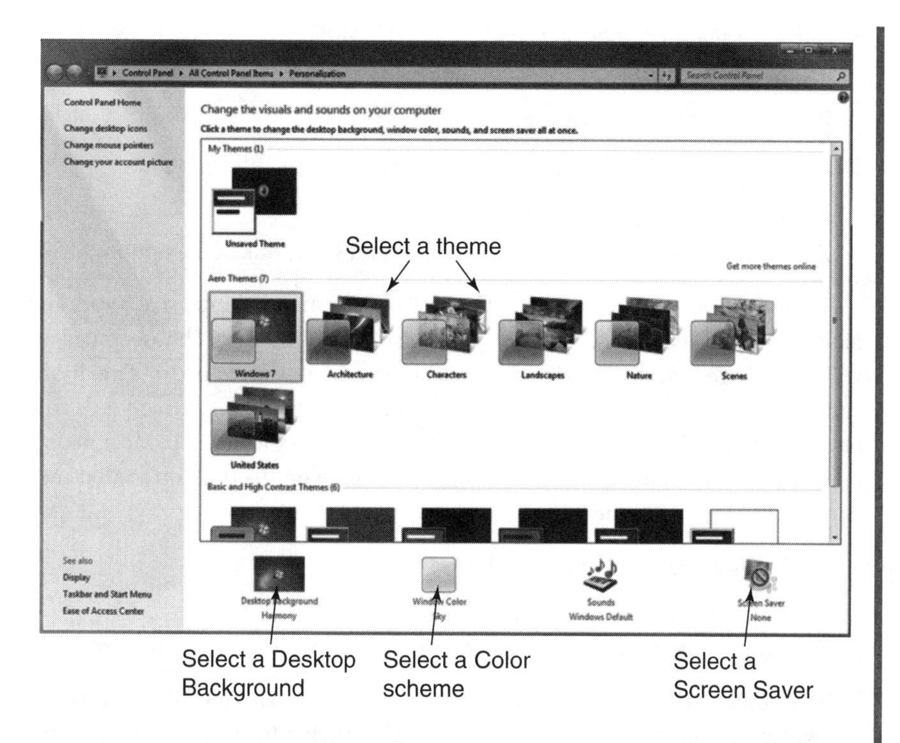

Figure 3-10 Changing the Window Color and Appearance, Desktop Background, and Theme

Moving Objects on the Desktop

Windows provides an option to change the location of any object on the desktop. The taskbar can be located on any of the four edges of the screen. The default is to place the taskbar on the bottom of the screen.

To change the location of the taskbar:

1. Place the mouse pointer on a **blank area** of the taskbar.
2. Drag the taskbar to the **left**, **right**, **bottom**, or **top** of the screen.
3. Release the **mouse button**.

NOTE: When you drag the taskbar, it initially appears not to move. Keep dragging the mouse toward the edge of the screen, and eventually the it moves unless it is locked in place. To unlock it, right-click a **blank area** of the taskbar and select **Lock the taskbar** from the menu to remove the check mark next to it.

To change the location of an icon, folder, shortcut, or file:

1. Select the **object**.
2. Drag it to the **new location**.

To arrange by name, size, type, and date modified:

1. Right-click a **blank area** of the desktop.
2. From the shortcut menu, select **Sort By** and select **one** of the options.

There are four choices in the Arrange Icons By menu: name, size, type, and date modified. (See **Figure 3-11**.) Depending on the option you choose, the icons will be arranged on the left side of the desktop in the selected order. The disadvantage of using this method of organizing icons is that every time you add a new object, the objects will appear in different spots on the desktop. Most people prefer their objects to be found in a consistent place on the desktop so that they do not need to spend time looking for them.

To align icons in a grid so they are evenly spaced:

1. Right-click a **blank area** of the desktop.
2. From the shortcut menu, select the **View, Align to Grid** option (Figure 3-11).

The objects (icons) will now be in the general area where you moved them, but will appear in a straight column or row. Underlying the screen is an invisible checkerboard. When you issue the command Align to Grid, the icons are snapped into the closest square to produce straight rows and columns. If the objects (icons) snap back into place when they should be moveable, right-click a **blank area** of the desktop, select **Arrange Icons By**, and click **Auto Arrange** to remove the check mark for that selection. (See Figure 3-11.) The check mark causes the icons to snap back into place.

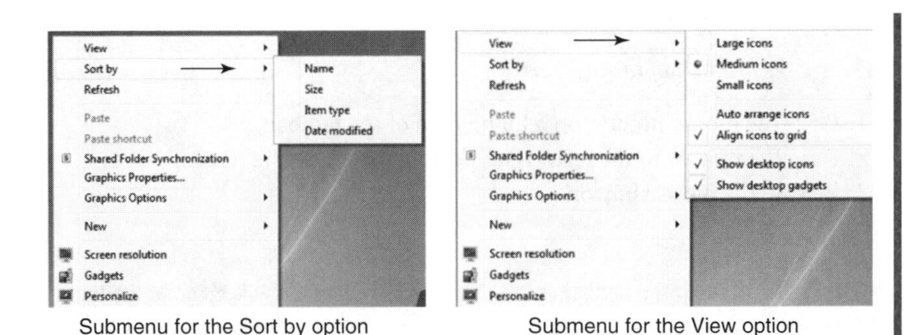

Figure 3-11 Arrangement of Icon Options

Choosing a Screen Saver

Screen savers are moving or static pictures displayed on the desktop when no activity takes place for a specified time. Screen savers were designed to protect the monitor from having images burned into it. Today, adding decoration seems to be their primary use in the home. In a healthcare setting screen savers have the added functionality of providing privacy. Many screen savers come with the operating system; others may be found on the Internet or in computer software stores. In addition, many people use a personal photo to create a screen saver. Make sure you pay attention to security issues when downloading anything from the Internet.

To set up a screen saver:

1. Right-click a **blank area** of the desktop.
2. Choose **Personalize** from the shortcut menu.
3. Click the **Screen Saver** option.
4. Click the **Screen Saver** down arrow, and select a **screen saver image**.
5. Set the **amount of time** to wait before activating the screen saver.
6. Click **Apply** and **OK**. See **Figure 3-12** for the **Screen Saver Settings** dialog box.

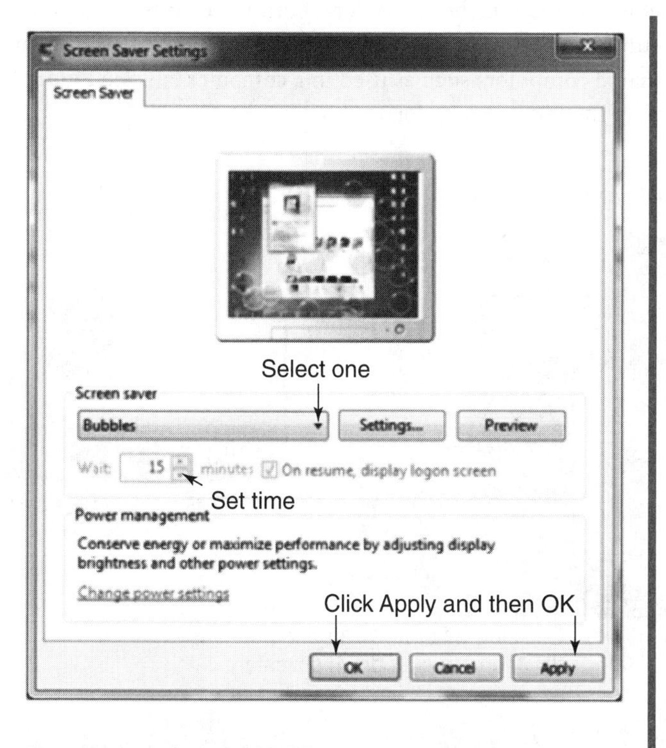

Figure 3-12 Screen Saver Settings Dialog Box

Working with Gadgets

Gadgets are small programs that run on the Windows desktop. They permit you to view information at a glance or to access frequently used tools.

To add a gadget:

1. Right-click a **blank area** of the desktop and select **Gadget** from the menu.
2. Double-click the **gadget** or right-click the gadget and click **Add**.

To use a gadget:

This depends on the gadget. For example, to use the currency gadget, you would select the currency you want to convert (US dollars) and the currency to which you want to convert it (Australian dollars), and accept the $1 or type in an amount.

To close a gadget:

Click the **Close** button (**X**) on the top right of the gadget.

Shutting Down the System

When you finish working with the computer, it is important to shut down the system before turning off the computer. Shutting down the computer saves the current settings and prevents the corruption of files. These directions are for networked, shared computers such as used in a computer lab. See **Figure 3-13** for a screen shot of the shutdown options.

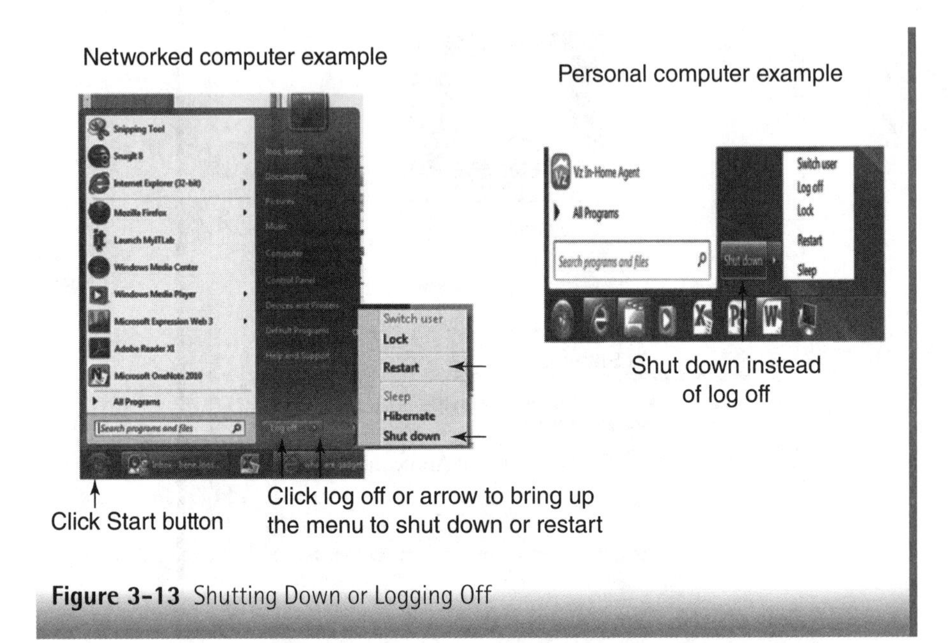

Figure 3-13 Shutting Down or Logging Off

To shut down the system and save your session:

1. Click the **Start** button on the taskbar.
2. Click the **arrow** to the right of the Log off button .
3. Select **Shut down** the system.

To log off and prepare the computer for another user:

1. Click the **Start** button on the taskbar.
2. Select the **Log off** option.

Most of the time, the appropriate option will be either Log off or Shut down. In most computer laboratories, the user logs off and does not turn off the computer. The computer saves all of the current user settings, closes all programs, and then prepares to receive another user. The computer remains turned on, and a login window appears with instructions (press **Ctrl+Alt+Del**) to log in. When the next user presses **Ctrl+Alt+Del**, the login screen appears. The user types their user ID and password. Some work environments ask you to log off but not to shut down the computer. They sometimes run updates during the night and if the computer is off, the updates do not run on that computer. At home, it is probably best to shut the computer down when not in use for a long time.

If more than one user account exists on a computer, you can switch between users using Fast User Switching. Both users' accounts remain open. Here you would select the Start button, click the arrow to the right of **Shut down**, and select **Switch User**. You can now switch between users by pressing **Ctrl+Alt+Delete**, and selecting the correct user. Save any open files because if another user shuts down the computer, you will lose your work.

The options you see on your computer may vary depending on how your system was configured. For example, in the network example in Figure 3-13 Switch User is disabled. Here are some additional options that may or may not be available.

- Hibernate or Sleep puts the computer into a low-power state, but will let the user quickly resume working. With this option, the computer looks like it is turned off, but the power lights remain on. To restart the computer, press the power button quickly on the computer or, in some laboratories, press the spacebar key. For some laptops, pressing the power button will wake up the computer if it is hibernating or in sleep mode.
- Lock prevents others from using the computer unless the user types the correct password.
- The Restart option restarts the computer. Use it primarily for updating or installing new programs.

Managing Windows

This section describes the layout of most application windows and the process of controlling the windows and changing the windows display options. Applications, files, and folders appear in a window, and each window shares similar attributes. To be able to work in the Windows world efficiently, users need to be able to manage the windows.

Common Windows Layout

Title Bar

Present in most windows, this horizontal bar is at the top of the window. The **title bar** contains the file or folder name and the program name. It may also include a path to a file or homepage in a browser window. In Office 2010, one can also pin commands to the Quick Access Toolbar on the left of the title bar. On the far right of the title bar are the window control buttons that minimize, maximize, and close the window. Some programs may also include a search box on the far right of the title bar. Use the title bar to move (drag) the window to another location on the desktop.

Tabs

In some newer versions of software like browsers and MS Office 2010, **tabs** are used instead of menu bars. They are part of the ribbon in Office 2010. They function just like menu bars by giving the user access to commands. Tabs will be described fully in later chapters.

Menu Bar

If the window has a **menu bar**, it contains names of available commands. (See **Figure 3-14**.) Use the menu or horizontal bar with words on it to obtain additional drop-down options. For example, clicking File brings up such choices as New, Open, Create shortcut, Delete, Rename, Properties, and Close, depending on the open program. Any command not available at this time appears dimmed.

To display the menu bar if it is not showing:

1. Right-click the **toolbar**, click **Menu bar** box to place an X there.
2. Alternatively, you can select **Tools** option down arrow on the toolbar, click **Toolbars**, and then click to place an **X** next to menu bar.

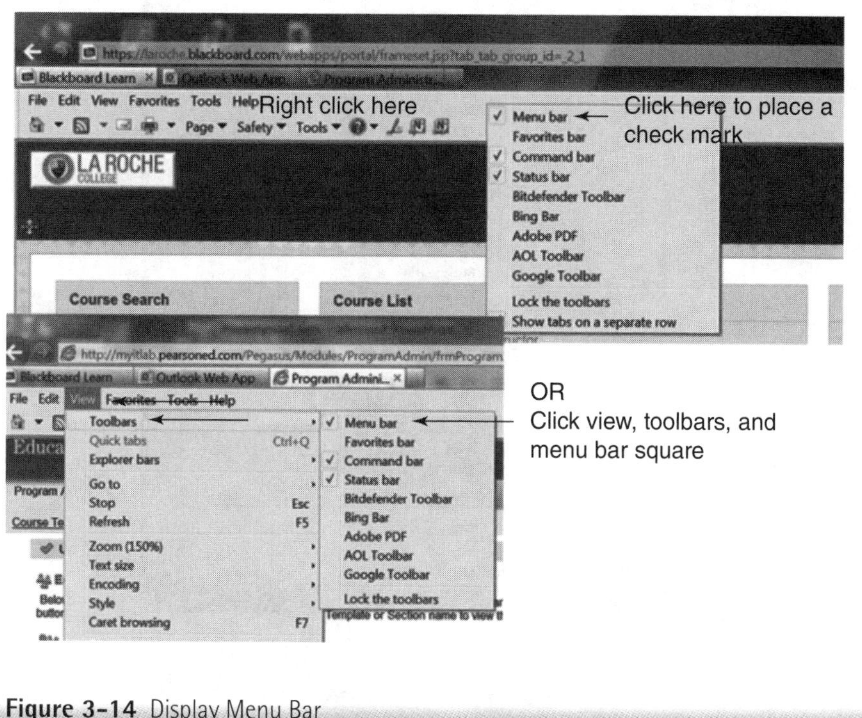

Figure 3-14 Display Menu Bar

If an option on a menu has three periods after it (ellipsis), a **dialog box** appears. A dialog box is a window that requests additional information from the user before it can implement the command. For example, in **Figure 3-15** the **Choose Details and Customize This Folder** commands bring up a dialog box. **Complete the information** as appropriate in the dialog box or accept the defaults. Click **OK** to execute the command.

If an option has a right arrow, another menu appears. In Figure 3-15, the commands Toolbars, Explorer Bar, Sort By, and so forth all open another menu. This additional menu is sometimes called a nested menu or a submenu.

Ribbons

In Office 2010, the ribbon is the control center for the application. It consists of Tabs, Groups, and Commands.

Toolbars

Some windows display one or more toolbars. The standard toolbar provides access to commonly used

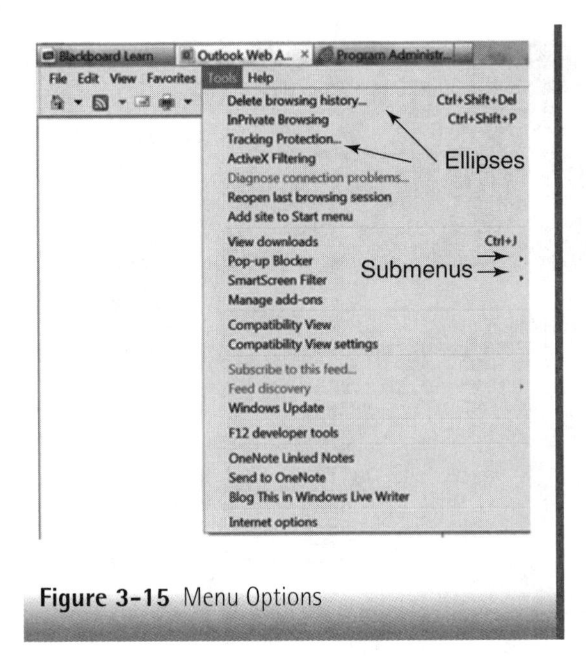

Figure 3-15 Menu Options

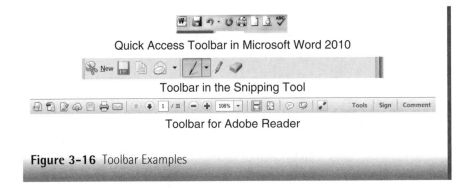

Figure 3-16 Toolbar Examples

commands such as Save, New, or Copy. depending on the application (see **Figure 3-16** for examples of toolbars). Additional or different commands may appear in some applications because of the nature of particular programs. For example, the Snipping Tool toolbar contains New, Save, Copy, Send, Pen, Highlighter, and Eraser on the toolbar.

If there is a second toolbar, it generally relates to specialty functions like formatting, ruler, and draw. The second toolbar provides quick access to commands associated with that task. Windows also gives the user the ability to display additional toolbars as necessary.

Status Bar

Some applications use a horizontal bar at the bottom of the window to display such things as the number of objects in the window, a description of menu commands, the number of pages in a document, the location of the cursor, and special **toggle** switches such as overwrite, num lock, and caps lock. Contents of the **status bar** depend on what is important in the application. For example, in Excel it displays the Cell Mode indicator, the View shortcut, the Zoom, and the Zoom slider, while in Word it indicates the current page number, the total number of pages, and the word count as well as the View shortcut, the Zoom, and the Zoom slider. By right-clicking the status bar, the Customize Status Bar menu appears. The check marks on this menu show the current features that are on and provide an opportunity to turn on other features of the status bar.

Scroll Bars

Located along the right and bottom of the window are the vertical and horizontal **scroll bars**. They appear when there is more data than can be displayed in the window. There are arrows at the top and bottom of the vertical scroll bar on the right and at the left and right for the horizontal scroll bar on the bottom, with a box somewhere between them. Clicking the arrow buttons moves the user slowly through the window. The box or elevator in the scroll shaft indicates the current location relative to the total document. Dragging the elevator in the scroll bar gives more control over viewing the contents of the window. You may also click on the elevator shaft to go to an approximate location in the document.

At the bottom of the vertical scroll bar are up and down chevrons 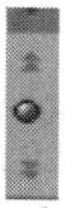 and a Select Browse Object button (a round circle). By default, the down chevron moves through the document one page at a time while the up chevron displays the previous page. The default can be changed by selecting the round circle and choosing a new option.

Opening a Window

You can open a window or program in several different ways:

- Double-click the **icon** representing the window.
- Right-click the **icon** representing the window to be opened, and select **Open** from the menu.

Once the window is open, the user can perform the appropriate tasks. Because more than one window may be opened at a time, the user will need to control the window display.

Jump Lists

Jump lists are shortcuts to files and commands that one uses frequently. These items change in accordance with what the user does. See **Figure 3-17** for some examples of jump lists. An item may also be pinned to the Jump List or removed from it.

To view a jump list:

- Right-click an **icon** on the taskbar or
- Click the **list arrow** to the right of a program icon on the Start menu.

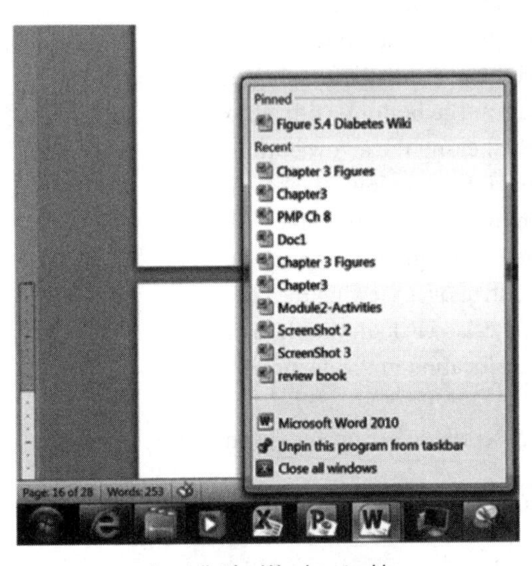

Jump list for Word on taskbar

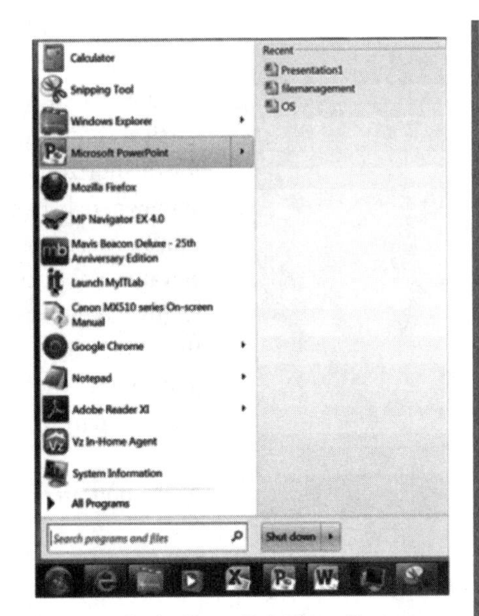

Jump list for PowerPoint from Start menu

Figure 3-17 Examples of Jump Lists

Controlling the Window Size and Placement

Several controls are available for working with windows. Use these controls to move a window to another location on the desktop, change the size of a window, or close a window. The resize features permit the user to control the actual size of the window. The Maximize and Minimize buttons use default standards to control the size of the window. Clicking the **Maximize button** expands the window to fill the screen. Clicking the **Minimize button** places a button for the application on the taskbar and removes the window from the desktop; with this option, the program remains open, but runs in the background. Clicking the **Restore button** returns the window to the size it was before it was maximized.

These buttons are helpful for controlling windows when the user is running multiple programs, opening multiple windows, or opening several files. They permit the user to view or work in each window while placing the others in the background.

In addition, the user may arrange windows on the desktop in cascade, stacked, or side-by-side style or use the new **Aero peek**. When many windows are open, the cascade option works well if it is necessary to see the open windows. With this option, open windows will cascade from the top of the screen down, with the title bar of each open window visible to the user. Use the **stacked and side-by-side** arrangements to partition the screen into quadrants depending on the number of open windows. These options are useful when the user wants to drag and drop data from one window to another. See **Figure 3-18** for examples of cascade and Aero 3D styles and **Table 3-1** for specific functions and directions.

Managing Folders and Files

This section deals with the management of files and folders. The file system is a key element for working efficiently and effectively with a computer. Consequently, knowing how to find, access, and manage files is important to managing the computer system as a whole. Use Computer to access files and folder options and to see all the folders and subfolders (which indicate the structure of the storage devices). **Figure 3-19** shows the Computer window without the folder option expanded on the left and with the folder option expanded on the right.

This section first introduces some basic file and folder management concepts. The specifics of creating, renaming, moving, copying, and deleting files and folders then follow.

Designating Default Disk Drives

The default drive is the drive that the program uses to find and save files unless told otherwise. Recall that the drive letter designation for the hard drive is generally C, and sometimes D; for a USB device and DVD or CD-ROMs, the default

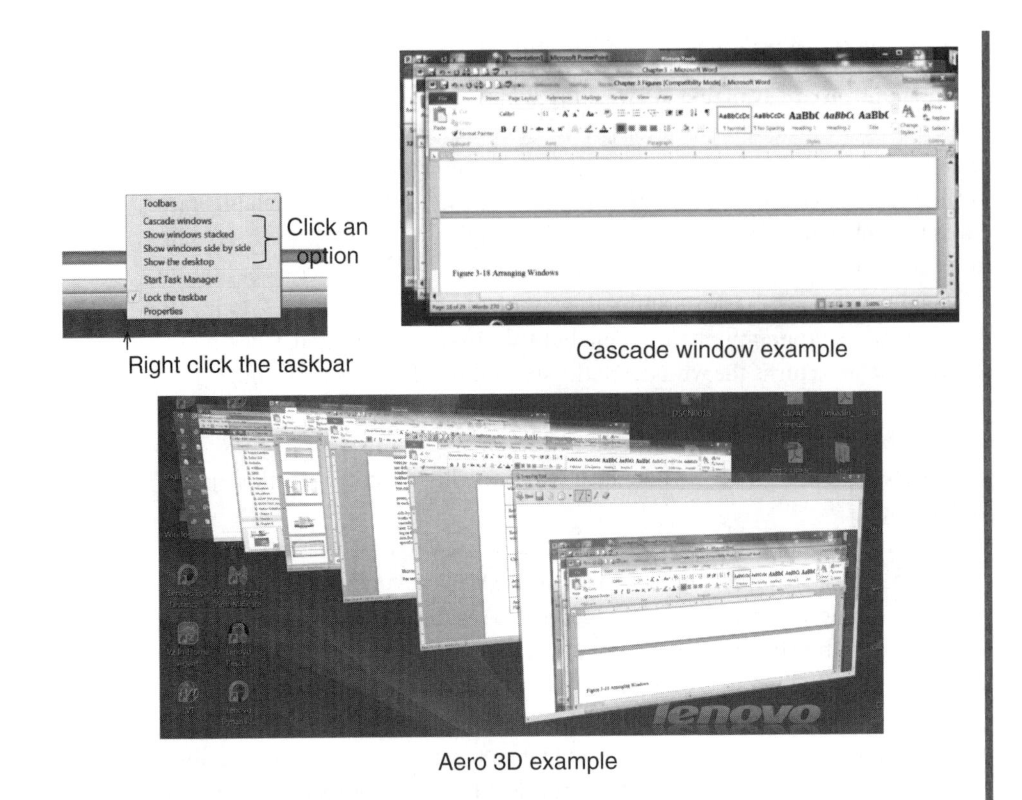

Figure 3-18 Arranging Windows – Cascade and Aero 3D Examples

letters are D, E, F, G, and so forth. Most programs use a default folder on the C drive to store newly created files. For example, Microsoft Office stores all Microsoft Office files in the Documents folder on the C drive under the user's account.

All programs provide the ability to change the default storage drive and folder. To do so, find the Preferences or Options command. This command is accessed from the File tab, Options icon, and Save command in Microsoft Office 2010; in other programs, this command may be located in the Tools menu or the Edit menu.

If you are not permitted to alter these settings (e.g., if you are working in a computer laboratory or restrictive work environment), use the File tab followed by the Save As command to change the location of files each time you access

TABLE 1-1 CONTROLLING WINDOW SIZE AND PLACEMENT

Function	Directions (make sure you have several open windows)
Move a window	Click a **blank area** in the title bar of the window to be moved. Hold down the mouse button while dragging the window to a **new location**, and then release the **mouse button**.
Resize a window	Select the window to resize by clicking its **title bar**. Point to a window **border** or **corner**. When the cursor becomes a double-headed arrow drag the **corner** or **border** until it is the desired size. Release the **mouse button**.
Enlarge a window	Select the window to enlarge by clicking its **title bar**. Click the **Maximize** button in the upper-right corner of the title bar. This button is a toggle switch and shares space with the Restore button.
Reduce a window	Select the window to reduce by clicking its **title bar**. Click the **Minimize** button in the upper-right corner of the title bar.
Restore a window	Select the window to restore by clicking its **title bar**. Click the **Restore** button in the upper-right corner of the title bar. This button is a toggle switch and shares space with the Maximize button.
Close a window	Select the window to close by clicking its **title bar**. Click the **Close** button in the upper-right corner of the title bar.
Arrange a window	Right-click a blank area of the **taskbar**. Select the arrange option: **Cascade**, **Stacked**, or **Side-by-Side**.
Aero Peek–Flip 3D	Hold down the **Windows key** and press the **tab** key to scroll through the open windows.

the program. In Office 2010 in the Save As dialog box, select the correct storage device or computer in the Navigation Pane.

Organizing Folders

Most users store files on removable storage media (USB storage devices or CDs and DVDs), on hard drives, on network file servers, or in the cloud. You must organize your files into folders to make it easier to locate and retrieve them. Organizing electronic files is analogous to the organization of filing cabinets. Electronic files are organized on the storage media in folders and subfolders.

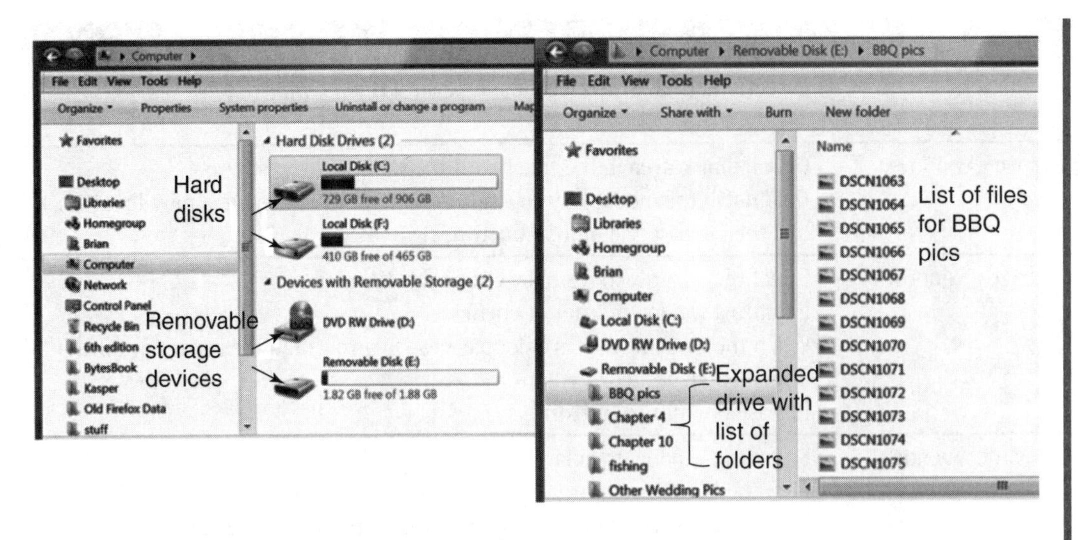

Figure 3-19 Computer Window without Folder Expanded and with Folder Expanded

Root Level — The "root" is the top level on which the folders reside. This level stores files the computer needs to access at start-up. A general rule is that a folder or file listing of the **root level** should not occupy more than one screen's worth of information.

Folders — Use **folders** to organize programs and data files. Before creating them, think about the nature of the work and the programs it requires. Most software programs automatically make a directory for their program files during the installation process. Be careful to ensure that these directories "fit" the organizational structure of the work world. Customize them during installation if necessary. A main folder might be the name of the project; in your case the name of your school.

Subfolders — **Subfolders** are contained within other folders. They provide further division or structure to the organization of files. Staying with the previous example, you may create subfolders for each semester and subfolders within them for each course.

Some rules/tips for creating and using the folder and subfolder structure are summarized here:

1. Select your organizational scheme carefully, keeping in mind the nature of how you work. At work you may not have a choice when working on project teams, but you may provide some suggestions.
2. Place each application suite in its own folder, with subfolders holding each application program. This structure makes installation of new versions, deletions of old versions, and maintenance of files easier and is done by default with some installations. Some suites also create subfolders for shared suite files and create the necessary structure automatically during the software installation process.
3. Place programs that don't belong to application suites in the Program Files folder in their own subfolder, with an appropriate name representing the application. For example, Adobe Acrobat Reader should have its own subfolder. Some users create a folder called Downloads and then create subfolders within it for each downloaded program. This is not the same as the downloads folder that is part of the Windows system. These subfolders are then backed up and used whenever needed. Other users also create a Utility folder off the root, and then place each utility program in its own subfolder within the Utility folder. For example, Norton AntiVirus, Norton Utilities, and WinZip would each have a subfolder in the Utility folder.
4. Create folders for storing data files. Never store data files on the root; this structure means that they will get mixed up with essential computer files. Instead, create a Data folder off the root. This will make it easy to back up your files. In the Data folder, create subfolders for each user on the system. Let each user then create the appropriate subfolders in his or her Data folder. While the hard drive contains Documents, Pictures, Music, and Games folders under a user account, most people prefer to create their own structure. On a networked computer, these folders are automatically created under the user's name. Computer labs or public spaces may enforce a different scheme.
5. Create a Graphic Library folder off the root or in the Data folder for storing graphic images. The Graphic Library folder could contain subfolders representing graphic file formats or categories. For example, you might create subfolders to hold JPEG and GIF graphic files or subfolders called Pets, Cities, and Computers. Some users also create a subfolder to hold photographs to facilitate the exchange of pictures with family and friends.
6. Use appropriate folder names. No two folders in the same level can have the same name, but subfolders within different folders can have the same name.

It is probably better not to name any folder on the computer with the same name as another folder. When folders have the same name it is very easy to forget which folder you are working in and to edit or delete the wrong file.

7. Watch out for long filenames. When using folders and subfolders, file names can become shorter.
8. Maintain the same structure on all your computers.

These are just a few tips; your work world may require all work to be stored on a file server on the network. Remember that files stored on the local hard drive may not be routinely backed up by the IT department. Others on the team will also not have access to files on the local hard drive.

Creating Folders

Users can organize and manage their files by creating folders and then saving their work in those folders. The best folder organization depends on what you want to do. For example, one folder might contain all files related to a specific course, another folder might contain personal items, and yet another folder might contain articles or publications. Storing files in the appropriate folders allows for easy retrieval and back up of data. Associating files with projects or tasks allows for easier cleanup upon completion of projects or tasks. By comparison, saving all files in Documents folders makes retrieving and deleting more difficult and time-consuming.

To create the folder:

1. Point to a **blank area** of the desktop or the open storage device window.
2. Click the **right mouse button**. A shortcut menu appears.
3. Click the menu item **New**. Another shortcut menu appears.
4. Click the menu item **Folder**. A new folder appears on the desktop or in the storage device window. The folder name is highlighted.
5. Type a **name** for the folder and press **Enter**. The folder now has the new name.

NOTE: When a storage device is displayed in the Computer or Documents window, you can create a new folder by clicking the **New Folder** New folder button on the toolbar and typing the name of the folder. When the menu option is present, select **File, New, Folder** from the menu. In addition, some applications include the New Folder button on a toolbar in the Save As dialog box. Use this same process to place folders within folders (subfolders) and further organize your work.

Naming Folders and Files

All folders and files have names. Generally, folder names reflect the essence of the files to be stored in them. For example, the project name mHealth. In the mHealth folder might be subfolders titled Policies, Minutes, References, Plan, and so forth. Folders do not take on a delimiter or extension.

There are three parts to the file nomenclature: the file name, a delimiter, and a file extension. For example, in "My Smiley Face.jpg," the file name is "My Smiley Face," the delimiter is a dot (period), and the file extension is "jpg."

File Name — In the preceding example, the portion to the left of the period ("My Smiley Face") is the file name. File names may include letters, numbers, or certain special characters, up to a maximum of 255 characters. Legal characters are letters of the alphabet (A–Z), digits (0–9), and all of the special characters except these: *, ?, < , >, \, /, ", :, and |. Although Windows permits the use of blank spaces between the characters of the file name to make the file name more readable and understandable, use blanks with caution: Some programs cannot handle file names with spaces or names longer than eight characters. File names are not case sensitive. You may type them in all lowercase, a combination of uppercase and lowercase, or all uppercase. Use a unique file name for each file; there can be no duplicate file names in the same folder.

Delimiter — The delimiter is the period that separates the file name from the extension. Its inclusion is optional; users do not need to use the delimiter unless they are typing an extension to the file name.

Extension — The portion of the file identifier found to the right of the delimiter is the extension. Extensions indicate the nature of the file and its associated application. For example, "docx" is the extension attached to files created with Word 2010. In most cases, the default option in the Windows environment is to hide the extensions. Therefore, the user does not need to type either the extension or the delimiter; instead, the application that creates the file assigns the extension by default. In this environment, Windows uses the extension to identify which application created the file. When the file name is double-clicked, the file opens inside the appropriate application. Users can use the extension to determine which application was used to create a specific file.

Before working with files, think about standards that you should apply when naming them for personal work, for a clinical area, or for a department. File names can be structured in many ways depending on the nature of the work, who does it, what users are sharing, how they are sharing it (on a network or hard drives), how they access it, and who retrieves it. The important point here is to use an understandable convention that will enable users to readily recognize what information the file holds over time—say, after 6 to 12 months have passed. In additon be sure you know and use any naming protocols required by your professor and never expect that the naming protocols will be consistent across professors

To name files, follow the directions given in **Table 3-2**. Folders are given names when they are created as noted in the previous section.

Viewing Folders and Files

Once the user creates and names the files and folders, the user will need to access them. In Windows, users view files and folders through the Computer window.

TABLE 3-2 NAMING FILES

Function	Directions
Name file (application)	Start an application such as Word or Excel. Create the **file**. Click the **File** tab or **File** command from a menu bar; **click Save** or click the **Diskette** icon on the Quick Access toolbar. Select a **location** from the Navigation Pane on the top or left or from the **Save in** text box. Type the **file name** in the File name text box. Click **Save**, **OK** or press **Enter** on the keyboard. You can also use the **Save as** command to give a file another name (For example, EthicsinNursing-draft or EthicsinNursing-draft2).
Name file (on desktop)	Right-click a **blank area** of the desktop or in a window. Select **New**. Select the **Type of file** (e.g., Word, Excel). Type the **file name.** Press **Enter**.

Double-clicking the Computer icon opens a window that displays the storage devices and folders stored on this computer (Figure 3-19). If the icon does not appear on the desktop, click the **Start** button, **Computer** option. The screen then divides into the left pane showing the organizational structure of each storage device. The default is to collapse the folders. A click on an object on the left changes the view of the main pane. The top pane shows the bread crumb (term used to show the path to the files) and one can use it to move up and down the folder structure. The main pane shows the storage device and when double-clicked files and folders display. Repeat the double-clicking action to display the correct file or folder.

The display of the icons in the window depends on the selected view. (See **Figure 3-20**.) There are multiple options for displaying icons in a window: extra-large, large, medium, small, tiles, list, details, and content. The view used is a matter of personal preference. Use the list and small icons options to see more of the information on the storage device; use the details view to see information about the size and type of file; and use the large, medium, and extra-large icons to see a thumbnail of the document.

To use Computer follow these directions:

1. Double-click the **Computer** icon on the desktop or click, **Start**, **Computer**.
2. Double-click the **storage device** where the file is located.
3. Double-click the **desired file** or double-click the **folders** until the correct file appears.
4. Double-click the **file**.

To change how files and folders look in the window:

1. Select the **View down arrow** from the toolbar bar.
2. Click the **desired view**.

You may also use the slider on the left side of the menu to change views. Clicking the View button will rotate the display through the view options. Which view you choose is a personal preference, although some views are better for specific tasks. For example, the detail view is better when you are looking for details about files or folders, such as date modified and size. The list view is best for seeing many files at one time without having to scroll through them.

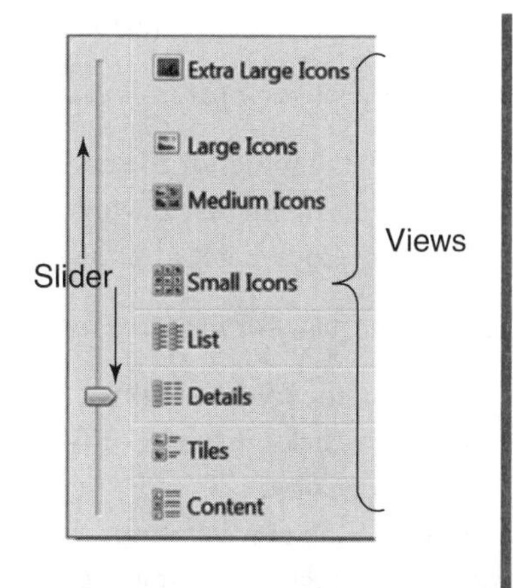

Figure 3-20 Computer Window Views

Copying Folders and Files

The Copy command copies one, several, or all of the folders or files from one place to another. That means there will be two copies of each folder or file. There are several ways to copy files and folders: menu systems, drag and drop, or the shortcut menu. The process for copying files and folders is the same. When using drag and drop from the F drive to another drive such as C, the default is to copy. When using drag and drop from the F drive to another folder in the F drive, the default is to move. You can override the default option by right-dragging the file. When dropping it in its new location, select Copy from the pop-up menu.

To copy one folder or file using a toolbar or menu bar:

1. Click the **folder** or **file** to be copied.
2. Select **Organize** from the toolbar, **Copy** from the menu, or **Edit, Copy** from the menu bar.
3. Navigate to the **new location** and click **there**.
4. Select **Organize, Paste** from the toolbar or **Edit, Paste** from the menu bar.

To copy one folder or file from one device to another device using drag and drop:

This works only when the file is being copied from one storage device to a different one.

1. Both the folder or file and the destination must be visible. Use what you learned about arranging windows.
2. Select the **folder** or **file**.
3. Drag it to its **new location**.
4. Release the **mouse button**.

To copy one folder or file from one folder to another folder on the same device:

1. Click the **folder** or **file** and then right-drag it to its **additional location**.
2. Release the **mouse button**.
3. Select **Copy** here from the shortcut menu.

To copy one folder or file using the shortcut menu:

1. Select the **folder** or **file**.
2. Right-click the **folder** or **file**.
3. Select **Copy**.
4. Go to the **new location**.
5. Right-click in the **new location**.
6. Select **Paste**.

To copy adjacent files:

1. Click the **first file** in the group.
2. Hold down the **Shift** key.
3. Click the **last file** in the group.
4. Release the **Shift** key.
5. Follow any of the first three sets of directions when all files to be copied have been selected.

NOTE: List view works best for implementing this technique.

To copy nonadjacent files:

1. Hold down the **Ctrl** key.
2. Click **each file** to be copied.
3. Release the **Ctrl** key.
4. Follow any of the first three sets of directions once all files to be copied have been selected.

NOTE: An alternative method for selecting multiple folders or files is to draw a box around them. To do so, go to the upper-left corner of the group of folders or files. Hold down the left mouse button. Drag the mouse to the opposite corner, and release the mouse button. Once the folders or files are highlighted, follow any of the first three sets of directions to copy them.

Moving Folders and Files

Moving files and folders is similar to copying files and folders. The Move command takes a file or folder from one place and puts it in another; it does not duplicate the file in the process. There are several ways to move files and folders: use menu systems, use drag and drop, or use the shortcut menu. When moving a file from one storage device to another storage device, use the right-drag option and select Move from the pop-up menu. Remember that the default for dragging and dropping a file between different storage devices is to copy the file. When moving a file from one place on the same storage drive to another place on the same storage drive, the default is to move the file.

To move one file using the toolbar or menu bar:

1. Select **Organize** from the toolbar, **Cut** from the menu that appears, or **Edit**, **Cut** from the menu bar.

2. Go to the **new location** and click **there**.
3. Select **Organize** from toolbar, **Paste** from the menu, or **Edit**, **Paste** from the menu bar.

To move one file using drag and drop:

1. Select the **file**.
2. Drag the file to its **new location**.
3. Release the **mouse button**.

NOTE: This method works only when the file is going from one folder on a storage device to a different one on the same storage device. Both the file and the destination must be visible.

If the file is to be moved from one storage device to another storage device, follow these directions.

1. Right-drag the **file** to its **new location**.
2. Release the **mouse button**.
3. Select **Move here** from the shortcut menu.

To move one file using the shortcut menu:

1. Select the **file.**
2. Right-click the **file.**
3. Select **Cut.**
4. Go to the **new location.**
5. Right-click in the **new location.**
6. Click **Paste**.

To move adjacent files:

1. Click the **first file** in the group.
2. Hold down the **Shift** key.
3. Click the **last file** in the group.
4. Release the **Shift** key.
5. Follow any of the first three sets of directions once all files to be moved have been selected.

To move nonadjacent files:

1. Hold down the **Ctrl** key.
2. Click each **file** to be moved.

3. Release the **Ctrl** key.
4. Follow any of the first three sets of directions once all files to be moved have been selected.

Deleting Folders and Files

The **Delete command** removes folders and files from the storage device. Use this command to clean storage devices and discard unneeded folders or files. Several versions of this command are available, as noted in this section.

When you delete files from a removable storage device such as a USB storage device, the system does not move them temporarily to the Recycle Bin but instead deletes them immediately. It only moves files temporarily to the Recycle Bin when you delete them from the hard drive. Thus, if a user accidentally deletes files from the hard drive, you may recover those files if you did not empty the Recycle Bin. Deleted folders appear as empty folders in the Recycle Bin but actually still contain the old files. Thus, when a user restores a folder from the Recycle Bin, it restores all of the original files as well.

To delete using the toolbar or menu bar:

1. Select the **file**.
2. Select **Organize** from the toolbar, **Delete** from the menu, or **File**, **Delete** from the menu.
3. Click **Yes** in response to the message "Are you sure you want to permanently delete this file?" or click **Yes** in response to the message "Are you sure you want to move this file to Recycle Bin?"

To delete using drag and drop:

1. Make both the **file** or **folder** and the **Recycle Bin** visible.
2. Drag the **file** or **folder** on top of the **Recycle Bin** icon.
3. When the icon turns greenish-blue, release the **left mouse button**.
4. If deleting the file or folder from a removable storage device, click **Yes** to confirm the deletion.

To delete using the delete key:

1. Click the **file or folder** to highlight it.
2. Press the **Delete** key.
3. Click **Yes** to confirm its deletion or its move to the **Recycle Bin**.

To delete using the shortcut menu:

1. Right-click the **file** or **folder** to be deleted.
2. Select **Delete** from the shortcut menu.
3. Click **Yes** to confirm the file or folder's deletion or move to the **Recycle Bin**.

You may select multiple files and folders, as noted in the earlier discussion of the copy and move operations. Use this same technique to delete multiple files or folders at once.

After files go to the Recycle Bin, you will periodically need to empty the Recycle Bin. How often you should empty it depends on how often you delete files and folders and how many files and folders you delete. Remember that deleted files and folders sitting in the recycle bin take up storage space.

To empty the Recycle Bin:

1. Double-click the **Recycle Bin** icon.
2. Select **Empty Recycle Bin** from the toolbar.
3. Click **Yes** to confirm the emptying of the Recycle Bin.

To restore a deleted file or folder:

1. Double-click the **Recycle Bin** icon.
2. Select the **files** or **folders** to restore (if you want to restore only selected items).
3. Select **Restore** all items from the toolbar.

NOTE: This command is not visible once you empty the recycle bin.

Renaming Folders and Files

The Rename command gives a file or folder a new name. Use this command to reorganize and change the names of files to be consistent with an organizational structure or to clarify the name because you create additional files or folders. You will not be able to rename a file if the file is currently open.

To rename a file or folder using the toolbar or menu bar:

1. Select the **file or folder** to rename.
2. Select **Organize** from the toolbar, **Rename** from the menu, or **File**, **Rename** from the menu bar.
3. Type the **new name** and press **Enter**.

To rename a file or folder using a shortcut menu:

1. Right-click the **file** or **folder** to rename.
2. Click **Rename** on the shortcut menu.
3. Type the **new name** and press **Enter**.

To rename a file or folder using the click-pause-click feature:

1. Click the **file** or **folder name**.

2. Pause, and click **again**.
3. Type the **new name** and press **Enter**.

Disk Management Concepts

This section covers a few disk management concepts that are critical to working with the computer and the operating system.

Copying a USB Storage Device

Once you create and organize your files and folders on your USB device, it is critical to make a copy of the disk. The simplest way to do so is to copy all files and folders on the storage device to another USB storage device, to a CD or DVD, to your network file server space, to your second hard drive or external hard drive, and/or to the cloud. Note here that this guidance applies to your personal data; the rules may be different for confidential data in a hospital setting where removable storage devices may not be allowed. When using cloud storage, follow the directions provided by that service. One advantage of the cloud is that most services have an option to automatically synchronize files between devices. Disadvantages may be that free file storage is limited and there may be potential security/privacy issues.

To copy a USB storage device or external portable hard drive:

1. Double-click the storage **device** in the **Computer** window.
2. Select all **files** and **folders** on the device (Ctrl+A), or select only those files and folders to which changes were made.
3. Either right-click the **selection**, select **Copy**, go to the backup location, and right-click to select **Paste** *or* **drag** the **selection** to the backup location.
4. Repeat Step 3 as needed to back up the files. When backing up files and folders to the same place the second time, you will be prompted to replace the existing files on the backup storage device. Select the **Copy and replace** option.

NOTE: If you are copying files and folders to a new CD/DVD, insert the disc into the writeable drive, select the **Burn files to disc** option, and type a **title** for the disc. The computer will then format the disc to prepare it to receive the files. You can then drag and drop the files onto the CD/DVD window. Use this option when you need to add/delete files regularly. The other option is Mastered, which can be used to burn once and paste many times. Each has its appropriate use. Here is Microsoft's URL for deciding on which format to use when burning files to a CD or DVD player: windows.microsoft.com/en-US/windows7/Which-CD-or-DVD-format-should-I-use.

Backing Up a Disk

Because of the size of hard drives today, most people no longer back them up. However, that practice will eventually cause the user problems because of hardware or software failures. The key question to ask is this: How important are the data? Although you can reinstall applications for the most part, data may be lost forever if a failure occurs and no backup exists. At the very least, users should back up all data files, including documents, images, pictures, and, in some cases, downloaded freeware. Back up anything that you cannot quickly reinstall or re-create. Data stored on the local drive of a networked computer are not routinely backed up when the network is backed up; instead, only data on the file server are backed up during this process.

Specific information about hardware, including storage devices such as tape drives, optical drives, removable hard drives, and the cloud, that people can use for backing up data is covered in Chapter 2. The user needs to seek answers to questions such as the following:

What type of data do I have that I cannot replace easily? How much data can I afford to lose?
What capacity do I need for the backup device?
How often do I need to back up my data?
How reliable is the backup medium?
How easy is it to use? Will it backup automatically?
What will it cost?
How secure is the data? Am I storing it in a different location?
If I use a cloud service, what protections are in place and what can they do with my data?

Ideally, system backup for large operations should be done automatically and on a regular basis. This backup does not include the data found on local hard drives on users' personal computers, however. For this reason, many organizations require users to store critical data on the network file **server** itself so that they routinely back up the data as part of the full system backup. Some organizations do not permit critical data to be saved on removable or local hard drives. Those users who do store some data on the local hard drive can regularly back up the data to their personal space on the file server or copy that data to a removable hard drive, CD/DVD, or USB removable storage device.

For a home computer or a small business, this kind of backup is more difficult to do without a managed network. Solutions to this dilemma might include use of a second hard drive installed internally or use of an external removable hard drive. With this approach, the user must remember to perform regular backups, set the timing for automated backups through the Windows Backup Wizard, or use software such as NovaBACKUP or DT Utilities PC Backup to automate the backup process. Automating the backup process requires that you leave the computer on. This backup is only secure, however, if you store it at a different location from the original. Some experts suggest having a third backup that you regularly place in a safety deposit box or off site in a secured place.

To backup your files in Windows 7:

1. Click the **Start** button.
2. Click **Control Panel**.
3. Click **System and Maintenance** option.
4. Click **Backup and Restore**.
5. If you have never used Windows Backup, click **Set up backup** and follow the Wizard steps. If you have used it before, click **Back up now** and follow the directions.

NOTE: Backed up files need to be restored if you need to access them.

Alternatively you can right-click the **hard drive** in Computer window, select **Properties** from the shortcut menu , click the **Tools** tab, click the **Backup now** button, and follow the directions in the Backup Wizard to set up the backup. Make sure the backup medium has enough space to hold the files.

Another solution is to use an online backup service. Several companies (e.g., myPCBackup.com, JustCloud.com, and Backup Genie) now offer backup services for a small monthly fee. Although this approach might sound like a great solution, it has some drawbacks. Some services discourage users from backing up certain types of files, such as MP3 files (music), and others limit how frequently the backups can occur. Some do not have easy-to-use interfaces. This approach requires a high-speed Internet connection, trust in the security of the servers used for backup, and confidence that the company will not go out of business or not secure your data. Each user must find a solution for backing up critical data that works for him or her.

Creating Shortcuts

Shortcuts can save time when you work in the Windows environment. Instead of forcing you to work with the Computer feature to try to find files, folders, or programs, shortcuts provide access to frequently used items on the desktop. Files, folders, application programs, and storage devices can all have shortcuts. Recall that a shortcut is a pointer to an object; it tells the computer where to find the object but is not the actual object. Double-clicking the shortcut opens the object that the shortcut "points to."

The general rule for using shortcuts is to create them for frequently used objects or as reminders to complete a task. Many people create shortcuts to their data files, the printer, Internet Explorer, and selected applications. Do not create shortcuts to infrequently used items, or your desktop will rapidly become overly cluttered. In some cases it might make more sense to pin the application to the Taskbar or Start menu.

A small curved arrow in the lower-left corner of an icon denotes that the icon is a shortcut. (See Figure 3-2.) Because it is simply a pointer to an actual object, deleting the shortcut deletes just the shortcut, not the actual object to which it is pointing.

To create a shortcut on the desktop:

1. Find the **executable file** to which the shortcut will point. An executable file is one that starts the application. For example, Word's executable file is winword.exe.
2. Right-click the **executable** file.
4. Select **Send to**.
5. Click **Desktop** (create shortcut) option.

In addition, some items on the start menu may have the option to Send to, Desktop (shortcut) by right-clicking the object, clicking **Send to**, and then selecting **Desktop (create shortcut).** For example, the objects Documents, Pictures, Computer, and Network Places located on the right side of the Start button menu can be placed on the desktop using the Send to option. Some people also place shortcuts to frequently used applications on the Quick Launch area of the taskbar to keep their desktop from getting too cluttered.

Managing Files with Disk Cleanup, Error-Checking (Scan Disk), and Defragmenter

Before running any of these programs, use the Disk Cleanup program to remove any unwanted files. This utility is available only for cleaning a hard drive; it is not applicable to removable storage devices except for external removable hard drives. The unwanted files include things such as temporary Internet files and downloaded program files; these files simply take up space and slow down the computer. Empty the Recycle Bin to free up even more disk space. Do this on a weekly basis.

To use the Disk Cleanup program:

1. Right-click the **Hard drive** icon in Computer.
2. Click the **Properties** option.
3. Click the **General** tab.
4. Click the **Disk Cleanup** button.

Alternatively, you can select **Start**, **All Programs**, **Accessories**, **System Tools**, and **Disk Cleanup**. Select just your files or all files on the computer, and then run the program.

Next, use an error-checking tool (Scan Disk) to check the file system for errors and bad sectors. Some technicians recommend using this tool once a week; others recommend using it once a month, and others recommend never unless you are a computer repair person. In reality, many users perform an Error-checking (Scan Disk) diagnostic once or twice a year. Close all programs including any program running in the background before running Error-checking (Scan Disk). For example, your antivirus program runs in the background. If a program is running, Error-checking (Scan Disk) will restart itself over and over. On networked computers, this tool may not be accessible unless the user is logged on as the administrator. **Figure 3-21** shows the Properties, Tools tab, and the Properties General tab. Depending on the size of the storage device, this program may take a while to do its job. Do not use the computer during this time.

To access this Error-checking tool:

1. Close **all files**.
2. Open the **Computer** window.

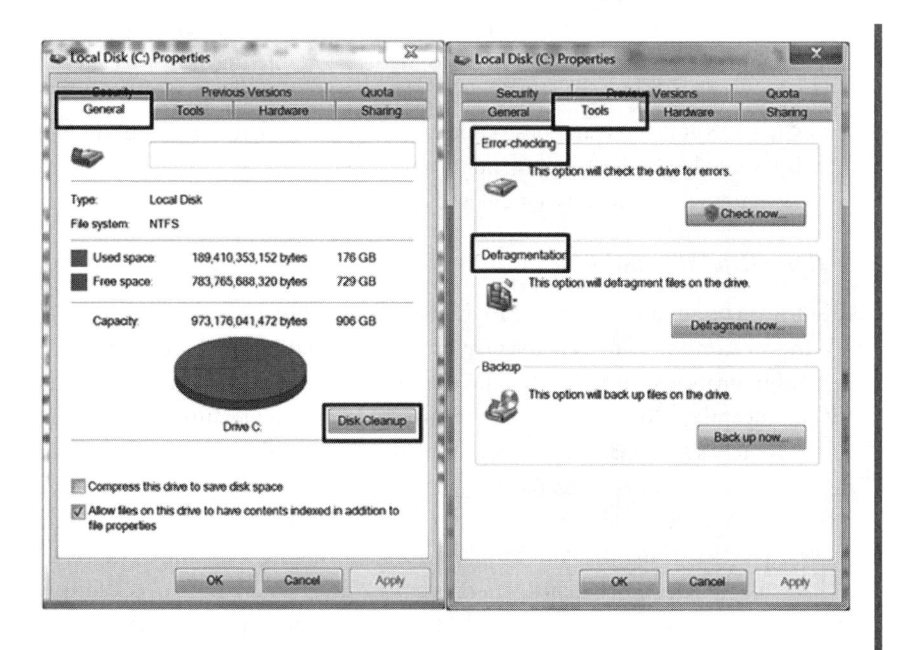

Figure 3-21 Disk Management Tools

3. Right-click the **storage device**.
4. Select **Properties** and the **Tools** tab.
5. Click the **Check now** button in the error-checking part of the screen (see Figure 3-21).
6. Place a check in the **Automatically fix file system errors** and **Scan for and attempt recovery of bad sectors** squares, and then click the **Start** button.

The last file management program discussed here is the Defragmentation utility. This program consolidates fragmented files and folders on the storage device so that each one is stored in a contiguous space. This consolidated structure provides for performance improvements in accessing files and folders. Once again, all programs must be closed before this utility is run, as this program checks and moves data. This tool should be run about two times per month, or more often if a user loads and deletes programs frequently.

To access the Defragmentation utility:

1. Close **all files**.
2. Open **Computer**.
3. Right-click the **storage device**.
4. Select **Properties**, and then select the **Tools** tab.
5. Click the **Defragment Now** button in the Defragmentation part of the screen (see Figure 3-21). A message appears stating either that your file system is fine and does not need to be defragmented now or that it is not okay and needs to be defragmented now.
6. Click **OK** if the system doesn't need attention or click the **Defragment Now** button to begin the defragmentation process.
7. Select the **drives** to defragment and click **OK**.

Applying Updates and Patches

All software programs—whether programs such as Word, operating systems such as Windows, or device drivers for printers, monitor, and other hardware such as the computer itself—involve periodic upgrades or **patches. Updates** are generally enhancements to the software that provide additional features or functions, whereas patches are generally fixes for problems discovered in the software after its original release. Many of these patches focus on fixing security problems inherent in the software that might make the user's computer vulnerable to hackers and viruses. The first thing that you should do after installing a software program is to check for updates and patches. Then, every so often, you need to check for new updates and patches. Some people make these checks once a month, while others check for updates and patches more frequently; others configure the program to check for such items automatically.

In Windows 7, the Start menu contains an option: Windows Update is either on the main menu or under All Programs. Clicking this option takes the user to Microsoft's Web site. Follow the directions for updating the Microsoft programs on the computer. After Microsoft scans the computer, it presents a list of updates or patches. These items are generally divided into Critical Updates, Windows 7 and Driver Updates, and so forth. Some are labeled not critical. Select the desired updates and download them to the computer. The computer must have an active Internet connection to complete this step. Note the size of the files before downloading them; some of them are quite large and may take substantial time to download depending on the time of day and speed of the connection. In addition, a message appears periodically on the right side of the taskbar reminding the user to check for updates. Most users today configure updates to run automatically. Windows Update will also update your Office programs.

To run Windows Update manually:

1. Click the **Start** button.
2. Click **All programs** (unless pinned to the start menu).
3. Click **Windows update**.
4. Click **Check for updates**.

Alternatively, you can go to the **Control Panel**, click **System and Security**, and then click **Windows Update**.

Summary

This chapter oriented you to the operating system and the Windows interface, including the common objects found on the desktop. Desktop management skills include setting screen savers, changing desktop colors, moving objects, and managing windows. File and folder management concepts are also essential knowledge for today's users. They need to know the commands to create, rename, move, copy, and delete files and folders to affect appropriate file and folder management. This chapter also presented some basic ideas about organizing files and folders and introduced a few utilities for managing the software.

Whether the operating system is proprietary, such as Windows, or open source, such Linux, one thing is certain: a user will always need a system for managing the hardware and interacting with the system. That system is not static, however, but will evolve to reflect changes in technology and in user needs.

Reference

Franklin, C. and Doustan, D. (n.d.). *How Operating Systems Work.* Retrieved from http://computer.howstuffworks.com/operating-system3.htm.

Resources

Microsoft's Web sites http://support.microsoft.com/ and http://windows.microsoft.com/en-US/windows7/help/getting-started contain many help guides and tutorials.

Hanson, M. (2011). Beginners guide to Windows 7. *Windows: The Official Magazine*, Issue 53 (March 27, 2011) is available online from TechRadar at www.techradar.com/us/news/software/operating-systems/beginners-guide-to-windows-7-937816

Exercises

EXERCISE 1 How Do I Manage a Desktop and Windows

Objectives

1. Identify and describe the desktop.
2. Apply a screen saver.
3. Add a gadget to the desktop.
4. Arrange the desktop to work efficiently and effectively.
5. Change the colors of the desktop.
6. Open, close, minimize, maximize, size, and arrange windows.
7. Switch between windows.

Activity

If necessary, make sure to turn on the computer and log in. You may also need to turn on the monitor.

1. Look at your desktop and answer these questions, but first press the **Print-Screen** button to capture your desktop. Open **Word** and press **Ctrl+V** to paste the screen shot in the Word document. Place your answers to these questions after the screen shot.
   a. How many icons are on the desktop? Describe what each one does.
   b. How many shortcuts are on the desktop? What do they do? What happens if you delete a shortcut?
   c. How many folders are on the desktop? What is the function of these folders?
   d. How many files are on the desktop? What type of file is each one?
   f. How many gadgets are on the desktop? Which ones?
   g. Is the taskbar displayed by default or is it hidden and shows when you place your cursor over it?
   h. What items are on the taskbar? Right-click an empty space on the taskbar. Is it locked?
2. Apply a screen saver.
   a. Right-click a **blank area** of the desktop.
   b. Choose **Personalize** from the shortcut menu.
   c. Click the **Screen Saver** option on the bottom right of the window.
   d. Click the **screen saver down arrow**, and select **3D Text**.
   e. Set the **amount of time** to wait before activating the screen saver to **20** minutes.
   f. Click **Apply** and then **OK**. **Figure 3-22** shows the screen saver dialog box.

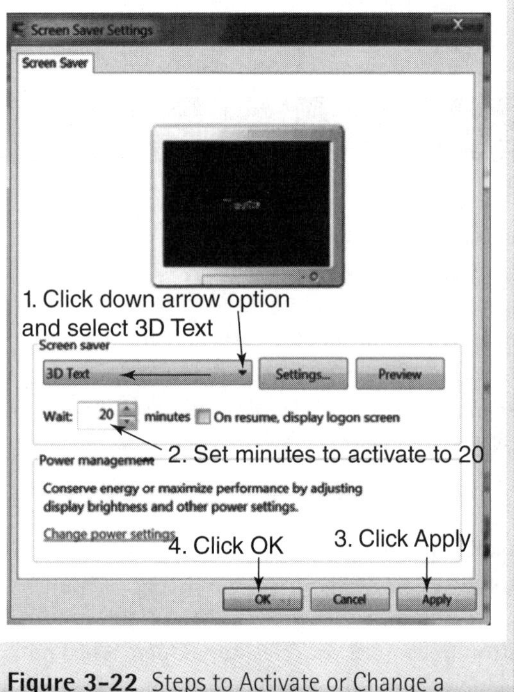

Figure 3-22 Steps to Activate or Change a Screen Saver

3. Add a gadget to the desktop. (See **Figure 3-23**.)
   a. Right-click a **blank area** of the desktop.
   b. Click the **Gadgets** Gadgets icon.
   c. Double-click the **Weather** gadget. It now appears on the desktop.
   d. Click the **Gadget** and then the **Options** button.
   e. Complete the dialog box for your city.

NOTE: Be cautious with using gadgets; there are some malicious ones out there. Use only ones from a trusted source. The Weather gadget is from Microsoft's Web site.

4. Move and arrange objects on the desktop.
   a. Drag the **Weather Gadget** to the top left of the desktop.
   b. Drag the **Recycle Bin** icon to the lower-left side of the desktop.
   c. Right-click a **blank area** of the desktop. Click **Sort by**, and then select **Name**.
   d. What happened to the icons?

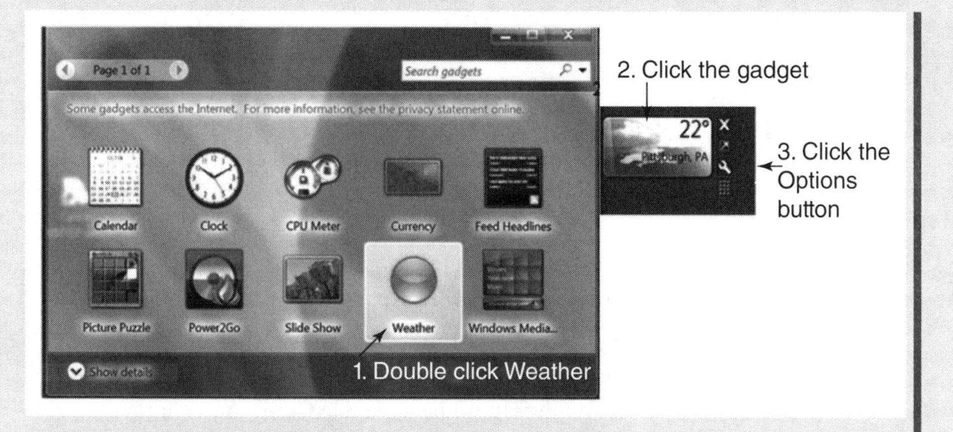

Figure 3-23 Steps to Add a Gadget

e. Drag the **Internet Explorer** icon to the upper-right side of the desktop.
f. Drag the **Weather Gadget** to the upper-right side of the desktop.
g. Right-click a **blank area** of the desktop. Select **View**, **Align icons to grid**.
h. What happened?
i. Drag the **taskbar** to the top of the screen.
j. Rearrange the desktop so the **taskbar** is back on the bottom, the **icons** are in a column on the left going from top to bottom, the **shortcuts** to the second column on the left, the **folders** are in the last column on the right, and **files** are to the left of the folders.

HINT: If the icons snap back into place, right-click a **blank area** of the desktop, select **View**, and then select **Auto arrange icons**. This series of actions removes the check mark next to the Auto arrange feature and permits you to move the icons. If the taskbar doesn't move, right-click the **taskbar** and select **Lock the Taskbar** to remove the check mark.

5. Change the desktop background.
   a. Right-click a **blank area** of the desktop and click **Personalize**.
   b. Click the **Desktop Background** option.
   c. Scroll to **Landscapes** and click a **landscape appropriate** for the season.
   d. Click the **Save Changes button** and then **Close** the window.
   e. To change the setup back to the default colors, repeat Steps a–d and select the **Windows 7** default.

6. Open, browse, and manage windows.
   a. Open the Computer window by double-clicking the **Computer** icon. If this icon is not on the desktop, click the **Start** button and select **Computer** from the menu.
   b. Using the title bar, drag the **Computer** window to the right approximately 3 inches and down from the top 3 inches. If it is set to fill the screen, use the **Restore** button to make it smaller.
   c. Now drag the window towards the top. What happened?
   d. Click the **Restore** button. What happened to the window?
   e. Click the **Minimize** button. What happened?
   f. Click the **Folder** icon on the taskbar.
   g. Place the pointer on the **right border** of the **Computer** window.
   h. With the double-headed arrow, drag the **window border** to the right 2 inches.
   i. Place the pointer on the lower-right corner of the **Computer** window.
   j. Drag the **window border up** and to the **left**, making the window approximately 3 inches square.
   k. Which additional bars appeared?
   l. Why might you need to know how to open and manage windows?
   m. Drag to enlarge the **Computer** window, making it approximately 6 inches square.
   n. Double-click the **Local Hard Drive** icon (usually C). Double-click the **Windows** folder. Notice that the default in Windows is to open each new folder in the same window.
   o. Click the **Back** button until the Computer window is open and the storage devices are showing.
7. Change the default folder option and switch between windows.
   a. In the Computer window, select **Organize** from the toolbar, **Folder and search options** from the menu, or **Tools**, **Folder options**. Alternatively, you can use the menu bar. Click **Tools, Folder Options**. (See **Figure 3-24**.)
   b. Click the **Open each folder in the same window** option under the **Browse** folders section of the dialog box.
   c. Click **Apply** and **OK**. Now each folder will open in its own window.
   d. At the main computer windows, click the **Change Folder Views** button.
   e. Select **Details.** What information appears about the files from this view?

HINT: If the menu bar is not visible, press the **Alt** key to display it.

   f. To try out the new setting, click **Start**, **Control Panel**, and **Appearance and Personalization**.

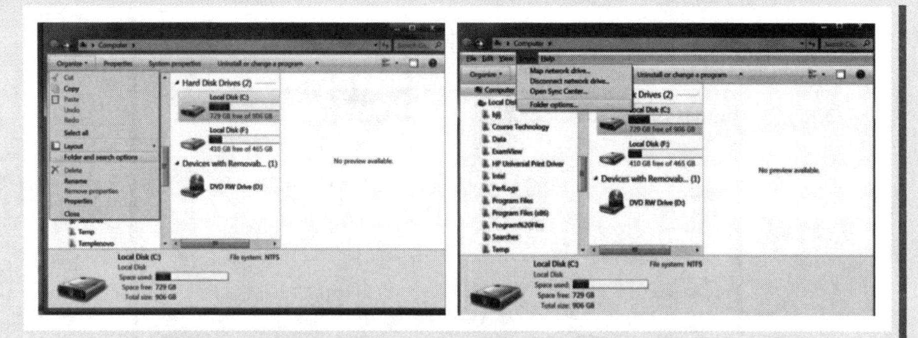

Figure 3-24 Changing Folder Options

g. Click **Display**. Notice how you have multiple windows open.
h. Move the **Computer** window so that the Control Panel window is visible.
i. Click anywhere in the **Control Panel** window.
j. Hold down the **Alt** key and press the **Tab** key. This brings up a window for switching between open applications. Use this feature to toggle between open windows.
k. Press the **Tab** key again while still holding down the **Alt** key.
l. Release the **Tab** and **Alt** keys. What happened?
m. Why might you want to switch between windows?
n. Click the **Close** buttons to close all open windows.

EXERCISE 2 How Do I Manage Folders and Files?

Objectives

1. Create folders and files.
2. Move, copy, and rename folders and files.
3. Delete files and folders.
4. Empty the Recycle Bin.

Activity

In this exercise, the term "USB storage device" refers to the flash drive. You may use any removable storage device for this activity.

1. Create a folder and subfolders on a removable storage device.
   a. Open the **Computer** window.
   b. Double-click the **USB storage device** icon. It should be labeled **Removable Disk** or USB Disk or some other label if you added a label to the drive, plus a letter such as G, H, or I, depending on the configuration of your computer. Alternatively, use your removable hard drive.

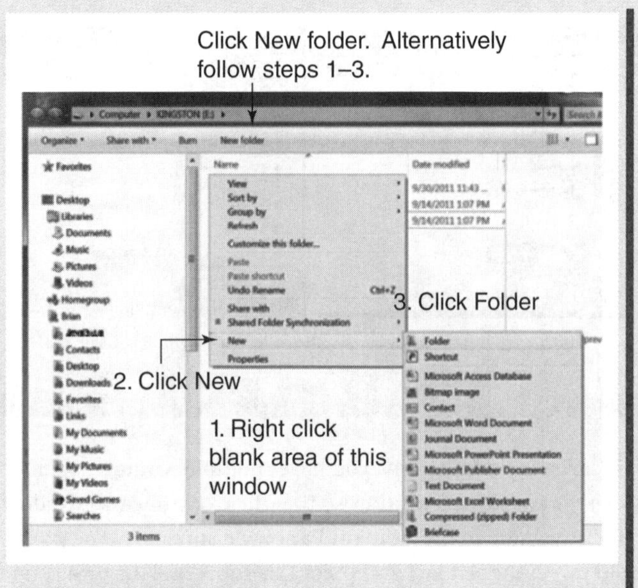

Figure 3-25 Creating a Folder

c. Click the **New Folder** [New folder] option on the toolbar. Alternatively, you may right-click a blank area of the device window, select **New, Folder**.
d. Type your current **Semester-Year** (for example Fall-2014) in the text box that appears and then press **Enter**.
e. Double-click the **Semester-Year** folder.
f. **Repeat the process in the Semester-Year** folder and create the following subfolders: **ENGL101**, **COMP101**, **CHEM111**, **PSYC100**, and **BIOL101**. You may substitute your real courses for these subfolders.
g. If the professor wants to see your work, submit the removable storage device or open the **Computer Class** folder displaying the subfolders, click **Print Screen**, open **Word**, type **your name**, and press **Ctrl+V** to paste the print screen image into the Word document. Print the Word file and submit it. The results should look like **Figure 3-26**.

2. Create files (empty files and files created in a document).
   a. Open the **Semester-Year** folder.
   b. Right-click a **blank area** of the **Semester-Year** folder. Select **New, Excel Worksheet.**
   c. Type **MyBudget2014-2015** and then press **Enter**.

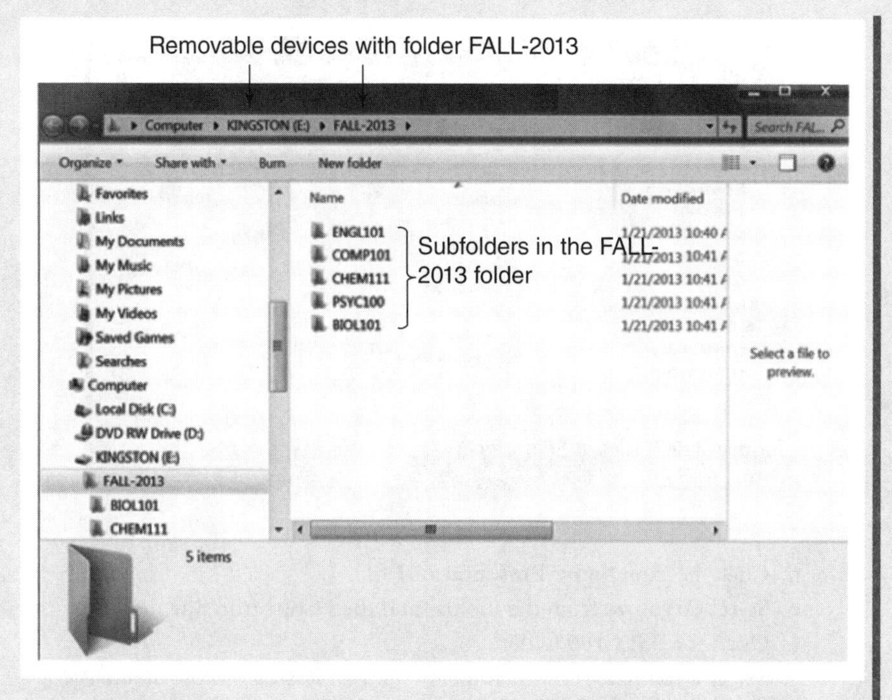

Figure 3-26 Screen Shot of Folder with Subfolders Displaying

d. Create two more files—one **Word document** and one **PowerPoint presentation**. Name them with an appropriate name such as Joos-Assign1 Joos-Presentation1 (Note: Use your name and not mine).

e. Open **WordPad** (Start, All programs, Accessories, and WordPad). Type **Isn't this fun. I never thought of organizing my work in folders.**

f. Click the **WordPad** [icon] icon equivalent to File. Click the **Save** command. In the Save as window, locate and select your **storage device**, double-click the **Semester-Year** folder (the one you named), click in the **file name text box**, type **WordPad-YourLastName**, and click **Save** button.

g. Submit a **print** of your work or your **USB device** as directed by the professor. See **Figure 3-27** for a sample of the work.

3. Copy, move, and rename folders and files.

Copy a file using the clipboard method:

a. Close all **open windows** except the **Computer** window.

b. Double-click your **removable storage** device.

c. Double-click the **Semester-Year** folder created earlier.

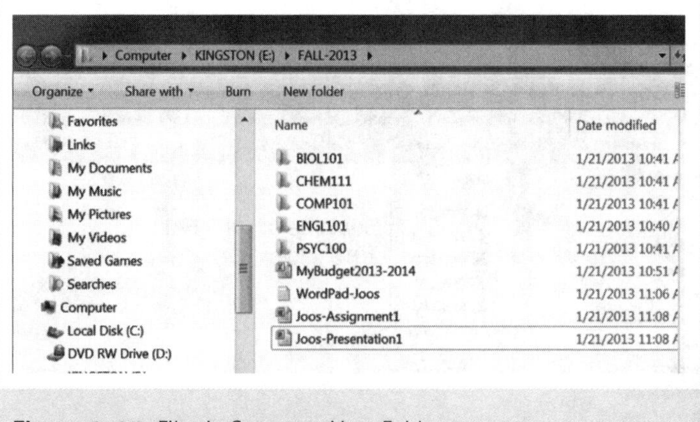

Figure 3-27 Files in Semester-Year Folder

d. Click the **YourName-Presentation1** file.
e. Select **Organize** from the toolbar and then **Copy** from the menu.
f. Open the **PSYC100** folder.
g. Select **Organize** from the toolbar and then **Paste** from the menu. A copy of the YourName-Presentation1 file is now in the Computer Class folder.

Alternately, you can right-click the file, select Copy from the menu, open the folder to which you intend to copy it, and click Paste.

Copy a file using the drag and drop method:

a. Open the **USB storage device** window if necessary.
b. Right-drag the **YourName-Assign1** Word file onto the ENGL101 folder and the **MyBudget2014-2015** file into the COMP101 folder.
c. Select **Copy** here from the shortcut menu. Notice that the YourName-Assign1 now exists in both folders.
d. Why do you need to right-drag the icon when copying from a file in USB storage device to the same USB storage device?

There are two ways to rename files and folders, and each process is the same for both files and folders. The first technique uses the command from the shortcut menu; the second uses the click–pause–click method.

Rename a file using the menu:

a. Right-click the **YourName-Presentation1** file in the SemesterYear folder.
b. Click **Rename.**
c. Type **YourName-Presentation2** and then press **Enter**. The file now has a new name.

Rename a file using the click–pause–click method:

a. Click on the file name **MyBudget2014-2015** in the Semester-Year folder **once**, and then click **again**. The text in the folder icon should be highlighted, but not the icon.
b. Type **MyBudget2015-2016** and then press **Enter**.

For the next task, the Computer window setting must be set to **Show each folder in its own window** (click **Organize, Folder and Search options**; check **Open each folder in its own window**; and click **OK**).

Move a file using the drag and drop method:

a. Drag the **YourName-Presentation2** file on top the PSYC100 folder.
b. What happened? Why?
c. Drag the **MyBudget2015-2016** file into the COMP101 folder. You now decide they don't belong in the COMP101 folder.
e. Create a **Budget** folder in the **SemesterYear** folder.
f. Open the **COMP101** and **Budget** folders. They should look like **Figure 3-28.**
g. Select both **files** in the COMP101 folder and drag to the **Budget** folder.

The default Copy or Move command can be overridden by right-dragging the file or folder and selecting the appropriate command. You can also use the Organize menu and select the correct command.

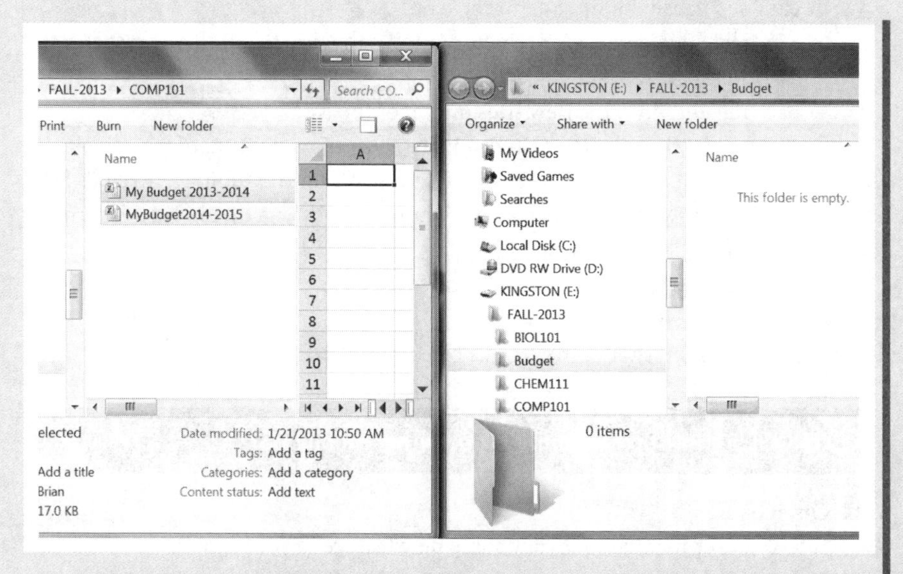

Figure 3-28 Dragging Between Two Open Windows

4. Delete files and folders.
   a. Click the **WordPad-YourName** file in the SemesterYear folder.
   b. Press the **Delete** key. Click **Yes** to confirm the deletion.
   c. Close all **open windows** except the Semester-Year folder. Make sure the view in the folder is **List**.
   d. Scroll on the left side of the window until you see the **Recycle Bin**.
   e. In the SemesterYear folder, click the **first folder** in the row or column. Hold down the **Shift** key, and click the **last item**. All of the objects (files and folders) are now selected.
   g. Drag the selected **folders** and **files** onto the Recycle Bin in the left pane.
   h. When the Recycle Bin turns greenish-blue, release the mouse button.
   i. Click **Yes** to confirm the permanent deletion of files and folders.
   j. Close **all windows**.

HINT: Files that are deleted from a USB storage device do not go to the Recycle Bin, which is why the question asking to confirm permanent deletion appears. Files from the desktop go to the Recycle Bin when they are deleted, so the question doesn't appear.

5. Empty the Recycle Bin.
   When you delete files from internal storage devices such as the C drive or desktop, you should empty the Recycle Bin periodically. In Windows 7, you can "see" trash building up in the icon.
   a. Create two blank **Word documents** on the desktop. Call one **test** and the other **test2**.
   b. Drag and drop the **new files** on top of the **Recycle Bin**.
   c. Double-click the **Recycle Bin** icon. A list of contents appears.
   d. Click the **Empty the Recycle Bin** button on the toolbar or select **File, Empty Recycle Bin** from the menu bar if it is displayed (Organize, Layout, click Menu bar).
   e. Click **Yes** to confirm the deletion.
   f. Close the **Recycle Bin** window.
   g. How often should the recycle bin be emptied?

EXERCISE 3 How Do I Organize Work with a Mobile OS?

■ **Objectives**

1. Use a user manual to review some new feature to your mobile device.
2. Locate a quality site for step-by-step instructions on file management on a mobile device.
3. Use those instructions to organize your mobile device.

■ **Activity**

1. Find out if there is a manual or help option on your mobile device. For example the iPad3 had a user's manual located at http://ipad3manual.com/. Select one new feature for your device that you didn't know was available or that you didn't know how to use. Try out the new feature.
2. Search the Internet for a quality site that provides step-by-step directions on how to create folders and manage files on your mobile device.
3. Discuss in class or in a discussion forum: Why would you trust that site? What makes it a reputable one? Were the directions easy to understand?
4. Now apply what you learned to organizing a few apps into one folder. For example, you have four healthcare-related apps. Organize them into one folder called health apps.

EXERCISE 4 How Do You Organize Data on the Computer?

■ **Objectives**

1. Develop an organizational scheme for data files.
2. Identify appropriate file naming conventions.
3. Support your work with resources.

■ **Activity A**

1. You are serving on a committee to develop the standards for file names that the committee will use when working on a strategic plan for implementation of an eHealth initiative at your organization. The charge to the committee also includes selecting how the committee will organize work on the file server that the committee will use. Some of the work will include obtaining reference materials, writing white or position papers, keeping minutes, developing a budget, and scheduling meetings.
2. Identify what other information you might collect or develop.
3. Develop a scheme for how the committee should organize the work on the file server. You will be presenting this to the committee for approval and acceptance. See **Figure 3-29** for an example of courses taught by one faculty member.
4. The next task is to decide on the file naming convention. Since the full committee will have access to this project folder, there needs to be agreement on how the committee members will name the files so all can easily locate the work.
5. Find two resources to place in the Library folder that talk about file naming conventions and their importance. Direct the committee members to review these before the discussions and vote.
6. Develop two sample naming-convention schemes for the committee to vote on.

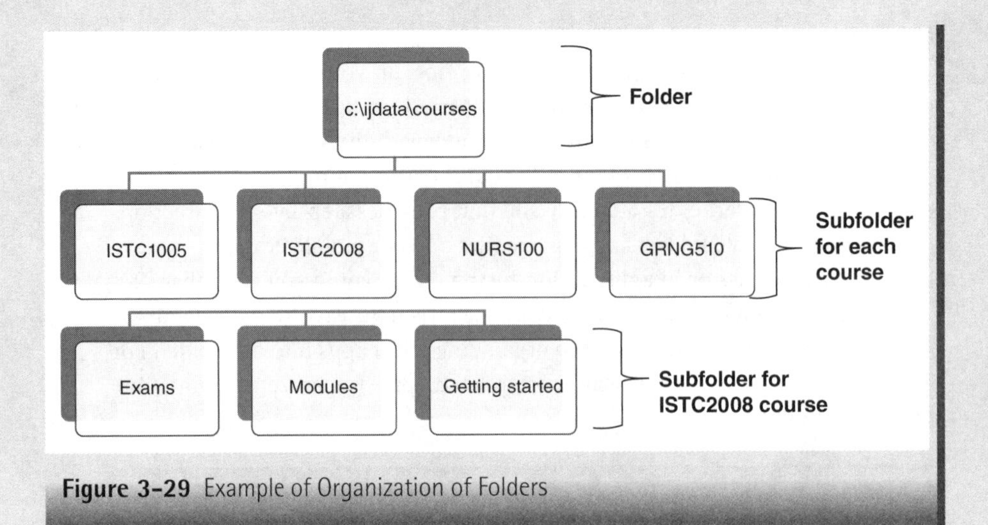

Figure 3-29 Example of Organization of Folders

Activity B

1. As a student just starting in your nursing program, you decide to organize your electronic files for easy access throughout your program of studies. You also want to give some thought to naming your files so you can retrieve them easily. In your senior year you will need to submit an e-portfolio as part of your graduation requirements.
2. You know you will have the following types of information: courses, finance, admissions, general college information, health library, etc. You also know you will be creating electronic files as part of your course work.
3. Develop a file structure for your time in school. Decide on file naming convention for your work. Share this scheme with your classmates to obtain feedback and suggestions. Provide feedback to at least two of your classmates on their structure and names.
4. Adjust your work based on your classmates' suggestions.
5. Create the structure and a few sample files.
6. Write a short description of your organization and the rationale behind it.
7. Zip the top-level folder and submit it to your professor.

EXERCISE 5 How Do I Customize My Start Menu and Taskbar?

Objectives

1. Alter the taskbar.
2. Alter the Start menu look.
3. Pin an item to the Start menu.

Some of these tasks may not be available in computer laboratories or in the work environment unless you are logged on as the administrator.

Directions

How to change the taskbar:

1. Right-click on a **blank area** of the taskbar and select **Properties**. The Taskbar and Start Menu properties dialog box appear.
2. Click the **square** to the left of Use Aero Peek to preview the desktop to place a check in the square. Click the **Apply** and **OK** buttons.
3. Add a few Microsoft Office icons to the **Quick Launch** area of the taskbar. Click the **Start** button, and select **All Programs, MS Office**. Right-click **MS Office Word 2010** and select **Pin to Taskbar**. The Word icon appears in the Quick Launch area, ready for you to start the program.

NOTE: If the program is open, right-click the program's button on the taskbar and click **Pin this program** to the taskbar.

4. Repeat Step 3 to add icons for other frequently used Microsoft Office programs to the Quick Launch area.

How to alter the Start menu:

1. Right-click the **Start** button and click **Properties**.
2. Click the **Start** Menu tab in the **Taskbar** and **Start Menu Properties** dialog box. If you do not like the new look, you can change it to an old look.
3. Click the **Customize** button next to the Start menu option.
4. Click to increase the number of programs to display on the Start menu size to **10**.
5. Scroll down until you see **Use large icons**. Click to **remove the check mark** next to this option.
6. Click **OK** and then **Apply**.
7. Click **OK** to apply the changes. Look at the changes to the Start menu: You should see small icons and a list of 10 applications.

HINT: Notice the Privacy area in the Taskbar and Start Menu Properties dialog box. If you do not want someone to see which programs were recently accessed on the computer or which files were recently opened, remove the check marks next to these options. Also review the Notification area in the Taskbar tab, which can be customized to change what it hides or what it shows.

How to pin an item to the Start menu:

1. Find **MS Office OneNote** in the All Programs menu. If you do not have this program, use another one.

2. Right-click the text and select **Pin to Start Menu**. The program now appears in the top-left pane of the Start menu; it can be accessed more easily from this location than by going through several layers. Use this feature for programs used regularly but not daily.

   Some users like to control the All Programs menu so that it does not become too unwieldy. Doing so requires thinking about how to organize the programs into appropriate categories and having administration rights on the computer. Here is one suggestion: Place all like programs together. For example, create a folder called Multimedia, and place all multimedia programs in that folder. Create a Utilities folder, and place all utilities in that folder.

How to organize the All Programs menu on the Start menu:

1. Click the **Start** menu.
2. Right-click on the **All Programs** option.
3. Click **Open**.
4. On the new window, double-click the **Programs** folder.
5. Create a **new folder** and move **Programs** into the new folder. For example, create a folder called **Browsers**. Now drag and drop all your browser applications into the Browsers folder.

Assignments

ASSIGNMENT 1 Where Do I Start with Organizing My Desktop?

■ Directions

1. First, think about how you work and what tools you want to have at your fingertips on the desktop. You must have at least one shortcut, one icon such as Computer, two folders, and two files. Alternatively, you can create the following objects on the desktop. Refer to the appropriate chapter discussions if you cannot remember how to create these objects.
   a. Shortcuts to the **Printer** and to the **Documents** folder
   b. A folder for information about your upcoming vacation including pictures for when you come back from vacation.
   c. A **Word** file named **FileManagement.**
   d. **Computer** icon on the desktop.
2. Next, rearrange the desktop, placing the **Taskbar** on the right, next to it the **folders**, and next to the folders, the **file**. Place the icon on the left side of the window with the shortcuts to the right of the icon.
3. Add a **Desktop Background** of your choice.
4. Select a **Screen Saver**.

5. Use the **Print Screen** button or the **Snipping** tool to capture these changes, open **WordPad**, and place them in the document.
6. Save the file as **Chap3-Assign1-LastName**- and submit to your professor according to the directions provided.
7. Restore the **desktop** and close all **open windows.**

ASSIGNMENT 2 Do I Understand Working with Files and Folders?

Directions

1. Create folders.
   a. Create a **folder** on your **USB storage device** named **Chap3-Assign2.**
   b. Open the **folder** and create a **Graphics** folder, a **Library** folder, a **Course** folder, and a **Newsletter** folder.
2. Find and copy files.
   a. Find a **JPEG file** on the hard drive. Click the **Start** button. Type ***.jpg** in the search box and press **Enter**.
   b. Copy **two of the files found** that have a .jpg extension to the **Chap3-Assign2** folder.
3. Create data files in the **Chap3-Assign2** folder.
   a. Create a **Word file** named **ANA Newsletter-June2013.**
   b. Create an **Excel file** named **Unit 5 Budget-2014.**
   c. Create a **PowerPoint** file named **Health Habits** for one of your courses.
4. Move files to the **correct folders**. Create any new folders that you believe are needed to complete this step.
5. Rename a file. Rename the **Health Habits** file to **My Nutrition100 Presentation.**
6. Zip the **Chap3-Assign2 folder** and submit to your professor according to the directions provided.

ASSIGNMENT 3 How Do I Organize Myself?

Directions

1. Develop an **appropriate structure** for storing your work this semester. Include folders representing the courses you are taking this semester as well as a few subfolders representing the work of each course. You may also complete this exercise using your personal or work environment.
2. Create your **structure** on your USB storage device under a folder with your last name.

3. Find **three files** created this semester and place them in the appropriate folders. List the files and their related folders here: ____________________ ____________________.
4. Create a folder called **Downloads**. Go to **www.adobe.com** and download **Adobe Reader file** to an appropriate folder on your USB storage device.
5. Write a short paragraph on why you selected this organization and store it under the main folder.
6. Compress the main folder (right-click the **folder**, select **Send To**, and then select **Compressed folder**). Submit to your professor according to the directions provided.

ASSIGNMENT 4 When Do I Upgrade to the Next Version of Windows?

Directions

1. Create a Word document and save as **Chap3-Assign4-LastName**.
2. Research the Windows 8 operating system and its new features.
3. Write a short paragraph on what you do on your computer and how each of the new features in Windows 8 may or may not be of help to you. Some questions to consider include:
   a. Will the next operating system run on my hardware?
   b. How easy is the interface to learn? Is it intuitive or will there be a large learning curve?
   c. What features are important to me? Why?
   d. Will my current programs function in the new operating system or will I have to upgrade all of them?
   e. Is the system easy to customize to my way of working?
   f. Does it support my peripheral devices such as printers, scanners, and mobile devices. That means are the Plug and Play features (i.e., device drives) compatible with my peripherals?
4. Save and submit the document and your analysis. Submit to your professor according to the directions provided.

c h a p t e r

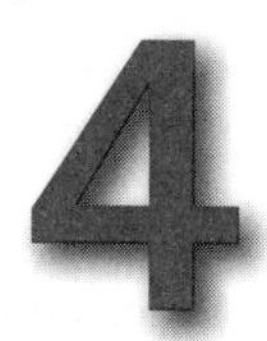

Software Applications: Common Tasks

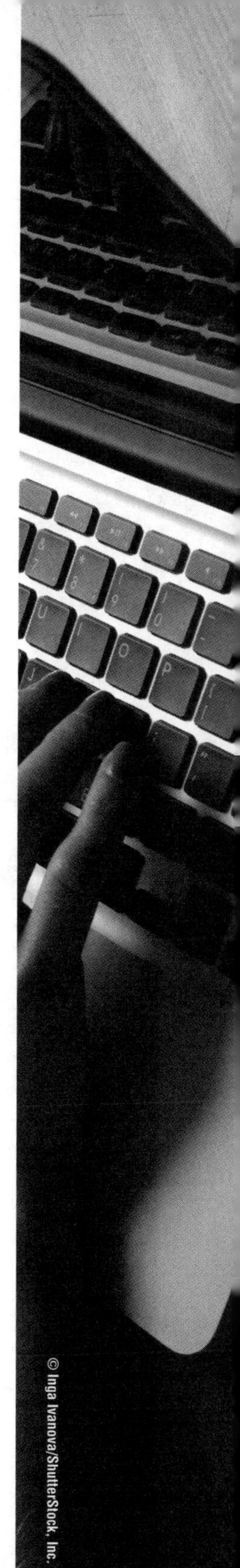

Objectives

1. Identify standards common to applications running in the Windows environment.
2. Describe and use the online help that the applications provide.
3. Use the MS Office ribbon and its tabs, groups, and commands.
4. Perform common tasks of opening, creating, closing, saving, finding, and printing files.
5. Use cut/copy/paste functions to move or copy data from within the same file or from one file to another.

Introduction

The focus of this chapter is to describe selected tasks that are used when working with **application programs** regardless of the application. In the Windows environment certain standards exist so that many applications share a common desktop environment. For example, **menus** provide the paths to action. Commands on a menu that are followed by an arrow result in the appearance of a submenu of related commands. Many applications display a title bar, a menu bar, one or more toolbars, a status bar, and graphical buttons. Microsoft Office 2010 fine-tunes previous Office versions with the goal of providing the appropriate tools at the time they are needed.

This chapter uses Microsoft Word 2010 on a Windows 7 computer to explain and demonstrate selected features and functions common to the 2010 Office suite.

Common Layout

MS Office 2010 improves on the previous Office version, Office 2007. The Office Button is gone. Instead the File tab, used in previous versions, returns and appears in the upper left corner of most applications. The File tab is blue in Word, green in Excel, and red in PowerPoint. When you click the File tab it defaults to Info and the **Backstage view** of the document appears. Backstage view helps you work with your document whereas the ribbon helps you work "in" your document. The file tab also provides access to document functions like open, save, close, help, print, exit, options, or share it. **Figure 4-1** shows the Backstage view in Word, Excel, and PowerPoint. Notice the info option for file management, such as permissions, sharing, versions, properties, author, that display by default when selecting the File tab.

Title Bar

In the center of the Title bar is the name of the file and the program used to create it. In addition, the left and right sides contain selected commands.

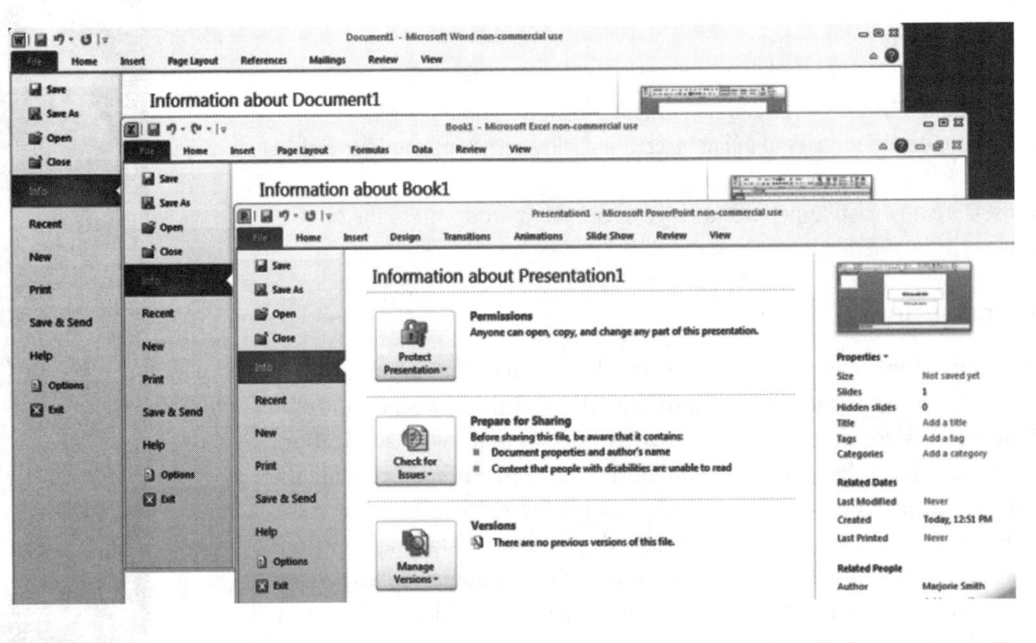

Figure 4-1 File Menus—Backstage View

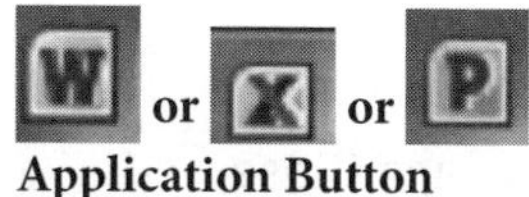

Application Button

A Word, Excel, or PowerPoint button appears on the far left of the title bar. Click this and a menu opens that allows you to resize the application window, move it, or close the program.

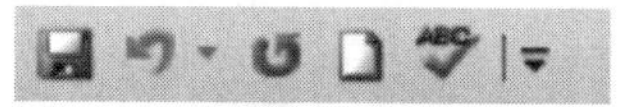

Quick Access Toolbar

To the right of the application button, the **Quick Access Toolbar** (QAT) remains visible no matter what tab you select. The standard items are Save, Undo, and Redo. New document and Spelling & Grammar have been added to this toolbar. To customize the toolbar click on the downward arrow; a menu appears with other commands as well as a submenu that offers more commands. The toolbar can also be moved below the ribbon. On public computers, however, you may not be allowed to alter this toolbar.

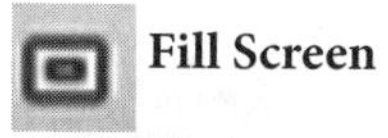

Fill Screen or Maximize

Use this button to fill the screen with the application window.

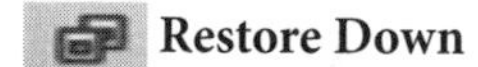

Restore Down

Use this button to resize the application window to its original size before it was maximized.

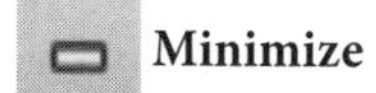

Minimize

Use this button to minimize the application window so that the desktop or other documents are visible.

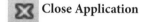

Close Application

Use this button to close the current application window or when you are finished with the application and have saved your work.

Ribbon

The **ribbon** is composed of task-oriented tabs, groups, and commands. It shows the most commonly used buttons associated with a certain task. The tab names resemble menu names and the groups resemble the toolbar, as in previous versions of Office. **Figure 4-2** shows the ribbons for Word, Excel, and PowerPoint with common features identified. Figure 4-2 also shows the command layout for WordPad and illustrates an interface that is common in other applications.

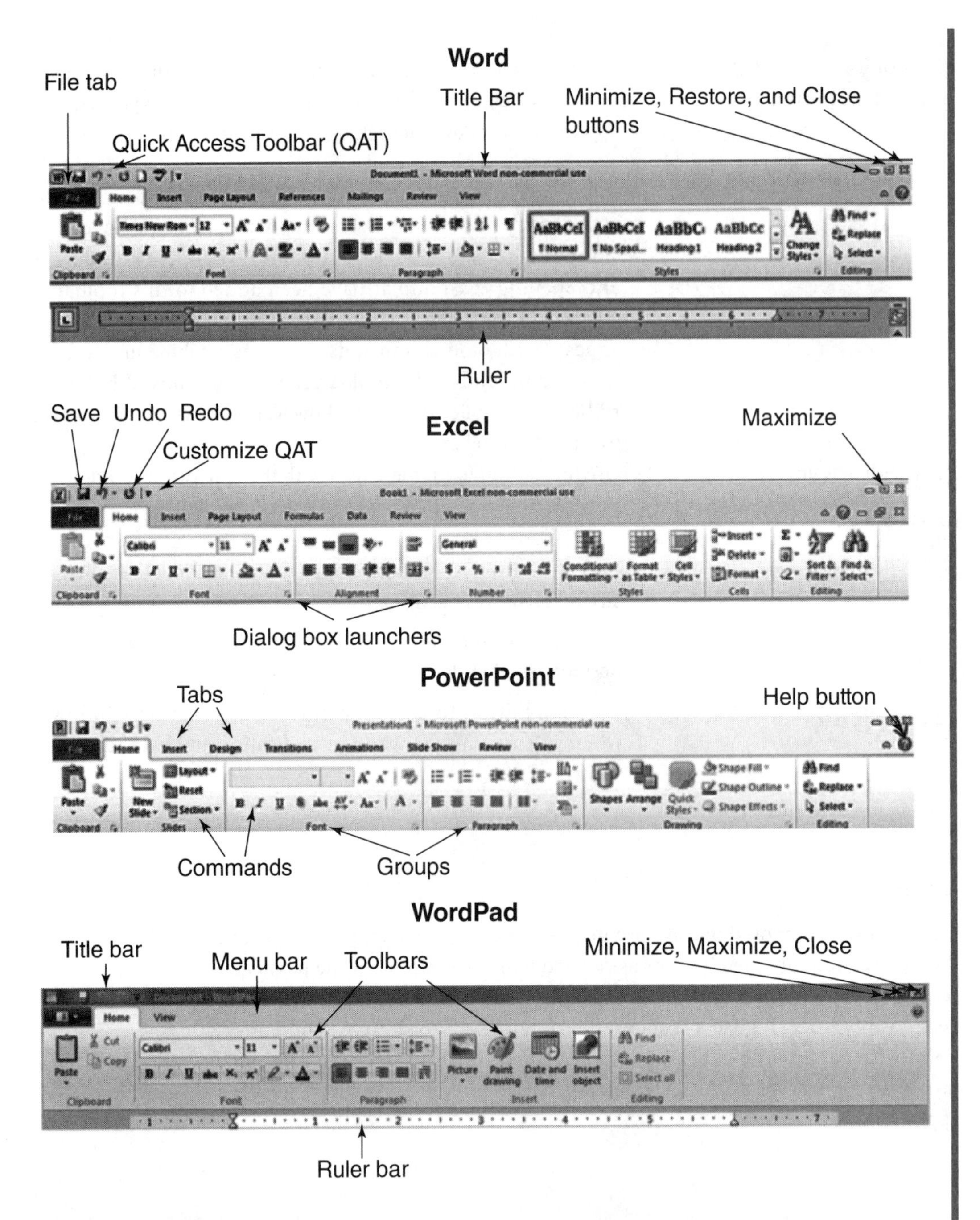

Figure 4-2 Sample Ribbons from Office 2010 and Command Layout for WordPad

These features shown in Figure 4-2 are described below.

File **File Button**	Click the File tab and a list of commands appear: Save, Save As, Open, Close, Info, Recent, New, Print, Save & Send, Help, Options, and Information about the document, book, or presentation.
Tabs	Tabs vary among applications, but all share File, Home, Insert, Review, and View. Some tabs like Home and View, are always available. Contextual tabs appear depending upon what you are doing. For example, the Table Tools tab appears when you are working in a table. Tabs function much like menu bars.
Groups	Each tab has several groups that show related items together. Groups function much like toolbars.
Help Button	The Help button opens a dialog box for Word, Excel, or PowerPoint help. Type the keyword or topic in the search box and click Search *or* Browse the Table of Contents listed in the dialog box.
Dialog Box Launcher	This button, located at the bottom right corner of selected groups, opens a dialog box with related commands and options.

Tabs and Groups

Basic task-oriented tabs appear across the top of the ribbon in Office 2010 applications. Tabs are broken into subsections called groups that further define the tasks associated with that group. (See **Figure 4-3**.) Clicking a tab shows tasks associated with that tab. For example, Page Layout allows you to define themes, set margins, add page breaks, and define indent and spacing parameters in Word.

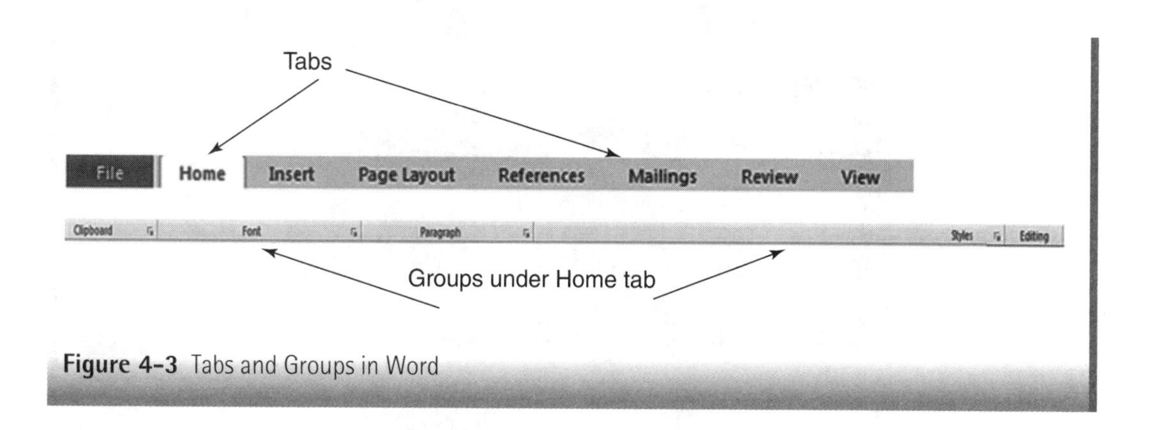

Figure 4-3 Tabs and Groups in Word

Clicking the **Dialog Box Launcher** in a group opens a dialog box in which further options are available. When a down arrow appears in a ribbon button it means more choices are available. When the mouse arrow is held over an option in the ribbon, a ScreenTip that describes its function appears. A **task pane** is a small window that displays additional options and commands for certain features while a **contextual tab** occurs in a window that is only available in a certain context or situation.

The File Tab

Figure 4-4 shows the menu and related commands that appear when New is selected on the File tab. These commands are described in more detail below using Word as an example. The functions are the same in PowerPoint and Excel; however, the options are for PowerPoint or Excel.

Save — **Save** file. If saving the file for the first time, you will be asked to name it and choose the location in which to save it. You can add a tag or specify its subject.

Save As — Clicking **Save As** brings up a window similar to Save. If the file has been saved before, you can rename it and select the place where it should be saved or change its file format.

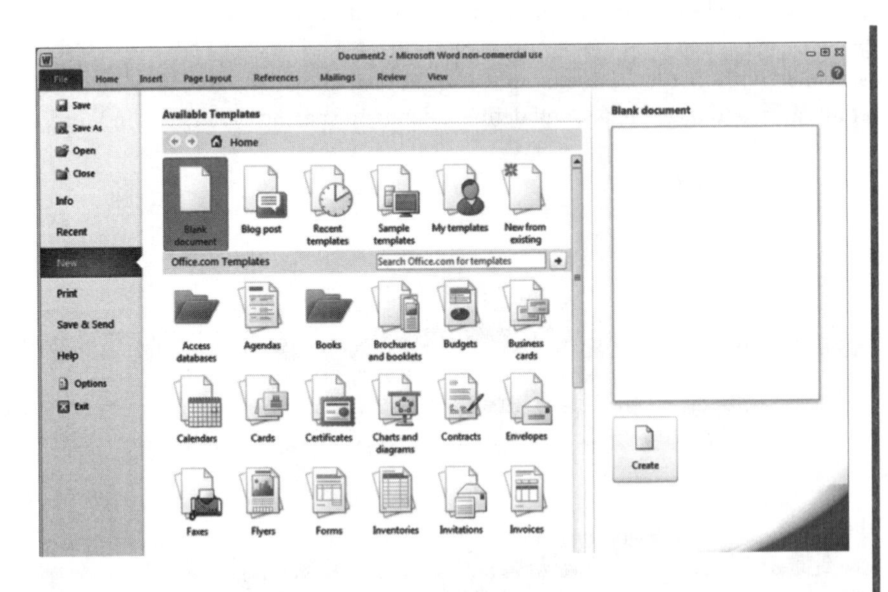

Figure 4-4 File Tab Menu in Word 2010—New Document Selected

Open Open allows you to select from the list of previously saved documents that appear on the right side of the window or click File, Open and look in other areas of the computer or storage devices for the file.

Close When you select Close, if you haven't saved the document previously a dialog box will open that will prompt you to choose Save, Don't Save, or Cancel. Select an option.

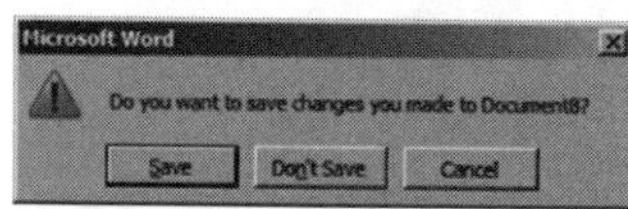

Info The Info command presents ways to protect your document, prepare it for sharing, or examine its properties.

Recent The Recent command provides a list of recently opened documents and places where they reside. You can "pin" a document here so it is always listed in the list of most recent documents no matter when it was written.

New You can open a new blank document or choose from a large selection of templates including agenda, brochure, calendar, envelopes, letter, memo, minutes, resume and CV, schedule, timesheets, and newsletters.

Print When printing, you can select the number of copies you need and which printer, settings, and page setup to use, among other options.

Prepare Preparing a document allows you to check its properties, add a digital signature, inspect or encrypt the document, and check for compatibility with earlier versions of the application.

Save & Send Use this to email a copy of the document, save it to the Web or SharePoint, or publish it as a blog post. You can also choose to send it as an attachment, a PDF, or a fax.

Help Selecting Help presents you with several choices, such as Microsoft Office Help, Getting Started, Tools for working with Office, or checking for updates.

Options Choosing Word Options opens a list with many choices that includes popular options for Word; how it is displayed; ways to proof, save, customize, and secure it; and resources. Some of these same options appear in the other Office applications.

Exit Exit will close the application. If the document is not saved, the same dialog box appears as that when Close is selected.

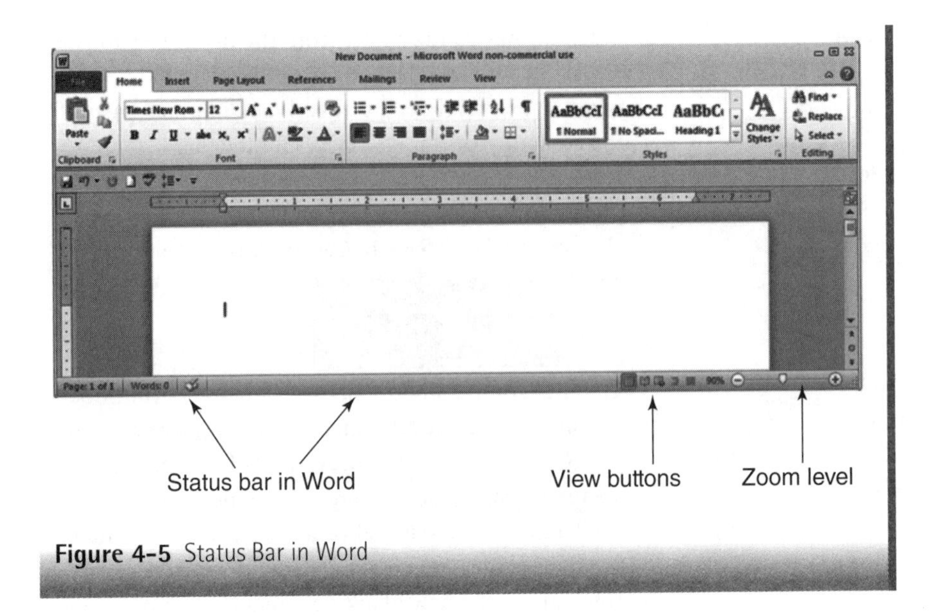

Figure 4-5 Status Bar in Word

The Status Bar

Figure 4-5 shows the **status bar** in Word. It shows the page number, number of words in the document (the document pictured is a new one), some view buttons, and the Zoom slider. **Zoom** allows you to examine a part of the document more closely or to see the complete page of the document. Setting the Zoom to page width can be helpful when working with a document in the landscape mode. Right-click on the status bar and a menu opens that allows you to customize it.

Keyboard Commands

Keyboard commands (access keys) make it easy to choose tasks in a ribbon. Press the Alt key to activate access keys and **KeyTip badges** (letters and numbers) appear. **Figure 4-6** shows what happens when the Alt key is pressed. If you press Alt and one of the letters shown, shortcut letters and numbers appear for the groups in that tab. For example, press **Alt+H** and you will see the KeyTip for **Bold**; then press **Alt+1** and the next thing typed will appear in Bold. If the **Cursor** is inside a word, that word will be changed to Bold. To cancel KeyTips, Press **Alt** again. The **F10** key will also show KeyTips.

If you press **Alt+F** in Word 2010, the drop-down menu for the File tab appears. Next to each command is the keyboard shortcut. For example, to Save press **S**. These letters work only when this particular drop-down menu is present, otherwise **Ctrl+S** is the keyboard shortcut for Save. These shortcuts work in all Office 2010 applications.

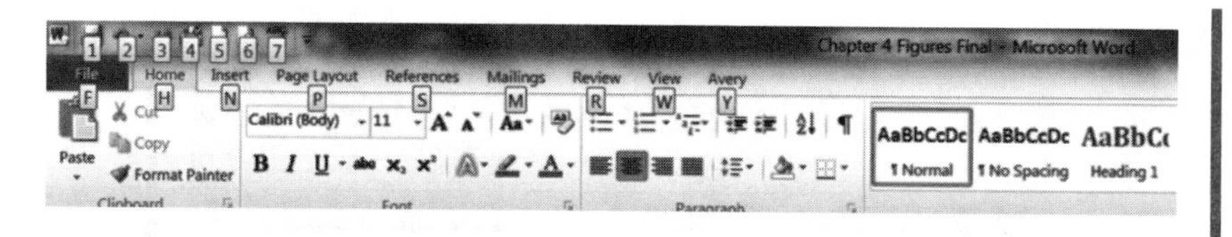

Figure 4-6 KeyTips (Shortcut Symbols) for Accessing Commands from the Keyboard

Common Tasks

This section describes selected common tasks that you can expect to use with all Office applications.

Obtaining Help

Access **Help** through the blue question mark on the ribbon or the Help option on a menu bar. Click the question mark and a Word Help screen appears. (See **Figure 4-7a**.) Topics describe what is available in Online Help; if offline, this symbol Offline is shown. For online help one must be connected to the Internet. If you hold the cursor over the symbols at the top of the window, a ScreenTip description of the object's function appears. Click this symbol and the Table of Contents appears. You can also search for help by typing an appropriate search term into the Search box under the symbols or by choosing "see all" under support.

Note the **dialog box** in the lower-right corner of Figure 4-7a. By clicking the green ball at the bottom right of the dialog box, the menu for choosing either online or offline help appears.

To select a help topic:

1. Click the **Help** button or press the **F1** key.
2. Open the **Table of Contents** if it is not open.
3. Click **Getting help** in the Table of Contents.
4. Click **Customize the Ribbon**.
5. Review the information provided.
6. Click **Getting help** to close that section.
7. Click the **Home** symbol at the top of Word Help window. You return to the original list of topics.

To select help with keyword:

1. Click the **Help** button or press the **F1** key.
2. In the **Search** text box , type **ScreenTips** (be sure to type it as one word).

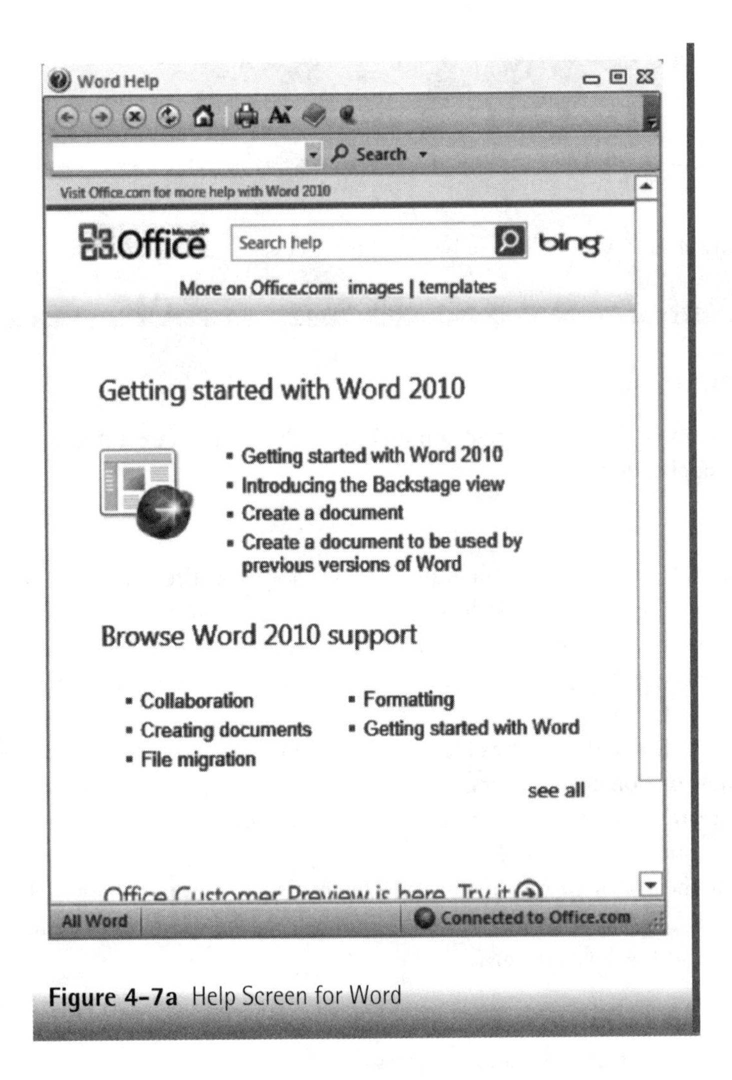

Figure 4-7a Help Screen for Word

3. Press the **Enter** key.
4. Choose **Show or hide ScreenTips.** You will see the screen shown in **Figure 4-7b**.

To select online help from Office.com:

1. Click the **Help** button or press the **F1** key.
2. Click the **Getting started with Word** symbol.
3. Go toward the bottom of the window and click the text **Getting Started with Microsoft Office 2010.** A new window appears. (See **Figure 4-7c**.)

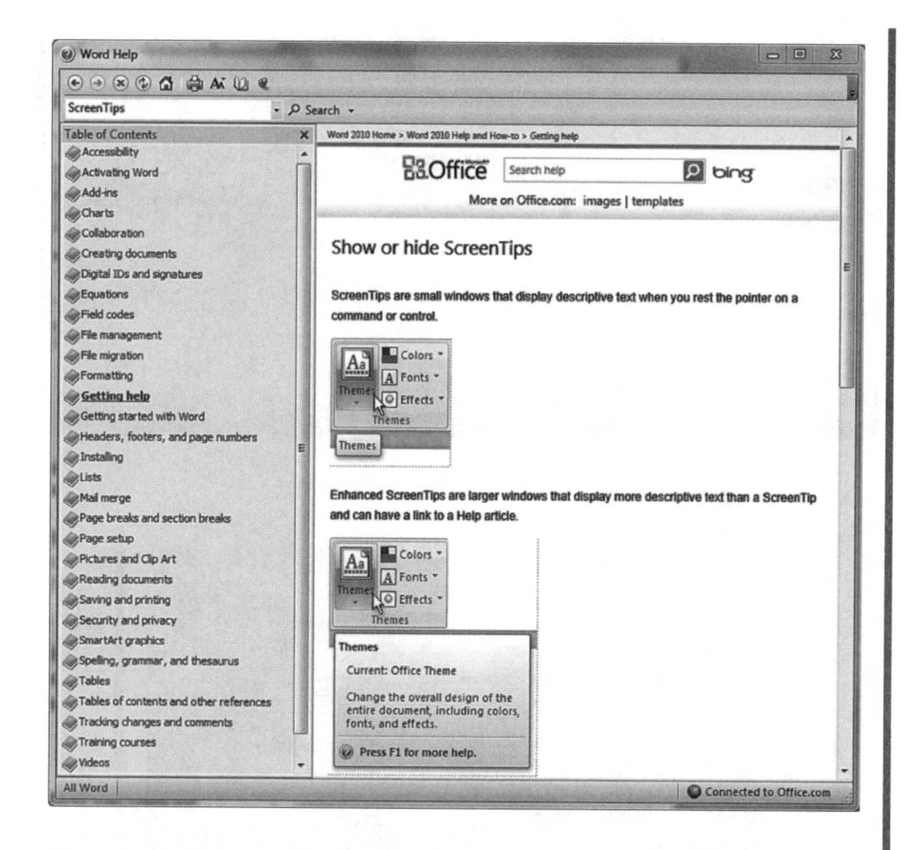

Figure 4-7b Show or Hide ScreenTips* Screen
*ScreenTips are small windows that display descriptive text when you rest the pointer on a command or control.

4. Click Word. Watch the video.
5. Choose another application of interest to review if you have time!

Creating a New Document

To start working in most applications, you must first create a new document, spreadsheet, database, or presentation. Most applications open to a new, blank document, spreadsheet, or presentation or present a series of dialog boxes asking the user to respond to questions. When PowerPoint is started, a blank title slide appears. In Excel a worksheet is opened. In this chapter the term document is used to represent a text document, a spreadsheet, a database, or a presentation.

When the computer is turned on, and you have a task to complete, you must first select the appropriate application. For this text we use Microsfot Office, but

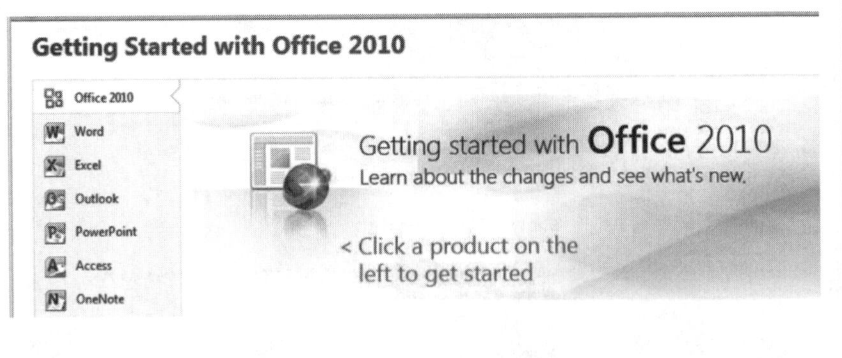

Figure 4-7c Getting Started with Office 2010

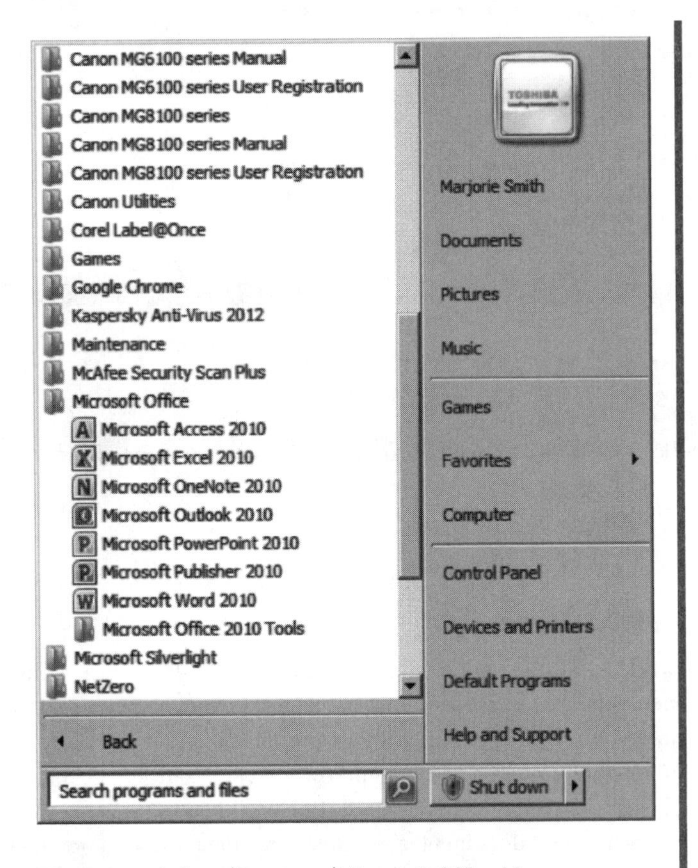

Figure 4-7d Start/Programs/Microsoft Office Menus

in some cases the application might be Publisher, Expression Web, and so forth. The key is to use the correct application for the task. For Microsoft Office click **Start**, select **All Programs**, and then select **Microsoft Office**; next select the correct application. (See **Figure 4-7d**.) A new document will open, such as the one shown in Figure 4-5.

One can also go to the Start button and open a Microsoft Office application from the Start Menu if it appears above Start or if you pinned it to the Start menu. Microsoft Office icons may also be placed on the Quick Launch Toolbar or on the desktop. Using this approach, the user clicks the correct button on the taskbar or double-click the shortcut icon on the desktop to launch the program. (See **Figure 4-8**.)

To start another document once the application is open:

1. Click **File** and choose **New**. Figure 4-4 shows the File menu with New Document highlighted.
2. Click the symbol for a **new blank document** if it has been added to the Quick Access Toolbar.
3. Alternatively, press **Ctrl+N** and a new blank document opens.

There are also several **templates** that you can use to minimize formatting time. Templates are either installed on the computer, made from previously constructed documents, or are available online.

To create a document using a template:

1. Click the **File** tab and choose **New**.
2. Click **Sample Templates**.
3. Select a **template** from the choices that appear by double-clicking on it. Alternatively, click **Download**.

All open documents will be accessible through the Word icon on the taskbar until they are closed. With Aero Peek if you hover over the Word icon on the taskbar, you can see all open Word documents.

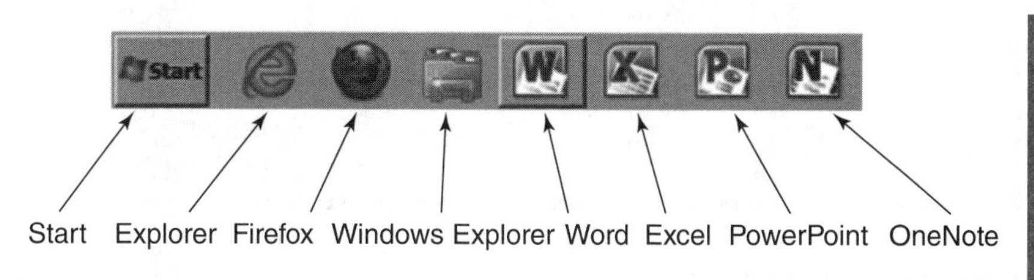

Figure 4-8 Taskbar in Windows 7

Opening, Minimizing, and Closing a File

Common to all applications is the function of opening and closing files. Once a document is created, it is saved and often reopened later for additions and/or corrections.

To open a file:
In the Windows world, a file can be opened in many ways. Because the focus here is on Office 2010, the Microsoft Office File tab is demonstrated.

1. Click **File** tab, then click **Open**. A list of documents/files appears on the right in the Documents library. (See **Figure 4-9**).
2. Double-click a **document** from that list or select **one** and click **Open**.

If the document is one on which you recently worked, select **File**, then **Recent**. **Figure 4-10** shows a list of recent documents and places on the computer. Each filename has a pushpin icon next to it. You can click on the icon to "pin" it to the Recent Documents list so it always stays there. To unpin the file, click on the blue pushpin icon.

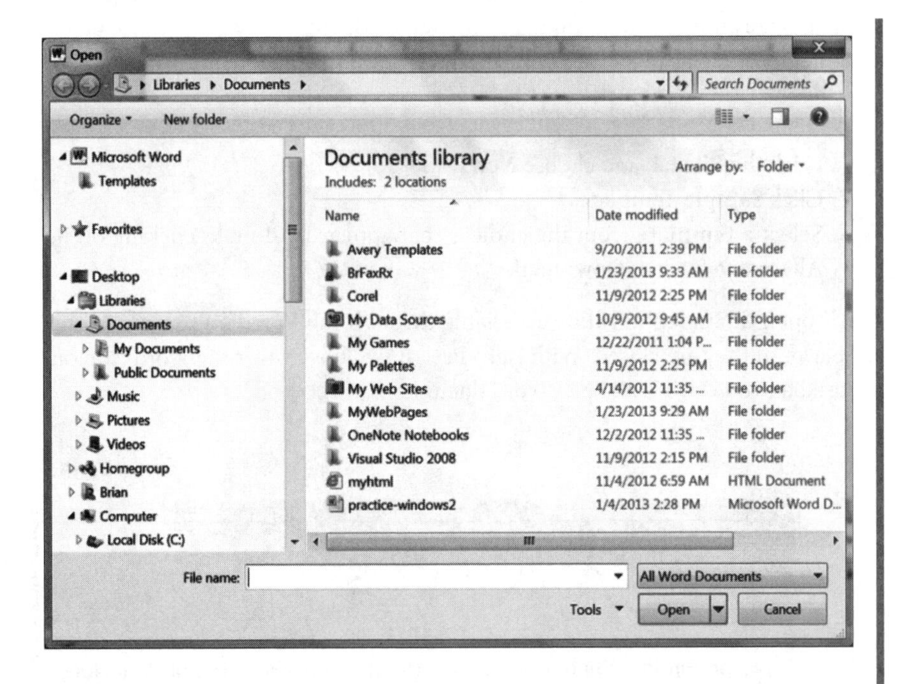

Figure 4-9 Documents Library

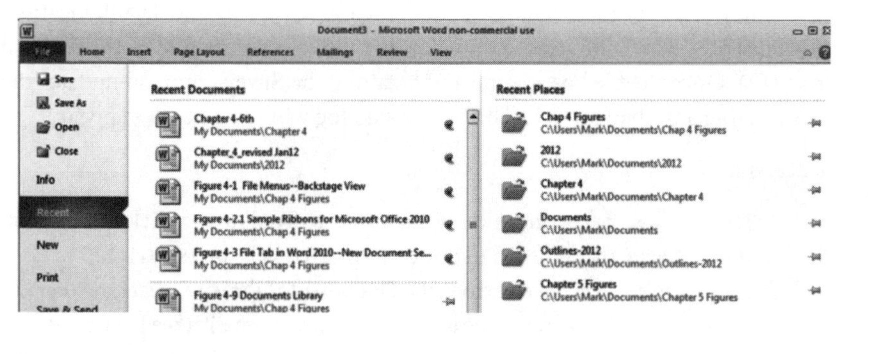

Figure 4-10 List of Recent Documents and Places

If the document is located on an external storage device or a network file server select **Computer** from the Start menu to see those devices. Files can be opened in many ways. Here are two more ways:

- In a window or on the desktop, **double-click** the file.
- In an application, press **Ctrl+O**.

To minimize a file:

Click the **Minimize** button in the upper-right corner of the window and the document will disappear but it will be available by clicking the Word Box at the bottom of the screen on the taskbar. Choose the document you desire.

To close a file:

1. Select the **File** tab, click the **Close** option .
2. If changes were made to the file and it was not saved, you will be prompted to save the file before closing it. Respond to the prompt.

Other options for closing a file include:

- Click the **Close** button in the upper-right corner of the window.
- Press **Ctrl+F4** on a traditional keyboard.

On some of the newer keyboards there is a Close button near where the F6 button is at the top of the keyboard.

Save Files

Once work begins on a file or document, it will need to be saved for future reference or revision. It is best to name and save your document when you first open it. Thereafter you can simply press **Ctrl+S** (or the Save button on newer keyboards) periodically to save your work to prevent loss of data. The first time that a file is saved a location and name must be specified (see Chapter 3 for file naming conventions). If a location is not specified, the file is saved in the default location. In Microsoft Office, the default location is the Documents folder on the hard drive (C:). Once the file has a name and location, the **Save** command updates the file by saving any changes to it. The **Save As** dialog window does not appear.

To access the Save command:

1. Click the **Save** icon on the Quick Access Toolbar, or click the **File** tab and select **Save** from the list of options. Alternatively, press **Ctrl+S.**
2. If the file has not been saved before, the **Documents Library** appears and the user must name the file and select the location in which to save it. (See Figure 4-9.)

To access the Save As option:

1. Click **File**, **Save As**.
2. Select a **location** to save the file.
3. Type a **name** for the file.
4. Select the **format** to save the file.
5. Click **Save** button.

When the **Save As** Save As button is selected a window similar to **Figure 4-11** appears. The file can be saved in the default format (Word 2010), as a template, in a Word 97–2003 format, or in other formats such as PDF. Other choices are available such as author, subject, add a tag, or company name. The Save As command can also be used to change the name or location of a document or to save a revised document while keeping the original as is. To use the keyboard to save a file, press **Ctrl+S** or the **Save** function key.

Your computer can be set to automatically save recovery information every 1 to 120 minutes in case there is a power failure or other problem with the computer.

To set the automatic save feature:

1. Select **Options** from the **File** menu.
2. Under **Word Options,** select **Save**.
3. Place a **check** in the box to the left of **Save AutoRecover information** and then set the time to 10 minutes or whatever time you choose. (See **Figure 4-12**.) The default location for saving files can be noted here or changed as desired. Note that this does not take the place of saving your document (**Ctrl+S**) every so often (every 10 minutes or so). On public computers you will not be able to alter these settings.

Printing Files

To print a file:

1. Click the **File** tab. Then click the **Print** Print button**. Figure 4-13** shows the Print dialog box that appears. **Ctrl+P** also opens the Print dialog box.

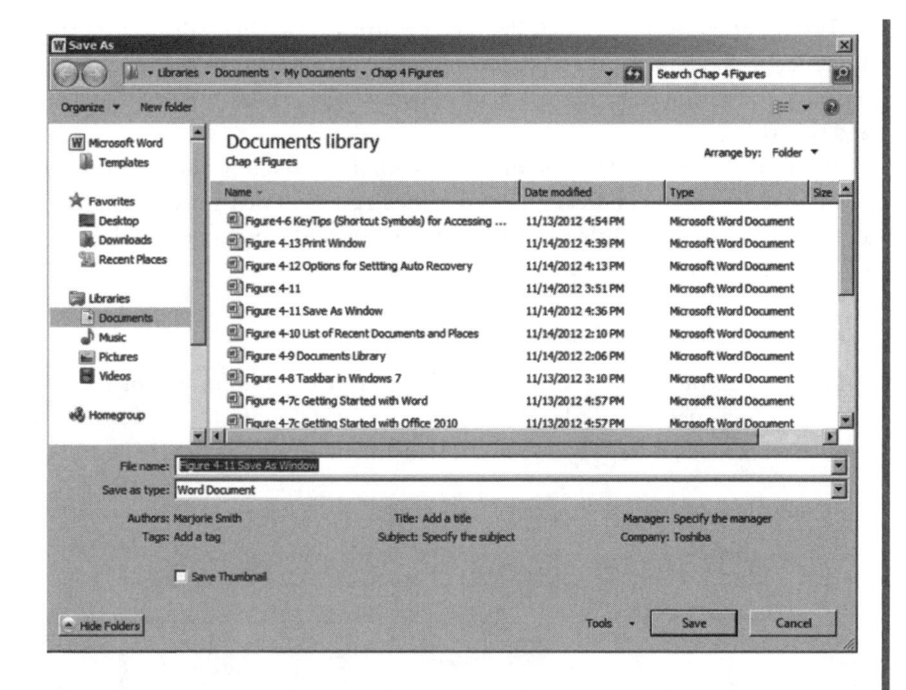

Figure 4-11 Save As Window

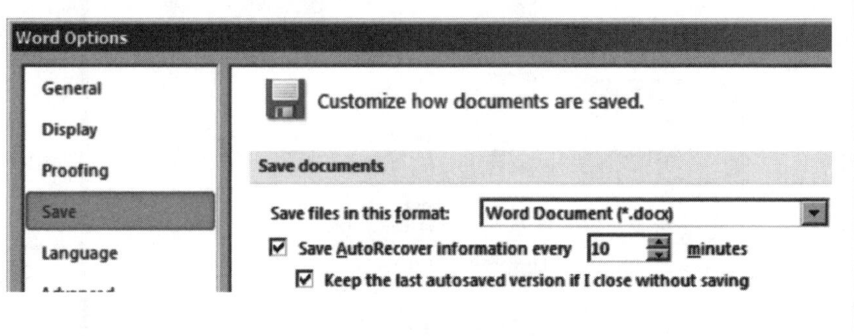

Figure 4-12 Option for Setting Recovery of Documents

2. Click the **Print** button.
3. Adjust the options as needed. There are several to choose from: changing the printer; choosing the number of copies to print; printing the total document, the current page, the selection, or selected pages; or collating multiple page documents. Adjust the options as needed.
4. Click **OK**.

Two other options are **Quick Print** or **Print Preview.** Quick Print prints the document without the dialog box showing and sends one copy of the current document to the default printer. There is no option to select number of pages, printer, and so forth.

Print Preview shows the document as it will look when printed. Some keyboards have a print function key located in the F12 area or that shares the F12 key. In that case, there is a toggle switch to move between F12 and Save, which brings up the Print dialog box.

Finding and Replacing Words

Another common task that computer users perform is the finding or finding and replacing specific words within a document. Suppose it is necessary to use a document that was previously created and now must be altered to fit the

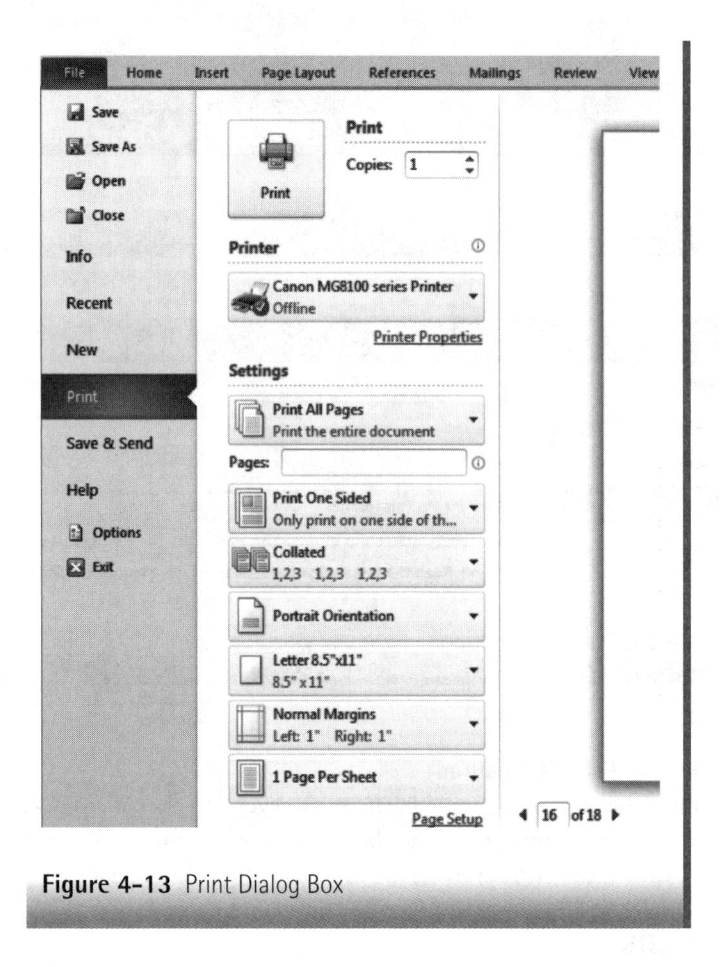

Figure 4-13 Print Dialog Box

current situation. It could also be a file or email that must be forwarded to someone else. Instead of manually searching for or replacing these words, let the computer do it.

To access the Find feature:
In some applications, you can select **Edit, Find**. In Office 2010, the command is on the Home tab in the Editing group on the far right.

1. Select the **Home** tab and choose **Find** from the Editing group. **Figure 4-14** shows the Navigation pane that appears to the left of the document.
2. With an open Navigation window, type the **word** in the Search Document window. You can choose "*Browse Headings*" or "*Browse Pages*" or just press **Enter**. All occurrences of the word will be located and bolded.
3. If there are more words that don't fit on the windows, continue clicking the down arrow until all instances of the word or file are found.
4. Click the **Close** button to close the navigation pane.

To find and replace text:
Most people find this feature more useful than the Find feature.

1. Click **Replace** in the Editing Group and the **Find and Replace** window shown in **Figure 4-15** appears.
2. Type the **text** or **word** in the search box.
3. Click the **Replace with** text box.
4. Type the **replacement text or word**, and click **Replace** .

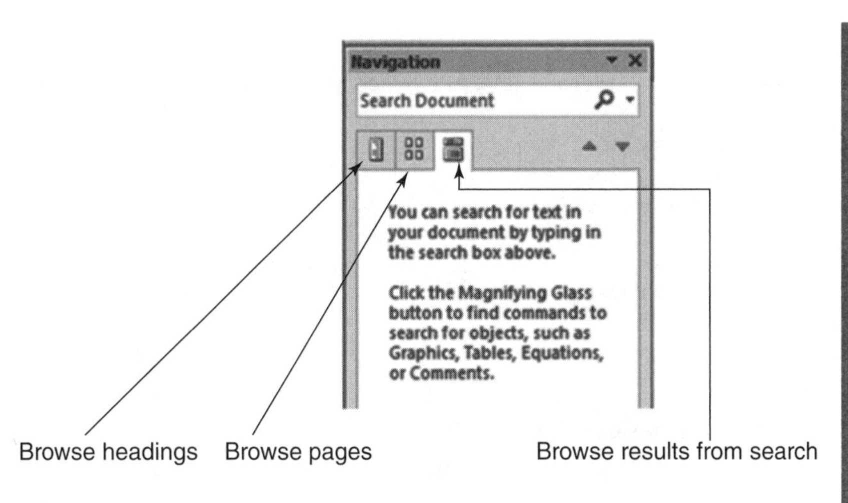

Figure 4-14 Navigation Pane for Searching Document

5. Continue clicking **Replace** until all of the instances of the word are either left alone or replaced.

Figure 4-15 shows the options available when More >> is clicked and match case is also selected. In this example, the word to find is *college*, and the replacement word is *university.* Be careful with the Replace All button. It automatically replaces all instances of *college* with *university*, which might not be desired. The find feature is not automatically case sensitive, although the option to match case was selected here. It is usually safer to use the Find Next option that requires you to confirm the replacement.

Selecting Text or Objects

Selecting text or objects means to highlight the text or object, such as a word or a cell in a spreadsheet. This is a common task when editing documents. Although it is fine to use the delete and backspace keys to complete minor editing tasks, it is not efficient for editing lines, sentences, paragraphs, columns, rows, cells,

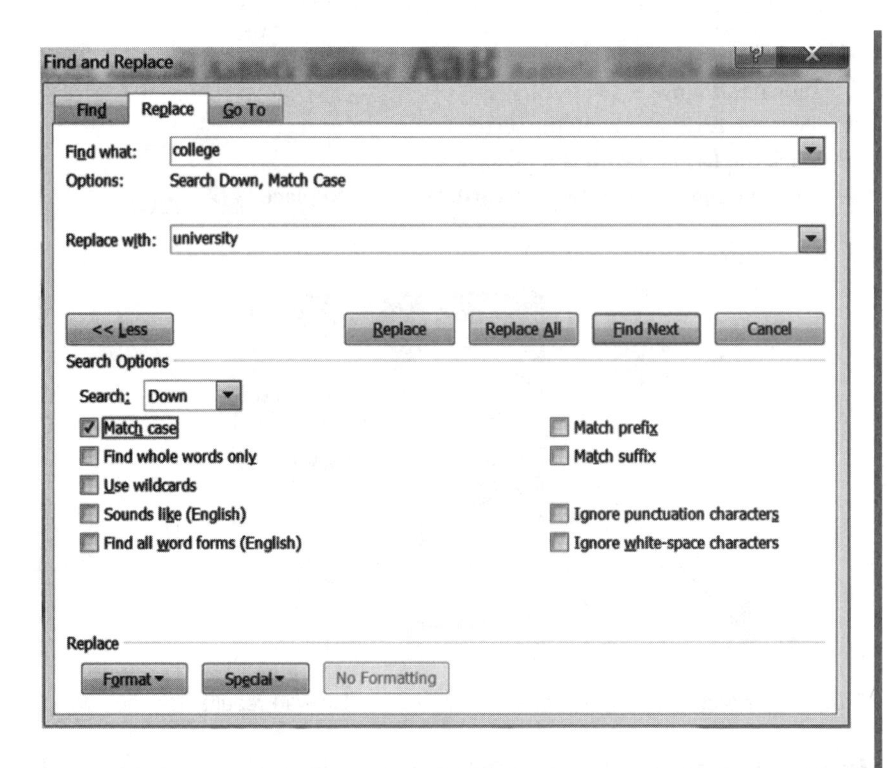

Figure 4-15 Find and Replace Dialog Box with "More >>" Selected

or an entire document. You can also use this feature when formatting documents. Once again, each item can be formatted separately, but this is very time consuming.

Each application has some minor variations for selecting or highlighting text and cells. Described here are some of the most common techniques for selecting them. Additional ones are presented in each application chapter as appropriate.

Select	Mouse Action
A word	Double-click the **word**.
Several words	Click and drag the mouse over the words or select the **first** word. Hold down the **Shift** key, and click the **last** word.
A sentence	Hold down the **Ctrl** key and click the **sentence**.
A line	Click in the **quick select area** (the cursor turns into a right slanted arrow when placed in the margin on the left side of the line).
A paragraph	Click in the **quick select area next to the paragraph** and double-click.
Entire document	Triple-click the **quick select area**. Use **Ctrl+A**.
A cell	Click the **cell**.
Multiple cells	Drag over the cells.

In addition to using mouse strokes, the keyboard can be used to select text. This is especially helpful when what must be selected spans greater distances or is on the edge of the document. For example, to select text that spans several pages, place the cursor at the beginning of the text to be selected. Hold down the shift key, and use the arrow keys to move down the document. As the cursor is moved, all of the text is highlighted. This technique also works in spreadsheets to select multiple cells.

If you need to select the entire document, press **Ctrl+A**. The entire document is now selected. You can also use the Editing group on the Home tab to select text. Click **Select** Select and the option to Select All appears.

Editing Text

Three basic editing features are used in applications: inserting, deleting, and replacing items.

Insert means to add new text, slides, rows, columns, and so forth. In word processing programs, insert is the default. When the user starts typing, the characters are placed at the insertion point. In applications for spreadsheets and graphics, commands must be used to insert rows, columns, or new slides. These commands are covered in each application chapter.

Delete means to remove text, a row, a column, or a slide from the document. Select what must be deleted and press the **Delete** key. If a mistake is made, go to the Quick Access Toolbar and choose the **Undo** button. In some applications, one would go to **Edit** and choose **Undo Typing**. Additional features available for deleting are covered in the appropriate application chapter. Note the difference between the Delete key and Backspace key. The Delete key deletes text to the right of the insertion point, whereas the Backspace key deletes text to the left of the insertion point.

Replace means to substitute one thing for another. In most cases it is not necessary to first delete the old text and then type the new. By highlighting or selecting the text it changes to the replace mode. This means that typing the replacement will delete what was highlighted. It is not necessary to delete it before typing.

Copying or Moving Text

The last of the common tasks presented in this chapter deals with copying or moving text from one place to another in the same document, from one document to another, or from one application to another. The most common method for doing this is using the **cut/copy/paste commands;** these use the concept of a clipboard as a temporary holding place for the cut or copied material. In Excel, PowerPoint, and Word these tools for cutting and copying can be found in the same place on the Ribbon—on the far left of the Home tab Paste Clipboard.

Another method for doing this is the **drag-and-drop** method. This method relies on selecting data and using the mouse to drag it to the new spot. The general rule for selecting the best method to use is based on distance to move or copy the material and how many times you want to paste the item. For short distances in the same document, use drag and drop. To copy or move data longer distances (to another page, to another document, or to another application), or to paste content multiple times, use the cut-and-paste clipboard strategy. To paste items multiple times, use the clipboard. Use the Format Painter to copy formatting from one place to another.

To copy data using the clipboard:

1. Select the **data** to be copied.
2. Click the **Copy** button.
3. Place the **insertion point** (cursor) where the data are to be copied.
4. Click the **Paste** Paste button.

To move data using the clipboard:

1. Select the **data** to be moved.
2. Click the **Cut** button.

3. Place the **insertion point** where the data are to be moved.
4. Click the **Paste** button.

It is important to know where the insertion point is because that is where the Paste command will place the data. The mouse pointer (I-beam) does not reflect where the data will go. If the data are moved to another document or application, you must use either the **File** tab, **filename** to access the other document in the application or by clicking on the application button from the Start menu to get to another application (refer to Chapter 3 if you are unsure about how to do this) or use **Aero Peek** to switch to the other document if it is open.

To collect items in the Office **Clipboard** the clipboard must be displayed. (See **Figure 4-16**.) Items that are cut or copied will appear there. Multiple data may be placed on the Office Clipboard at one time and may be used in any other documents. The Clipboard task pane will show how many items are on the clipboard with the last item copied at the top. You have the choice of pasting one or more of these items into a new document or clear the clipboard. The clipboard can hold 24 items at one time. When the 25th item is added, the first one is deleted. The last item added to the Office Clipboard is also sent to the system clipboard. When you close an application, you will be reminded that there is a large amount of content on the clipboard; then you will be asked if you want the content available to other applications after you quit Word or whatever application you are using.

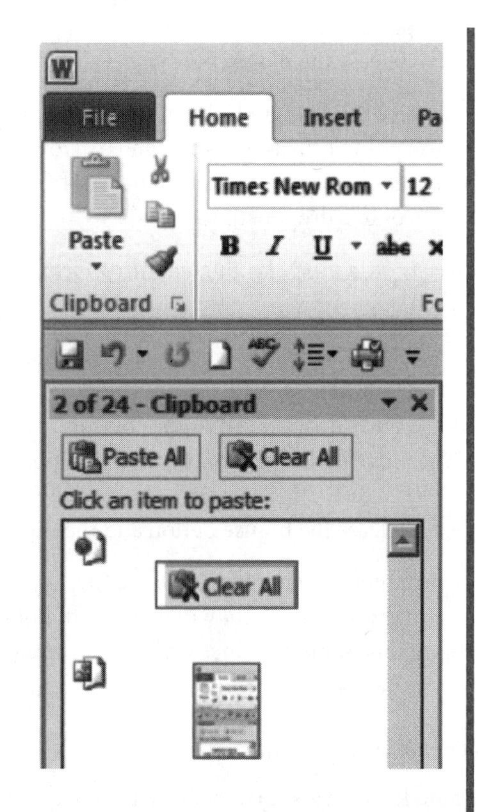

Figure 4-16 The Clipboard Task Pane

To paste the contents of the Office Clipboard into a new document:

1. Open a **New** document.
2. Click the **Clipboard Dialog Box Launcher** to display the **Office Clipboard**. The clipboard task pane appears.
3. Click the **items** to add to the new document.

A new document can be created from multiple items on the Office Clipboard. When using the Paste command, the system clipboard is used, not the Office Clipboard. Items stay in the Office Clipboard until the user exits Microsoft Office or clicks the Clear All button Clear All in the clipboard task pane. When clearing the Office Clipboard, the system clipboard is also cleared.

The cut/copy/paste commands can also be accessed through the keyboard. After selecting the text, press **Ctrl+X** for cut, **Ctrl+C** for copy, and **Ctrl+V** for paste. The keys for these commands are in the same order on the bottom row of the keyboard as are the icons on the ribbon going from top to bottom. On some keyboards the X, C, and V keys are marked Cut, Copy, and Paste.

To move data using the drag-and-drop method:

1. Highlight the data to be moved.
2. Place the pointer on the **selected area**.
3. Hold down the **left mouse** button.
4. Move the **mouse** so the insertion point (broken vertical bar) is in the new place.
5. Release the **mouse** button.

Notice the changing look of the mouse pointer when using drag and drop. The mouse pointer turns to a left-slanted arrow with a box below it, and the insertion point turns to a broken vertical bar. **Cut (move)** is the default option when using the drag-and-drop method.

To copy data using the drag-and-drop method:

1. Select the **data** to be moved.
2. Place the pointer on the **selected area**.
3. Hold down the **Ctrl** key.
4. Hold down the **left mouse** button.
5. Move the **mouse** so the insertion point (broken vertical bar) is in the new place.
6. Release the **mouse** button and then the **Ctrl** key.

It is important not to release the Ctrl key until after releasing the mouse button or else the selected data will be moved, not copied. When copying, the pointer appears the same as it does when cutting except that there is a plus sign in the box below the pointer.

Keyboard Shortcuts

Some keyboard shortcuts have been explained in earlier parts of this chapter. **Table 4-1** lists the common shortcut keys for Office 2010. They will work in most Office applications.

TABLE 4-1 SHORTCUT KEYS FOR OFFICE 2010

Command	Shortcut
Select **A**ll	Ctrl+**A**
Bold	Ctrl+**B**
Copy	Ctrl+**C**
Delete	Ctrl+**D**
C**e**nter	Ctrl+**E**
Find	Ctrl+**F**
Go to	Ctrl+**G**
Replace	Ctrl+**H**
Italics	Ctrl+**I**
Justify (Full **J**ustify)	Ctrl+**J**
Insert Hyperlin**k**	Ctrl+**K**
Left Align (**L**eft Justify)	Ctrl+**L**
Indent	Ctrl+**M**
New Page	Ctrl+**N**
Open a Document	Ctrl+**O**
Print	Ctrl+**P**
Right Align (**R**ight Justify)	Ctrl+**R**
Save	Ctrl+**S**
Tab	Ctrl+**T**
Underline–**U**nderscore	Ctrl+**U**
Paste (**V**elcro)	Ctrl+**V**
"Do You **W**ant to Save Changes?"	Ctrl+**W**
Cut	Ctrl+**X**
Redo	Ctrl+**Y**
Undo	Ctrl+**Z**

Additional Common Office Tasks

Office has some additional common tasks that cross all applications and that are covered in the chapter on Word. These tasks relate to the Insert, **Page Layout,** and **Review tabs** and include such items as spelling and grammar checker, thesaurus, comments, page orientation, margins, and inserting clip art and pictures.

Summary

This chapter presented some standard commands that are used in applications in the Windows 7—Office 2010 environment. It described the online help provided in applications. Common tab and group commands were presented that show how to perform such tasks as opening, creating, closing, saving, finding and replacing words, and printing files. In addition, the cut/copy/paste and drag-and-drop functions to move or copy data from one file to another in the same and different applications were presented. These commands and tasks cross applications and provide some consistency when working in this environment.

Exercises 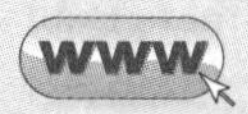

EXERCISE 1 Using Online Help in an Application

Objectives

1. Use the various forms of Help available in application programs.
2. Navigate through the Help screens.
3. Compare different ways of using online Help.

Activity

1. Find help in Microsoft Office Word 2010.
   a. Start **Word**. Make sure you are connected to the Internet for this exercise to work.
   b. Click the **Help** button on right of the tabs on the ribbon. The Word Help window appears.
   c. Click **Create a document**.
   d. Look for the option **Start a document from a template**.
   e. **Click** it and read the material provided.
   f. Click the **Home** button on the toolbar. The original window appears.
   g. Type **open document from template** in the Search text box.
   h. Click **Search.** A list of topics appears.
   i. Click **Create a memo**. Instructions for creating a memo appear.
   j. Click **Start a memo from a template**.
   k. Review the information.
   l. Click the **Home** button on the toolbar.
   m. Click the **arrow** in the Search box. Review the list of past searches there.
   n. Close the **Help** screen.

Do you prefer looking at a list of topics or did you prefer using the search bar for the information needed? Why?

2. Find help in Excel 2010.
   a. Start **Excel**.
   b. Click the **Help** button on the far right of the tabs bar.
   c. Click the **Table of Contents** button on the toolbar. A table of contents appears. Note that if the book icon is open the Table of Contents pane should already be open on the left side of the screen.
   d. Click **Getting started with Excel 2010**.
   e. Click **What's New in Excel 2010**. A summary of an article appears.
   f. Click **Microsoft Office Backstage view.** Review the material.
   g. Close the Table of Contents task pane by clicking the **open book**.
   h. Type **create a workbook** in the Search text box and click the **Search** button.

i. Click **Video: Create a workbook**. Make sure there is an active Internet connection. Click the **Start** button.
j. Listen to the video. Click the **Close** button.
k. Close the Overview-Training window by clicking the **Close** button.
l. Close the **Help** window and then close **Excel**.

What were the similarities between this Help command and the one from Activity 1 with Word?

3. Obtain additional help without using the Help button.
   a. Open **Word**.
   b. Place the mouse pointer over the Line spacing button in the **Paragraph** group in the **Home** tab. Do *not* click.

What happens after a few seconds? What is this called? When would you use this feature?

4. Have more practice in finding additional help in Word.
   a. Open **Word** if necessary.
   b. Click the **Help** button on the far right of the tabs bar. Make sure there is an active Internet connection. The Help window appears.
   c. Type **format a document** in the Search text box and click **Search**. Your results are displayed.
   d. Click **Word 2010 Formatting** Text – Lesson 3. Review the four pages and watch the video.
   e. Close **Help**.
   f. Close online help.
5. Use Office Online for Training (Figure 4-7a).
   a. Make sure Word **Help** is open.
   b. Click the **Table of Contents** button.
   c. Click **Training courses** in the Table of Contents. You will need to scroll down to find it.
   d. Click **Word 2010 tips and tricks.**
   e. **Click** the **Start this course** Start this course →.
   f. Print the **Quick Reference Card** at the end of the lesson. Review the contents.
   g. Close all **open windows.**

EXERCISE 2 Common Tasks: Create, Open, Close, Find, Print, Save

■ **Objectives**

1. Create a new document using the File tab, New option or the New button on the Quick Access Toolbar.
2. Use the commands from the File tab menu and the Quick Access Toolbar to open, close, print, and save a file.

3. Use the Find and Replace command to replace text and the Windows Find command to locate a file.

■ Activity

1. Start an application.
   a. Click **Start**, **All Programs**, **Microsoft Office**, and **Microsoft Office Word 2010**. Other methods may be used to open Word. Use the technique that is appropriate for the computer being used.
   b. Type **I'm learning how to create a new word processing document using Word 2010**.
   c. Click the **File** tab.
   d. Click **Save** button Save.
   e. Select **Documents** or whatever folder and storage device are used for this class. (This could be a folder created for another chapter with the name of your course.)
   f. In the File name text box, type **Learning Word**.
   g. Click **Save**.
2. Open and save another document.
   a. Click **New** in the Quick Access Toolbar (If the button is not there, right-click the **File** tab and choose **Customize Quick Access Toolbar**. Then click **New**, **Add**, and **OK**.)
   b. Type: **I'm creating this second document to tell you about why I entered the healthcare field**.
   c. Press **Ctrl+S**.
   d. Select the appropriate folder and storage device as directed by the professor.
   e. In the File name text box, type **Choosing a Healthcare Profession**.
   f. Click **Save** or press **Enter**.
3. Open, edit, and save an existing document.
   a. Click the **File** tab.
   b. Click **Learning Word** under Recent Documents. (If this file is not visible, make sure that the correct storage device and folder are selected.)
   c. Edit the document by adding a sentence or two stating what you want to learn about Word.
   d. Click **Save** under the **File** tab or press **Ctrl+S**. Notice the Save As dialog box did not appear because the file already has a name and location. The file was just updated. The file remains open.
4. Print the document.
   a. Click the **File** tab and move the pointer to **Print**. What are your choices?
   b. Select **Print** from the menu. What happened?

5. Open and edit the second document.
   a. Click the **File** tab
   b. Click **Choosing a Healthcare Profession** under Recent Documents. (If this file is not visible, make sure the correct storage device and folder are selected.)
   c. Click the **File** tab and then **Save As**. The Save As window appears.
   d. Type **Nursing** or your healthcare major in the File name text box and press **Enter** or click **Save**. The file now has a new name.
6. Find and replace text.
   a. Make sure the **Choosing a Healthcare Profession** file is open.
   b. Click **Replace** in the **Editing** group on the **Home** tab.
   c. Click **More** [More >>].
   d. Type the words **healthcare field** in the Find what text box.
   e. Tab to the Replace with box.
   f. Type the lowercase word **nursing** or your **healthcare major** in the Replace with text box.
   g. Click **Find Next** in the dialog box.
   h. Click **Replace**. (Be very careful when using Replace All. Undesired things can happen to the document.) A message appears stating that Word has finished searching the document.
   i. Click **OK** and then click **Close** in the dialog box. Notice what happened to the Word document.
   j. Click **Save** to save the file.
7. To close a document.
   a. Click the **File** tab, then click **Close** or click the **Close** button at the top of the window to close the document. You will also exit Word if this is the only Word document that is open.
8. Find a file using the Windows search feature.
   Sometimes it is easier to locate a file by using the Windows search feature.

On the hard drive:

   a. Click the **Start** button. The Start menu opens.
   b. Type **Learning Word** in the Search text box. As you type, files appear above the Search text box.
   c. Click the **Learning Word** document. The document opens provided it was stored on the hard drive during Activity 1.

On a removable storage device:

   a. Double-click **Computer**, which should be located on the desktop, or from the **Start button, Computer** option.
   b. Click the **removable storage device** where you are storing your files.

c. Type **Learning Word** in the Search text box.
d. Click the **Date modified down arrow** key on the contextual toolbar and select today's date. Note the other options available.
e. Double-click the **Learning Word** document. The document opens provided it was stored on the removable storage device during Activity 1e.
f. Close all **open windows.**

EXERCISE 3 Copy and Move Data Using Cut/Copy/Paste and Drag and Drop

Objectives

1. Copy and move text from one place in the document to another using the clipboard.
2. Copy and move text from one place in the document to another using drag and drop.
3. Copy text from one document to another.

Activity

1. Start the program and enter text or retrieve a file.
   a. Start Microsoft Office Word 2010. Select **Start**, **Programs**, **Microsoft Office**, and then **Microsoft Office Word**. Use the default Word setting for font (Calibri, 11 points).
   b. *If you are not using the Copy-Move file from the textbook Web site (Chapter4-Exercise3-Physicians.docx), use the following to create your document: If using the Copy-Move file, go to 1e.* Type **Understanding how to copy and move data is an important skill that can save the user time.**
   c. Press the **Enter** key twice.
   d. Type the **following text**, pressing the **Tab** key between items and the **Enter** key at the end of the row.
   Below is a list of physicians and their associated specialty. Please use the beeper number to access these physicians during off-hours.

Dr. M. Smith	**Orthopedics**	***4567**	**Monday/Wednesday/Friday**
Dr. K. Bones	**Orthopedics**	***4512**	**Tuesday/Thursday/Saturday**
Dr. P. Roberts	**Oncology**	***5678**	**Sunday**
Dr. Z. White	**Internal Med**	***3489**	**All week**

   e. If you created the file, click the **Save** button and name the file **Chap4-Exercise4-CM with Drag** or if you opened the Copy-Move file from the textbook Web site, rename the file **Chap4-Exercise3-CM with Drag** using the **Save As** command.

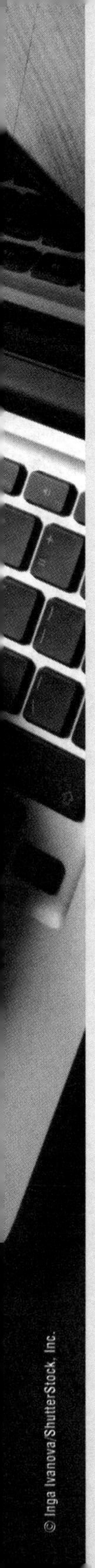

2. Move text using drag and drop.
   a. Select the **Dr. Smith** line. (The quickest way to do this is to place the pointer in the Quick Select area. Place the pointer out at the margin across from Dr. M. Smith; when the pointer is a right-slanted arrow, **click**.)
   b. Place the pointer on the **highlighted** area. Hold down the left mouse button and drag the selection to the **blank line below the "D" in "Dr. Z. White."** Release the mouse button. If the Enter key was not pressed after the last line, you will not be able to move to the line below "Dr. White." Place your cursor to the right of "k" in "week" and place text there. **Click** to the left of the "D" in "Dr. M. Smith," and press **Enter**. "Dr. M. Smith" is now at the end of the list.
3. Move text using the clipboard.
   a. Select the second line of text in the list, which begins with Dr. P. Roberts.
   b. Click the **Cut** button .
   c. Click to the left of **"Dr. M. Smith"** so the blinking vertical line is to the left of the "D." Do not select the entire line.
   d. With the insertion point to the left of the "D" in "Dr. M. Smith," click the **Paste** button Paste. The list should now look like the one shown in **Figure 4-17**.
4. Copy text using drag and drop.
   a. Go to the **end** of the document (Press **Ctrl+End.**).
   b. Press the **Enter** key twice to create two blank lines.
   c. Type the **following information**, remembering to use the Tab key between items and the Enter key to go to the next line.

Chris Walker	**Nursing Assistant**
Mary Robb	**Registered Nurse**
Lee Dock	**Nurse Practitioner**

   d. Click the **Save** button .
   e. Select the **first line of text** in this list (**"Chris Walker"** through **"Assistant"**).

Dr. K. Bones	Orthopedics	*4512	Tuesday/Thursday/Saturday
Dr. Z. White	Internal Med	*3489	All week
Dr. P. Roberts	Oncology	*5678	Sunday
Dr. M. Smith	Orthopedics	*4567	Monday/Wednesday/Friday

Figure 4-17 Results of Moving Text with Drag and Drop

f. Place the pointer over the **selected text**.
g. Hold down the **Ctrl** key and the **left mouse button**, and drag the text so that the broken vertical bar is to the left of "**Mary**."
h. Release the **mouse button** and then the **Ctrl** key. The text is copied.
i. Highlight **Chris** in the second row, and type **Brian**.

5. Copy text using the clipboard.
   a. Select the text from "**Mary Robb**" through "**Registered Nurse**."
   b. Click the **Copy** button.
   c. Move the pointer to the left of the "L" in "Lee Dock" and click. Do not highlight the text.
   d. Click the **Paste** button.
   e. Highlight the second **Mary** and type **Nancy**.
   f. Click the **Save** button to save the document.
6. Copy text from one document to another.
   a. Select all the **text** from "**Chris**" through "**Practitioner**."
   b. Click the **Copy** button.
   c. Click the **New** document button on the Quick Access Toolbar or the Office button menu.
   d. Click the **Paste** button. The text is now inserted into a new Word document.
   e. Save the document as **Chap4-Exercise3-CMwithClipboard2**.
7. Copy text from one application to another.
   a. Click **Start**, **All Programs**, **Microsoft Office**, **Excel** (or use one of the shortcut techniques to open Excel).
   b. Click the **Paste** button. The contents of the clipboard are now inserted into an Excel worksheet. Columns will need to be enlarged to see all the data. Names should be in column A and Job title in column B unless you added two tabs between items forcing the Job title to column C. There is more on tabs and their settings in the Word chapter.
8. Close all **files** and **programs**. There is no need to save anything again unless requested to do so by your professor.

EXERCISE 4 Customizing the Quick Access Toolbar

Objective

1. Customize the Quick Access Toolbar to contain tools you need.

Activity

1. Click the **Customize Quick Access Toolbar** down arrow to the right of the QAT.
2. Think about what commands you use frequently and that are sometimes difficult to find.

3. Add two more commands to the QAT. For example, add the spelling and grammar command and print preview.
4. Open **Excel**. Where are those commands found on the QAT in Excel? What does this mean? How would you go about finding additional commands not on the drop-down menu?

Assignments

ASSIGNMENT 1 Using Help

■ **Directions**

1. Use the Excel online Help feature to learn about charts in Excel. Click "**Charts**" under "**Browse Excel 2010 support**" and review the material. Review any other feature in which you are interested.
2. Print one or two appropriate Help screens for future reference.
3. Using Word, Excel, or PowerPoint, find out how to insert a SmartArt diagram in a Word document, Excel spreadsheet, or PowerPoint presentation. Use the online Help feature to learn how to complete this task in each application.
4. Open **WordPad** (**Start**, **All Programs**, **Accessories**, and **WordPad**). Copy and paste the directions for inserting SmartArt from the Help screen into the WordPad document. Make a note regarding the source of this material. Save the document as **Insert SmartArt** and print it.
5. Submit the printouts from Steps 2 and 4.

ASSIGNMENT 2 Finding Additional Help

■ **Directions**

1. Sometimes Office Help does not provide information in a manner understandable to the user. Select a topic from this chapter (or something you always wanted to know how to do in Office). Use the Internet to search for a user guide, directions, or a video, on the selected topic. Do not use Microsoft's Web site.
2. Provide your classmates with the URL (link) to the directions you found and a reason why this is a great source for learning that concept.
3. Submit your work following the directions provided by the professor.

ASSIGNMENT 3 Copy and Move Text

Directions

1. Create a one-page document describing how to perform the following tasks. Each description should take the form of its own paragraph in the document. Type your name on the document.
   - Save a document.
   - Print a document.
   - Create a new document.
   - Move text in a document.
2. Save the original document as **Chap4-Assign3-CM-LastName** and then print it.
3. Using the move text feature of the program, rearrange the text as follows:
   - Create a new document.
   - Move text in a document.
   - Save a document.
   - Print a document.
4. Save the document as **Chap4-Assign3-CMRev-LastName**. Print the revised document. Submit both documents in either print or electronic form.

chapter

5

Introduction to Word Processing

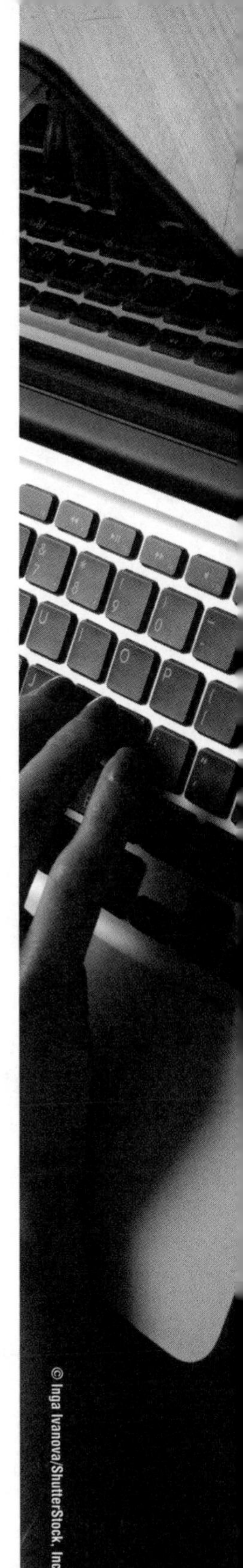

Objectives

1. Describe the basic functions of a word processing program and the types of projects that are best managed by using it.
2. Define common terms related to word processing.
3. Use appropriate keyboard shortcuts to speed up document creation and editing.
4. Describe the basic Word window and related navigational functions.
5. Create, format, edit, save, spell check, and print Word documents.
6. Use the appropriate features when creating Word documents.

Introduction

A word processing program permits us to manipulate text and related objects such as pictures. If the need to use mathematical processes to manipulate numbers or to manage data, then a word processing program is not the correct application to use. The main purpose of a word processing program is to permit the user to create text documents, edit (insert, delete, and replace) text and objects, format the document to increase readability and appearance, print a copy of the document, and save the document for future use or reference. This chapter provides the basics of word processing using Microsoft Word 2010.

Definitions

Understanding some of the common concepts related to text manipulation makes using the help system easier and increases your problem-solving skills when things go wrong.

Block — A **block** is a selected (highlighted) section of text that the program treats as a unit. You can apply most individual formatting functions, such as bold and underline, to blocks of text, thereby making formatting and editing functions more efficient.

Clipboard — A **clipboard** is a holding area or buffer for copied or cut data for later use. You can place data onto a clipboard and then paste it into another document, another application, or another location within the original document. In Office 2010, the Office Clipboard can hold as many as 24 items at a time (see Chapter 4 for details).

Format — **Formatting** is the process of editing the appearance of a document by altering the look of fonts and using indentations, margins, tabs, justification, and pagination; format conditions affect the document appearance. In Word, format features vary depending on whether you are formatting characters (font, size, emphasis, and special effects such as highlight or superscript/subscript), paragraphs (tabs, alignment, indentation, line spacing, and line breaks), or pages (headers, footers, margins, paper size, and orientation).

Hard Return — The **hard return** is a code that you insert in the document by pressing the Enter key. A hard return usually marks the end of a paragraph. In Word, the paragraph mark is ¶. Users may toggle the paragraph markers on to show marks in the document when typing or toggle them off by clicking the Show/Hide button ¶ in the Paragraph group of the Home tab. To always show the Show/Hide feature click **File** tab, **Options**, **Display**, and place a check in the **Always show Paragraph marks** check box.

Insert — To **insert** means to add characters in the text at the point of the cursor, thereby moving all other text to the right. Insert mode is the opposite of overtype mode and is the default in most word processing programs. In Office 2010, the Insert tab is next to the Home tab on the ribbon; use it to insert pages, tables, illustrations, links, and so forth.

Move — **Move** is a function in word processing programs that permits the user to relocate text or graphics to another place in the document or to another document.

Outliner — **Outliner** is a feature of many word processing programs that enables the user to plan and rearrange large documents in an outline form.

Overtype — **Overtype** means to replace the character under the cursor by the character typed. To turn it off, click the **File** tab, click **Options,** click **Advanced,** and clear the **Use the Insert Key** and **Use Overtype Mode** check boxes.

ScreenTips — **ScreenTips** are small windows that display descriptive text when you rest the pointer on a command or icon. Office 2010 offers enhanced ScreenTips with larger windows and more text.

Scrolling — **Scrolling** is the process of moving around a document to view a specific portion of a page of text when the entire document does not fit on the screen. This navigation process does not change the location of the insertion point until the user clicks elsewhere in the document.

SmartArt — **SmartArt** is a feature in Office 2010 that permits you to easily create a visual representation of your information. It is commonly used to display the organizational structure of an organization.

Soft Return — A **soft return** is the code that the program inserts in the document automatically when the typed line reaches the right margin.

Template — A **template** contains predesigned formats and structure. It creates a copy of itself when you open it. When you select **File, New** you will see a list of templates with more available online at Office.com. Some commons ones are budgets, calendars, memos, and resumes.

Toggle	Toggling switches from one mode of operation to another mode: on or off. For example, a user might **toggle** from insert mode to replace/overtype mode.
Word Wrap	This feature automatically carries words over to the next line if they extend beyond the margin.

Data Exchange

Word processing software saves documents in file formats that are unique to that software program. Office 2010 documents, worksheets, and presentations are saved in XML with extensions that end in *x* or *m*. The *x* indicates an XML file that has no macros. An *m* indicates the file contains a macro. Many word processing programs allow the option of saving documents under another file format by using the Save As feature. For example, you can save a Microsoft Word 2010 document in several ways, such as a Word 2010 document (docx), Word template (dotx), rich text format (rtf), Word 97–2003 (doc), PDF (pdf), or Word XML (xml). This feature permits you to exchange a file with others who are working with different word processing programs, versions, or systems. It also permits you to save a word processing file as a Web page (htm or html). Other file formats are also available. By default, Word 2010 uses the *docx* format.

Saving Work

Every person probably has at least one horror story that he or she can tell about lost data or documents. To avoid accidental loss of data, follow these tips:

1. Periodically save your work. When typing a document, the computer holds that document temporarily in **random-access memory (RAM)**. Once you instruct the program to save the document on a storage device, the document exists both in RAM and on the storage device. If power goes off (even temporarily), you lose all the data in RAM. While you can set your Office programs to use the **AutoRecover** feature, this is not a substitute for regularly saving your work through the Save command. AutoRecover does not replace the Save command; it is only effective for unplanned disruptions, such as a power outage or a crash. AutoRecover files are not designed to be saved when you close the program in an orderly fashion. Conversely, you do not lose data stored on secondary storage devices unless that medium gets corrupted.
2. Pay attention to software warnings. These warnings are hints to remind you that doing certain things will have a predetermined result. For example, saving a document with the same name as another one results in a message

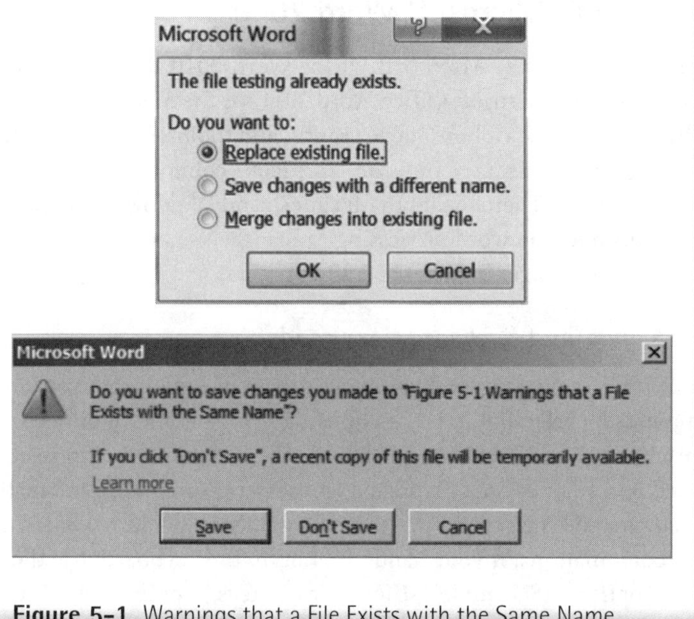

Figure 5-1 Warnings that a File Exists with the Same Name

asking whether the file is to be replaced (**Figure 5-1**). Do not respond with "Replace existing file" unless you have no need for the original document.

3. Always keep a backup or duplicate copy of a document. That backup could consist of a CD, USB storage device, or another hard drive. Store the backup in a different place. If something happens to the original document or the computer, the backup copy will then be available for restoring the data. A particularly valuable document, such as a thesis or research paper, should have a backup that you keep in a different location from the primary document. Many options for automatic backup are available today from places like MozyHome, MediaFire, or SkyDrive. If you select an online backup service, do your homework first. Some people will also send a copy of the document to themselves as an email attachment thereby having it in another place, the mail server.
4. Word 2010 AutoSaves a document as a draft for four days when you choose Don't Save or exit without saving. To find it click File, Recent, and click the box **Recover Unsaved Documents** at the bottom of the page. Again, these files may not be perfect or as you remembered them when you retrieve them.

Introduction to Microsoft Word 2010

Examples in this text use Microsoft Office Word 2010 for Windows 7. (See **Figure 5-2a**.) Using Microsoft Office Word 2011 for the Macintosh, however, is essentially the same; the ribbons, tabs, groups, and toolbars include most of the same headings and icons. (See **Figure 5-2b**.) Icons common to all applications appear on the ribbon. Therefore, both Macintosh and Windows users can use the chapters in this book on word processing, spreadsheets, and graphics presentation with very few changes between operating systems.

Ribbons, Menus, and Keyboard Commands

Most word processing programs are menu driven, meaning that you can carry out commands by selecting icons or choosing from a menu of options. Menu-driven programs provide you with two options—use the mouse to select items from the **ribbon** (menus) and command icons or use keystroke combinations to issue the command. The general rule is if your hands are on the keyboard, use the keystroke combinations; if your hands are not on the keyboard, use the mouse and ribbons options. (See **Table 4-1** for shortcut keys.) For example, **Ctrl+Enter** inserts a hard page break in a document. In the Macintosh operating system, the Apple key (or command key), which is next to the space bar, acts like the Ctrl key in the Windows system.

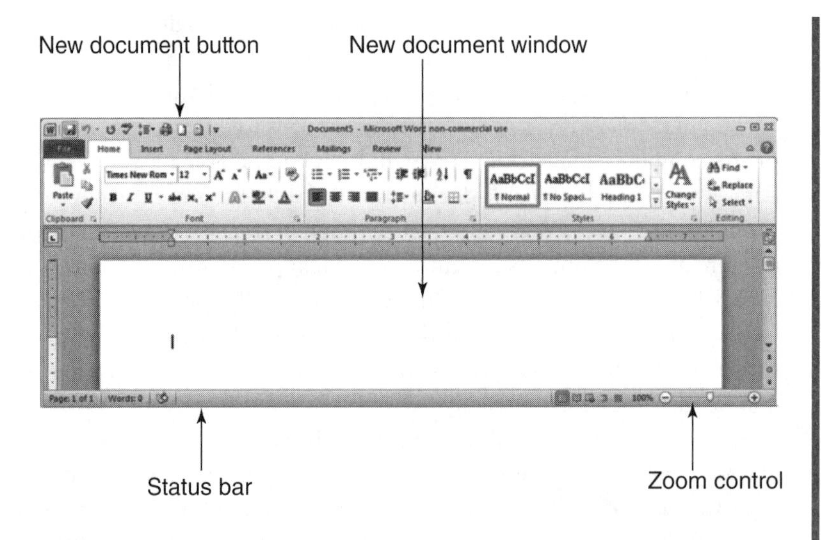

Figure 5-2a Microsoft Office Word 2010 Window, Home Tab Selected

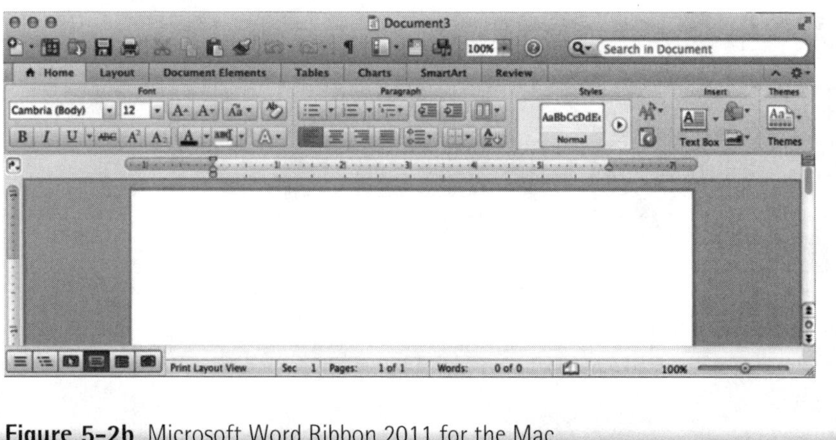

Figure 5-2b Microsoft Word Ribbon 2011 for the Mac

Starting Word

As with all Windows programs, there are many ways to start Word including the following. Chapter 4 also described several ways of opening a new or existing Word document.

1. Click **Start**, **Programs**. Select **Microsoft Office**, and then choose **MS Office Word** from the available options (Figure 4-7d).
2. Click the **Word** icon on the Quick Launch area of the taskbar if it appears there (Figure 4-8).

Creating a New Document

After starting Word, a new blank document opens by default. At this point, you can simply type and format the text as desired. Two methods to create a new document once you open Word follow:

1. Click the **File** tab and then **New**. A window appears (**Figure 5-3**). Click **Blank document** and a new document appears formatted using the normal template. Note the choices available for a new document under Templates.
2. Add the **New** document button to the Quick Access Toolbar. Click the **File** tab, choose **Options, Quick Access Toolbar, New, Add** Add >>, and **OK**. Alternatively, you can click the **arrow** to the right of the Quick Access Toolbar. Click **New**. Now the New document button shows on the Quick Access Toolbar. Click the New button and the new document window appears. (See Figure 5-2a.)

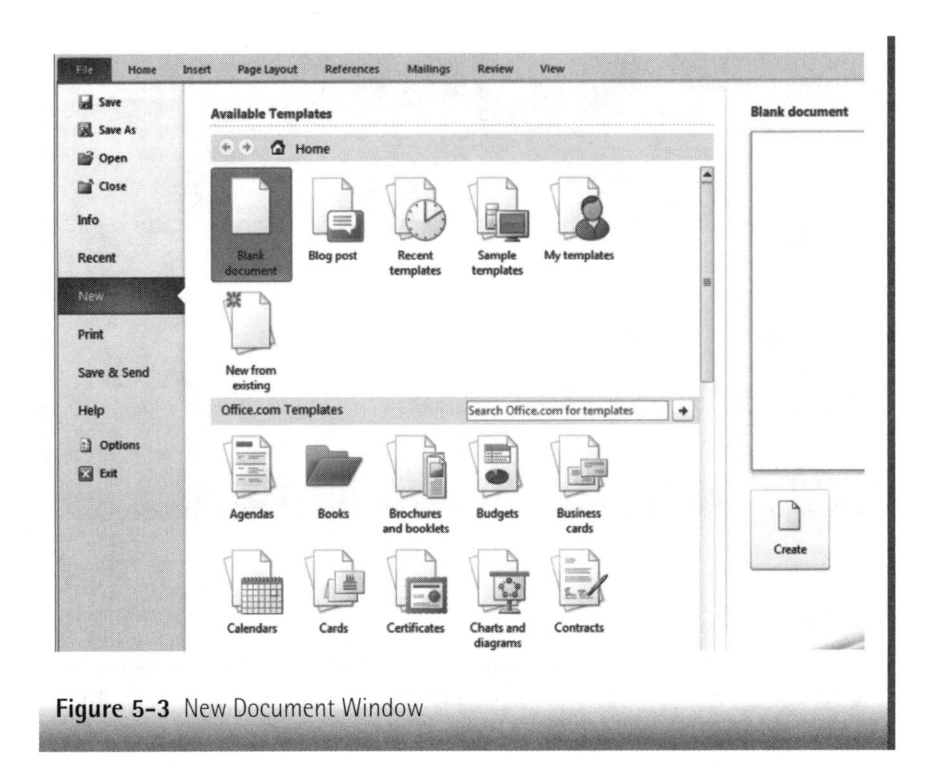

Figure 5-3 New Document Window

For each document, Word presents a screen with the ribbon at the top, a blank window or document workplace in the center, a scroll bar on the right side, and the status bar on the bottom. A blinking vertical bar, or insertion point marker, represents the position of the cursor in the document. In Figure 5-2a the cursor appears at the beginning of the document.

Opening a Previously Saved Document

When changes or additions are necessary in a document, several options are available for opening the document again after you saved it (see Chapter 4 for additional ways to open existing documents).

If the application is not open:

1. Start **Word** and click the **File** tab A list of Recent Documents appears on the right. Click the **desired document**.
2. Start **Word**, click the **File** tab, and choose **Open**. The Open dialog box appears (Figure 4-10) with a list of documents. Note that you can also choose Recently Changed; this choice brings up a complete list that includes the name of each document as well as its size, type, and date modified.
3. Go to the **location** of the file and double-click the **file** you want to open.

If Word is open:

1. Click the **File** tab and **Recent**. A list of Recent Documents appears (Figure 4-10).
2. If the file is not in the list of Recent Documents, click the **Open** button in File tab. The Open dialog box appears, allowing you to search and select the file to open (Figure 4-9).

The Ribbon in Word: Microsoft's "Fluent User Interface"

The Microsoft Word 2010 **ribbon** contains a series of task-oriented **tabs** and **groups** organized to keep like tasks together. (See **Figure 5-4**.) Each tab contains a different group of commands or tasks that help you to use Word. Use the Quick Access Toolbar to add frequently used commands like New, Spelling & Grammar check, and so forth. Following is a brief description of each tab and its groups in Word 2010. Note that the ribbon shows the groups by default. If you turned that option off and only see the tabs, click the Expand the Ribbon button on the far right of the Tabs.

Home	**Figure 5-4** shows the Home tab and its groups: Clipboard, Font, Paragraph, Styles, and Editing. These groups allow you to format the document by (1) cutting, copying, or pasting items to the clipboard; (2) selecting a font style, size, and color; (3) setting indents and spacing, adding bullets or numbers to a list, and adjusting text alignment; (4) selecting a document style; and (5) using Find and Replace.
Insert	The Insert tab (**Figure 5-5a**) has groups such as Pages, Tables, Illustrations, Links, Header & Footer, Text, and Symbols. You can add a cover page or insert a blank page, page break, table, chart, SmartArt, or clip art using this tab.

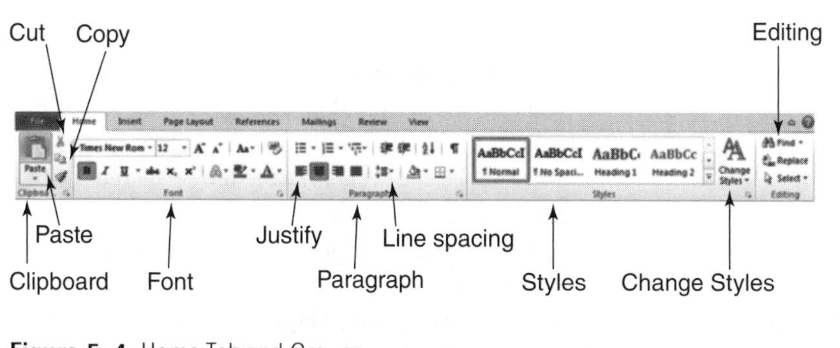

Figure 5-4 Home Tab and Groups

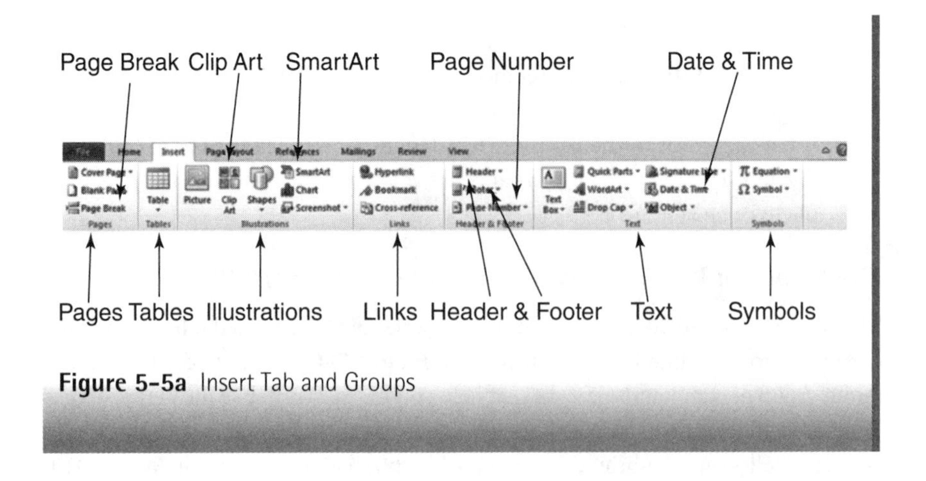

Figure 5-5a Insert Tab and Groups

Figure 5-5b shows the menu for adding a page number in a footer. Among other things you can use this ribbon to add a hyperlink, bookmark, text box, or the date and time.

Page Layout — **Figure 5-6** shows the **Page Layout tab** and its groups: Themes, Page Setup, Page Background, Paragraph, and Arrange. These groups help you select the font style and color, margins, page orientation, paragraph indents and spacing, and allow you to add watermarks, add a page border, or change the page color or arrangement.

References — The groups under the References tab (**Figure 5-7**) are: Table of Contents, Footnotes, Citations & Bibliography, Captions, Index, and Table of Authorities (cases, statutes). These groups help you add endnotes, footnotes, citations, index, and tables (content and authorities), and then update these items as necessary. For example, you can manage citation sources such as books, journals, or Web sites, insert the citation in the document, and choose the style for the source such as APA or MLA. In addition, you can automate the creation and updating of a table of contents for documents that require them.

Mailings — The Mailings groups (**Figure 5-8**) help you prepare envelopes, labels, mail merge letters, and recipient lists.

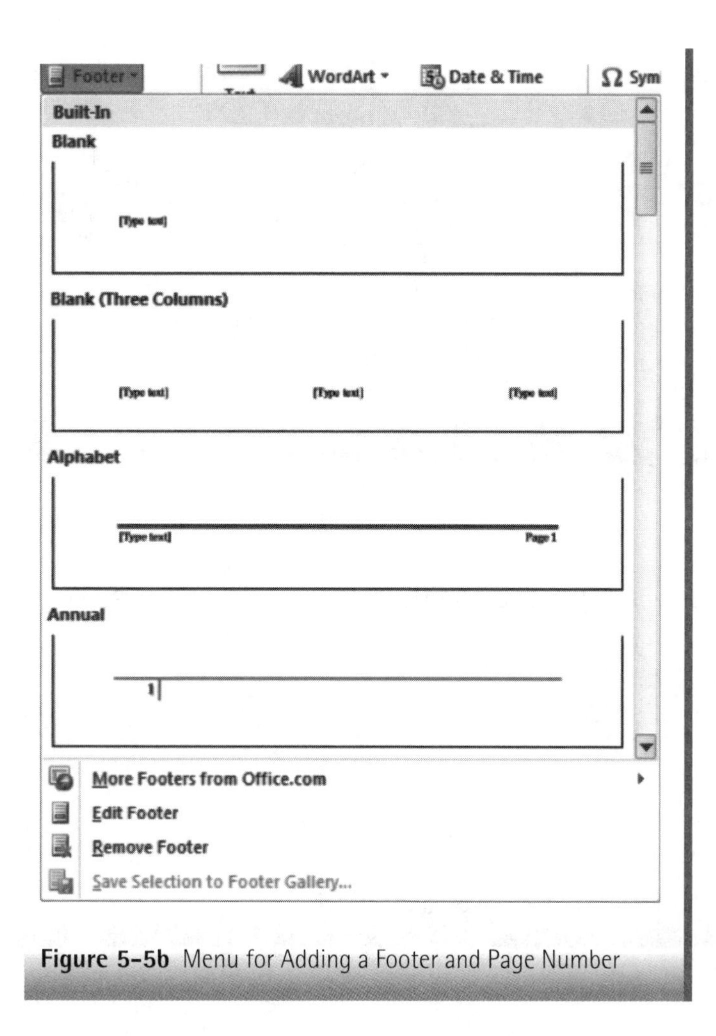

Figure 5-5b Menu for Adding a Footer and Page Number

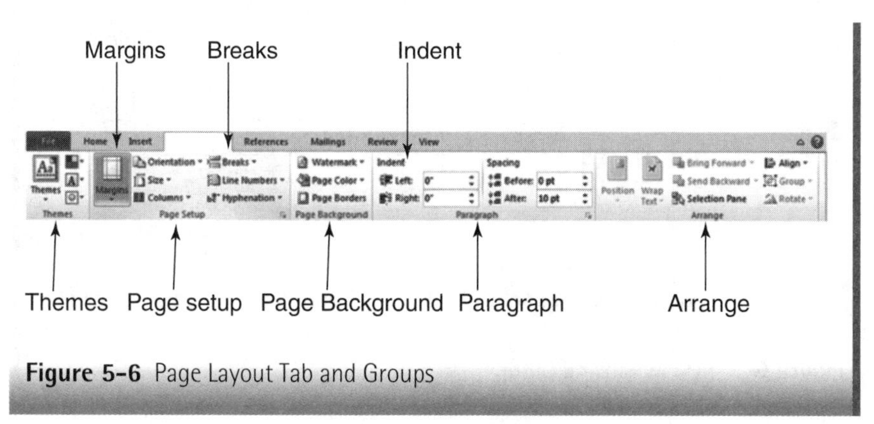

Figure 5-6 Page Layout Tab and Groups

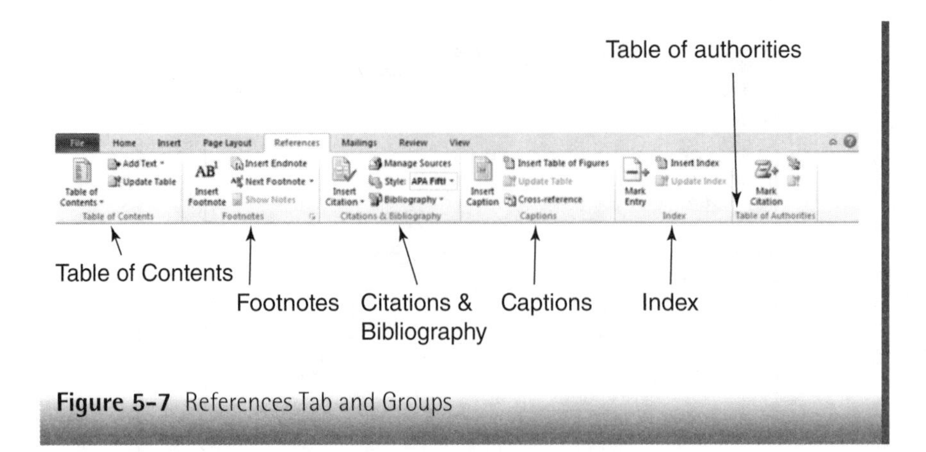

Figure 5-7 References Tab and Groups

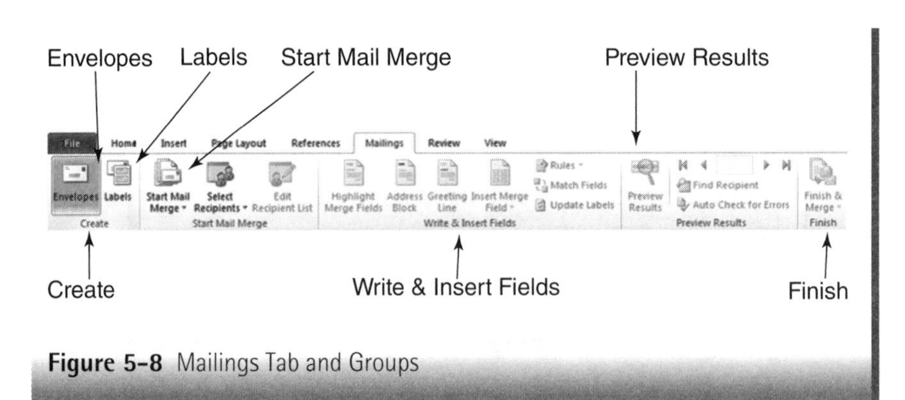

Figure 5-8 Mailings Tab and Groups

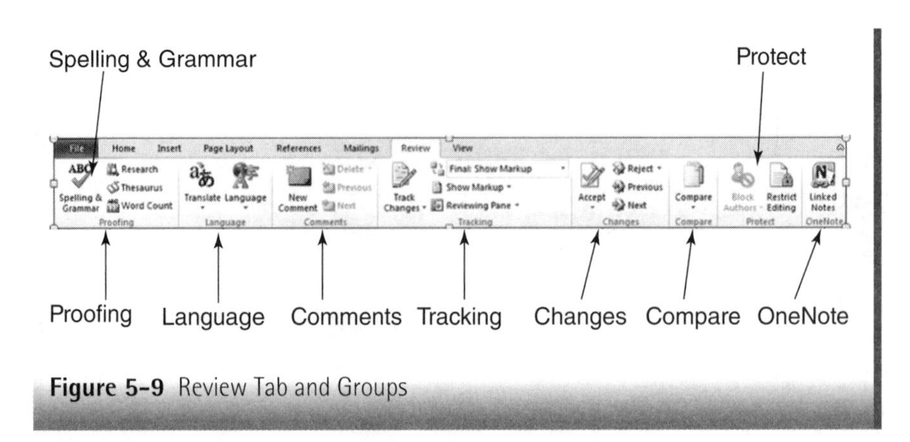

Figure 5-9 Review Tab and Groups

Review

You can use the Review tab for proofing a document (**Figure 5-9**); for example, these groups help you check spelling and grammar, do a word count, track changes, insert comments, enable ScreenTips for showing a word in another language, or protect a document from changes by someone else.

While not part of the Review tab, you may also use a readability index to test the readability level of the document. To set this option, click **File** tab, **Options**, **Proofing**, and **Show readability statistics**. Now, when you check the spelling and grammar of the document, a readability index will also appear. This consideration is very important when developing patient-education materials, however, this approach is not sufficient for measuring the health literacy level needed to understand the document. Chapter 14 further explains health literacy.

View

The **View tab** includes commands that allow you to view the document in print layout, full screen reading, Web layout, outline, or draft form. (See **Figure 5-10**.) The next group has commands to show or hide various items in Word, such as the ruler, gridlines, the message bar, the document map, and thumbnails. Zoom controls are in the Zoom group or on the status bar at the bottom of the window (Figure 5-2a). Options also allow you to view one or two pages of the document. The next group focuses on the window and provides ways to view a document or to switch between windows. The last group is Macros; a **macro** is an automated sequence of operations that can prove useful for repetitive tasks.

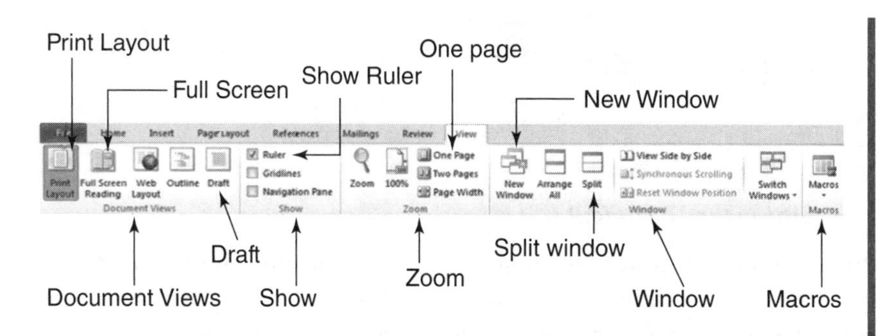

Figure 5-10 View Tab and Groups

Moving Around the Document

There are several ways to move around a document.

Arrow keys	Move the insertion point one line or letter at a time.
Ctrl + arrow keys	Move one word, section, or paragraph at a time.
Home key	Moves the cursor to the beginning of the line.
End key	Moves the cursor to the end of the line.
Ctrl+Home	Moves the cursor to the beginning of the document.
Ctrl+End	Moves the cursor to the end of the document.
Page Up and Page Down Keys	Move the cursor quickly through the document one screen at a time.
Ctrl+PageUp	Moves the cursor to the previous page.
Ctrl+PageDown	Moves the cursor to the next page.

At the right side of the document window is a **scroll bar** (Figure 5-2a). The View Ruler icon, at the top of the vertical scroll bar, toggles the ruler bar off and on. Dragging the elevator in the scroll bar moves you up or down the scroll line as quickly as desired. The single arrow in the scroll bar is used to move up or down one line at a time, but does not alter the location of the insertion point. Clicking the double arrows (chevrons) up or down moves you through the document a page at a time like the Crtl+PageUp and Crtl+PageDown keys. Clicking and dragging the dotted triangle on the lower-right corner of the window (when the window doesn't fill the screen) allows you to change the dimensions of the window as do the double-headed arrows on a window border. If you click on the title bar and drag, you can move the window around the screen.

NOTE: A scroll wheel on a mouse will also let you scroll through a document by moving the wheel back and forth.

Formatting the Document

By using formatting-related commands, the document can be made to look professional at the same time it makes the message in the document more understandable. There are four components to formatting—character, paragraph, page, and document.

Character Formatting

The following terms describe the components of fonts and the options for character formatting.

Font — A **font** defines a descriptive look or shape (font face or typeface), size, and style of a group of characters or symbols. For example, one font is Times Roman, 12 point, Bold, Italic. Another font is Calibri, 10 point, Italic. The default font for Word 2010 is Calibri. The general rule is to limit the number of different fonts in one document to three. Use serif fonts (fonts with little feet) for text documents; this makes the document easier to read.

Size refers to the height of the characters and is measured in 72 points per inch. Normal sizes for business documents are 10 to 12 points; Word's default is 11 points.

Style or attributes include bold, italics, and condensed. Use these attributes for emphasis—not for the whole document.

Spacing — Proportional or fixed pitch spacing. Proportional means a variable amount of space is allotted for each character depending on the character width. Fixed space or monospace means a set space is provided for each character regardless of the character width. For example, an *I* is allowed the same amount of space as a *W*.

Special Effects — Word provides the user with the ability to apply special effects to characters. Some of these special effects are: superscript, subscript, strikethrough, highlight, color, and small caps. Use these as appropriate for the document and the message. Use color only when printing on a color printer or moving the document around electronically. A black and white printer needs to interpret the colors, sometimes making them not easily readable in black and white.

Symbol Set — The characters and symbols that make up the font is called the **symbol set**.

Typeface — A **typeface** is the specific design of a character or symbol, commonly referred to as the font face. For example, Helvetica, Courier, Times Roman, Times Roman Bold, and Times Roman Italic are all different typefaces.

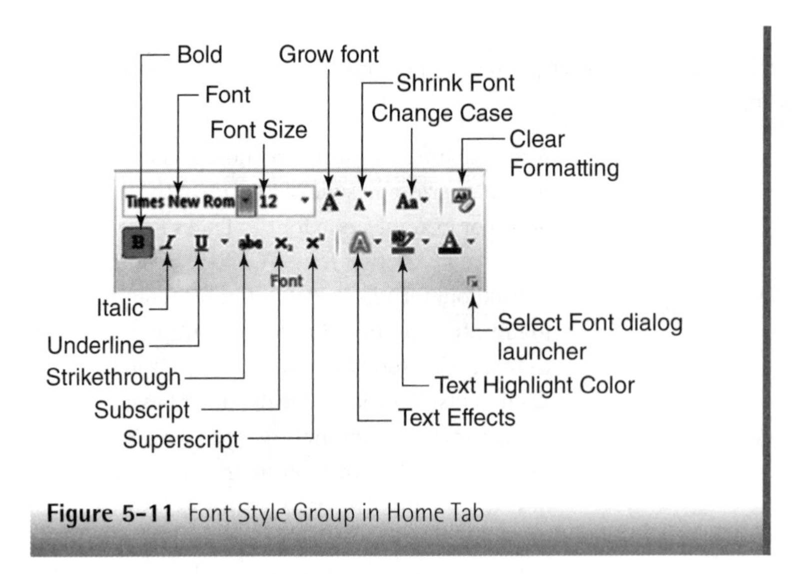

Figure 5-11 Font Style Group in Home Tab

To format a character—font size and style

As in previous examples, you can choose the font size and style in several different ways.

- Select the **text** to apply the font and size. Click the **Home** tab. Choose a **font** and **size** from the Font group (**Figure 5-11**).
- Click the **dialog launcher** in the Font group and the Font dialog box appears (**Figure 5-12**). You can select a font, font style, size, effects, color, and character spacing in this dialog box. You can also choose a default font style and size that will be the default style for all documents. By default, the font size for business documents is 10 to 12 points, but you may also choose a larger size that can be easily read on the screen if you like. Later, you can change the font if necessary. For example, you can highlight the entire document by choosing **Select** in the **Editing** group and then **Select All** (or press **Ctrl+A**) and reduce the print size before printing by choosing another font size or print style or both.
- Style buttons are available in the Font group for bold, italic, and underline (Figure 5-11).

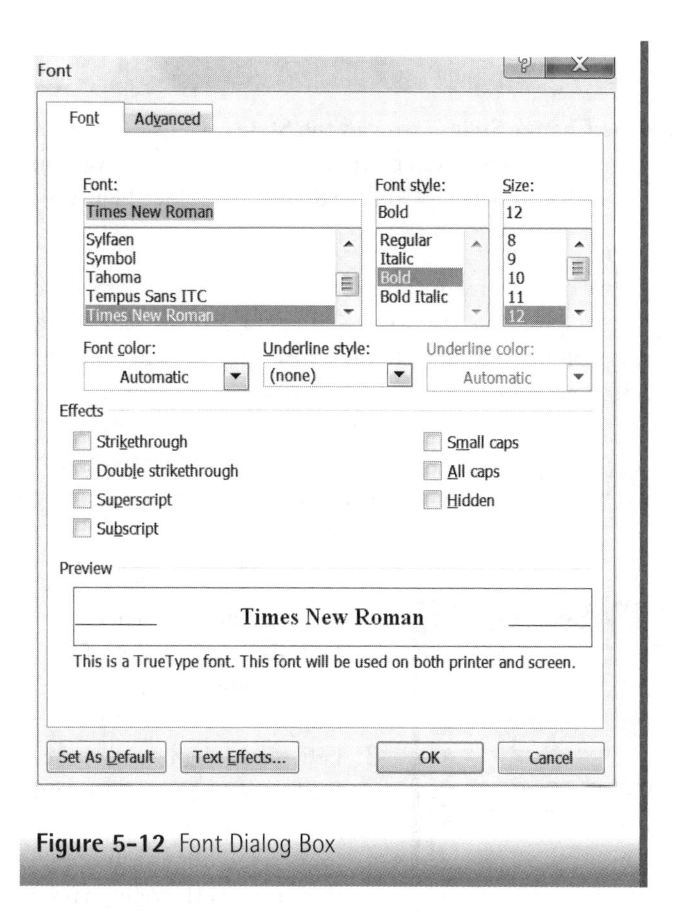

Figure 5-12 Font Dialog Box

To use the Style buttons for bold, italic, and underline:

1. Highlight a **word** or **section of text**.
2. Click the desired **Style** button that appears. You can use the **Style** button in the **Font** group to change style attributes. Alternatively, when you highlight a word, a small toolbar will appear as you hold the mouse arrow over the highlighted word; you can then choose bold, italic, or another font size from among the other choices on the toolbar.
3. Clicking a **Style button** again will change the style back to its previous style. You can turn these attributes on or off by pressing **Ctrl+B** (bold), **Ctrl+I** (italic), or **Ctrl+U** (underline). Note also that the underline button underlines all the highlighted text. To access variations of underlining, use the Font dialog launcher and select the desired underlining.

4. Click the **Change Styles** arrow in the **Styles** group to select a style, color, and font for text. Even more styles and choices are available when you click the dialog launcher in the **Styles** group. (See **Figure 5-13**.)

Paragraph Formatting

Just as there are options for formatting the characters, there are options for formatting paragraphs. Note that we define a paragraph by the ending paragraph mark ¶. Paragraph formatting includes justification, indents, lists, line spacing, borders, shading, and tabs.

Alignment Justified text is aligned relative to the left and right margins. There are four options for justification:

1. Center places the paragraph equidistant from both margins.
2. Full is alignment of the paragraph flush against both the left and right margins.
3. Left is alignment of the paragraph flush against the left margin and staggered on the right.
4. Right is alignment of the paragraph flush against the right margin and staggered on the left.

Borders Word provides you with the option to place a **border** around a paragraph to highlight or make that paragraph stand out. One can choose a line style, width, or color for the border.

Indent To **indent** text means to establish tab settings that place subsequent lines of text the same number of

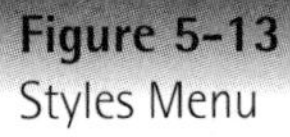

Figure 5-13
Styles Menu

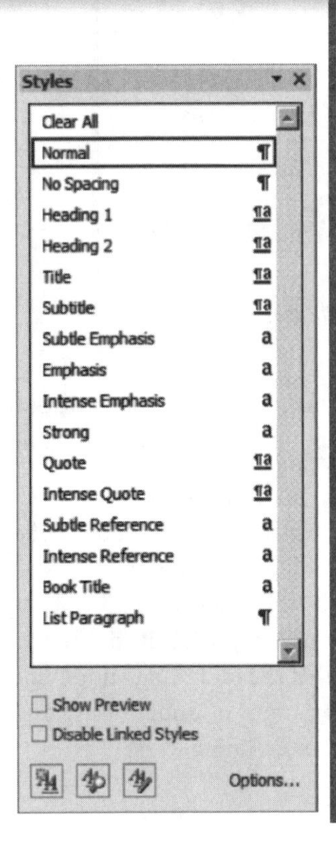

spaces from the margin until the next hard return. Word has four indents: first line, left, right, and hanging (**Figure 5-14**). The ruler displays these indent markers. Dragging the top indent marker to the right (first line indent) indents the first line of a paragraph; pressing the Tab key does the same thing. The middle marker is the left indent marker; use it to indent all lines of the paragraph except the first one. The top and middle markers will move together with the bottom marker when you select and move it. The middle marker is the hanging indent when you place it to the right of the first line indent marker. To apply a hanging indent (to the right of the first line), drag the middle marker to the right of the first line indent marker. A hanging indent will indent all lines of a paragraph except the first line.

Line Spacing

Line spacing is the space between lines or the space before or after each paragraph. By default Word assigns line spacing of 1.15 and 10 points after a paragraph. Most style manuals require double spacing for lines of text.

Lists

Word provides for bulleted, numbered, and multilevel **lists** that can turn your text into lists of items. Automatic bulleting and numbering can be helpful—and frustrating! For example, you might want to stop the list and then start another list later in the document. Word will pick up the previous number and continue numbering from it until you adjust the settings.

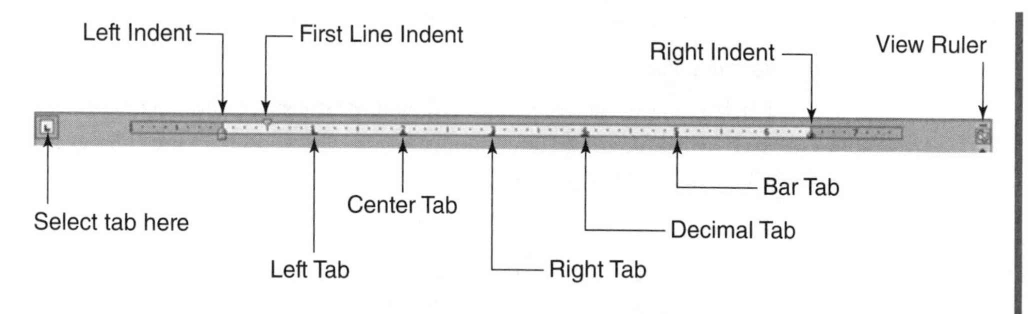

Figure 5-14 Ruler with Indents and Tabs

Shading	**Shading** means to set a paragraph in a color. Use it to highlight an important paragraph or give a box look to the paragraph.
Tab	A **tab** is a setting that places the subsequent text on that line a certain number of spaces or inches in from the left margin. Tab settings by default are five spaces (0.5 inch) although they are not visible to you. These settings can be changed, however. Five styles of tabs are available—left ( ), right ( ), center ( ), decimal ( ), and bar ( ). All deal with the alignment of the text around the tab mark. (See Figure 5-14.) You can adjust and place tabs on the ruler using the mouse. Never use the space bar to move text around; use the tab key. There should be only one tab between items; to line up text properly, adjust the tab location.

To set the indents:

1. Place the **insertion point** in the paragraph that you will indent. Alternatively, highlight multiple paragraphs if you want to indent more than one paragraph.
2. Drag the **appropriate marker** to the chosen tick mark on the ruler bar. You may also access the indents under the Page Layout tab, Paragraph group or by clicking the dialog launcher in that group.

To set the tabs:

1. Click the **Left Tab** button on the ruler bar until the correct tab mark appears.
2. Click the ruler bar location where the tab should be set. (The ruler bar must be showing to use this option.) You may adjust and apply additional features through the Page Layout tab, Paragraph group dialog launcher, and then Tabs Tabs... at the bottom of the dialog box.

To remove a tab(s):

1. Click a **tab** on the ruler bar and drag it **off the ruler** into the document.
2. To clear all the tab settings at once, double-click a **tab** on the ruler and click **Clear All** Clear All button.

To create a bulleted list:

1. Type the **text** to be bulleted.
2. Highlight the **text**.
3. Click the **bulleted list** icon in the Paragraph group of the Home tab or click the **down arrow** and select a different type of **bullet**.

You may also click the bullet button and start typing the list. To modify the appearance of numbers and bullets, click the arrow in the button and choose an appropriate style.

To create a numbered list from existing text:

1. Type the **text** to be numbered. Make sure the Home tab is active.
2. Highlight the **text**.
3. Click the **numbered list** icon in the Paragraph group of the Home tab or click the **down arrow** and select a **numbering style**.

To create a numbered list from scratch:

1. Select the **Home** tab.
2. Place the cursor in the **document** where you intend for the list to begin.
3. Click the **Numbering** icon in the Paragraph group (**Figure 5-15**).
4. Type the **list**, pressing the **Enter** key at the end of each item.
5. When you have finished typing your list, press the **Enter** key **twice** or click the **Numbering** icon to turn off the automatic numbering.

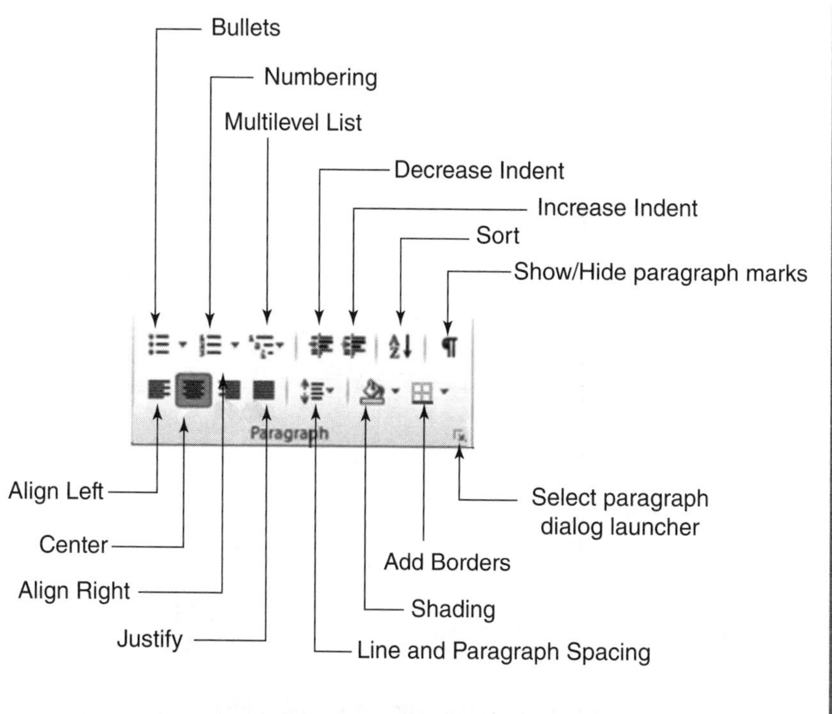

Figure 5-15 Paragraph Group in Home Tab

Alternatively, you can type the first number and press the **Enter** key; for the next item, Word will automatically add the 2. When your list is complete, simply backspace to get rid of the next number or press the **Enter** key twice.

Page and Document Formatting

Page and document formatting alters the appearance of the page and the document. It includes such features as headers/footers, page break, margins, page orientation, pagination, section breaks, and columns. **Figure 5-16** shows the Page Setup dialog box.

Footer The **footer** is an information area that appears consistently at the bottom of each page or section of a document. It can indicate the name of the document, the page number, the date, or any information that is helpful.

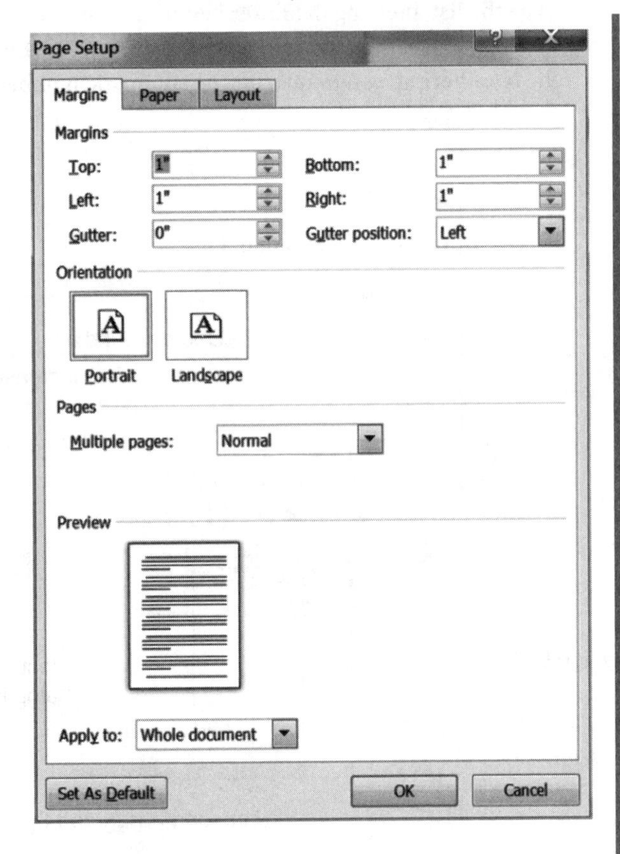

Figure 5-16 Page Setup Dialog Box

Header	The **header** is an information area that appears consistently at the top of each page or section of a document. It can hold the name of the document, page number, date, or other identifying information. If you use section breaks, you can have several different headers.
Line Breaks	To force lines and paragraphs to move as desired, use the appropriate pagination options of Keep lines with next and Keep lines together. Access this feature from the Paragraph dialog box.
Margins	Margins are the distance between the text and the edge of the paper. By default, Word sets the margins to 1 inch at top, bottom, left, and right.
Page break	A **page break** is the place where Word ends the text on one page before it continues text on the next page. You can manually insert a page break by going to the Insert tab and selecting Page Break from the Pages group or by pressing Ctrl+Enter. The program then places the break at the cursor or insertion point location. It is a good idea to review your finished document to determine where page breaks are necessary. Use this feature cautiously until you make all the necessary document revisions. You can also insert a page break from the Page Layout tab in Word; choose Page Layout and then click Breaks. A list of choices appears. You may also select column, text wrapping around objects, and section breaks here.
Page Orientation	**Page orientation** refers to the layout of the paper. **Portrait** means the paper is upright, longer than it is wide; **landscape** means the page is sideways, wider than it is long.
Pagination	**Pagination** simply refers to the process of assigning page numbers to your document. Word processing programs automatically keep track of your pagination, but if you want the numbers to appear in your document you need to select that option in the Header & Footer group on the Insert tab. Simply click on Page Number and choose the placement option that suits you.
Section Break	Section breaks permit you to apply several different formats in a single document, such as one format for a preface using roman numerals for page numbers, and

another for chapters using arabic numerals. By default, a document is one section so page and document formatting applies to the total document. When applying a section break, you can format each section differently. For example, preface material may have *i, ii, iii* page numbering while the body of the document has 1, 2, 3, and so forth.

To open the Page Setup dialog box:

1. Open a **New** document.
2. Choose the **Page Layout** tab.
3. Click the **dialog launcher** at the lower-right corner of the Page Setup group. The Page Setup dialog box appears (Figure 5-16). Use it to adjust the document's margins and decide on paper orientation (portrait or landscape), paper size, and layout. In this example, margins are set 1 inch at the top and bottom of the page and on the left and right sides of the page. Vertical centering of the text can also be set in this dialog box; use this feature to center a title page.

To change the margins:

1. Click **PageLayout** tab and **Margins** icon.
2. Select the **margin** necessary.
3. To change the margins of a section of the document, choose the **Page Layout** tab and click **Margins**; choose **Custom Margins** at the bottom of the box and do what is necessary and then select **This point forward** from the **Apply to** options.

To set a page break:

1. Go to the **place** in the document where you want to place the page break.
2. Press **Ctrl+Enter** or select the **Insert** tab and **Page Break** from the Pages group (Figure 5-5a). Use this feature cautiously; use the lines and page break feature in the paragraph dialog box to keep lines together. For example, use this feature to keep a paragraph from splitting between pages or a title from being separated from its related paragraph. Use the page break feature to separate the reference list from the body of the paper.

To add a header or footer to a document:

1. Choose the **Insert** tab and select **Header** or **Footer** from the Header & Footer group (Figure 5-5a).
2. Select either **header** or **footer**. See Figure 5-5b for footer and page number choices.
3. Select one of the **style options**. (See **Figure 5-17a**.)

(a)

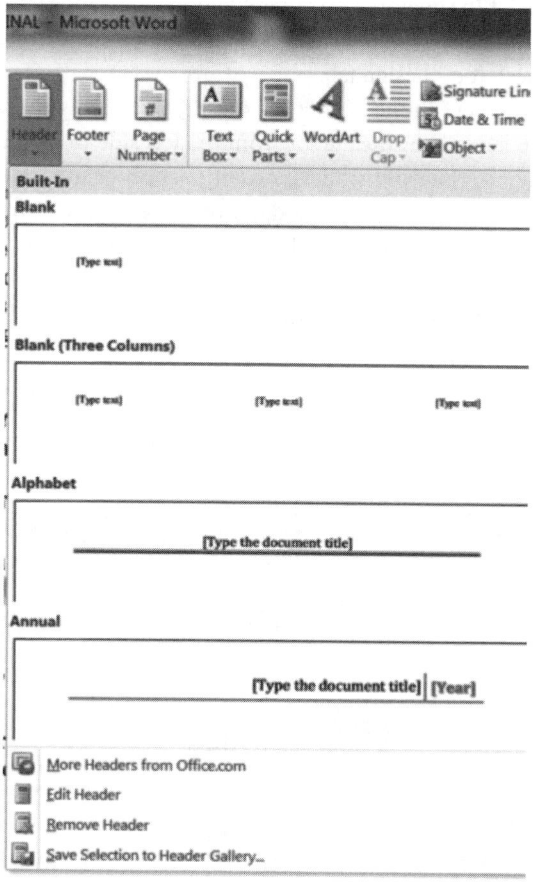

(b)

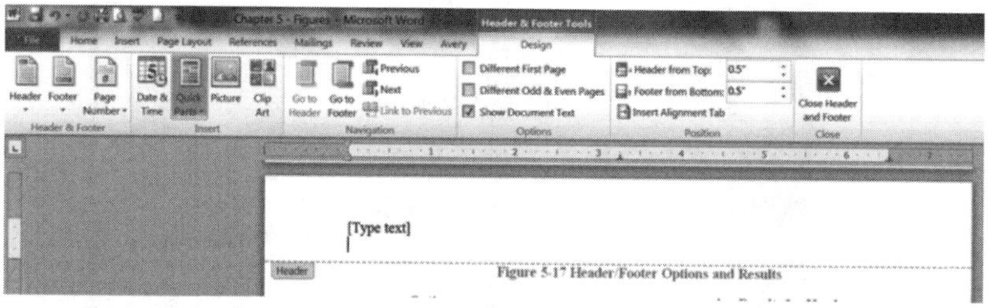

Figure 5-17 Header/Footer Options and Results

4. **Figure 5-17b** shows the document window that appears after you select the Header Header option. Note the addition on the ribbon of the Header & Footers Tools design tab.
5. Type your **text** in the header (or footer) box by highlighting **[Type Text]**. The tab key moves the cursor from the left side to the middle of the page, and then to the right side. Choose the appropriate spot for inserting the name of the document, the date, or page number. You can also select options from the groups such as Page number, Date & Time, Options, or Position.
6. Click the **Close Header and Footer** button Close Header and Footer Close when you finish (Figure 5-17b).

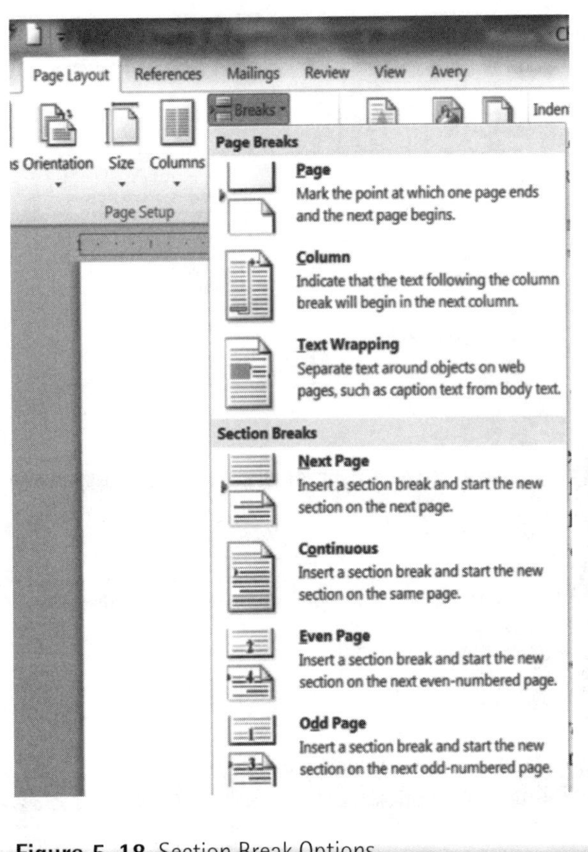

Figure 5-18 Section Break Options

To add a section break to a document:

1. Go to the **place in the document** where you want to place the section break.
2. Click **Page Layout** tab.
3. Click the **Breaks** option Breaks in the Page Setup group.
4. Select an **option** from the Section Breaks part of the menu (**Figure 5-18**).

Preparing a Document

The previous section explained some of the key concepts in formatting your document. This section addresses the process you might use. You can prepare the formatting for a document in three ways: (1) by setting the formatting before you begin to type the text, (2) by typing the text and then formatting the document, or (3) by selecting a preformatted template. Personal preference should determine how to proceed; remember, however, that the idea is to create and format the document efficiently and effectively.

The process we describe here focuses on setting the formats before you create the document.

- Set the margins. By default they are 1 inch all around. If you intend to bind your document, a left margin of at least 1.5 inches is necessary. If you plan to print the document on letterhead, measure the letterhead's height. You may need a margin of as much as 2.4 inches to make sure that the body of the letter begins below the letterhead.
- Select the font type and size.
- Apply styles if necessary. If this is a formal paper, you may want to apply heading styles to the titles of the document parts, such as Introduction or Definitions. This will also permit you to generate a table of contents.
- Set paragraph formatting. The Paragraph dialog box appears as shown in **Figure 5-19**. Many institutions require that you submit your paper in APA style, so you would need to change the line spacing using the dialog box shown in Figure 5-19. You can also select line spacing by clicking the arrow next to the line spacing box in the Paragraph group. On a computer screen, it may be easier to work on a document that uses 1.5 or single spacing. Later, you can change this option to whatever spacing is required or preferred for the final product. You can also highlight the entire document (**Ctrl+A**) and change its spacing by pressing one of the following key combinations:
  - **Ctrl+1** to create single-spaced lines
  - **Ctrl+5** to create 1.5-spaced lines
  - **Ctrl+2** to create double-spaced lines
- Use the Show/Hide feature to check that your formatting is done properly.
- Select the Print Layout view when working on the document. This shows you how the document will look when you print it.

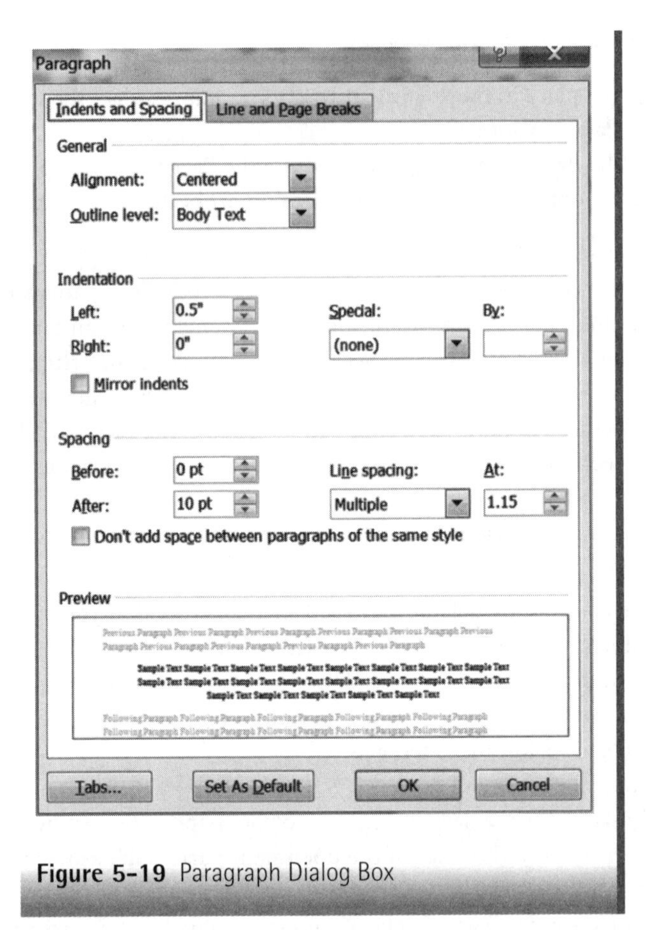

Figure 5-19 Paragraph Dialog Box

- Type your document!
- Check your spelling and grammar.
- Save your work periodically and know where you are saving it.

Viewing a Document

Word provides several ways to view a document on the screen. Here are your choices.

- The most common option is Print Layout. Print Layout shows the document as it will look when you print it. This is usually the best view for preparing a document.
- Full Screen Reading view maximizes the space available for reading. This view hides the ribbon and status bar to provide the maximum viewing area on the screen.

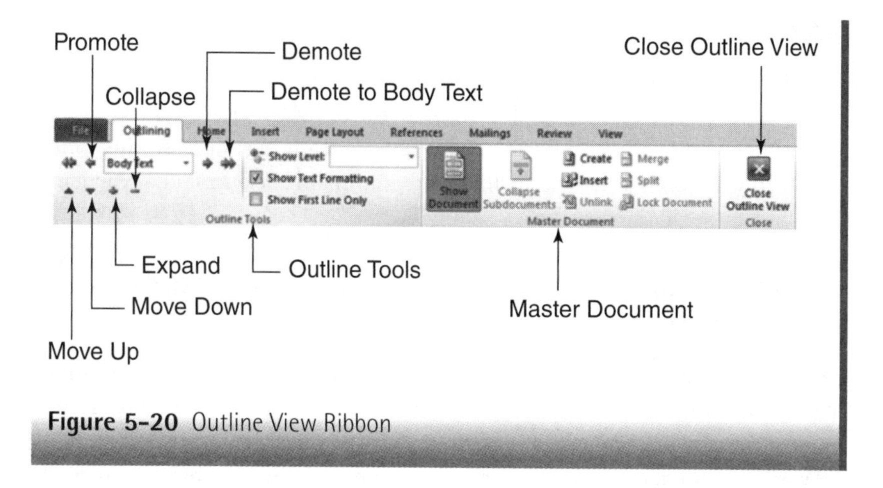

Figure 5-20 Outline View Ribbon

- Web Layout view shows how the document will look when you display it in a browser.
- Outline view provides an outline view of the document. Click **Outline** and the outlining ribbon appears (**Figure 5-20**). An outline provides a map to guide the writing process for a document. It can also help when you want to arrange pictures or columns and so on. Word uses its built-in heading styles for outlines (Heading 1, Heading 2, and so forth) by default.
- Draft view displays text only with very large print.

You can also access these views from the Status bar in Word. Other groups in the View tab are Show (as in ruler or gridlines), Zoom, which allows for viewing the document as one page or two pages, Window, and Macros.

To change a view:

1. Select the **View** tab.
2. Click the **View Option** desired from the choices in **Document Views** or click one of the icons in the **Zoom** group that corresponds to the view desired (Figure 5-10).

Checking Spelling, Grammar, Readability, and Word Counts

Word 2010 includes spelling and grammar checks, translation, and thesaurus tools under the Review tab (Figure 5-9). Word automatically checks spelling and grammar as you type. If you misspell a word, a wavy red line appears under the word. If the program detects a grammar error, the wavy line is green. Because wavy lines distract some people, Word provides an option to turn this feature off.

To turn the spelling and grammar checker off:

1. Click **File** tab and then **Options.**
2. Click **Proofing.** Remove the check marks in "Mark grammar errors as you type" and "Check spelling as you type." Changing these settings means you will need to run the spelling and grammar checker manually when you finish the document.
3. Click **OK**.
4. After you set this option, to check spelling and grammar click the **Spelling & Grammar** icon under the Review tab.

Most programs come with a built-in spell checker, which is a program that checks words for correct spelling. Word combines the spelling and grammar checker. A wavy red line under a word means that it is misspelled or that it is not in Word's dictionary. The spell checker only checks for words that are misspelled, not misused.

A grammar checker (an add-in that often comes with word processing programs) provides feedback to the user about errors in grammar. For example, using "there" when "their" is appropriate or using subjects and verbs that do not agree will result in a wavy green (grammar) line to appear under the offending sentence or phrase. Within the grammar checker, you can select several settings and styles. By default, this feature shows the errors as the user types.

A thesaurus is a built-in feature that helps you search for alternative words. In Word 2010, the Thesaurus appears in the Proofing group under the Review tab.

To correct spelling and grammar errors with the checker set to default:

1. Right-click the **error**.
2. Select a **correction**, choose to **ignore it,** or **add the word** to the spelling dictionary. **Figure 5-21** shows the menu that appears when "error" is misspelled.

To run the spelling and grammar checker with default off:

1. Click the **Review** tab.
2. Click **Spelling & Grammar** icon.
3. Select a **correction**, choose to **ignore it,** or **add the word** to the spelling dictionary. Figure 5-21 shows the menu that appears when "error" is misspelled.

When adding a word to the dictionary, be sure that it is spelled correctly. The spelling dictionary is stored on the hard drive, so it is available only on the computer to which it was added. Some computer labs may refresh the computer image each time a new user logs in; in such a case, any words added to the dictionary will not be permanent.

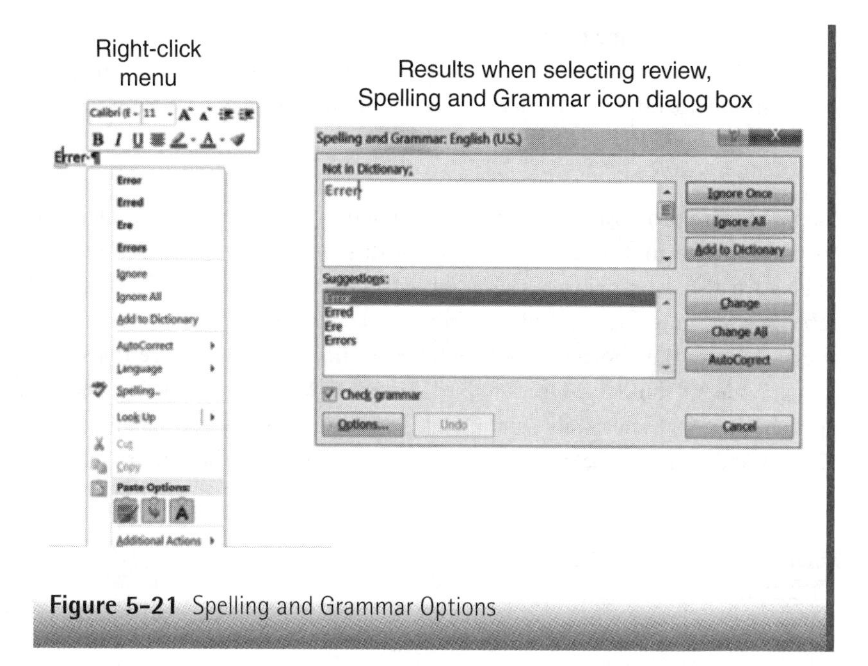

Figure 5-21 Spelling and Grammar Options

Readability statistics provide information about the reading level required to understand the document. The readability level of the document should match the reading ability of the audience for whom the document is intended. It is best to perform grammar, spelling, and readability checks after you have finished the document. While these tools are helpful in improving your document, you will still need to proofread it. Word will not find all the misspellings, wrong terms, or grammar problems that might exist. This is especially true if you have used a correctly spelled word, but it is not the word you intended to use. For example, you may have meant to type the word *explore,* but actually typed the word *explode.*

To run the readability option:

1. First, set the option to **run** with the spelling and grammar checker.
   a. Click **File** tab, and **Options.**
   b. Click **Proofing**, and then click **Show readability statistics**.
2. Place your cursor at the **beginning** of the document.
3. Run the **Spelling & Grammar** checker. At the end, the readability dialog box appears with the results.

Also under the Review tab is the Word Count icon **Word Count**, which appears in the Proofing group (Figure 5-9). Performing a word count is helpful when you are writing an abstract or paper that has a word or character count limit.

You can also determine the number of pages, words, lines, paragraphs, or characters in a document by using this option. Note also that Word lists the number of words in the document in the left part of the status bar next to Page number.

Creating a Table

Tables in word processing have many uses. For example, they help you set columns for recording minutes of a meeting or for organizing any kind of information. Tables are also essential to research reports. It is a good idea to plan the kind of table needed in terms of number of rows and columns required before selecting them. Among the choices for a new table in the Tables group are Insert Table, Draw Table, or (built-in) Quick Tables. **Figure 5-22** shows the dialog boxes that appear when you select Table and Quick Tables under the Insert tab. **Figure 5-23** shows the dialog box that appears when you select Insert Table (under the grid).

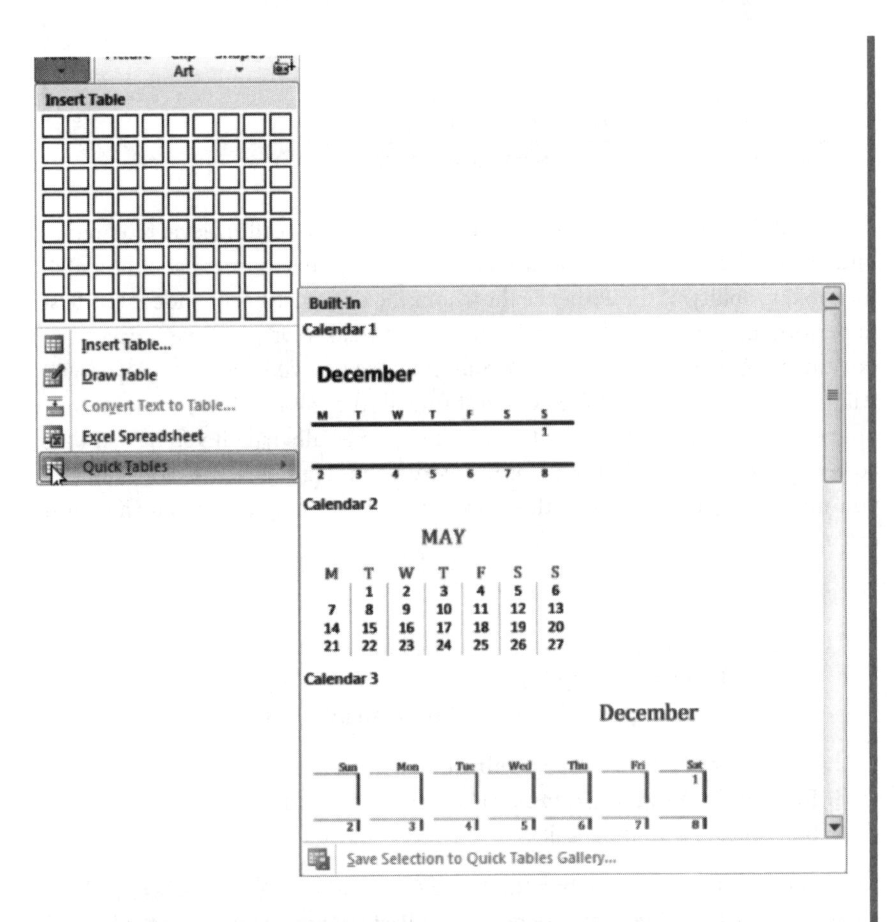

Figure 5-22 Table Menu Plus a Quick Table Example

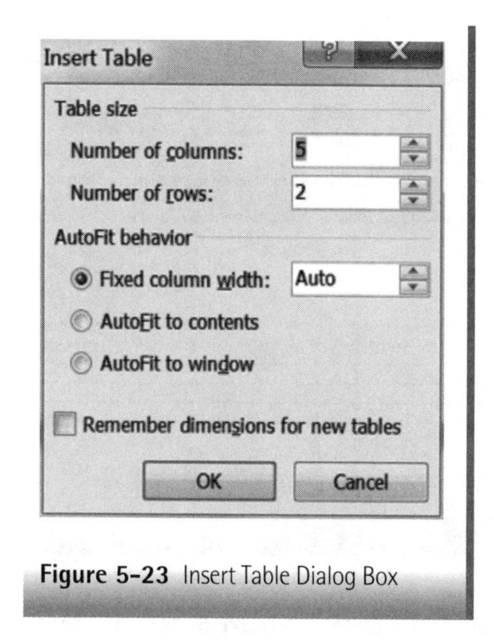

Figure 5-23 Insert Table Dialog Box

To create a table:

1. Place the **insertion point** where the table should appear in the document.
2. Click the **Insert** tab, the **Table** icon, and **Insert Table.**
3. Select the number of **rows** and **columns** and click **OK** or, if using the mouse, drag over the cells for the number of rows and columns desired. Remember that a row is necessary for headers. Insert additional rows or columns if necessary.

To create a table by dragging:

1. Click the **Table** icon on the Insert tab.
2. Place the mouse over the **grid** and drag to highlight the **number of rows and columns** needed. Keep dragging until you create the correct size for the table.

To insert a row:

1. Right-click in a **row**.
2. From the menu, select **Insert** and select **Insert Rows Above** or **Insert Rows Below.**
3. You may also insert multiple rows at one time by selecting the **number of rows** to be inserted using the quick select area in the left margin, and right-clicking the selection. Follow the directions from the shortcut menu. Insert columns the same way.

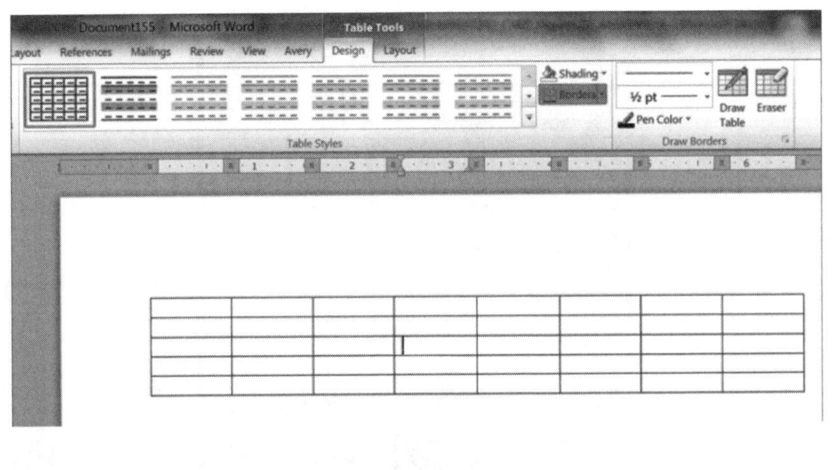

Figure 5-24 Table Tools Tab

The Table Tools tab appears (**Figure 5-24**) once the table is in place and selected. Use the **Table** tab to adjust the table and enhance it. For example, you can change the width or height of a row or column, alter the style of the table, or delete grid lines.

To delete a table:

1. Click the **four-headed arrow** on the top left of the table to select the table.
2. Right-click the **table** and select **Delete Table.**

Creating an Outline

Sometimes people need to submit an outline before they start work on the actual content of the document. This provides you with a reminder of what should be in the document and how it might need to be organized. Outlines are based on heading styles; they can include a maximum of nine levels of headings. **Figure 5-25** shows a multilevel outline of this chapter. While shown in this figure, the title of the chapter is not generally included in the outline levels. It is better to use the heading styles for major content areas of the document, not the document title.

To make an outline:

1. To create an outline before you start the document, choose **View**, then **Outline**.
2. Type the **first line** in the Outline. It will show as Level 1.

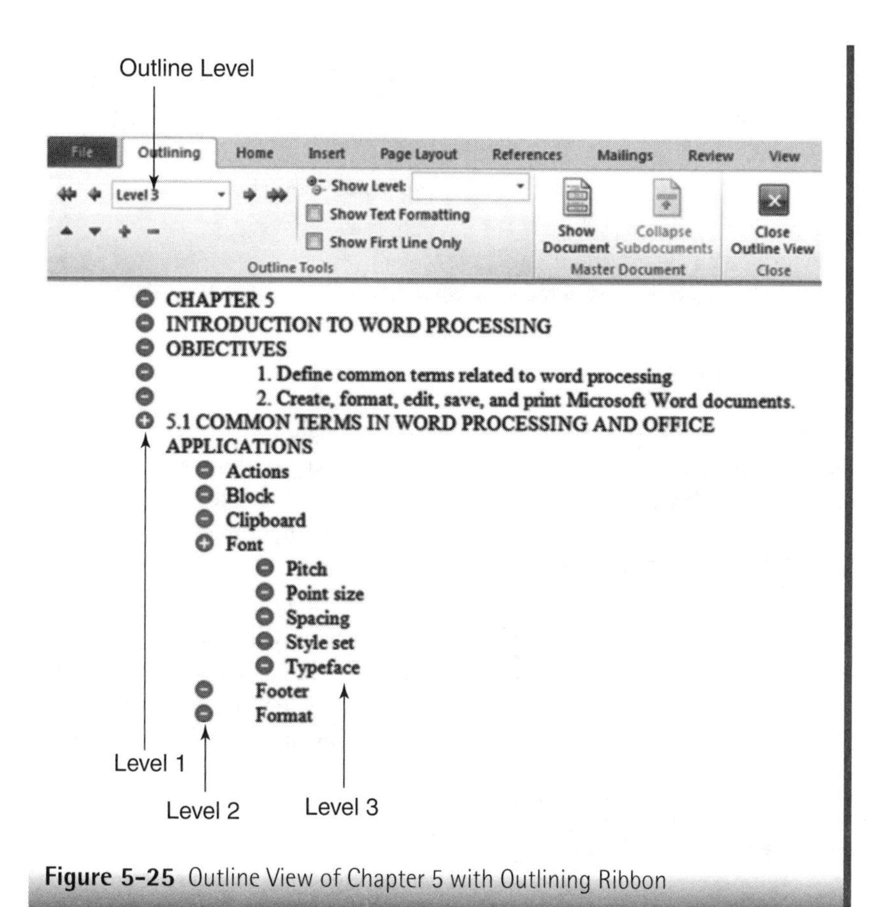

Figure 5-25 Outline View of Chapter 5 with Outlining Ribbon

3. Press **Enter**. Another line at the same level will appear.
4. Type the **next line of text** or press the **Tab** key. The Tab key demotes the next line to the Level 2. Note that a plus symbol appears in front of the first line; this symbol indicates that there is a heading below it. If the minus symbol appears, then there are no subordinates. To promote a level, press **Shift+Tab**.

If you want to create an outline after you write a document, be sure to apply the appropriate heading styles to the headings in your document. If you don't want to use the preset styles that come with Word (**Figure 5-26**), you can redefine the formula for the default heading styles or apply a different style by choosing the Styles group dialog launcher, selecting the level to change, right-clicking, and making the desired changes. (See **Figure 5-27**.)

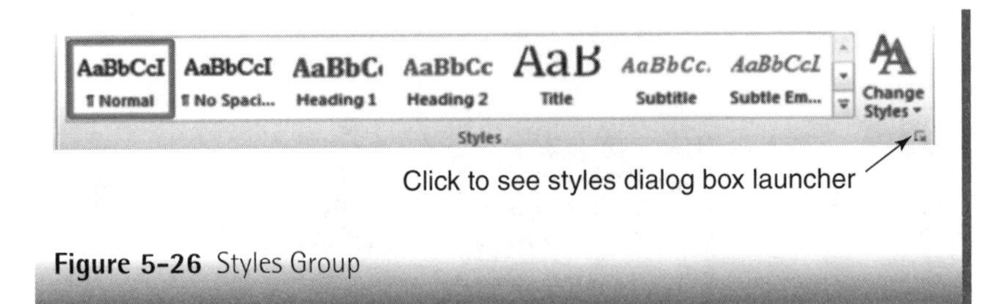

Figure 5-26 Styles Group

Creating a Table of Contents

A table of contents (TOC) usually appears at the beginning of a document after the title page and provides a list of headings from a certain level along with their page numbers. **Figure 5-28** shows a partial table of contents for Chapter 7. Each head in the document that you want to display in the Table of Contents must have a heading level assigned to it. The Table of Contents feature will save you time when you edit and change the document. All you have to do is regenerate it and the table of contents will update to reflect your changes.

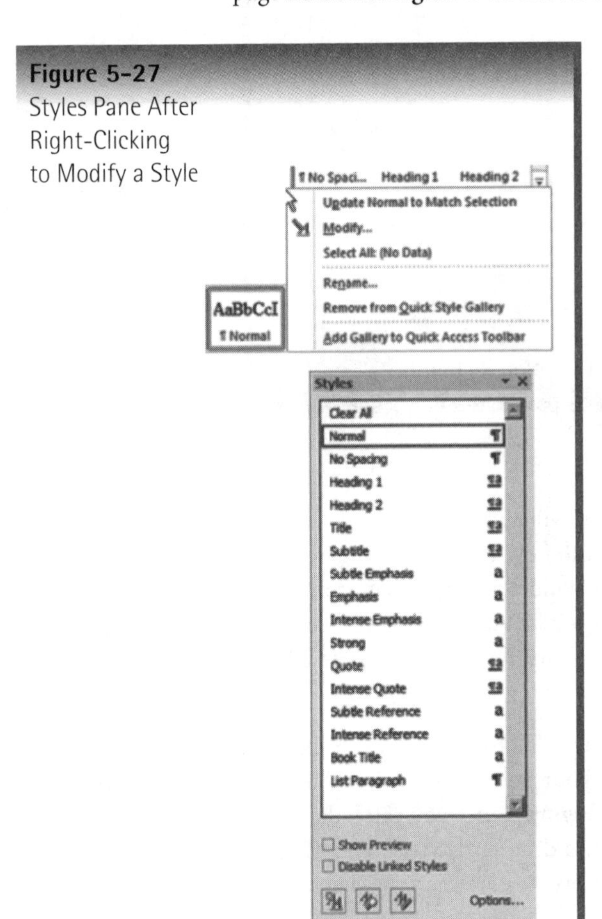

Figure 5-27 Styles Pane After Right-Clicking to Modify a Style

To create a table of contents once you create the document:

1. Go through your document and assign a **style** to each heading. For example, **Heading 1** for major headings, **Heading 2** for minor headings, and so forth. Most of the time we use from one to three levels of headings.
2. Place the insertion point on the **page** where you will generate the Table of Contents. This is usually after the title page. It should begin on its own page, which means insert a page break after the title page.
3. Click the **Reference** tab, then the **Table of Contents** icon.
4. Select a **predesigned table of contents** style (See **Figure 5-29a**) or click **Insert Table of Contents** (See **Figure 5-29b**).

Chapter 7 Introduction to Spreadsheets

Contents

Objectives.. 1
Common Spreadsheet Terms 1
Rows.. 2
Columns 2
Spreadsheet Screen Display.. 3
Current Cell Address.. 3
Formula Toolbar 3
Getting Ready to Use a Spreadsheet.. 3
Accomplishing Tasks in the Worksheet 4
Entering Data.. 4
To enter data: 4

Figure 5-28 Table of Contents Example

Insert Table of Contents gives you the option to customize the look of the Table of Contents. Figure 5-29b shows you the custom options in the dialog box.

To update the table of contents once you make changes to the document:

1. Click the **Table of Contents.**
2. Click the **Update Table** Update Table... icon that appears at the top left.
3. Select **Update page numbers only** or **Update entire table** and click **OK.** The table will update based on the selection you made.

Creating Merged Documents

Word has features that will help you create envelopes, form letters, and print personalized copies of both for each person on a list. Word replaces merge fields from a main document with information from a data source. As with many other Word functions there is more than one way to send a form letter to a list of people. We use the Step by Step Mail Merge Wizard to prepare the documents in the example in this section.

A mail merge requires the creation of two documents. A data source document contains the name, address, and any other necessary individualized data for

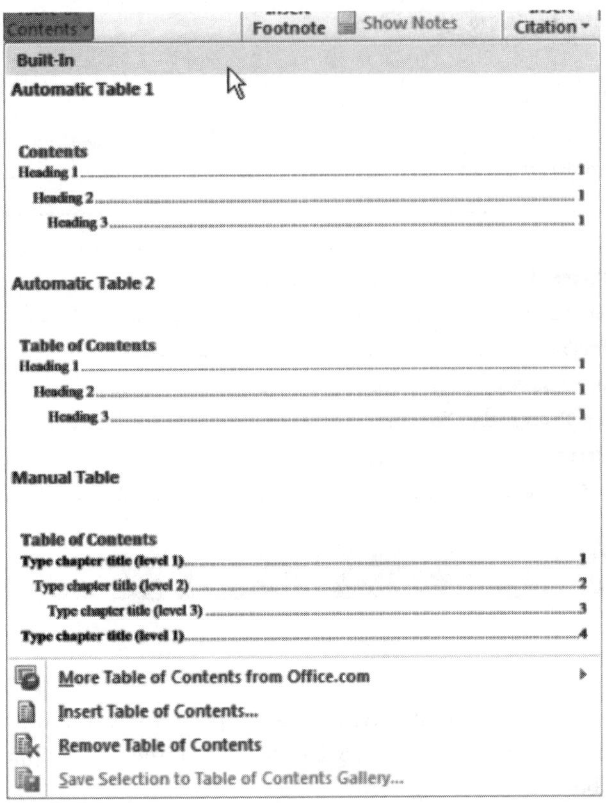

Contents Footnote Show Notes Citation

Built-In

Automatic Table 1

Contents
Heading 1 1
Heading 2 1
Heading 3 1

Automatic Table 2

Table of Contents
Heading 1 1
Heading 2 1
Heading 3 1

Manual Table

Table of Contents
Type chapter title (level 1) 1
Type chapter title (level 2) 2
Type chapter title (level 3) 3
Type chapter title (level 1) 4

More Table of Contents from Office.com
Insert Table of Contents...
Remove Table of Contents
Save Selection to Table of Contents Gallery...

Figure 5-29a Table of Contents Dialog Box

each letter. The data source can be an Outlook address book, an Access database, an Excel spreadsheet with column headings, or a Word table. In this example, the data source is a Word table. Every data source consists of three parts: records, fields, and field headers. Each row in a data source is a **record**, and each column is a **field**. You must plan the data source carefully so that it does what you want it to do. A main document contains the same text that will appear in each letter and the field code from which to insert the personalized data from the data source.

To perform a step by step mail merge:

1. Open a **New** document.
2. Select the **Mailings** group, then click **Start Mail Merge** (**Figure 5-30**).
3. Click **Step by Step Mail Merge Wizard** 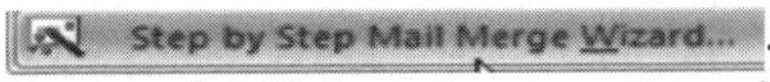 Step by Step Mail Merge Wizard... . The next screen that appears shows Step 1 of 6 (**Select document type**) (**Figure 5-31**).

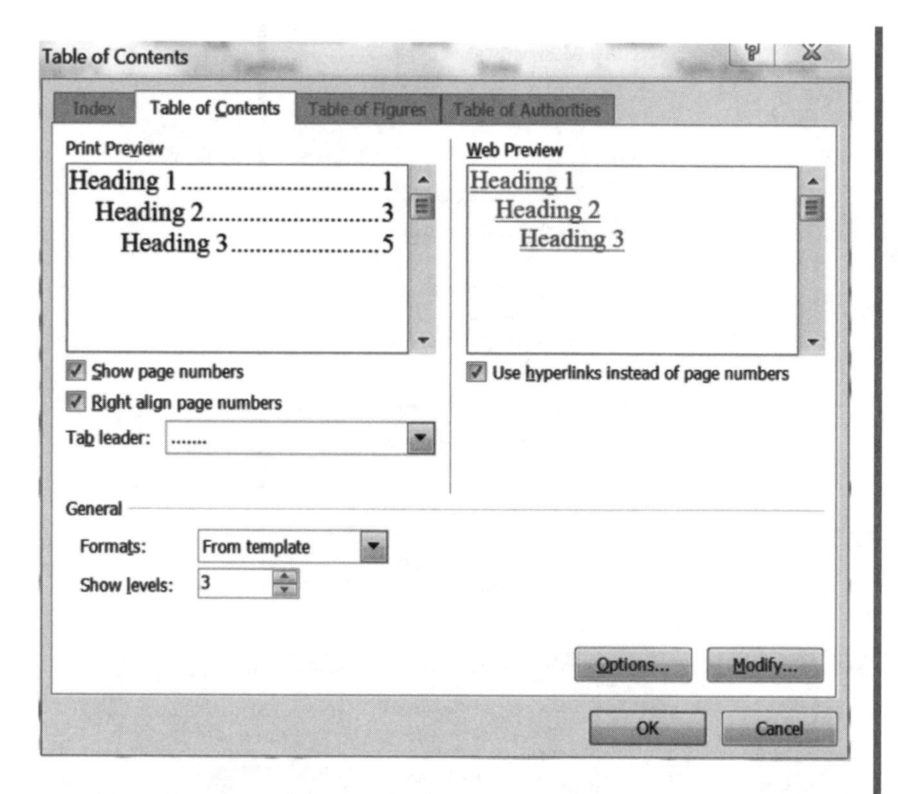

Figure 5-29b Dialog Box that Appears When You Select Insert Table of Contents

4. Choose **Letters** [Letters].
5. Click **Next: Starting document** [Next: Starting document].
6. Choose **Start from a template**, and then click **Select template** [Select template...].
7. Click the **Letters** tab in the Select template window and select the **type of letter** (**Figure 5-32**).
8. Click **OK**. **Figure 5-33** shows part of the letter that appears. Because the computer we used to prepare this example belongs to Marjorie Smith, that name appears automatically at the top of the letter.
9. Click **Next: Select recipients**.
10. Select **Type a new list** and then click **Create**.
11. Type the **Title, First Name, Last Name, Address, City, State, and Zip Code** for the first recipient. (Use the Tab key to move between the address fields.) Some fields may be hidden, and the table must be enlarged left to right.

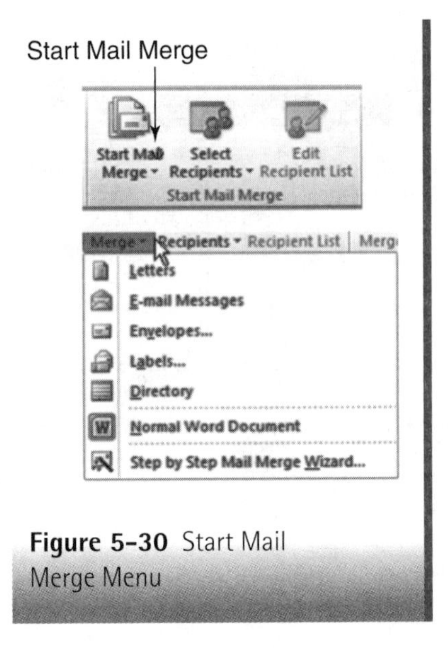

Figure 5-30 Start Mail Merge Menu

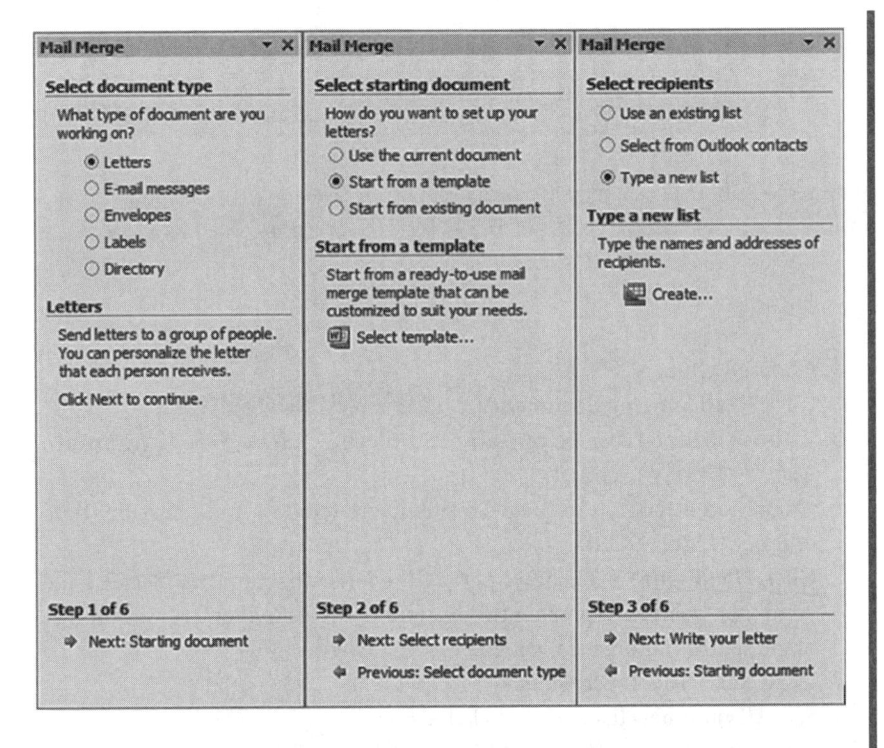

Figure 5-31 Steps 1-3 of Mail Merge Wizard

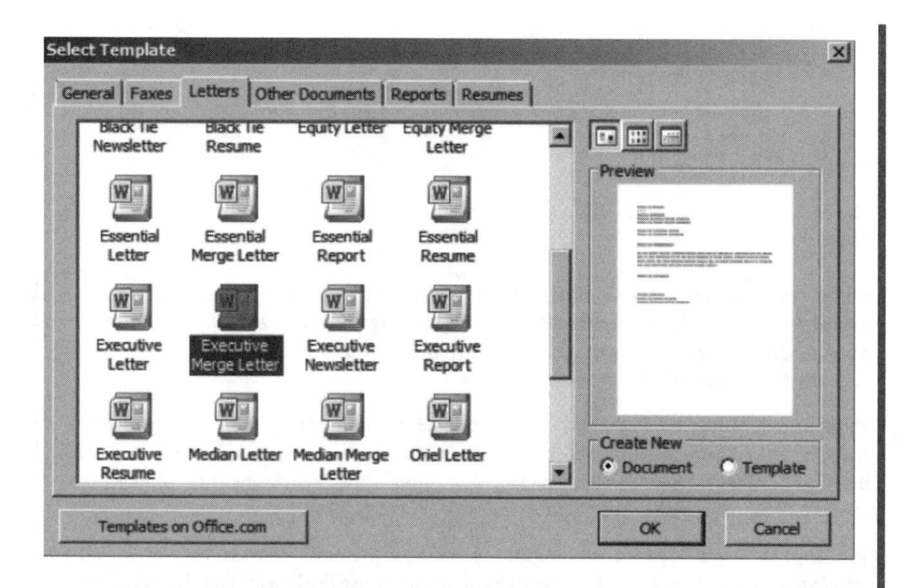

Figure 5-32 Dialog Window for Selecting a Letter Template

12. Click **New Entry** and add a **second recipient**. **Figure 5-34** shows the New Address List window that appears after you add street names. Add two or three more recipients.
13. Click **OK** at the bottom of the window. The program will prompt you to name your list and save it in My Data Sources. Type a **name**, click **Save**, and then **OK**. **Figure 5-35** shows a Mail Merge Recipient List that is ready for mail merge.
14. Click **Next: Write your letter** in Step 3. Step 4, "Write your letter," appears. See **Figure 5-36** for Steps 4–6.
15. Click the **Pick the date** down arrow at the top of the letter and select **TODAY**.
16. Type a **name** in the upper right if it isn't there. Add an **address** and a **phone number**.
17. Leave the **Address** and **Greeting** fields as is. If you desire to change the Greeting line, **Figure 5-37** shows the dialog box for choosing the type of greeting line you desire. Click **OK** when you are finished.
18. Highlight the **body of the letter** and type a **message**.
19. Click **[Type the closing]** and type **Sincerely**.
20. Add **your name** and **appropriate informatio**n at the bottom of the letter.
21. Click **Next: Preview your letters**in Step 4 (Figure 5-36).
22. Preview the letters by clicking **Recipient 1**, **Recipient 2**, and so on in the right pane.

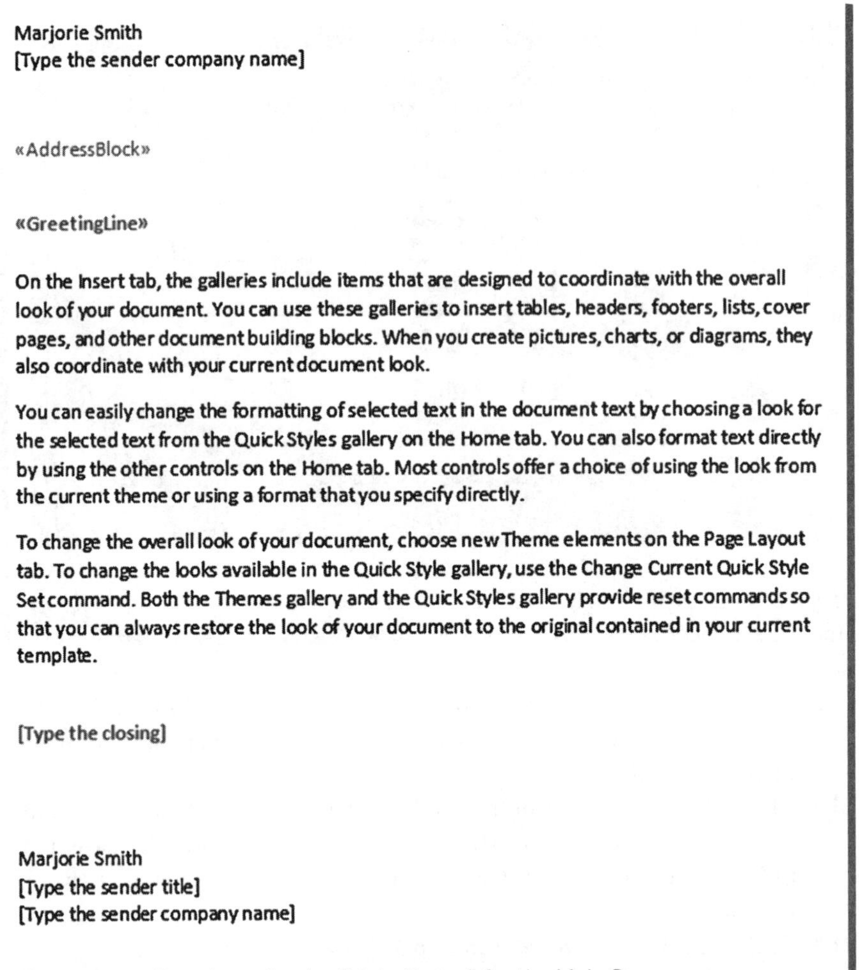

Marjorie Smith
[Type the sender company name]

«AddressBlock»

«GreetingLine»

On the Insert tab, the galleries include items that are designed to coordinate with the overall look of your document. You can use these galleries to insert tables, headers, footers, lists, cover pages, and other document building blocks. When you create pictures, charts, or diagrams, they also coordinate with your current document look.

You can easily change the formatting of selected text in the document text by choosing a look for the selected text from the Quick Styles gallery on the Home tab. You can also format text directly by using the other controls on the Home tab. Most controls offer a choice of using the look from the current theme or using a format that you specify directly.

To change the overall look of your document, choose new Theme elements on the Page Layout tab. To change the looks available in the Quick Style gallery, use the Change Current Quick Style Set command. Both the Themes gallery and the Quick Styles gallery provide reset commands so that you can always restore the look of your document to the original contained in your current template.

[Type the closing]

Marjorie Smith
[Type the sender title]
[Type the sender company name]

Figure 5-33 Templates for the Origin "Letter" for the Main Document

23. When you are satisfied with the way the letters look, click **Next: Complete the merge** in Step 5.
24. In Step 6, choose **Print**. A dialog box appears (**Figure 5-38**).
25. Choose to **print all of the letters**, the **current record**, or those records between selected numbers.

Using Bibliography Options

One of the features in Word 2010 is the ability to automatically generate bibliographies in several formats. The Citations & Bibliography tools in Word work well if you set the style before you enter the source. Even if you change your mind later, you won't have to reenter all your source information. Once you enter

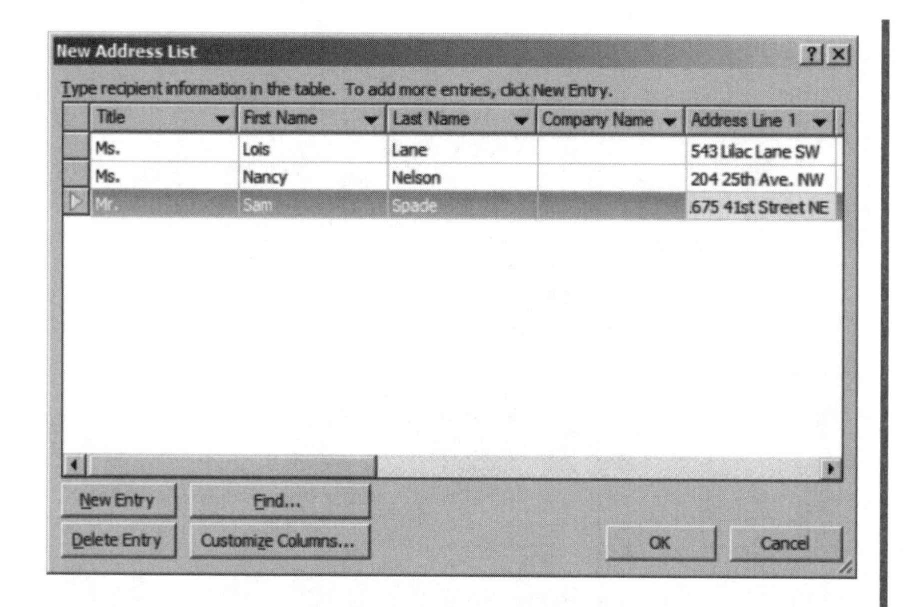

Figure 5-34 New Address List for the Data Source

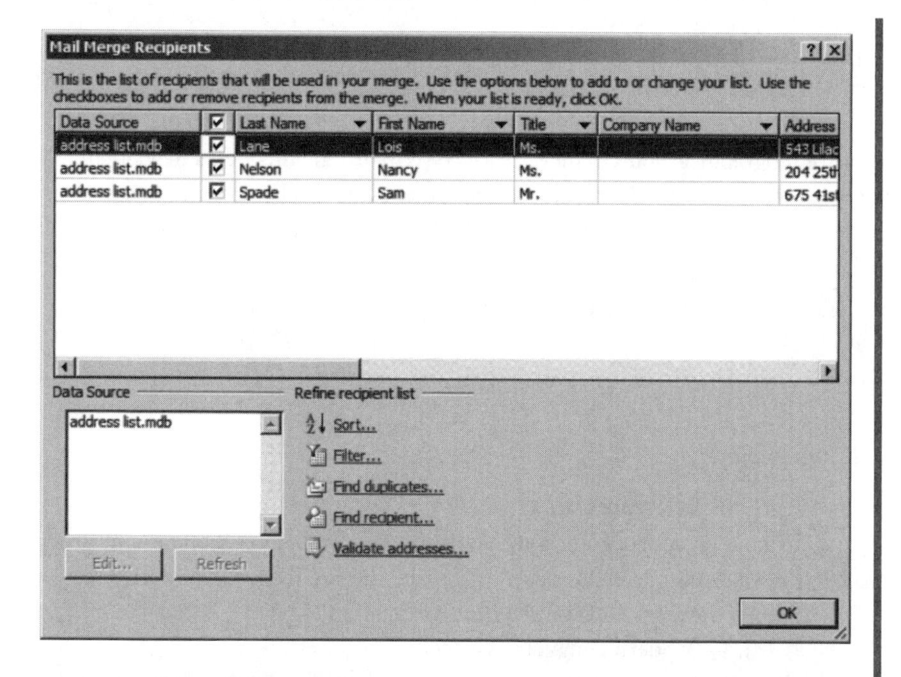

Figure 5-35 Mail Merge Recipients List

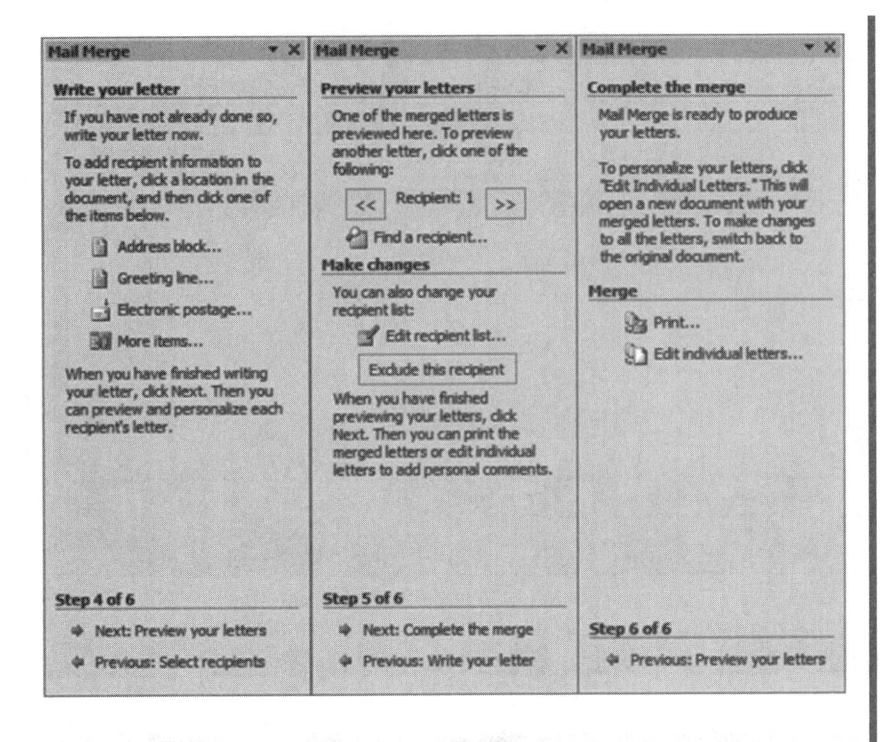

Figure 5-36 Steps 4–6 of Mail Merge Wizard

the bibliographical sources they are saved by Word. If you open a new document, sources that you used for a previous document can also be used in the new document. You are most likely to use one of two specific styles as is discussed below.

> NOTE: If you are using this function for a course assignment, be sure you use the specific format and version of that format that is acceptable to the faculty who will grade your paper.

To add a source:

1. Click the **References** tab.
2. Choose an **appropriate style** in the Citations & Bibliography group. For this example, APA is used. These are the two most common styles.
   - APA—American Psychological Association
   - MLA—Modern Language Association
3. Choose **Manage Sources**. The Source Manager dialog box opens (**Figure 5-39**).

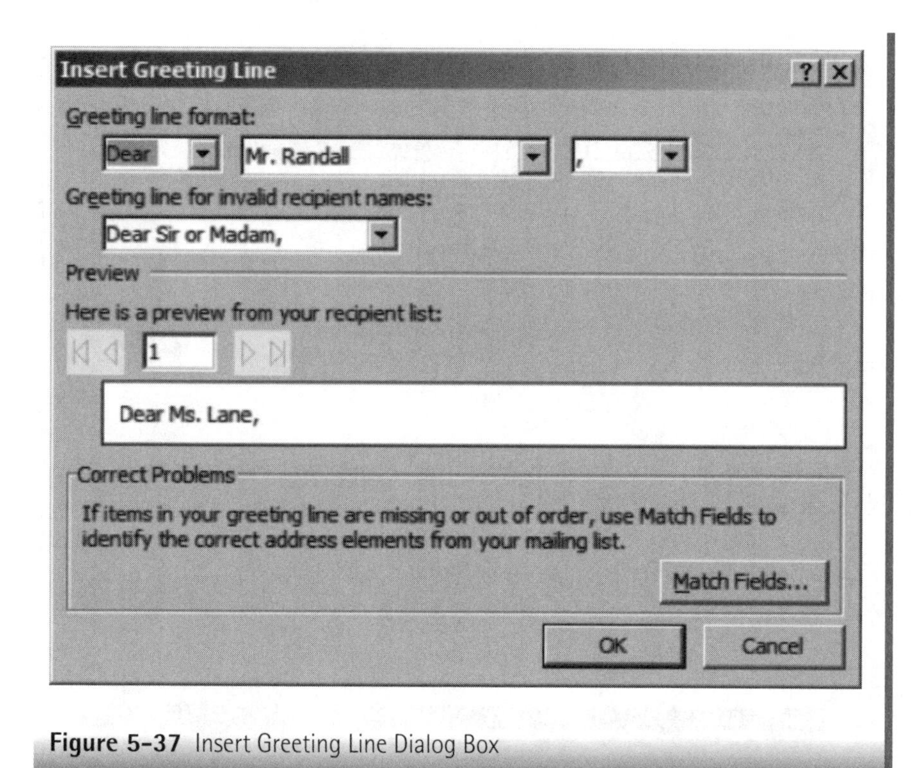

Figure 5-37 Insert Greeting Line Dialog Box

4. Click the **New** button. The Create Source dialog box opens (**Figure 5-40a**).
5. Choose **Book**.
6. Type the **author's name**, the **book title**, **year of publication**, **city** where published, and **publisher**. If the book has more than one author, click **Edit**. Type the information for the first author, click **Add**, type the **second author's name**, and repeat until you have added all authors. Click **OK**. The entry will appear in both the Master and Current lists in the Source Manager dialog box. You can add additional citations at this time or later. **Figure 5-40b** shows the Create Source dialog box that appears when you chose a **Journal Article** as Type and select **Show All Bibliography Fields**.

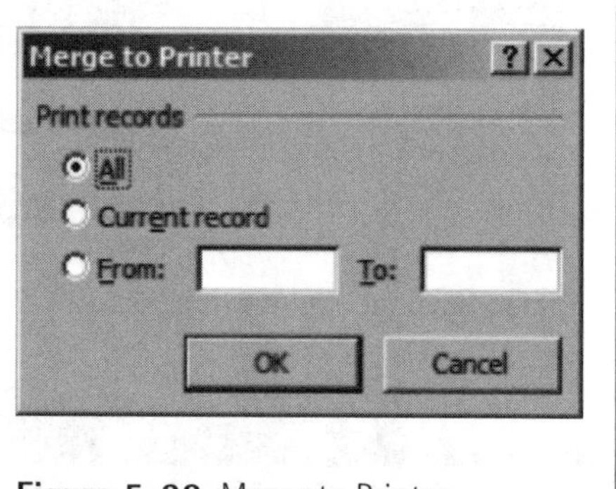

Figure 5-38 Merge to Printer Dialog Box

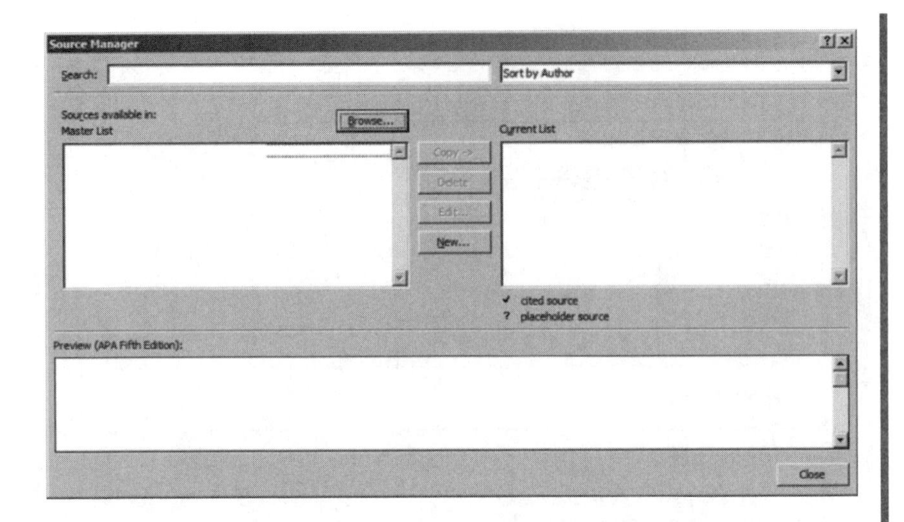

Figure 5-39 Source Manager Dialog Box for a Bibliography

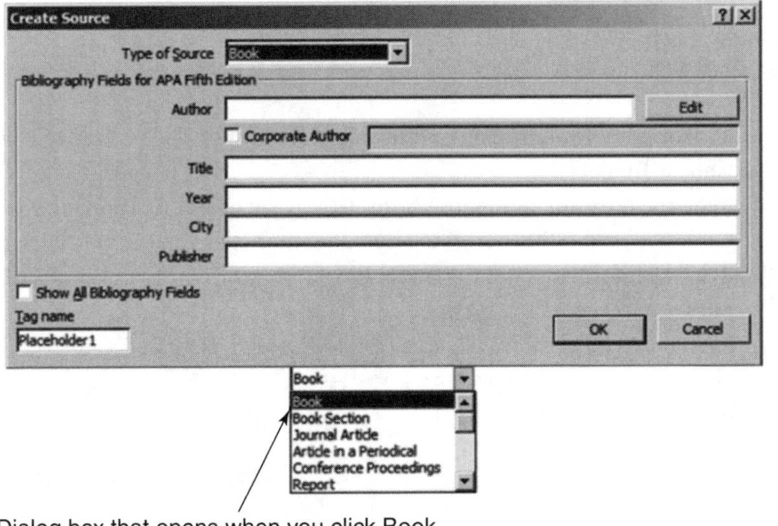

Figure 5-40a Dialog Box for Creating One Source and Editing One Name

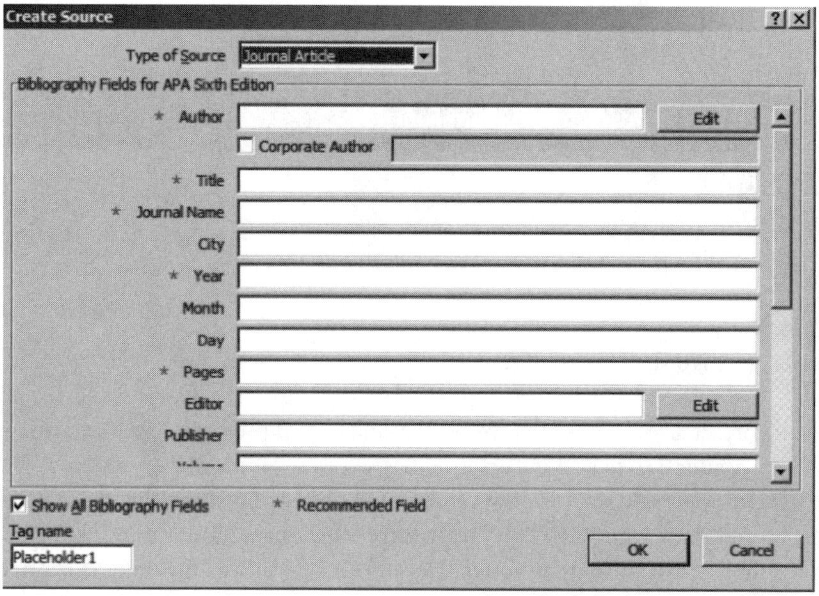

Figure 5-40b Dialog Box Showing All Bibliography Fields for Journal Article

Summary

Word provides unlimited possibilities for creating custom documents. This chapter described some of the basic skills necessary to begin using Word features effectively and efficiently. These include saving and opening documents; moving around Word; viewing documents; formatting characters, paragraphs, pages, and documents; using the spelling and grammar checker; doing readability and word counts, and creating a table. Additional features you might want to investigate include creating an index or bibliography, working with clip art and SmartArt, making newsletters, writing blogs, addressing envelopes, and customizing and optimizing Word. To develop additional skills use one of the many Word reference books available or go to Office.com and take advantage of the many assistance and training opportunities available. Of course, much time and diligent work will be necessary before you can take advantage of all of the program's features. However, once you learn the basic features you will discover it is easier to learn new functions and to adapt to the newer versions of the application that arrive every few years.

Exercises

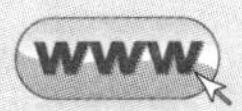

EXERCISE 1 Basic Microsoft Word Functions

■ **Objectives**

1. Perform selected word processing functions.
2. Explain basic word processing terms and functions.

■ **Activity**

1. Start **Word**. (This exercise can be done using any word processing program.)
2. Create a **New** document. Type the following text as fast as possible. Do not correct any mistakes that you make, and do not press the Enter key. Do not pay attention to spelling errors.
   Outcomes-based reimbursement will change how health care is delivered. It is important for healthcare workers to understand what this may mean to their practice. Here are a few things that might change: (1) Payment will be based on outcomes and not volume. (2) Healthcare informatics and electronic health records will be critical to quality care. (3) Continuity of patient care will increase, and (4) Wireless technologies will facilitate capturing critical information when needed.
3. Correct the document. Make sure you are at the top of the document. Click the **Spelling & Grammar** icon on the Quick Access Toolbar or click the **Review** tab, and the **Spelling & Grammar icon**. Make any corrections necessary. Click the **Change** button if the highlighted selection is correct and the **Ignore** button to ignore a correctly spelled word. If no suggestion is given or incorrect words are suggested, Word doesn't recognize the word so can't give a correct spelling. Use an appropriate dictionary for the correct spelling and type it manually if not spelled correctly. Word will announce the completion of the spelling and grammar check and provide readability statistics if you have chosen that option under the **Proofing** section of **Word Options**.
4. Save the document.
   a. Click the **File** tab and then click **Save**, or press **Ctrl+S**.
   b. Type **Chap5-Exercise1-LastName** in the highlighted File name text box.
   c. In the Location text box at the top of the Save As dialog box, select the correct **location** and click **Save**. (See Figure 4-11 for further help.) Alternatively, you can save the document by clicking the **Save** icon on the Quick Access Toolbar. Once the document has a name and location, clicking the **Save** icon (or pressing **Ctrl+S**) will update the file and not display the Save As dialog box.

5. Move around the document.
   a. Practice moving around the document.
   b. Use the **arrow keys** and **Page Up** and **Page Down** keys.
6. Edit text.
   a. Highlight the **text** (or press **Ctrl+A**).
   b. Click **Copy** Copy on the Home tab (or press **Ctrl+C**).
   c. Press **Ctrl+End** to position the insertion point below the original paragraph.
   d. Press **Enter** twice.
   e. Click **Paste** (or **press Ctrl+V**). Now there are two copies of the text.
   f. Click **Undo** icon on the Quick Access Toolbar.
   g. Try doing the same thing using the **Cut** Cut and **Paste** icons in the Clipboard group. If there is more than one copy left, delete the extra copies ending with one copy.
   h. Go back to the Quick Access Toolbar and click the **Repeat paste** icon.
   i. Go to the clipboard. Click the **dialog launcher** button. A list of what you copied appears on the clipboard.
   j. End this task with the document containing two of the same paragraphs.
7. Align text.
   a. Highlight the **second copy** of the text. Click the **Align Text Right** icon in the **Paragraph** group of the **Home** tab. Note what happens.
   b. To use both right and left alignment click the **Justify** icon. All sentences appear flush at both margins except for the last sentence.
   c. Click the **Align Text Left** icon .
8. Edit the document.
   a. Delete any **extra copies** of the text, leaving only one copy.
   b. Use the **Tab**, **Indent**, and **Enter** keys to create a document that looks like this:

      Outcomes-based reimbursement will change how health care is delivered. It is important for healthcare workers to understand what this may mean to their practice.

      Here are a few things that might change:

(1) **Payment will be based on outcomes and not volume.**
(2) **Healthcare informatics and electronic health records will be critical to quality care.**
(3) **Continuity of patient care will increase, and**
(4) **Wireless technologies will facilitate capturing critical information when needed.**

9. Format the document.
   a. Type **Ctrl+Home**, type **Implications of Outcomes-Based Reimbursement**, and press the **Enter** key twice.

Implications of Outcomes-Based Reimbursement

Outcomes-based reimbursement will change how health care is delivered. It is important for healthcare workers to understand what this may mean to their practice.

Here are a few things that might change:
(1) Payment will be based on outcomes and not volume,
(2) Healthcare informatics and electronic health records will be critical to quality care,
(3) Continuity of patient care will increase, and
(4) Wireless technologies will facilitate capturing critical information when needed

Figure 5-41 Finished Exercise 1

b. Highlight the **title**.
c. Click the **Bold** B icon, and the **Center Text** icon.
d. Click *in the text* to deselect the title. See **Figure 5-41** for the finished result.

10. Print the document.
a. Click the **File** tab, select **Print**, and choose an option.
b. Alternatively, press **Ctrl+P** or click the **Printer** icon on the Quick Access Toolbar.

11. Close and save the document.
a. **Click** the **Save** icon or press **Ctrl+S** to save the document. This will update the file saved earlier.
b. Click **Close** X on the Word application title bar, or **File** tab, **Close** Close .

EXERCISE 2 Character Formatting

■ **Objectives:**
1. Apply the appropriate typeface to a selection of characters.
2. Change the font size of selected text.
3. Apply font attributes to selected text.
4. Apply special effects to selected text.
5. Use the change case feature to change text case.

■ **Activity**
1. Type Face. This refers to the look of the characters.
a. Download and open the document **Chap5-Exercise2-Character-formatting**.
b. Select the **two lines** immediately following the word "Arial" by placing the pointer in the margin across from the two lines and double-clicking

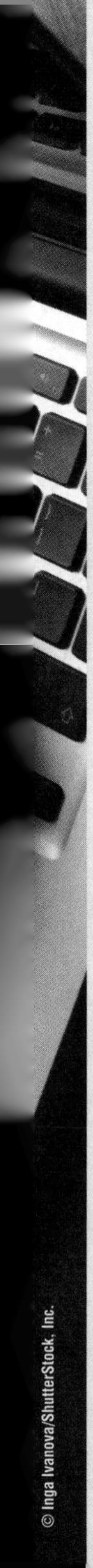

and/or holding down the left mouse button while dragging the mouse to the end of the text. Let go of the mouse button before moving on to the next step.

c. Click the **font down arrow** Times New Ron in the Font group of the Home tab. Click **Arial**. Repeat these directions for the remaining three fonts. *Notice the little feet on the "i" and "h" for Courier and Times New Roman. These are serif fonts; the other two are sans serif fonts.* Use serif fonts for word processing.

2. Font Size. This refers to the height of the characters.
   a. Select the line beginning with **18 Point** like in the exercise above.
   b. Click the **down arrow** 12 next to the current size (12) in the Font group of the Home tab. Select **18 points**. You may also right-click the selection and click on font from the shortcut menu. Select the correct size in the dialog window.
   c. Repeat these directions for the remaining points in the exercise. In the healthcare field why would you want to use some of the larger fonts? Type your answer under font size section.
3. Font Attributes and Special Effects
   a. Select the first "**I am going to be an excellent healthcare provider and Word user**" sentence.
   b. Right click the **selection** and select **Font** from the shortcut menu.
   c. At the bottom of the tab, under Effects, there are boxes with options such as Strikethrough, Small caps, and All caps. Select the box to the left of the **Strikethrough** option. Click **OK**.
   d. Repeat the same steps for the next three sentences, choosing the **Superscript**, **Subscript,** and **Small Caps** options.
   e. Select the **fifth** sentence. Click **Bold** on the Font group in the Home tab.
   f. Select the **sixth** sentence. Right-click the selection and select **Font** from the shortcut menu. In the Underline styles options, choose the **words only** option.
   g. Select the **seventh** sentence and click the **italic** icon on the Font group in the Home tab.
   h. Select the **eighth** sentence. Click the down arrow to the right of the **Font Color** icon in the font group. Under the font color menu, choose any color. The sentences should now display eight different font attributes and/or special effects.
   i. Write a sentence next to each sentence as to the conditions under which you might use this effect.
   j. Select the text in parentheses that reads **cHANGE cASE**. Click the **Change Case down arrow** Aa in the Font group then select **tOGGLE cASE**.
4. Save this file as **Chap5-Exercise2-LastName**. Submit as directed by your professor.

EXERCISE 3 Paragraph Formatting—Tabs, Indents, and Justification

Objectives

1. Apply the appropriate tab for the text.
2. Apply left, right, hanging, and first line indents to selected text.
3. Apply center, justify, left, and right alignment to selected text.

Activity

Working with Tabs

Imagine that you are nearly finished with your college degree and are ready to start practicing in the healthcare field. Much to your chagrin, your advisor tells you that you've forgotten to fulfill a general literature requirement and that the only appropriate course with seats available is Readings in Contemporary Poetry. So there you are, in this poetry class, when your professor tells you that there's no book to buy at the bookstore and that you're going to create the book yourself. She hands each student the name of a poet and tells him or her to pick that poet's ten best poems and copy them into a neat anthology for the class. You've been handed Nicholas Christopher and you've already selected your poems. But the professor keeps saying that the anthologies *must* look nice. "Remember that this is our textbook," she keeps saying. The anthology's appearance is 40% of your grade, so you want your list of poems and their related pages to look nice. What do you do?

1. Download and open the document **Chap5-Exercise3-LeftTabsandDot-Leaders**.
2. Select all text in the **Part 1** list.
3. Look at the ruler above the document. To its left is a box with a short L in it [L]. If there isn't a plain, short L facing the right way, click the **tab** box until there is. The L means that Word is ready for you to set standard left tabs.
4. Click just below the **half-inch** mark on the ruler, but just above the gray, which separates the ruler from the document.
5. Click the **tab** box on the left of the ruler bar, until a **right** tab appears. [⅃]
6. Set a right tab at **5.5"**.
7. The titles in boldface are the books from which the poems come, and the other titles are the poems themselves. Move the cursor in front of "Reflections on a Bowl of Kumquats, 1936," the first poem title, and press the **tab** key once. Repeat this step for each of the rest of the poem titles.
8. There is still one more thing that can be done. Select **all the text** in the list again. Double-click the right [⅃] tab.
9. In the Tabs dialog box on the left of the Tabs window, select the **5.5"** tab.

10. In the same window, under Leader, select **2**, which is a series of dots. Click the **Set** button.
11. Click **OK**.
12. Part 2: Your employer has a Word document in which the content listed in part 2 of the Left Tabs and Dot Leaders file. He is stumped as to how to align the words so they look nice. What he wants to do is insert multiple tabs to move the text over to align properly, but knows there must be a better way. He asks you to format them properly.
13. Turn on the **Show/Hide mark** (Click the **Show/Hide** ¶ icon in the paragraph group of the Home tab. Check to make sure there is only one tab mark between the items.
14. Select the **first line** of text. That would be student number, year, exam 1 and exam 2.
15. Make sure the left tab displays on the far left of the toolbar (if not, click it until the left tab marker displays).
16. Place tabs stops at the **1.5**, **2.5**, and **3.5** marks on the ruler bar.
17. Select the **next two lines** of text. Place a left tab stop at **1.5** on the ruler bar.
18. Change the tab to display a **decimal align** tab. Place a decimal align tab on the sixth **tab** stop between the 2" and 3" marks on the ruler bar and then on the sixth **tab** stop between the 3" and 4" marks.
19. What other feature could you use to create the list of poems?

Working with Indents

1. Download and open the document **Chap5-Exercise3-Indents**.
2. Select the **text** below Left Indent, starting with *this* and ending with *spaces*.
3. Press the **Tab** key. The paragraph should now be indented from the left margin. You can also use the ruler bar and drag the indent marker as a unit . Under what conditions do you use the left indent?
4. Select the **text** below Right Indent, starting with *right* and ending with *toolbar*.
5. On the ruler near the top of the screen, there is a triangle pointing up at 6". Click that triangle and drag it to 5" . Your paragraph is now right indented. Under what conditions is the right indent paragraph formatting feature used?
6. Place the insertion point to the left of *this* and press the **Tab** key ." The first line of the paragraph is now indented. You may also drag the top indent marker to the .5" mark on the ruler bar. Some style manuals require the first line of a paragraph to be indented a half inch from the left margin.
7. Select the **text** below Hanging, starting with *depending* and ending with *spaces*.

8. Click the **Paragraph Dialog Box Launcher**. This time, from the "Special" box, select **Hanging**. Now your paragraph has a hanging indent. Under what circumstances is the hanging paragraph used?

Working with Justification

1. Download and open the document **Chap5-Exercise3-Justification.**
2. Select the **title My Story—A Brush with Death** immediately following Here is an example under Center Justification.
3. Click **Center** in the Paragraph group. What happens to the text? Why would you use center alignment?
4. Select the **text** "This is a paragraph... in the paragraph" following the justification description.
5. Click **Justify** in the paragraph group. The text is now flush at both the left and right margins. The words are spread out to make the text flush. Under what conditions would you use this justification?
6. Left alignment is the default. There is no need to select this paragraph because it is already left aligned.
7. Select the **text Title of My Paper through Name: Irene Joos** following the right alignment description.
8. Click **Align Text Right** in the paragraph group. The text is now flush at the right margin. Under what conditions would you use this justification?
9. If directed by the professor, save these files by adding your name to the end of the file name and submitting as directed.

EXERCISE 4 Merge and Find Functions

Objectives

1. Create main, data source, and merged documents.
2. Use the find and replace function.
3. Print created letters.

Activity

1. Create the documents.
   a. Create the main and data source documents like those at the end of this exercise. Use the directions given earlier in this chapter for creating the mail merge documents. Save the files **Chap5-Exercise4-Doc1DM** and **Chap5-Exercise4-DataDM.**
2. Use the find and replace function and replace all occurrences of DM with **diabetes mellitus,** September 25, 2013 with **January 25, 2014**, and medications with **insulin.**

3. Merge the documents.
   a. Use the mail merge feature to generate and print the individual letters.
   b. Check the letters for accuracy.
   c. Save the results as **Chap5-Exercise4-3-LastName.**

   The appearance of the fields depends on the word processor used. The fields may be indicated with the name of the field, a number with a hyphen (-), or something else.

Main Document

Figure 5-42 shows the sample main document. Make sure you use the insert field feature; do NOT type the fields and the related chevron into the document.

DATA SOURCE

Title	First Name	Last Name	Address	City	ST	ZIP
Ms.	Mary	Jones	325 First Street	Carnegie	PA	15102
Mr.	Robert	Tutor	45 Software Ave.	Milford	PA	15102
Dr.	Susan	Master	8997 Default Lane	Eagan	MN	55123

<<Title>> <<FirstName>> <<LastName>>

<<Address>>

<<City> <<State>> <<PostalCode>>

(Use the automatic date function to place date with this style: Month Day, Year.)

Dear <<FirstName>>:

We invite you to attend a patient education program on adult-onset DM. The date of the program is September 25, 2013. The program time takes place from 1 to 3 p.m. in the Patient Education Conference Room, 4th floor, Computerville Hospital. We designed this program for newly diagnosed diabetics. The program will address adjusting to diabetes, diet and exercise, and medications. The guest speaker is Nellie Netscape, Nurse Practitioner. Please notify us at 624-3333 if you plan to attend. There is no charge for this program. We look forward to seeing you.

Sincerely,
Chris Data. PhD. RN

Figure 5-42 Sample Main Document

4. Using the information from the letter, make a flyer that you can post in the clinic where other patients might see it.
   a. Choose an **Event flyer** from Office.com under **Templates, Flyers**.
   b. Include **clip art** that is appropriate for the document.
   c. Save the flyer as **Chap5-Exercise4b-LastName.**
5. Place all work in a folder titled Chap5-Exercise4-LastName. Zip the folder and submit as directed by the professor.

Assignments

ASSIGNMENT 1 Preparing a Résumé

You will need Microsoft Word and an Internet connection for this assignment.

Directions

A résumé that summarizes educational and professional accomplishments is necessary when you apply for a job. This assignment uses the registered nurse résumé, but you may select another if you desire.

1. Obtain a want ad from the paper (preferably in the health field).
2. Compose a résumé using a Word résumé template.
   a. Click **File** tab and then **New**.
   b. Under **Templates** and **Office.com** (you will need to have an authorized MS Word application on your computer to do this and an Internet connection):
      i. Click **Resumes and CVs**.
      ii. Click **Job-Specific resumes** and select the **Registered nurse resume** or another of your liking.
      iii. Click the **Download** button.
      iv. Complete the template by replacing the text placeholders with your own information. Delete any extra placeholders. Remember that this template uses tables to hold the data, so you will need to work with tables to add or delete rows. Make sure the résumé includes the following information:
         - Information about the person: name, address (city, state, ZIP code), phone number, and email address
         - Summary of your professional skills
         - Listing of your professional credentials, such as registration and certifications
         - Education (school, degree, date, major)
         - Professional experience as a health professional/nurse (begin with your most recent position and include the year, name of position, and type of unit)

- Affiliations, such as professional associations, and any offices held
- Community service activities

c. Use uppercase and lowercase.
d. Spell check your document.
e. Save the résumé as **Chap5-Assign1-LastName**.

3. Compose and revise a cover letter applying for the position.
   a. Open the résume file **Chap5-Assign1-LastName;** if necessary, go to the **end of the file**, and **create a page break**. Type the **cover letter**. Save the **file.**
   b. Run the cover letter through the **spelling and grammar checker** including a **word count** and **reading level**. Make **spelling and grammar corrections.** Use the snipping tool to **capture the readability statistics** dialog box results (**Start, All Programs, Accessories, Snipping Tool, New down arrow** , and select **Window Snip**). Copy the image in the snipping window to the end of the résumé file.
   c. Insert a copy of the original cover letter page after the readability statistics page. Make appropriate revisions in the cover letter using the results of the spelling and grammar check.
4. Save the **file** as **Chap5-Assign1-LastName.** Submit the **advertisement**, a **letter of application** (original and revised), and the **résumé** as directed by the professor.

ASSIGNMENT 2 Creating a Table

Directions

1. Select a topic that lends itself to a table. For example, a list of nurses with contact information, a list of items with a description and price, budget items you would like to request along with descriptions, number, and cost, and so forth. Use content that means something to you.
2. Create a table using the following directions.
   a. Create at least five columns.
   b. Add at least five records.
   c. Format the table using one of the design auto format features.
   d. Copy the table to a new separate page in this document (insert a page break and place the table on next page).
   e. Sort the first table by name from A–Z.
   f. Sort the second table by data in another column. Format it with a different design.
3. Save the file as **Chap5-Assign2-LastName**. Submit as directed by the professor.

ASSIGNMENT 3 Preparing a Newsletter (a Challenge to Show What You've Learned)

Directions

1. Use the following features to create a one-page newsletter.
   a. Use WordArt to create the title – Eating Healthy. Size it to span 6 inches across the page and apply a text effect. (Commands are on the Insert tab.)

HINT: Press the Enter key twice and anchor the WordArt on the first paragraph mark.

   b. Insert a section break, continuous, at the second paragraph mark.
   c. Create two columns for the second section.
   d. Type at least five subtitles and add content about each.
   e. Make the first letter of the content under each subtitle a drop cap.
   f. Add at least one clip art image in an appropriate place(s).
   g. Place a border around the page.
2. Save this assignment as **Chap5-Assign3-LastName**. Submit it to the professor as directed.

ASSIGNMENT 4 Formatting a Formal Paper

Directions

Assignment 4 has you working with a formal paper that includes a title page, table of contents, headers, table, and bibliography. You will use APA style 6th edition for the paper.

1. Use a paper you have written for another class or one provided by your professor.
2. Create a title page.
3. Insert a header and the page number according to APA style.
4. Apply the appropriate heading styles to enable later generation of the table of contents.
5. Add a relevant table.
6. Format the table attractively.
7. Add appropriate clip art, pictures, or SmartArt appropriate to enhance the message.
8. Generate the table of contents.
9. Create a reference list.
10. Save the file as **Chap5-Assign4-LastName**. Submit following the directions of your professor.

chapter

6

Introduction to Presentation Graphics

Objectives 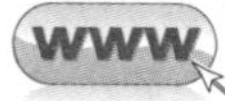

1. Define basic terminology related to presentation graphics.
2. Describe selective uses of presentation graphics software.
3. Recognize components of a quality slide presentation.
4. Develop quality PowerPoint and poster presentations.

Introduction

Healthcare professionals and students use presentation graphics programs when presenting at conferences, in educational institutions, on social media sites, and in mobile situations. In many courses, students must use presentation graphics software for their in-class and distance education presentations; healthcare professionals use the software for presentations at conferences as well as for preparation of patient education materials; and educators use it during face-to-face and distance education courses. In today's mobile world, we use presentation graphics to present patient educational materials on mobile devices. Presentation graphics software makes it possible to view data visually through charts/graphs that help users to "see" the data and use it to make decisions. Microsoft PowerPoint is one of the most commonly used presentation graphics programs while Keynote is very popular for Apple mobile products. Applications such as word processing and spreadsheet programs typically contain some graphics capabilities, but none of them has the power inherent in **presentation graphics programs** to prepare and deliver quality presentations.

Graphics programs include presentation software like PowerPoint, drawing programs like CorelDRAW and OpenOffice Draw, and computer-aided design (CAD) programs like AutoCAD and MicroStation. Most presentation programs include capabilities for text handling, outlining, drawing, graphing, inserting clip art and pictures, and adding special effects. They allow for the production of high-quality presentation slides, transparencies, handouts, posters, or electronic slide shows. Drawing programs help users produce clip art and images that they can then incorporate into presentation programs or other applications where images might enhance the message. Computer-aided design programs are used by draftsmen, engineers, and architects to produce design plans and drawings. New to the presentation arena are programs like Brainshark that aid in the conversion of PowerPoint presentations into mobile video presentations, and Prezi (http://prezi.com/), which is a software as a service (SaaS) cloud-based presentation software and storytelling tool that is growing in popularity.

This chapter focuses on presentation graphics using PowerPoint. Users employ PowerPoint and similar presentation graphics programs to present information in a pleasing visual fashion to facilitate decision making and to communicate a message. The inclusion of visuals that sustain the audience's interest, highlight content, and disseminate information clearly enhances the effectiveness of presentations.

Presentation

Presentation graphics programs support presentations by demonstrating the ideas and concepts within the presentation through graphics or images.

Professional Guidelines

This section presents guidelines for creating professional presentations.

- Clearly define the purpose or message of the presentation. A clearly defined purpose assists in determining the content and message to convey.
- Define the target audience. This will aid in the design of the presentation and the selection of images to use. The same design and images appropriate for children would not be acceptable for a professional audience.
- Outline or organize the message. Remember this step outlines the content for the presentation and helps in organizing the content. List the key points or message that each slide is to convey. Watch that you do not use the outline to create all text or bulleted list slides. The outline should focus only on the message to be conveyed.
- Decide on the best medium for the presentation. This decision requires knowledge of both the environment where the presentation will occur and the equipment that will be available. For example, if you are giving

a presentation in a classroom you might be presenting your materials using an interactive whiteboard, but at a conference you might have a data projector designed for use with a large screen in an auditorium. You will also want to use the selected medium to its best advantage. There are also differences in designing a presentation for delivery through distance education courses when the speaker is not present.

- When developing a presentation for a course, be sure to follow the guidelines from the professor. The same concept is true when presenting for a patient or staff education program or for a professional conference. That is—be sure to follow the guidelines from the sponsoring organization.
- Follow the general guidelines under preparing a presentation in this chapter.

Presenters commonly use a variety of media for their presentations—namely, **handouts, slide shows, transparencies**, and **posters**. With the current technology, presenters rarely use 35mm slides; this text will not discuss them.

Output Types

Handouts

Sometimes presenters provide handouts to the audience to outline the presentation, define selected terms, or present complex information. Use the presentation program's handout feature when you want to provide printed copies of the slides or speaker notes for yourself or for the audience. It is easy to develop appropriate handouts and notes that go with the presentation. To prepare notes or reference lists that will not be covered in the presentation or reference lists, use a word processing program. No special equipment is needed to manage handouts during the presentation, but handouts can be expensive depending on the needed number and the printing process (including whether or not the handouts are printed in color). To avoid the cost of printing, some speakers will offer to email a copy of the slides to participants after the conference. If you elect to distribute handouts in this way, it is best to save the slides as a PDF file before sending to avoid modification of your original slides. Some presenters and conference sponsors now provide those handouts on their Web sites or in the conference proceedings. In these cases it is common practice for the conference sponsors to request that you transfer the copyright of the presentation slides to the conference sponsors.

Slide Shows

Using a **data projector** connected to a computer, you can project the presentation on a large screen or smart board. You can create the slides in PowerPoint, and then add special effects. Adding sound is especially effective, but should only be done if it is appropriate to the subject and audience and if an adequate sound system is available.

PowerPoint slide shows make it easy to adapt a presentation to different audiences and time slots without incurring additional expenses. Data projection systems are generally available in educational and healthcare institutions as well as at convention centers. Newer models are portable, less expensive than traditional devices, and project high-quality images in regular lighting.

Always have a backup plan should something happen to the data projection system, such as a burned-out light bulb or a network issue. Make sure that the appropriate software is in place and that you use the "package presentation for CD" option (**File**, **Save & Send**, and **Package Presentation for CD**) to avoid compatibility issues. With the latter approach, Microsoft Office PowerPoint Viewer and any linked files (such as movies or sounds) are copied as well as the presentation itself; by doing this, the presentation does not depend on the availability of the correct version of PowerPoint (in earlier versions of PowerPoint, this capability was called the "pack and go" option). Note the other options available in Save & Send, such as saving and sending to SharePoint (a Microsoft software program that makes it easier for people to work together by sharing information, managing documents, and publishing reports), broadcasting a slideshow, creating a video, or publishing to the Web. Finally, always try to test your presentation on the equipment that will be used in the setting where it will be used well before the presentation date.

Transparencies

Some presenters opt for transparencies because they are easy to prepare and use, although the necessary projection equipment is disappearing. **Document cameras**, which can also show transparencies, are slowly but surely replacing overhead projectors. If you are planning to use transparencies always check to be sure you will have access to the necessary equipment such as an overhead projector or document camera. You can use transparencies in rooms with normal lighting, which facilitates note taking. Because most printers can print them, transparencies are easier and less expensive to produce than slides and might work better at less technologically advanced sites. Use of laser and color printers can also enhance the effectiveness of transparencies. Transparencies, however, are not as easy to revise as electronic slide shows because it requires reprinting the transparencies.

Posters

Posters are useful to present the results of a research study or to communicate ideas. The poster holds the presentation while the presenter stands nearby, ready to field questions. A poster is a static, visual medium that is usually prepared in color. Custom PowerPoint Poster templates let you add content and color to the presentation and print it on large paper for mounting on a poster board, but this can be expensive. It is wise to check these details before beginning the poster development. While PowerPoint provides a quick and easy way to create the poster through custom poster templates there might be other requirements at your institution.

Podcasts

You can turn a PowerPoint presentation into a **podcast** for uploading and sharing with others. Once you create the presentation, use the record narration feature, and then save it as a PowerPoint slideshow. Upload the podcast to a Web site, YouTube, or a podcast hosting service such as Podbean (http://podbean.com/), libsyn (http://libsyn.com/), or PodOmatic (www.podomatic.com/).

Videos

When you want to provide your classmates, professors, and others with a high fidelity version of your presentation, consider turning it into a video. PowerPoint has a function to save and play it as a video. The default format is Windows Media Video (.wmv), but there are also third-party utilities that will convert the file into formats such as .avi, and .mov.

Once you complete the planning process, develop a presentation outline, and select the output medium, the next step is to create the graphic presentation.

Key Points in Creating Graphic Presentations and Posters

Nothing is worse than using a graphics presentation that detracts from the message the speaker is trying to convey or that presents nothing but text on the screen. For poster presentations, nothing is worse than trying to cram in too much information in too small a font for the size of the poster. A program such as PowerPoint will never be a substitute for a well-prepared and organized speaker, a speaker who speaks well, and a speaker who can adjust the presentation to the needs of the audience. Likewise, a poster presenter must be knowledgeable about the topic and able to answer questions. PowerPoint will not make the speaker a great speaker, nor will a great poster presenter turn you into a great presenter. Instead, the graphics program is simply a tool to aid in the development of the presentation or poster.

This section outlines some basic guidelines for preparing a graphic presentation or poster and for delivering the presentation. You should adjust these guidelines based on the message and intent of the slide or poster.

Preparing a Presentation

- Begin the presentation with a title slide. The content of this slide should orient the audience to the topic of the presentation and to the identity of the presenter and/or company. Add a subtitle, date, or clip art if desired.
- Select a design theme and apply it to the presentation. PowerPoint comes with many preset design templates; even more options are available online from Office.com. Other templates are available for purchase from

independent providers. The conference sponsor might also provide guidelines for what will work well with their equipment, including screen ratios and font types.

- Use an easy-to-read font. This means a simple upright font without swirls and scripts. Recommended fonts include Times New Roman, Arial, and Garamond.
- Obey the 44/32 guideline. Font sizes for titles should be between 40 and 44 points, whereas font sizes for text should be between 24 to 32 points. It is better to err by making the font too large than to run the risk of making it so small people cannot read the slides from the back of the room.
- Use a maximum of three different fonts in a presentation. Use of too many different fonts will prove distracting to the audience.
- Use both uppercase and lowercase letters for most text. Text that appears in all-capital letters is more difficult to read, although a title or word can be placed in all uppercase letters for emphasis.
- Use no more than five to seven words across the slide and five to seven lines down the slide—a guideline that translates to "use phrases and not complete sentences." Use two slides if you need to include more than seven items. Be aware that speakers have a tendency to read the slides if they use complete sentences.
- Limit the use of italics. While pretty, words in italics are more difficult to read.
- Apply bold and shadow attributes to the text. Boldface increases the stroke weight and projects the words better than plain text. Shadowing fonts put a crisp edge around the text. In some design templates, however, shadowing the font may produce a blurred image.
- Use bulleted lists to organize the points for the audience. Left align bulleted lists; don't center them. Use no more than three bulleted list slides in a row. The presentation becomes very boring if all slides are bulleted list slides.
- Use clip art, shapes, and SmartArt to add interest to the slides. Make sure that these graphic elements "fit" with the message that the slide is conveying and that the graphic elements are an integral part of the slide. For example, place a definition in the "callout" shape or a list of items inside a pyramid.
- Use diagrams instead of complete sentences to describe processes. For example, you might use shapes or SmartArt features to present the diagnostic process instead of bulleted lists. People tend to remember things when visuals are part of the slide.
- Use an interesting image to signal a break for questions and answers during the presentation.
- Keep special effects and sound to a minimum unless they enhance the presentation. If using special effects or sounds, make sure the equipment that

you use for the presentation can handle these options. It can be very distracting when a speaker stops the presentation to try to deal with a special effect that is not functioning. In this case, the best option is to simply to state that a special effect is not working and move on with the presentation.
- Use the spell checker for all slide, poster, and online presentations.
- Be sure to proofread the slides one final time after using the spell checker.

Preparing an Online Presentation

For an online presentation, follow the general guidelines for a quality presentation, albeit with some alterations:

- Use a white background template with colored objects. This design results in a smaller file size than do busy, highly colored background templates; smaller files, in turn, speed up the download process.
- Keep image and picture sizes smaller for quicker download and viewing.
- Include speaker notes or narration to elaborate on the content. Remember that adding sound will increase the file size.
- Save the file as a PowerPoint slide show, PDF (Portable Document Format) file with speaker notes, packaged for CD, and/or Web page. The choice of how you save the file depends on the nature of the presentation and the method of delivery.
- If recording your voice, keep the microphone no more than 5 inches away from your mouth and use a normal speaking voice.
- If recording, speak slowly and clearly.

Delivering a Presentation

Preparing to deliver a presentation requires the speaker to take some steps to ensure that the presentation will go smoothly and achieve its purpose:

- Know the topic and presentation well. Speak about topics on which you are knowledgeable, and practice the presentation so you are familiar with the sequence of slides. Prepare speaker notes to help keep yourself focused on what you intend to say about the slide.
- Face the audience and talk to the audence; don't read your slides or speaker notes, but refer to them as needed to reinforce your points. Novice presenters sometimes face the whiteboard or screen and talk to it instead of addressing the audience. If you need to, look at the monitor at the speaker podium instead of turning your back to the audience. The key point here is *look*—do not *read* from the monitor.
- Be prepared to present your materials with a limited view of your slides. Sometimes the slides will appear over your shoulder (i.e., behind you) and

not on the monitor in front of you. If your slides appear on the monitor, remember that the audience is looking at the projected slides. Often the projected slides are not as sharp and clear as the ones on the monitor. If the slides are behind you, look at the slides and use a laser pointer to direct the audience's attention to key points on the slides. With this approach, you and the audience are looking at the slides together.

- Use the speaker preparation rooms or student practice rooms to become comfortable with the technology that you will use. The technology—in this case, a PowerPoint presentation, computer, and data projection system—should be transparent to the audience. Remember that the technology is there to enhance the presentation, not to detract from it.
- Slow down and speak up. Nothing loses the audience more quickly than someone who talks too fast or too softly. Practicing the presentation before its actual delivery will help hone these skills.
- Have a backup plan. Technology sometimes fails, so be prepared.
- Keep to the time limit. Most presentations will have a set time for you to present your topic. Practice the timing so you aren't rushed at the end or finish too soon.

Delivering a Poster Presentation

For poster presentations, follow these guidelines:

- Arrive during the scheduled time to arrange your poster in the poster area. Make sure you have mounting supplies in case the conference or organization does not provide them.
- Be present during the time scheduled for poster presentations and be ready to answer questions that viewers may ask.
- Provide handouts to further explain the project. Make sure the handouts contain your contact information. You should also have business cards available for viewers who want additional information. These are easy to produce using Word and a laser printer with business card paper or can be printed at a copy business.

Delivering an Online Presentation

With online courses and social media, many of you will "post" your presentation either in a course management program or on a social media site. Remember that PowerPoint is a presentation graphic program, meaning there should be a presenter. Here are some guidelines to consider when posting your presentation online without the presenter.

- At minimum, include speaker notes as part of the presentation. This will tell the viewer what you would be saying about each slide. If converting to a PDF for upload, make sure you adjust the publish option to Notes Page so viewers can see the notes. Don't waste time with animations as the PDF file will not show those.

- Add voice narration to the presentation and use the laser pointer feature. Save it as a podcast or video.
- Make sure the intended audience has access to the file. This can be done through embedded links in social media sites or in the learning management system.
- If the uploaded site provides a comment option, respond professionally to comments made by others.

Presentation Graphics Terminology

General Terms

General terms that apply to discussions of presentation graphics software are as follows:

Analytic Graphics	**Analytic graphics** present data in graph form for analysis, understanding, and decision making. Presentation graphics, spreadsheet, or statistics programs can be used to create these graphs.
Density per Inch (DPI)	**Density per Inch (DPI)** DPI indicates the pixel density—that is, the number of dots (pixels) per inch. Resolution quality increases with a larger DPI.
File Format	The **file format** is how the program stores the graphic or image—an important consideration for importing data and developing slides. PowerPoint supports several popular graphic file formats, such as Enhanced Metafile (.emf), Windows Metafile (.wmf), 97-2003 PowerPoint (.ppt), Windows Media Video (.wmv), and so forth. It also permits users to import multimedia file types such as audio video interleave (.avi) and Waveform (.wav) for audio and video files.
Handles	**Handles** are the squares that surround a selected image or block of text seen on the screen. Use the handles to move, enlarge, or shrink the image or text block.
Landscape	**Landscape orientation** presents a slide in a wide or horizontal view. Use this orientation for onscreen presentations.
Pixels	**Pixels**—more formally, picture elements—are the tiny dots that make up the screen image. The more pixels, the sharper the image (resolution).

Portrait	**Portrait orientation** presents a slide in an upright or vertical view. Use this orientation for overhead transparencies and (sometimes) for poster presentations.
Presentation	A **presentation** is the group of slides that makes up the actual material for viewing. It can vary from an unlimited number of slides to only a few. Remember that more slides are not necessarily better. The general guideline is to use one slide for every 1–3 minutes of a presentation.
Resolution	**Resolution** is the number of pixels on the screen.
Slides	**Slides** are the individual screens that make up a presentation.
Slide Layout	**Slide layout** refers to the way in which you arrange the placeholders for the text and images on the slide. Many different slide layouts are available in PowerPoint.

Graphics and Multimedia Terms

The terms in this section are used to describe and work with graphics or clip art.

Audio	Sound files in a variety of formats that will play in a PowerPoint presentation. Some of these file formats are .mp3, .wav, .wma, and .au.
Bullet	A **bullet** is a graphic that appears to the left of a text list. Different symbols are available for bullets, such as a dot, arrow, block, or check mark.
Bitmaps	**Bitmapped graphics** images are stored and represented as pixels (tiny dots). Bitmaps are commonly used for clip art images. Examples include the .gif, .pcx, and .tif formats.
Clip Art	**Clip art** is a library of symbols (images) prepared by others for use with specific graphics programs. You can obtain additional clip art online at Office.com or at other image sites. When downloading clip art from Web sites for use in your own presentations, you must obey the applicable copyright laws.
Pictures	**Pictures** are digital photographs that can be imported and used in a graphic presentation. They are generally in .jpg file format.
Shapes	**Shapes** are predesigned forms used to enhance the look of the slide. Use them in place of bulleted lists or to show processes. Shapes include rectangles, circles, arrows, and callouts.

SmartArt	**SmartArt** graphics are visual representation of information and ideas. Use SmartArt to create graphic lists, show a process, or demonstrate hierarchies. SmartArt adds color and visual interest to slides.
Symbols	**Symbols** are small images, such as dingbats and special characters, that are available within, or can be imported into, a presentation program.
Themes	**Themes** (also called presentation styles in some programs) are professionally designed format and color schemes for a presentation.
Vector Graphics	**Vector graphics** are images created with lines, arcs, circles, and squares. This file format stores images as vector points. Examples include .ai, .chr6, and .wmf.
Video	Videos may be embedded in a PowerPoint presentation, linked to a video file on your storage devices, or linked to a Web site like YouTube.

Slide Layouts

Slide layout refers to the text or content placeholders that appear on a slide as well as the way in which these elements are arranged and formatted on the slide. PowerPoint 2010 includes nine predesigned layouts (See **Figure 6-1**). When the slide layout uses the term "content placeholder," the content to be added can include a title, subtitle, table, SmartArt, picture, clip art, media file, or chart.

Slide Layout Schemes

Common slide layout schemes are described here.

Title Slides	Use title slides to introduce the presentation and to separate sections within the presentation. These kinds of slides are a helpful tool for orienting the audience to the topic and its parts. Title slides can have one or two placeholders.
Title and Content	This slide layout includes one text placeholder, usually for the title, and one content placeholder for items like a bulleted list, a table, or a graph.
Section Header	A section header has two text placeholders. Use this layout when you have to break a presentation into separate parts.
Two Content	This slide layout includes one text placeholder for the title and two side-by-side content placeholders.
Comparison	This slide layout includes a title placeholder, two text placeholders below it, and two content placeholders below them.

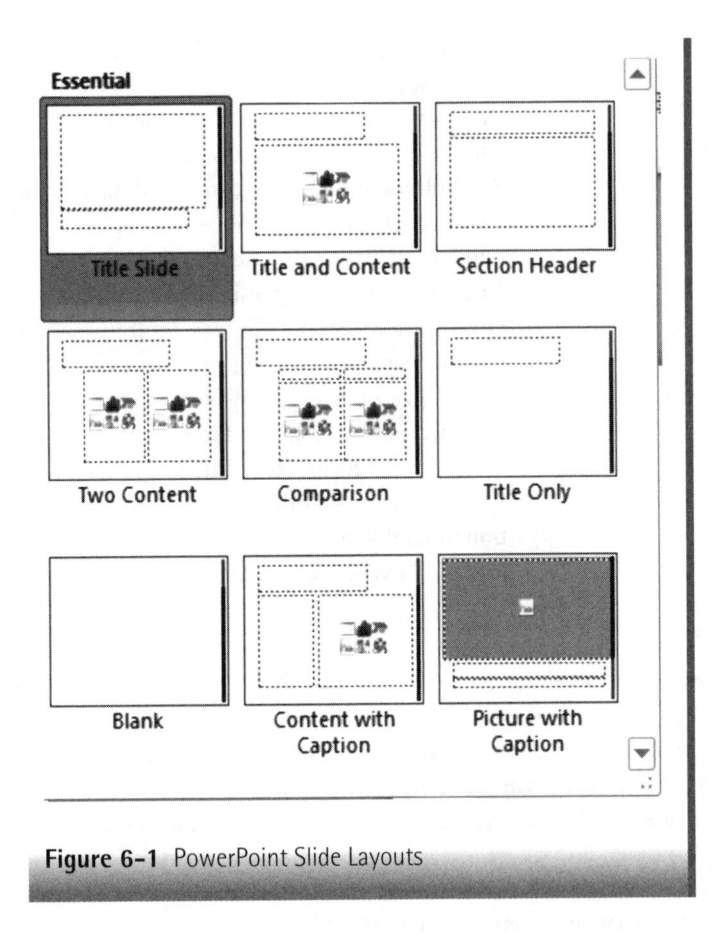

Figure 6-1 PowerPoint Slide Layouts

Title Only	Use this slide when you want to have a title placeholder but the rest of the slide with custom image or picture.
Blank	There are no placeholders in this slide.
Content with Caption	This slide layout features two text placeholders, one for a title and one for explanatory text. The third placeholder is intended to hold content.
Picture with Caption	This slide layout includes two text placeholders and one content placeholder that will accept only pictures.

Charts

PowerPoint has 11 types of charts and many variations of each, plus other types of graphic elements such as organizational charts. Use charts to represent numbers pictorially for ease in interpreting the data. The most important point to consider when using charts in your presentation is to pick the correct type of chart—one

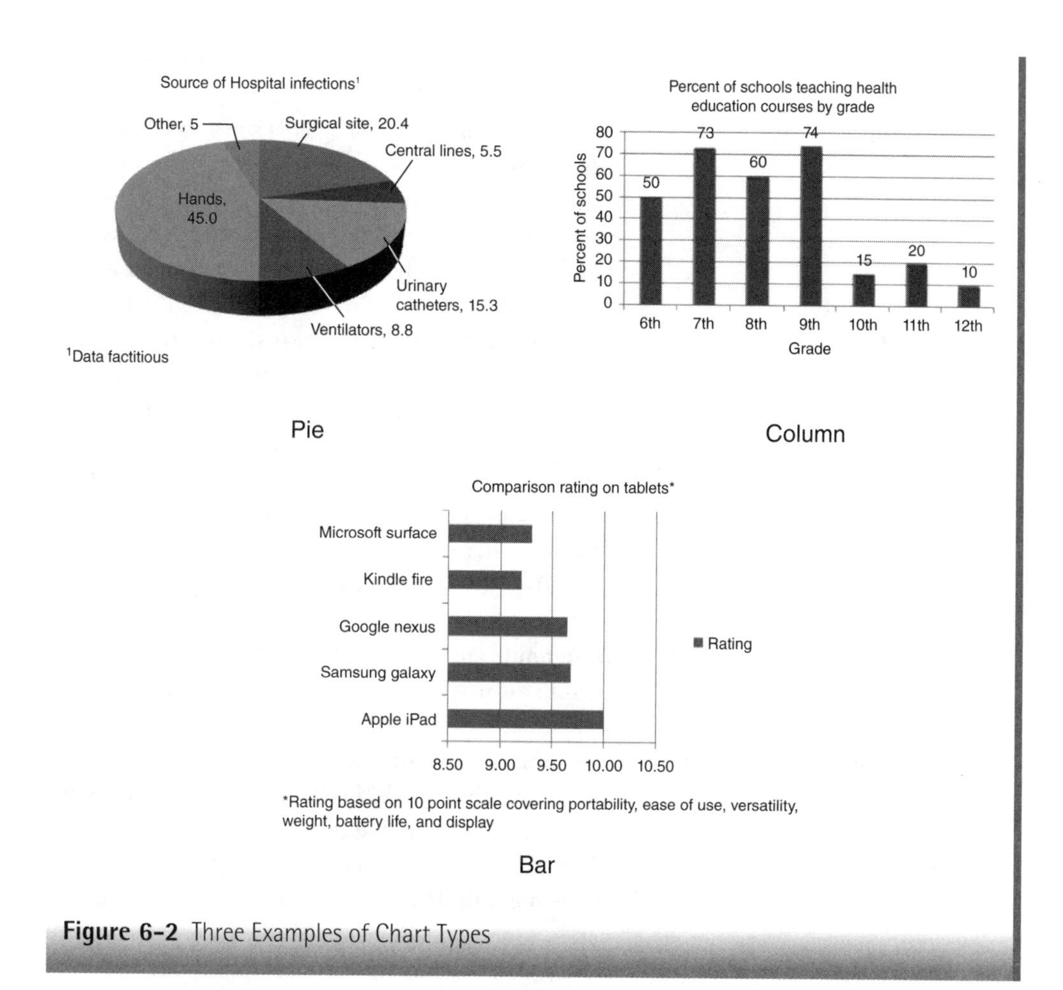

Figure 6-2 Three Examples of Chart Types

that visually and accurately conveys the data. The most commonly used types of charts are listed below; see **Figure 6-2** for some example charts.

Chart Types

The types of charts one might elect to use in a presentation are the same **chart types** available in Excel. In fact, you can import Excel charts into a PowerPoint presentation.

Area — **Area charts** present or emphasize the total quantity (volume) of several items over time. It draws a line from the last plot point to the current one and the entire area below the plot line is filled with color. Use an area chart when you want to show trends over time among related attributes.

Bar	**Bar graphs** compare data against some value at a specific point in time. The categories (similar to types of antibiotics) are arranged vertically in a column on the *y*-axis, whereas the values (rating effectiveness) are arranged horizontally on the *x*-axis. The emphasis with this type of chart is on the comparison, not time.
Bubble	**Bubble charts** shows relationships among three values by using bubbles. You must arrange data in three columns so that *x* values are in the first column, followed by *y* values, and then bubble size values.
Column	**Column graphs** show data changes over time or illustrate comparisons. The data or values are presented vertically (*y*-axis), whereas the categories appear horizontally (*x*-axis)—the reverse of bar charts. Many variations of column charts exist.
Doughnut	**Doughnuts** are variations of pie charts. They compare parts to the whole but can combine more than one data series.
Line	**Line graphs** present a large amount of data to show trends over time. In the healthcare field, vital signs are sometimes shown in line charts.
Pie	**Pie charts** compare parts to a whole or several values at one point in time. They also emphasize a particular part or to show relationships between sets of items.
Radar	**Radar charts** compare the aggregate values of multiple data series (data series: Related data points that are plotted in a chart. Each data series in a chart has a unique color or pattern and is represented in the chart legend. You can plot one or more data series in a chart. Pie charts have only one data series). For example, use a radar chart to compare objects or corporations that have similar quantifiable attributes, such as healthcare institutions and their death rates, patient length of stay, hospital-acquired infection rates, and complication rates. Radar charts (also called spider or star charts) plot the values of each category along a separate axis that starts in the center of the chart and ends on the outer ring.
Scatter (XY)	**Scatter graphs** show trends or statistics, such as averages, frequency, regression, or distribution.

Stock — **Stock charts** show the high, low, opening, and closing prices for individual stocks over time. Data must be arranged in columns or rows in a specific order to create a stock chart. While stock charts are generally used to represent fluctuation in stock prices, they can be used for scientific data. The way stock chart data is organized in the worksheet is very important. For example, to create a simple high-low-close stock chart, you should arrange your data with High, Low, and Close entered as column headings, in that order.

Surface — Use a **surface chart** when you want to find optimum combinations between two sets of values.

Chart Terms

Charts are used to visually represent data in a meaningful fashion. The following chart terms describe the components that one uses when creating charts.

Chart Styles — Each **chart style** offers a range of predefined combinations of formatting elements to control the appearance of the chart. For example, 3D, stacked, and clustered.

Datasheet — The table that provides the underlying data for a chart. This is generally an Excel spreadsheet.

Labels — **Labels** refer to the groups that represent the content of graph slides. They help the user to understand the graph (e.g., the names given to each pie wedge or bar).

Legend — A **legend** is a box used to identify the various series plotted on the chart.

Series — A **series** is a collection of related numbers located in a column or row under a common heading such as Month or Quarter.

Title — A title is a brief description of what the chart represents.

x-Axis — The ***x*-axis** refers to the horizontal reference lines or coordinates of a graph.

y-Axis — The ***y*-axis** refers to the vertical reference lines or coordinates of a graph.

Introduction to PowerPoint

PowerPoint is the graphic presentation program in the Microsoft Office suite. It provides the user with the ability to design, create, and edit presentations. You can display these presentations to the target audience in several ways: as transparencies, using computer screens, as Web pages, as handouts or notes, as posters,

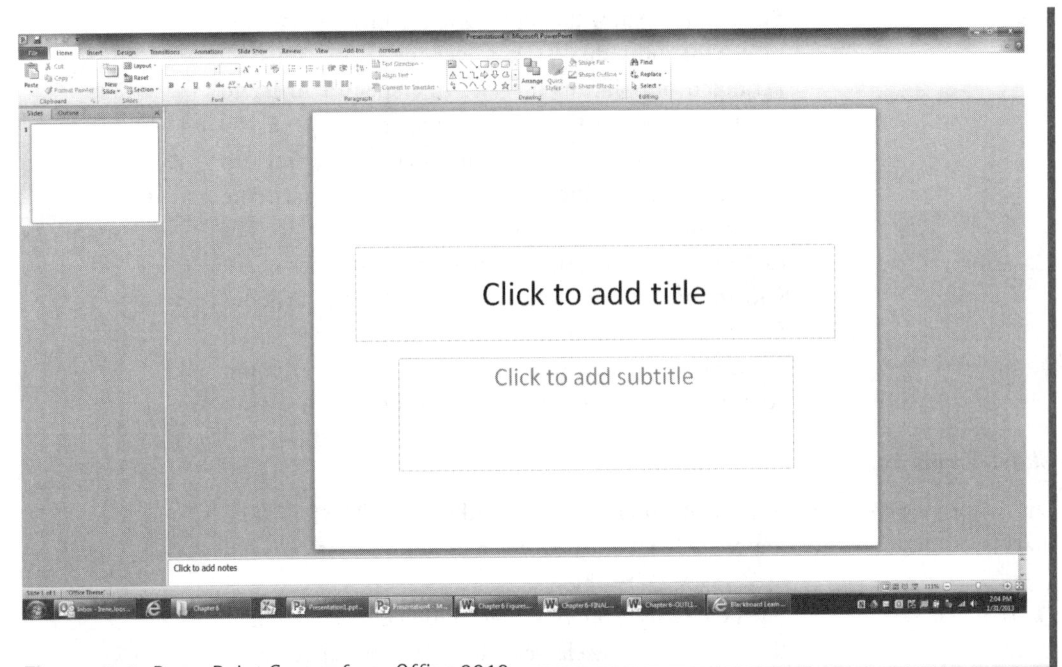

Figure 6-3 PowerPoint Screen from Office 2010

and even as workbooks. **Figure 6-3** shows the PowerPoint screen for Microsoft Office 2010.

PowerPoint screens are similar to Word and Excel screens, especially in terms of the title bar, ribbon, and groups. For a quick overview of creating presentations, click the Help icon on the right side of the screen and type "create a presentation." Select the appropriate hypertext link for creating a presentation. Much of the help is now available only online at Office.com, so make sure your Internet connection is active.

Starting PowerPoint

Here are three ways to start PowerPoint presentation.

1. Click the **Start** button on the taskbar. Select **All Programs**, **Microsoft Office**, and then click **Microsoft PowerPoint 2010**. Some systems place PowerPoint on the Start menu in the pin area.
2. Click the **PowerPoint** icon in the Quick Launch area of the taskbar.
3. Double-click the **icon** of a previously prepared **PowerPoint presentation** or **PowerPoint shortcut** on the desktop.

The main PowerPoint ribbon with the Home tab selected is shown in **Figure 6-4**. Comparing Figure 6-4 with the corresponding Figure 5-4 from the Word chapter and Figure 7-3 from the Excel chapter demonstrates how similar the ribbon is. When you position the pointer over one of the ribbon buttons, a box appears with the name of the command that the button represents. These floating toolbar button descriptions are called tooltips or **ScreenTips.**

The first two tabs (Home and Insert) and last two tabs (Review and View) are the same for PowerPoint, Word, and Excel. The middle tabs—Design, Transitions, Animation, and Slide Show—relate to PowerPoint features. You may also see context-sensitive tabs on the right side when using certain features like Charts (chart tools), or Picture (picture tools). There may also be a few tabs if add-ons have been installed. The most common add-on is Acrobat.

As in Word and Excel, you can customize the Quick Access Toolbar to add commonly used commands such as print, print preview, save, and spell check.

PowerPoint Ribbon Options

Home

The Home tab contains commands that are similar to those available in other Microsoft applications. They include groups such as Clipboard, Font, Paragraph, and Editing that are like those in Word and Excel. In addition, there are groups specific to Slides that deal with slide layouts, creation of new slides, and so forth. The Drawing group is similar to the Insert, Shapes option in Word. (See Figure 6-4.)

Insert

The Insert tab provides options for inserting tables; images such as pictures and clip art; illustrations such as shapes, SmartArt; links (hyperlinks); text such as text boxes, headers and footers, and WordArt; symbols; and media such as video and audio. (See **Figure 6-5**.)

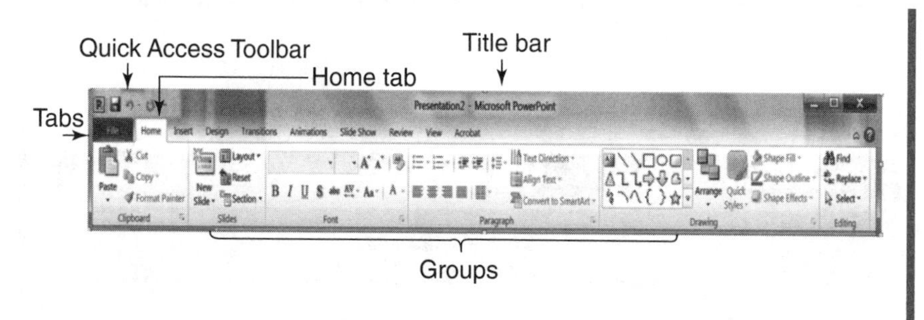

Figure 6-4 PowerPoint Ribbon with Home Tab and Groups

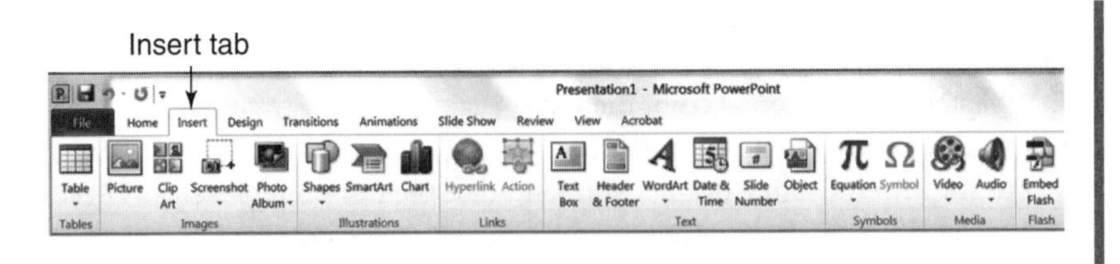

Figure 6-5 PowerPoint Insert Tab on the Ribbon

Design

The **Design tab** contains options for changing the page setup, themes, and background. (See **Figure 6-6**.)

Transitions

The **Transitions tab** permits the developer to add transitions to each slide in the presentation. You can then preview the transitions and add timing to the slide. Transitions determine how slides will come on and off in a slide show. (See **Figure 6-7**.)

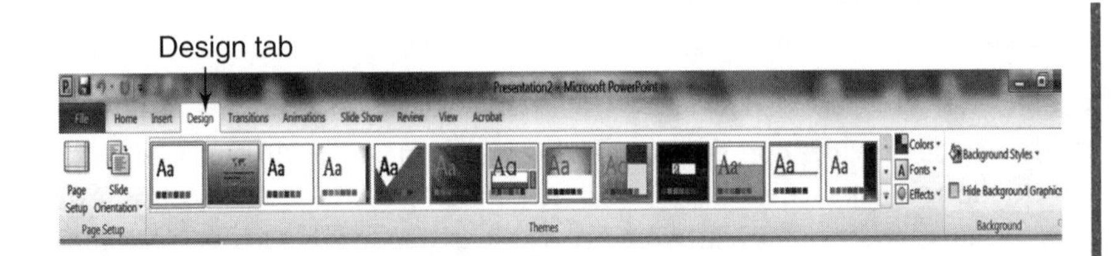

Figure 6-6 PowerPoint Design Tab on the Ribbon

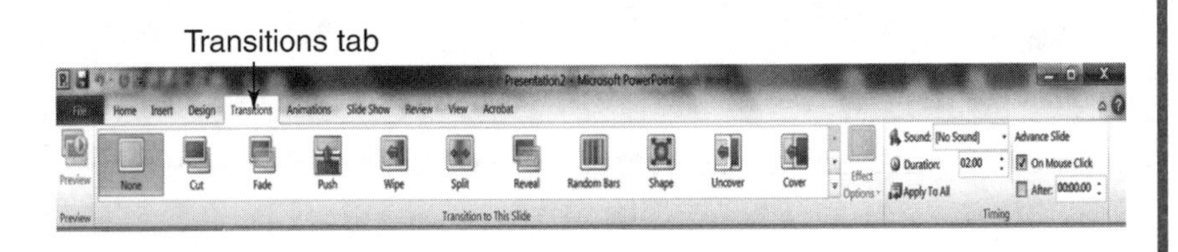

Figure 6-7 PowerPoint Transitions Tab on the Ribbon

Animations

The **Animations tab** also contains commands to control entrances and exits and changes in color or movement. It contains a preview option, animation and advanced animation commands, and timing options. Note that the main difference between the Transition and Animations tabs is that the former affects the total slide, whereas the latter affects objects on the slide. New to PowerPoint 2010 is the animation painter in the Advanced Group. It works like the format painter except that it copies the animation formatting from one object to another. (See **Figure 6-8**.)

Slide Show

The **Slide Show tab** has options for starting the presentation, setting it up, and determining how it will display. The commands on the Set Up Slide Show group provide for selecting show type, show options, pen color, and how to advance the slides. (See **Figure 6-9**.)

Review

The **Review tab** is similar to the tab in Word but includes only proofing, language, comments, compare, and OneNote commands.

View

The **View tab** is also similar to Word's View tab but includes presentation and master slide views instead of a document view, as well as show, zoom, window, and macros options. It also contains a group of commands for changing the color to gray scale and black and white.

Like Word and Excel, PowerPoint includes additional tabs that appear during certain functions, such as when you use the table and drawing/picture tools.

Creating a New Presentation

Now that you have a basic understanding of the interface, you are ready to begin creating a presentation. Before beginning a new presentation, consider your audience, think about what information you want to share with them, and decide

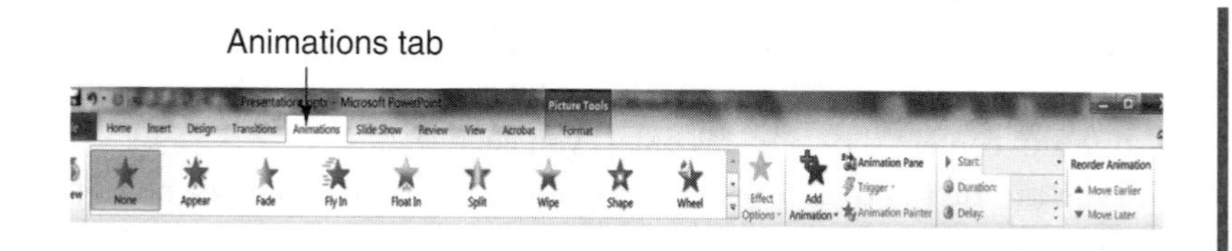

Figure 6-8 PowerPoint Animations Tab on the Ribbon

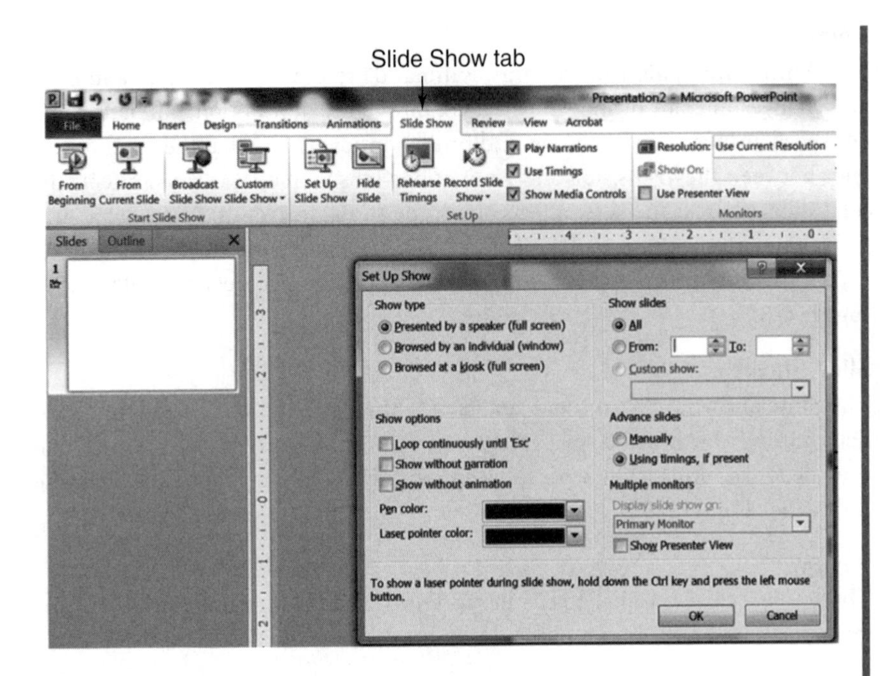

Figure 6-9 PowerPoint Slide Show Tab with Set Up Slide Show Selected

the best way to present that information. Create an outline of the major points that you want to cover. Once you have completed this you are ready to work in PowerPoint.

1. Start **PowerPoint**. The PowerPoint main screen opens. By default (clicking the New Slide icon), a title slide layout screen using a blank presentation template appears (**Figure 6-10**).
2. Click the **Title** placeholder, and type the **title** of the presentation.
3. Click the **Subtitle** placeholder, and type the **subtitle** for the presentation.
4. Click the **New Slide** button down arrow on the Home tab, Slides group.
5. Select a **layout** from the pop up menu (See Figure 6-1). If you click the New Slide button, the next slide will be a title and content slide. If you click the down arrow you see the layout options from which to pick, but the default title and content slide remains unless you change it.
6. Type the **text** and continue adding new slides until the presentation is complete.

PowerPoint has many templates and themes. To access them, click **File**, and then click **New** on the menu that appears. Some of the options available are blank and recent templates, sample templates, themes, my templates, and templates

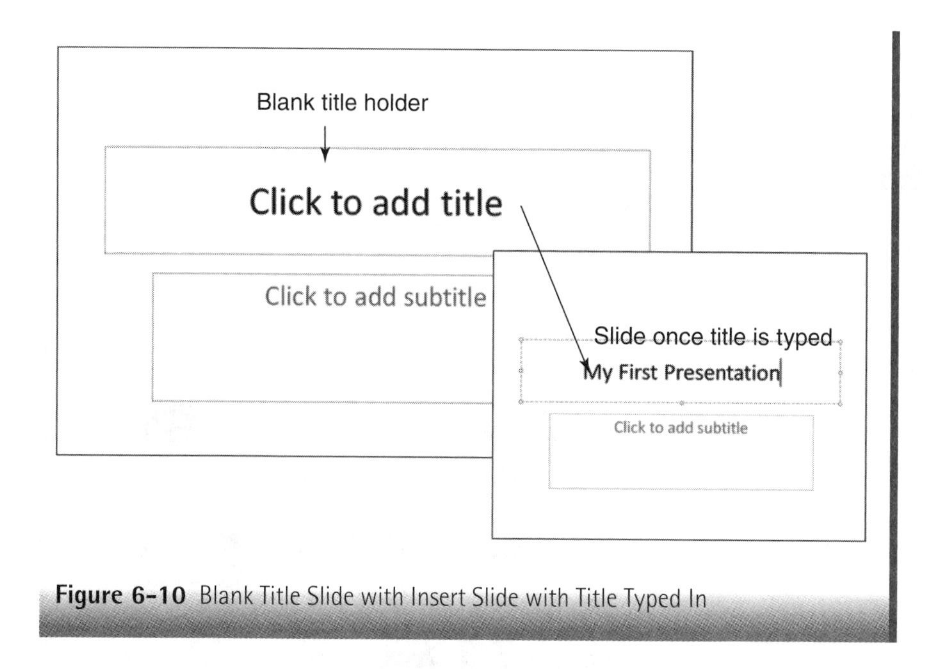

Figure 6-10 Blank Title Slide with Insert Slide with Title Typed In

available from Office.com. See **Figure 6-11** for an example of the results of typing healthcare in the search box for Office.com online templates.

Blank Presentation

This is the default template that appears when PowerPoint opens. Slides that use this template have minimal design and no color. Replace the text in the title and subtitle placeholders with appropriate content, and then click the **New Slide** button to continue adding slides. The ribbon provides options to change the design, layout, and background of the presentation and/or slides as well as options to add and format graphics and apply transitions and animation.

Template

This option presents a variety of **templates** to apply to the presentation. Think of it as a "starter document." A template is a pattern or blueprint of a slide or group of slides that you can save as a .potx file and reuse. **Figure 6-12** shows examples of the templates available from Office.com under the PowerPoint presentations and slides option on the Available Templates and Themes window with the Academic presentations selected. There are many helpful templates available on Office.com, so make sure you have an active Internet connection and a legal copy of the software to access them.

Templates generally include layouts, a theme color and fonts, background styles, and, in some cases, suggested content. Every template has a theme. Users

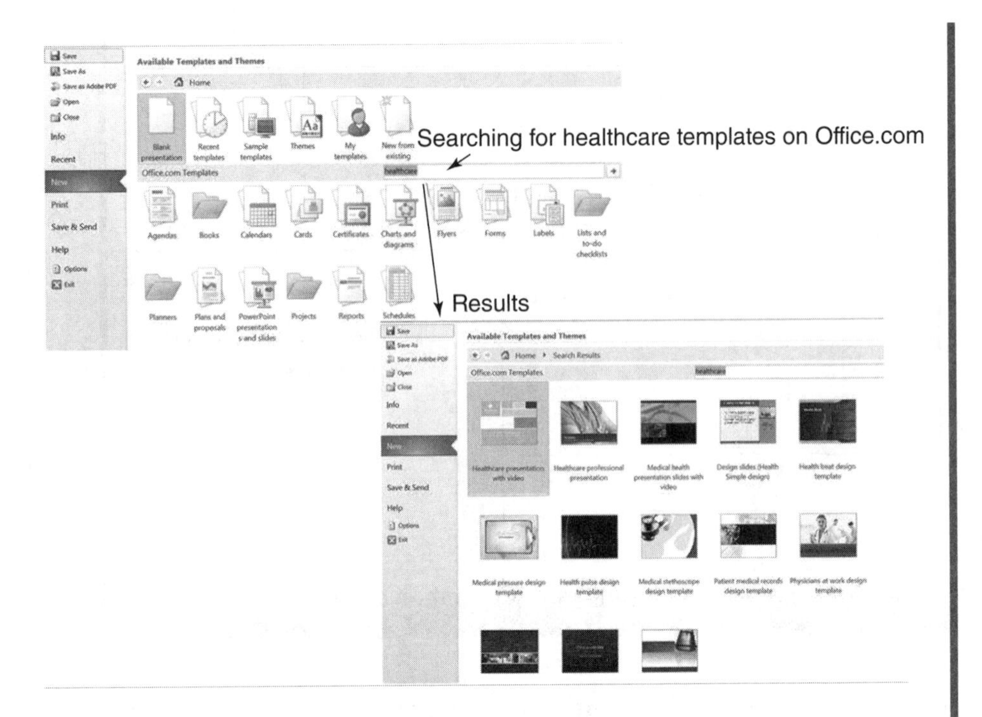

Figure 6-11 Results for Options for Healthcare Templates and Themes from Office.com

can also design their own template or use one that their institution has created. Note that there are also a few poster templates available on Office.com. No matter which template you select, it should not be too busy or distracting. The template should match the topic of the presentation, be appropriate for the target audience, and reinforce the topics presented.

Themes

A theme tells PowerPoint what color to use for the text in the slides, the background look, size and style of fonts, what graphic effects to use, and so forth. Themes are displayed in the Themes gallery in the Design tab. Every document created in PowerPoint 2010 has a theme attached to it. Themes do not contain text or data, but rather certain colors, fonts, or effects that are applied to each slide. They contain multiple master slides for title slides, speaker notes, and audience handouts. Unlike a template, it does not offer a custom slide layout or suggest content.

Reuse Slides

This option imports an existing presentation or selected slides into an existing or new presentation while preserving the original presentation. The user is free to change

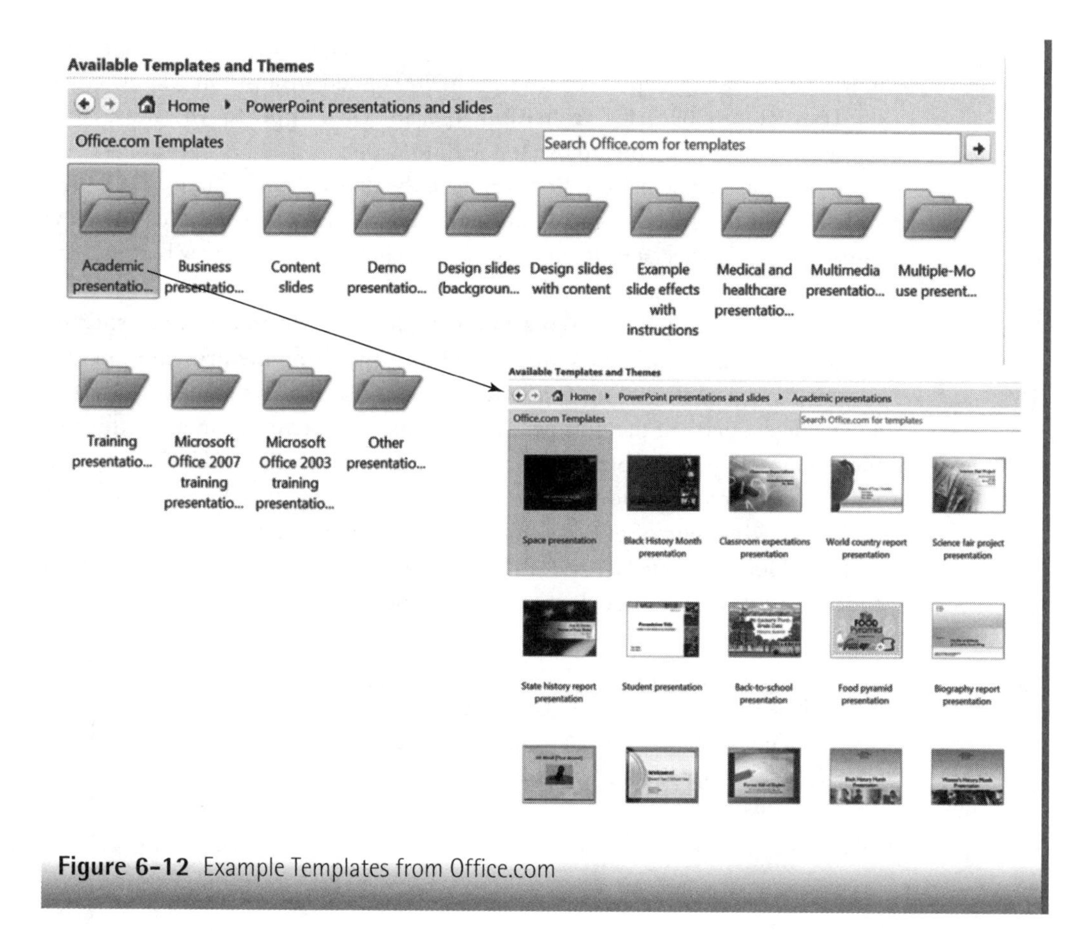

Figure 6-12 Example Templates from Office.com

the design, delete or add new slides, or change the content of existing slides. With the current presentation open, select the **Home** tab, click **New Slide down arrow**, and then click **Reuse Slides** . In the pane that opens on the right side of the screen, click **Browse** and **Browse File** to select the presentation from which the slides will be taken. To select one slide, click it. To select all the slides, right-click any slide and click **Insert All Slides**. To keep the source formatting, check the **source formatting box** before inserting the slides, (otherwise, they will assume the formatting of the destination presentation). Another option for using slides from a previous presentation is to open both presentations, click **View**, and **Arrange All**. Now drag and drop the slides from one presentation to the other presentation.

Developing a Presentation

Most users will start with a blank presentation or select a template from the gallery of templates on the computer or available online. After clicking the desired template, the user can also choose to change the color scheme of that template (click the **Design** tab, and then click a **Theme**) or add a transition scheme (click the **Transitions** tab, click a **Transition** type, and click **Apply to All**). Most users select the template and then move to the slide layout.

To develop a presentation, first complete the title slide information, and then click **New Slide**. To apply the default layout (title and content), click the **New Slide** button. To select a different slide layout, click the **down arrow** button. Pick one of the layouts from the menu of options.

Now begin typing the presentation by typing directly on the actual slide or in outline view. Outline view works well for organizing the presentation and ensuring a logical flow of ideas. If you choose the second approach, it is easy to add or delete parts of the outline. The decrease and increase indent buttons in the Paragraph group promote and demote content or slides. The Tab key and Shift+Tab key combination also do the same thing. If you right-click a slide in outline view, a menu of options appears for working with slides and slide content; see **Figure 6-13** for a list of the commands. You may also reorder or delete slides. Objects on the slide do not appear in outline view, nor does text created

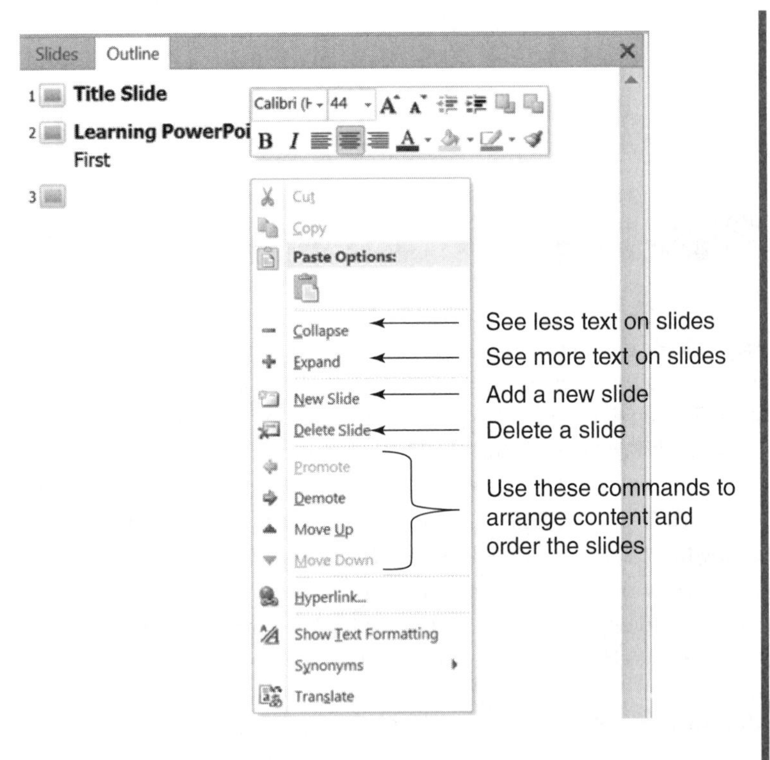

Figure 6-13 Shortcut Menu When Working in Outline View

as an object or with WordArt. The only text that shows in this view is text in placeholders. Beware that outline view may lead you to use all text slides, which violates good design guidelines.

As you continue to develop the presentation, you may find that you need to use the table, chart, or graphic slide layouts.

To change or select a new slide layout:

1. Click the **New Slide** icon and the default slide layout (title with content) appears. Select the correct option from the content tools. These options represent tables, charts, SmartArt, pictures, clip art, and media clips. (See **Figure 6-14**.)
2. Alternatively, select the correct slide layout from the **Layout** button in the Slides group of the Home tab. The screen shown in Figure 6-1 appears, and you may choose the correct slide layout.

You can also move back and forth between the Outline and Slides tabs. In fact, after typing an outline segment, you can go to the tab and review the entire slide presentation. View buttons make this easy to do.

View Buttons

The view buttons at the lower-right side of the screen are used to scroll through the different views of the slide presentation. These choices (and a few others) can also be found under the View tab in the Presentation group. Use these buttons to move between different views of the presentation.

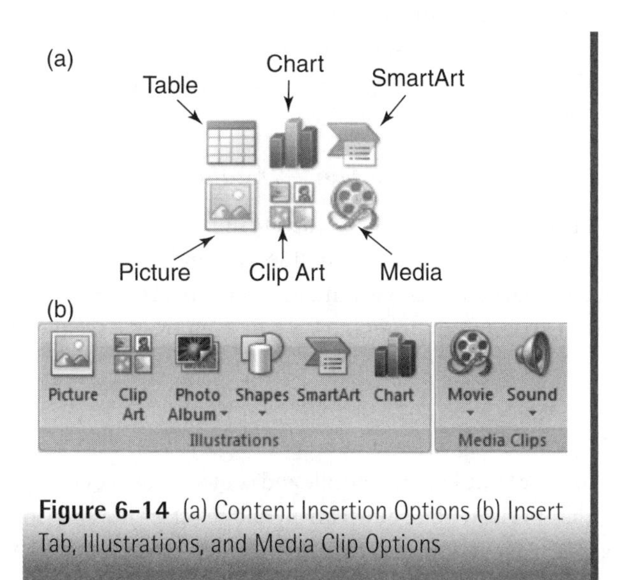

Figure 6-14 (a) Content Insertion Options (b) Insert Tab, Illustrations, and Media Clip Options

The **Normal** view is the default view. It contains three parts: the slide, the notes pane at the bottom, and the left pane for seeing all the slides or outline view. The user works on one slide at a time in this view. The chevron keys at the bottom of the right scroll bar allow you to go back and forth between slides.

The **Slide Sorter** view displays the entire presentation so that you may easily rearrange slides. This view gives you an opportunity to view the presentation in its entirety. To move a slide, simply click it and drag it to a new location. You may also select and easily duplicate slides in this view. Add Transition effects in the slide sorter view.

The **Reading** view displays one slide at a time, much like flipping the pages of a book. Use it to deliver your presentation to someone viewing your presentation on his or her own computer or to see the presentation on a full screen without the additional features of Slide Show.

The **Slide Show** view is the best way to view the slide show. You can easily see transitions from one slide to another or any special effects or sounds in this view. Press the **Esc** key or right-click the mouse to end the slide show.

To access the **Outline** view, click the **Outline** tab in the left pane of the window; access the notes page view at the bottom part of the screen. Use the notes section of the normal view to create and edit the presentation speaker's notes.

To see and edit the total **Notes page** view, select the **View** tab, **Notes page** Notes Page option. At this point, the slide may be made smaller, making more room available for notes. You can also enlarge the text placeholder, making it easier to see. Similarly, you may enlarge the font.

The **View** tab also contains the **Presentation** and **Master** view options. Use the Presentation group to alter the master slide; it includes both a title slide and subsequent slides. Altering the Master view affects all the slides in the presentation. If you want to alter all of the notes pages or handout pages, click those options in the Master Views group of the View tab.

Adding Clip Art, Pictures, and Movies/Audio

PowerPoint includes several hundred clip art images as well as some sounds and movies; thousands more are available online. A Search feature is available that can help you locate a particular clip art image. You may also add pictures to the Art Gallery from CD collections, from the Web, or even from a scanned photo.

Clip Art

To add clip art:

1. Click the **New Slide** button. The title and content slide should appear by default. If not, click the **New Slide down arrow** and select a **Title and Content** option.
2. Click the **Insert Clip Art image** in the add text placeholder (Figure 6-14b); the Clip Art task pane opens on the right side of the screen.

3. Type the **word** that represents the clip art in the search box, and click **Go**. Either a gallery of clip art or a message saying "No results found" appears.

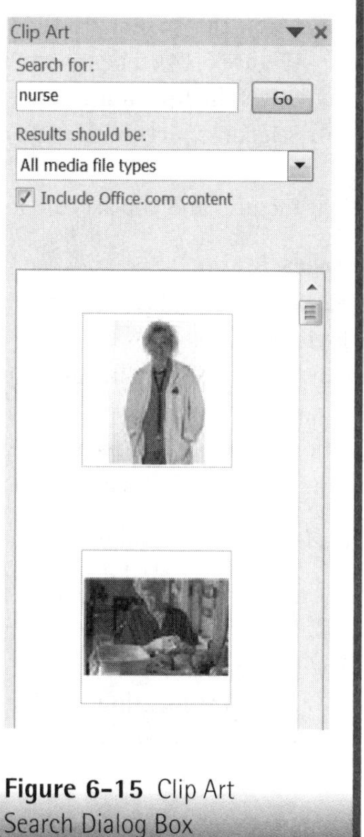

Figure 6-15 Clip Art Search Dialog Box

Clip art and pictures may also be inserted in the normal view from the Insert tab when they are not to be placed in an object placeholder. In the normal view, select the **Insert** tab, and then choose **Picture** or **Clip Art** from the Images group. When using the Clip Art Gallery for the first time, PowerPoint must create a clip art database; to do so, click **Yes** in the dialog box if it comes up. Type the name that might represent the image for which you are looking such as "nurse" (See **Figure 6-15**); all clip art of a nurse will then appear.

Finally, you can find clip art on the Internet, but always pay attention to copyright issues when selecting clip art online. You may insert clip art found on Web sites by using the Insert tab and selecting the appropriate pictures: Locate the **picture**, click **it**, and then click **Insert**. You may insert clip art from any file into PowerPoint as long as you save the graphic in a compatible graphic file format.

Pictures

Digital pictures may also be inserted into PowerPoint presentations. To do so, follow the same procedure used to insert clip art from a Web site. Save these files before you try to insert them into the presentation. Be aware that digital pictures can dramatically increase the size of the presentation. Pictures may also be inserted in current slides by clicking the **Insert** tab, and selecting **Picture** in the Images group.

To add pictures:

1. Click the **New Slide** button. The title and content slide should appear by default. If not, click the **New Slide down arrow** and select a **Title and Content** option.

2. Click the **Insert Picture** image on the Insert object placeholder (Figure 6-14). The Insert Picture dialog box appears.
3. Select the **location** and **file** that contains the picture.
4. Select the **picture file** and click **Insert**. The picture is now inserted into the slide.
5. Pictures and clip art can be moved and resized.

Movies/Audio

You can insert and play movies and audio sounds in a PowerPoint presentation. Movies are video files that have extensions such as .avi, .mov, .mp4, .mpv2, and .wmv. Animated files include motion; they carry a .gif file extension. These files contain multiple images that are streamed together to produce the effect of animation. Although not technically a movie, animations can demonstrate a process or motion. Sound files carry extensions like .adts, .aif, .au, .mid, .pm3, and .wav.

To add a movie or audio:

1. Display the **slide** in which to add the sound or movie.
2. Select the **Insert** tab and then either **Movie** or **Audio** from the Media Clips group.
3. Select the **location** and **file** that contains the movie or audio.
4. Use the content-sensitive tab to make adjustments to how the movie or audio will display and play. (See **Figure 6-16**.)

You can also insert movie and audio files from the content area in the title and content, two content, content with caption, and comparison layout options.

A few sounds and animated .gif files come with the installed version of PowerPoint. Find others at Office.com or on the Internet. Embed movie and audio files in the presentation or link them to the files on the storage device. When you link files in the presentation, you must copy those files along with the presentation if another computer will be used for the presentation.

Adding Tables

Use tables to summarize data, place information in categories, show research results, or help the viewer make comparisons between items.

To add a table:

1. Click the **New Slide** button in the Slides group of the Home tab. A new title and content slide appears.
2. Click the **Insert** table option in the new slide. **Figure 6-17** shows the Insert Table dialog box.

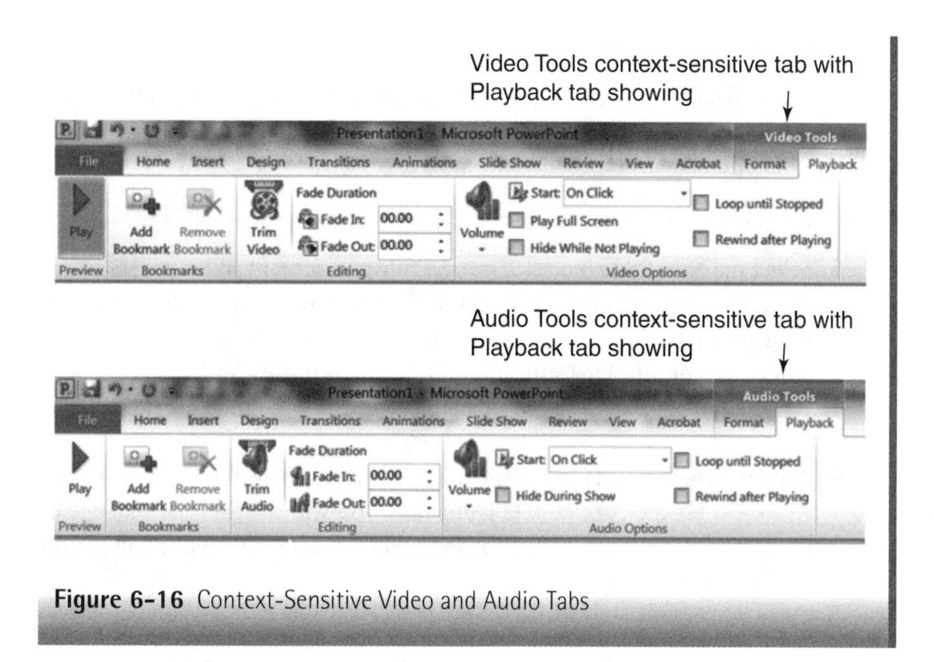

Figure 6-16 Context-Sensitive Video and Audio Tabs

3. Type in the **number of columns** or use the arrows to select a number.
4. Press the **Tab** key and type the **number of rows**, or use the arrows to select a number.
5. Click **OK** when you have finished.
6. Type the **data** in the table cells.
7. When the table contents are complete, click **outside the table** on the slide.
8. Select the **Title** placeholder and type the **title of the slide**.

You can also insert a table from the content area in the title and content, two content, content with caption, or comparison layout options.

A table created in PowerPoint functions just like a table created in a Word document. That means you can use the Tab key (or Shift+Tab) to move around the table. When working in the table, a context-sensitive Table Tools tab appears with two additional tabs: Design and Layout. You add rows and columns to the PowerPoint table in the same way you would do so in Word. Remember, however, that a slide contains a limited amount of space. Having too many rows or columns in a table will render its contents unreadable.

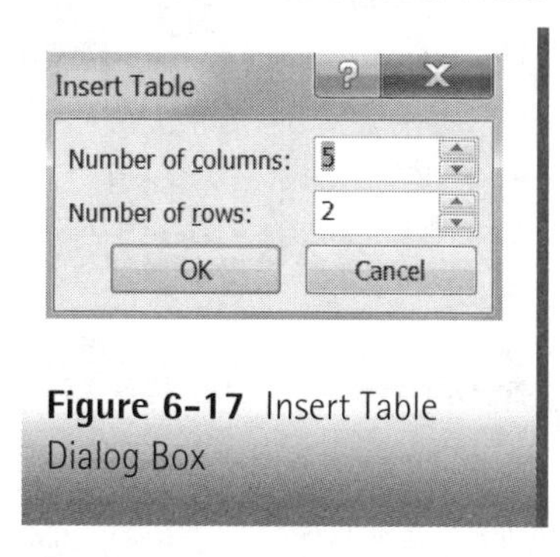

Figure 6-17 Insert Table Dialog Box

Adding a Chart (Graph)

As mentioned earlier in this chapter, charts are pictorial representations of data. In PowerPoint (unlike in Excel), you choose the type of chart you want first and then either add data or import data from Excel.

To add a chart or graph:

1. Select the **New Slide** button. The new title and content slide appears.
2. Click the **Insert Chart** option in the new slide. The window in **Figure 6-18** appears, allowing you to select the type of chart to insert.
3. Select a type of chart and click **OK**. The window splits in two, with PowerPoint appearing on the left and a spreadsheet on the right. (See **Figure 6-19**.)
4. Type the **correct data** in the spreadsheet screen, replacing the default data. As you enter the correct data and labels, you will see the chart change on the left side of the screen. Filling in the data sheet is much like completing an Excel spreadsheet.
5. Once you enter the data, delete any unnecessary rows and columns.

Alternatively, you can insert a graph from the content area in the title and content, two content, content with caption, or comparison layout options.

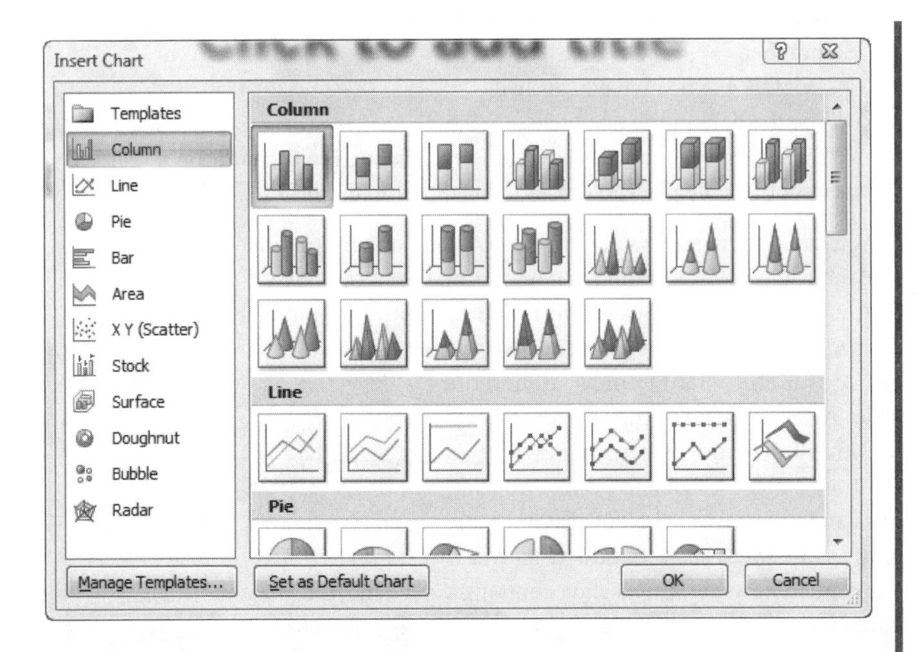

Figure 6-18 Types of Charts in Insert Chart Dialog Window

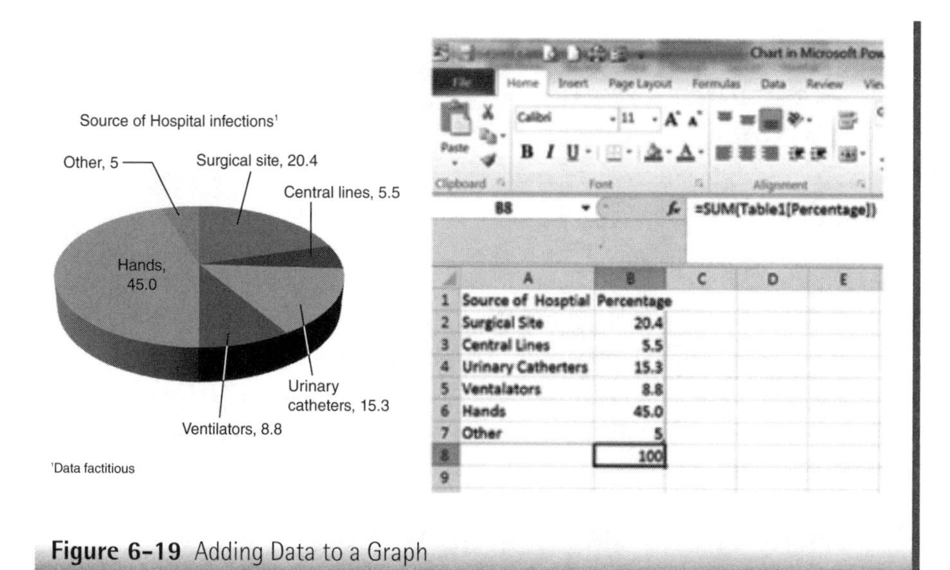

Figure 6-19 Adding Data to a Graph

Pie charts are good choices for comparing parts to the whole. Bar and column charts compare different items over time. Line charts show progress over time or multiple data sets.

When you single-click the graph, you can then move or size it as desired. Right-click the graph and select **Edit Data** option or select the **Design** tab, **Edit Data** option to make the data sheet return. Note that three additional tabs are available under the Chart tools tab—Design, Layout, and Format—that enable you to adjust the graph. There is much more to learn about graphs and charts, of course. Be sure to look at the documentation that comes with PowerPoint and keep experimenting!

Adding a Hyperlink

Hyperlinks take the user to another location or provide additional information about a topic. PowerPoint permits the use of hyperlinks to go directly to a specific slide within the presentation or to a Web site.

To add a hyperlink:

1. Select the **text or object** for which the hyperlink will be created.
2. Select the **Insert** tab, **Hyperlink** option in the Links group. **Figure 6-20** shows the Insert Hyperlink dialog box with the file or Web page selected.
3. Make the appropriate selections and click **OK**.

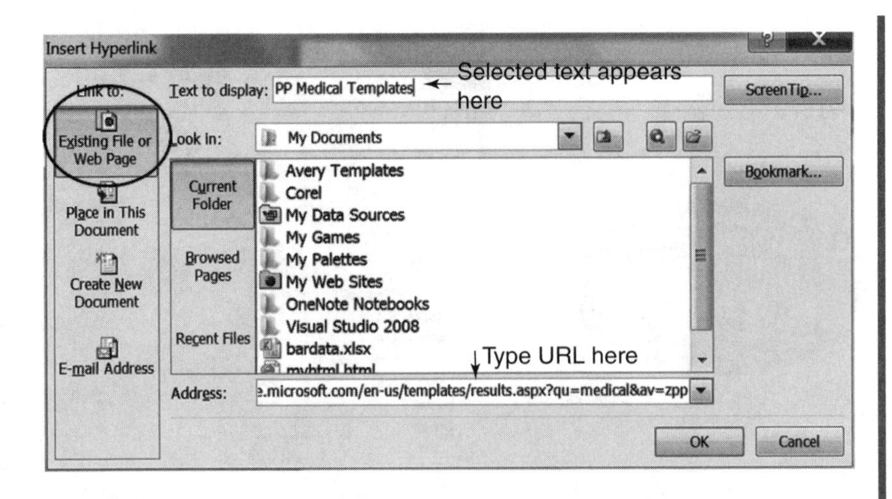

Figure 6-20 Inserting a Hyperlink to File or Web Page

NOTE: The hyperlink will not work unless you are in slide show view; if the hyperlink goes to an Internet site, you must also have an active Internet connection. You can also create a link to other slides in the presentation from the Insert Hyperlink dialog box.

Adding SmartArt

SmartArt graphics add visual representations of information and ideas. The many different layouts provide a quick way to communicate a message without a lot of text. Such illustrations and graphics help the audience understand and remember the information better than text-only presentations can. They are also more visually interesting. **Figure 6-21** shows some of the SmartArt options. You do not need to spend time creating these illustrations; simply select the appropriate one and type in the content.

To create a SmartArt graphic:

1. Click the **New Slide** button. A new title and content slide appears. Click the **SmartArt Graphics option** in the content area of the slide. Alternatively, click the **Insert** tab, **SmartArt** button in the Illustrations group. Figure 6-21 shows the Choose a SmartArt Graphic dialog box.
2. Select the **type** and **layout** of the SmartArt to be inserted and click **OK.**

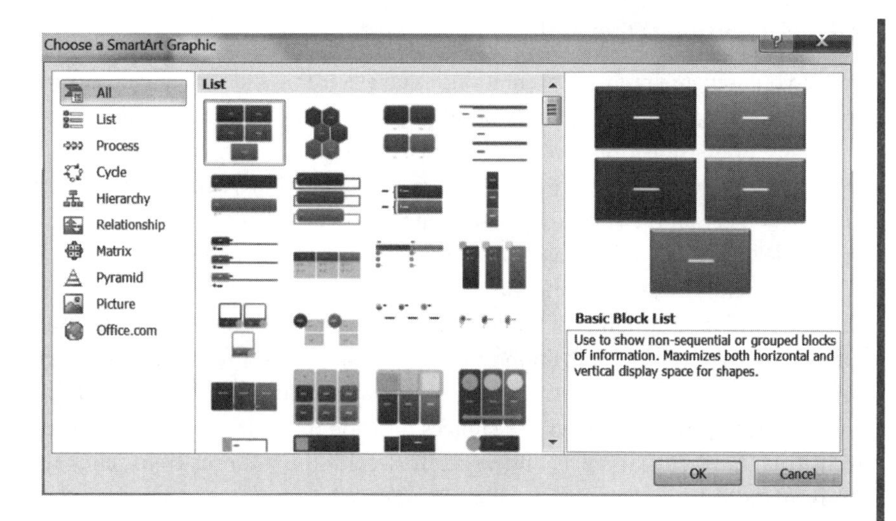

Figure 6-21 SmartArt Graphic Options

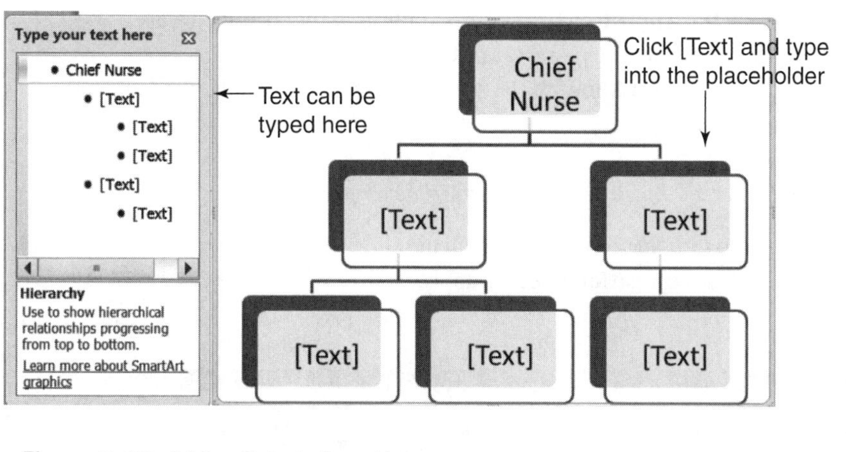

Figure 6-22 Adding Data to SmartArt

3. Enter the text either by clicking in a shape and typing the text or by clicking the **[text]** placeholder in the text pane and typing or pasting the text. You may also copy and paste text from another program and paste it into the text pane. See **Figure 6-22** as an example of adding data.

Adding Transitions to a Slide Show

When you prepare graphic presentations as an electronic slide show, you can add transitions or animations to parts or all of the slide show to make it flow more smoothly. Slide transitions are animation-like effects that appear when moving from one slide to the next during an onscreen presentation. A custom animation lets each object on the slide appear separately. You can also control the speed of each slide transition and any associated sound as well.

As a general rule, transitions should move the presentation along without distracting from the key points of the presentation. For this reason, it is usually more effective to use the same transition or complementary transitions throughout the presentation unless it is necessary to use a specific transition to reinforce a specific point. **Figure 6-23** shows the choices for slide transitions. They include no transition, fade, cut, dissolve, and wipe. To see additional transitions, click the **More** arrow [▾].

To add the same slide transition to all slides in the presentation:

1. With the presentation open, select the **Transitions** tab.
2. Click the **transition effect** to apply.
3. Click the **Apply to All** [Apply To All] button in the **Timing** group.
4. Make any other necessary adjustments in the **Timing** group.
5. Click the **Slide Show** [icon] button to see the results. Make any adjustments as necessary.

To add different transitions to a specific slide or group of slides:

1. In the slide sorter view [icon], click the **slide** to which the transition will apply.
2. Click the **transition** effect to apply.

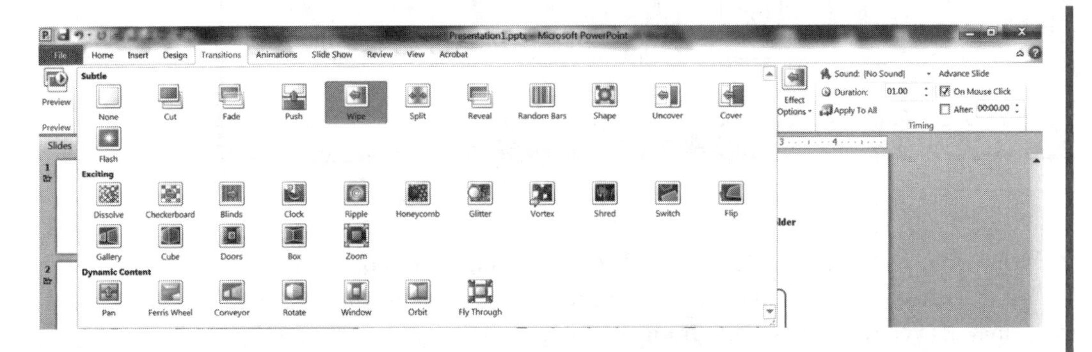

Figure 6-23 Slide Transitions

3. Click the **next slide** to which to apply a transition.
4. Click the **transition** effect to apply.
5. Repeat this process until all slides that need a transition have one.

Adding Custom Animations

Custom animations apply a special visual effect or sound to text or other objects on the slide, such as diagrams, clip art, and charts. For example, each bulleted item may appear in an animation by "flying in" or "dissolving in," giving you an opportunity to discuss the point before the next bulleted item appears.

You can apply custom animations using a preset animation scheme or you can apply them to each item individually on the slide. (See **Figure 6-24**.) Be careful to ensure that any animation used adds clarity to the message, rather than detracts from it. Most users carefully select items for custom animations and do not apply them to the total presentation. This provides some variety and interest to the presentation.

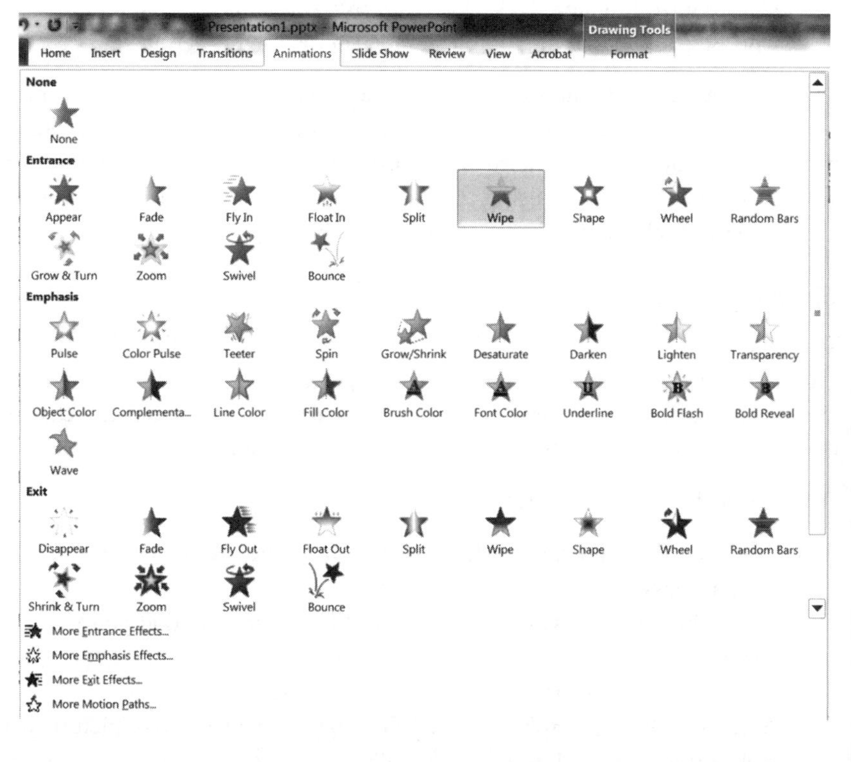

Figure 6-24 Custom Animation Options

To activate the custom animation option:

1. Select the part of the slide to animate by clicking the object, such as a bulleted list or clip art.
2. Click the **Animations** tab.
3. Click the desired **Animation**.
4. Select an **Effect option** Effect Options or leave the default.
5. Make any timing adjustments or leave the default.

Some of the many animation choices include options for playing a sound, adding one letter at a time, and adjusting the speed of the animation. In addition, you may dim previous bulleted items as each new item appears.

Changing a Presentation Design

The theme of a presentation can always be changed to fit the situation.

With the presentation open, to change the theme:

1. Click the **Design** tab.
2. Choose **another theme** from the options in the **Themes** group.

When you place the mouse pointer over a different theme and hold it there without clicking, the slide displays the new look. You can check out all the possibilities before choosing the one you like. Also note that you may change the color scheme for your designs by using the theme colors Colors option. There are also a variety of other options to customize your selection.

Changing the Master Slides

To change text or objects for all slides in the presentation, use the Slide Master. The master template affects all the slides in the presentation. Use the master slides to add items such as corporate or university logos to all slides. You can also change the text properties of all slides by modifying the master slides.

To change text or objects for all slides:

1. Select the **View** tab, then **Slide Master** Slide Master from the **Master Views** group.
2. Click the **first slide** in from the left pane.
3. Select the **text** or **text placeholder** on the master slide that you want to change.
4. Change the **text properties** (e.g., bold, shadow, font size, color).
5. Adjust or **add any graphics** desired. For example, add a logo or picture that will appear on each slide.
6. Click the **Close Master View** button Close Master View Close to exit the slide master view.

You can also make an adjustment to a specific master slide by clicking it and making the adjustment. For example, you may remove the date from a specific layout that will affect only those slides using that layout.

Printing with PowerPoint

PowerPoint has many options for printing various parts of the presentation.

To print overheads, audience handouts, notes, or a presentation outline:

1. With the presentation open, click **File** and then **Print**. **Figure 6-25** shows the Print dialog box with the full page option selected.
2. Select the option you want: **Slides**, **Handouts**, **Notes Pages,** or **Outline**.
3. Check the other settings to make sure that they are correct, and then click **OK**.

The Print All Slides option prints the entire presentation using one page per slide. The default option uses 8½ × 11-inch paper. The **Handouts** option prints a smaller version of the slides, with the number of slides selected per page (i.e., 1, 2, 3, 4, 6, or 9 slides per page). The **Notes Pages** option prints a slide at the top of the page, with the notes appearing on the bottom half of the page; this option prints one slide per page. The **Outline** option prints all the text shown in the outline view. Expand the outline to see all the text in the outline. This option does not print any text from inserted text boxes or graphics.

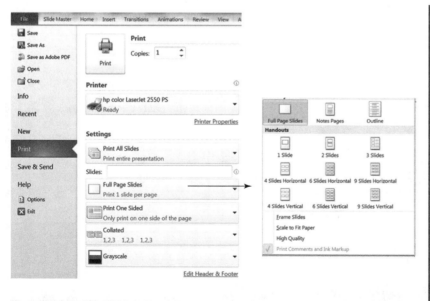

Figure 6-25 Print Dialog Box

Be sure to choose the correct option before printing so that you only print what is necessary. If you are printing handouts, print one page of three or six slides to a page to decide which format will work the best for your audience. Avoid printing handouts before you complete the presentation and make all necessary revisions. It can be very confusing if the printed handout is different from the presented slides, even if all you've done is reorganize a few slides. Always run the spell checker, and consider using AutoCorrect to handle misspellings as you work. Again, proof your slides after you run the spell checker.

Developing a Poster Presentation Using PowerPoint

Since poster presentations are sometimes used at conferences, utilize PowerPoint to develop professional-level poster presentations. Make sure you follow the guidelines given earlier in the chapter when doing so.

To create a poster from a template:

1. Open **PowerPoint**.
2. Click **File**, and then **New**. **Figure 6-26** shows a poster search and the results.
3. Select a **poster template**. (A message may appear stating that only legitimate users can access the templates. Click **Continue** and follow any screen prompts to confirm that your copy of PowerPoint is legal.)
4. Select the **text placeholders**, and type appropriate **text** or add **graphics** to replace them.
5. Save the **file**.
6. Print the **poster** to a printer that will print in color and handle larger paper.

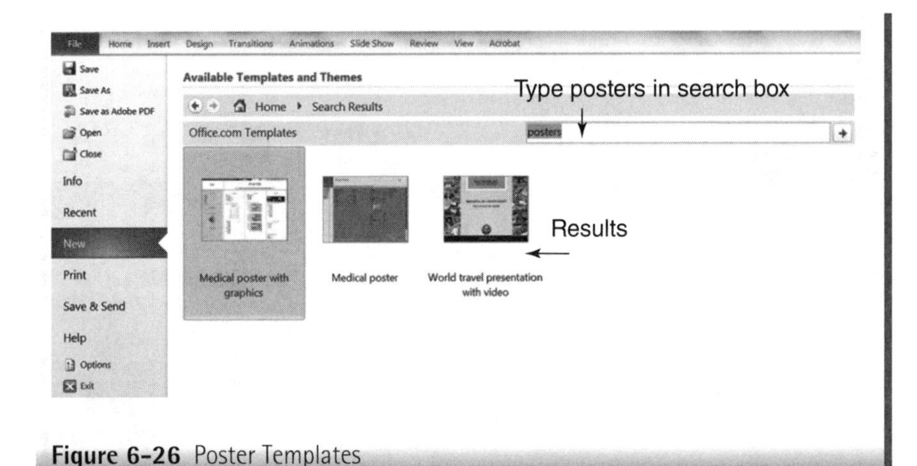

Figure 6-26 Poster Templates

Other poster templates are also available on the Internet. Many institutions also have poster templates that its research or public relations departments have created. Some templates, as noted in the zoom area, are presented at 13% to 18% of their actual size so that you can see the total layout and design of the template. When working on the actual poster, set the zoom level higher so that you can see the text placeholders.

You can create a custom poster size and layout by opening a blank presentation, selecting the blank layout, setting the page setup to the width and height desired (**Design** tab, **Page Setup** option), and showing the gridlines (**View** tab, **Gridlines** option). Use options in the Drawing group to insert text boxes and format them as desired. Be aware that creating such a customized poster will be much more time-consuming than simply finding and adjusting an existing poster template.

Summary

PowerPoint is a powerful program that can help you produce professional presentations and posters that effectively reach your audience. This chapter outlined the beginning steps you need to follow to produce a PowerPoint slide presentation or poster. As you continue to learn about PowerPoint you can progress to more advanced features.

References

National Cancer Institute (NCI)(2011). Making Data Talk: A Workbook. NIH Publication Number 11-7724. Bethesda, MD: NCI. Retrieved from http://www.cancer.gov/cancertopics/cancerlibrary/MDT-Workbook.pdf

Resources

Blakesley, D. and Brizee, A. Designing Research Posters. Purdue University Writing Lab Indiana Department of Transportation Workshop Series http://owl.english.purdue.edu/media/pdf/20080626013023_727.pdf is a handout of tips for designing research posters.

CustomGuide. http://www.customguide.com/computer-training/quick-references provides a series of quick reference guides (2 pages) for PowerPoint and many of the other Office products. Requires you to sign up for the free guides.

Microsoft. http://office.microsoft.com/en-us/help/training-FX101782702.aspx offers many help guides and tutorials including PowerPoint.

Free PowerPoint Templates. http://www.free-power-point-templates.com/category/ppt-by-topics/medicine-health/. A site that provides free healthcare-related templates.

Exercises

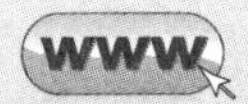

EXERCISE 1 A Basic Presentation—Where to Start?

Objectives

1. Apply a design to a presentation.
2. Create a title slide and edit it by inserting a graphic.
3. Create a bulleted list slide with and without clip art.
4. Edit slides by altering the formatting and placement of objects.
5. Insert and adjust clip art from the clip organizer and from Office.com
6. Enhance the slides.
7. Save the presentation.

Activity

1. Create the title slide and apply a design.
   a. Start **PowerPoint**.
   b. Click the **Design** Design tab.
   c. Scroll until you find **Technic** design and click it.
   d. Click the **title text placeholder** (this means click the words Click to add title) and type **Professional Presentations – Tips**.
   e. Click the **subtitle text placeholder**. Type **your name**.
2. Edit the title slide.
   Sometimes the placeholders and text need to be altered or moved to fit your style.
   a. Click the **title placeholder** and move the mouse over the border of the placeholder until the four-headed cursor appears. Drag the title **placeholder 1 inch from the top**. (Turn on your rulers in the View tab.) Click the **Home** tab and the **center** alignment icon.
   b. Move the **subtitle placeholder** 2 inches from the bottom following the same directions as above. Click **inside the subtitle placeholder** before your name and type **By** and press the **Enter** key.
   c. Click the **Insert** Insert tab and **Clip Art** Clip Art icon. In the Clip Art task pane on the right type people in the search box and press **Enter**. Scroll down until you find an image that you feel represents a presentation. Click the **selected clip art**. Move the clip art to the left side of the slide. See **Figure 6-27** as an example of a finished exercise.

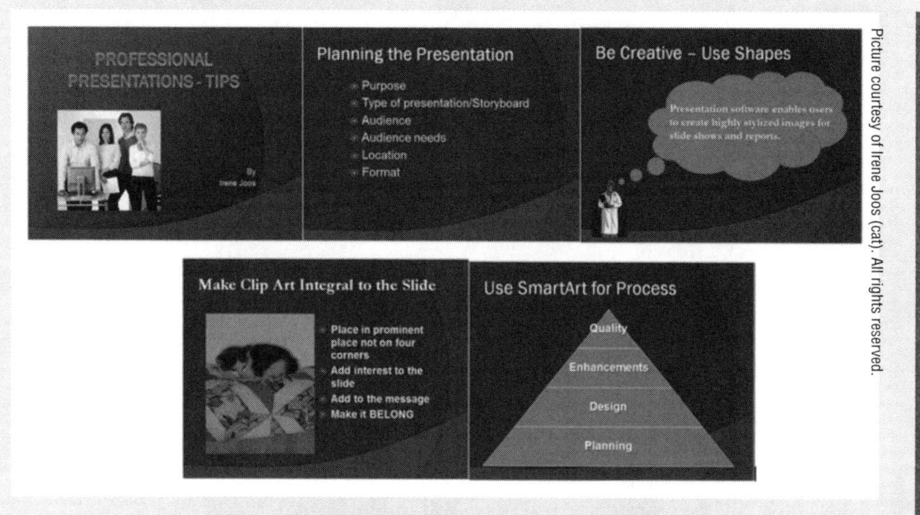

Figure 6-27 Finished Presentation Exercise 1

3. Create a bulleted list slide.
   a. Click the **New Slide** icon on the Home tab, Slides group.
   b. Click **title placeholder** and type **Planning the Presentation**.
   c. Click the **Click to add text** placeholder and type the following items pressing **Enter** after each but the last one: **Purpose**, **Type of Presentation**, **Audience**, **Audience needs**, **Location**, and **Format**.
4. Edit the bulleted list.
   a. Click the **text placeholder border.**
   b. Drag the text placeholder to the right so the bullets are 1.5 to 2 inches from the left slide of the slide.
5. Insert a shape, add clip art, and text.
   a. Click the **New Slide** icon on the Home tab, Slides group.
   b. Click the **Layout** icon on the Home tab, Slides group and click **Title Only** layout.
   c. Click the **title placeholder** and type **Be Creative – Use Shapes**.
   d. Click the **Insert** tab and click the **Shapes** icon in the Illustrations group. Select the **Cloud Callout** in the Callouts group (fourth from the left). Starting at the lower left of the slide, drag to the upper right. Click the yellow diamond on the bottom of the cloud and drag to the left.
   e. On the Insert tab, Text group, click **Text Box** icon. Click in the cloud and type **Presentation software enables users to create highly**

stylized images for slide shows and reports. Click the **text box border** and change the font to **Garamond, 28 points, shadow** and **bold.**

f. On the Insert tab, click **Clip Art** icon, type **person** in the search box and press **Enter**. Select an appropriate image and click it. Click the image and drag the sizing handles until it is about 1 to 2 inches in size. Move the image to the bottom left of the slide. (See Figure 6-27.)

6. Insert a mixed slide.
   a. Click the **New Slide** icon on the Home tab, Slides group.
   b. Click the **Layout** icon on the Home tab, Slides group and click **Two Content** layout.
   c. Click the **title placeholder** and type **Make Clip Art Integral to the Slide.**
   d. Click the left Content placeholder **Clip Art** icon. Type **funny** in the clip art search box and press **Enter**. Click any image.
   e. Click in the **Right Content placeholder** and type:
      Place in prominent place not on four corners and press **Enter.**
      Add interest to the slide and press **Enter.**
      Add to the message and press **Enter.**
      Make it BELONG.
   f. Center the bulleted list between the top and bottom of the image.
7. Insert an AutoShape.
   a. Click the **New Slide** icon on the Home tab, Slides group.
   b. Click the **Slide Layout** icon on the Home tab, Slides group and click **Title and Content** layout.
   c. Click the **title placeholder** and type **Use SmartArt for Process.**
   d. Click the **SmartArt Graphics** icon in the content placeholder.
   e. Select Pyramid and the **first one** on the left.
   f. Type the following text:
      Quality and press **Enter**
      Enhancements and press **Enter**
      Design and press **Enter**
      Planning
   g. Make any **font** (such as bold and shadow) and **size** adjustments.
8. Save the presentation.
   a. Click the **Save** button on the Quick Access Toolbar or click **File, Save.**
   b. Click the **location** to save the file on the left side of the window (such as a USB storage device) and type **Chap6-Exercise1-LastName.**
   c. Click the **Save** button.
9. After looking at slide 5, you decide a better approach than the pyramid might be another SmartArt option that shows the information as a cycle.

Add a sixth slide using one of the cycle options. Save the presentation. Now examine whether slide 5 or 6 represents the information better. Explain your rationale.

EXERCISE 2 How Do I Use a Picture and Print Handouts?

Objectives

1. Import a picture and add it to a slide.
2. Use both a picture and clip art on a slide.
3. Add speaker notes.
4. Print handouts and speaker notes.

Activity

1. Import a picture to a slide.
   a. Open PowerPoint to a **New** presentation.
   b. Click the words **Click to add title** and type **My School**.
   c. Click the words **Click to add subtitle** and type **By** and press **Enter**. Type **your name**.
   d. Click the **Design** tab and select **Aspect** theme.
   e. Click the **New Slide down arrow** button on the Home tab and select the **Picture with Caption** layout.
   f. Click the **Picture** icon in the content placeholder.
   g. Select the **Storage Device** and **Folder** where you placed the .jpg picture. If you don't have a picture of your school, take one and upload it to your storage device. Click the **picture** and click **Insert** Insert button.
   h. Click the words **Click to add title** and type the **College Name.**
   i. In the right slide of the slide, click the words **Click to add text** and type a **caption** for the picture. This could name the building, describe what is offered in that building, or describe the location of the picture.

NOTE: Make sure you have permission to use a photo you didn't take.

2. Add a picture and clip art to a slide.
   a. Click the **New Slide** New Slide icon on the Home tab, Slides group.
   b. Click the **Layout** Layout icon on the Home tab, Slides group and click **Title only**.
   c. Click the **title placeholder** and type **Location of My School**.

d. On the **Insert** tab, click the **Clip Art** icon, type the **name of your state** (or country) in the search for box and press **Enter**. Click the **clip art** of your state (or country).
e. Size the image by **dragging the sizing** handles so that the image is about 4 inches. Move the image to the **bottom left** of the slide.
f. Click the **Text Box** icon on the Insert tab, Text group. Click and drag the **textbox placeholder** in the approximate location of your school on the image. Type an **X**. If needed enlarge the X.
g. Now, insert another picture (**Insert**, **Picture**, **locate picture**, and click **Insert**) of your school or the city in which the school resides on the slide. Move the picture to the top right of the slide.
h. Click the **picture** and then the **Format** tab under the Picture Tools tab opens.
i. Click the **More** button in the pictures styles group. Click **Bevel Rectangle** option.
j. Click the **Insert** tab, **Shapes** icon. Click the **Line** tool and draw a line from the **X** to the **picture**. (See **Figure 6-28**.)
k. Click **File**, **Save**. Select a **location** for the file and name the presentation **Chap6-Exercise2-LastName**.

3. Add speaker notes.
   a. Click **Slide 1** to make it the active slide.
   b. At the bottom of the slide click the words **Click to add notes**.
   c. Type **Hi and Welcome to my presentation about NAME OF SCHOOL. My name is (TYPE YOUR NAME and something about yourself)**.
   d. Click **Slide 2**. Click the words **Click to add notes** and type what you might say about this slide.
   e. Repeat the process for **Slide 3**.
   f. Save the presentation.
4. Print handouts.
   a. Open the **presentation** created in Exercise 1.
   b. Select **File**, **Print**.
   c. Click the **down arrow** next to Full Page Slides.
   d. Click **3 Slides** per page. This will provide the user with an area to take notes.
   e. Make sure it says **Grayscale** unless you are printing to a color printer.
   f. Click the **Print** button. (See Figure 6-25.)

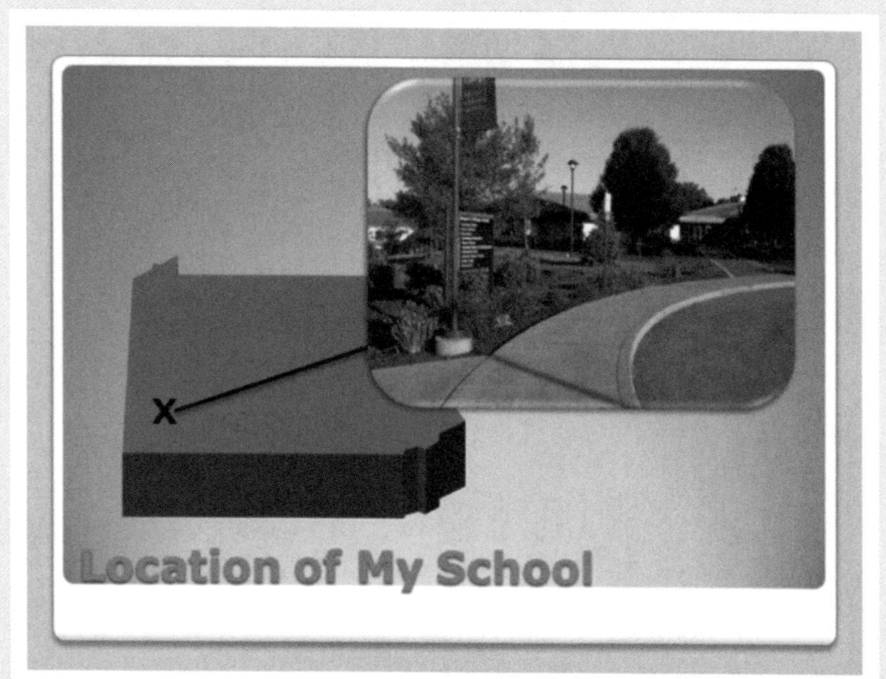

Figure 6-28 Finished Mixed Clip Art, Shape and Picture - Exercise 2

5. Print a presentation with speaker notes.
   a. Open the presentation about your school titled—**Chap6-Exercise2-LastName.**
   b. Select **File**, **Print**.
   c. Click the **down arrow** next to Full Page Slides.
   d. Click **Note Pages** option. This will place one slide at the top of a page with room for notes.
   e. Make sure it says **Grayscale** unless you are printing to a color printer.
   f. Click the **Print** button.

NOTE: If you click the printer icon on the standard toolbar, you will use the default setting, which is one copy of all the slides in slide view sent to the default printer. That means that the printer will print each slide on a page, filling up the page with the slide.

EXERCISE 3 How Do I Display Data for Easier Interpretation?

This exercise can also be done with Excel, although our preference is to have you practice with PowerPoint at this point rather than linking a spreadsheet to a graph in PowerPoint. The table can also be created in Word.

Objectives

1. Create a table to display data in a PowerPoint presentation.
2. Create a pie and a column graph for use in PowerPoint presentations.
3. Save the presentation.

Activity

1. Create a table.
   a. Open **PowerPoint** and create a **New** presentation.
   b. Click the words **Click to add title** in the title placeholder and type **Displaying Data in Tables and Charts.**
   c. Click the words **Click to add subtitle** in the subtitle placeholder and type **By** and press **Enter**. Type **your name.**
   d. Click the **Design** tab and apply the **Verve** style.
   e. Click the **New Slide** New Slide icon on the Home tab.
   f. Click the words **Click to add title** in the placeholder and type **Using a Table.**
   g. Click the **Table** icon in the content placeholder.
   h. Type **3** in the column box and **11** in the row box. Click **OK.**
   i. Go to www.cdc.gov/injury/wisqars/pdf/10LCID_All_Deaths_By_Age_Group_2010-a.pdf and enter the data using Rank for the first column, Condition for the second, and Total for the last column. Use the total column (last column) for the numbers not the age groups.
   j. Select the **first row** of the table and **center** the words. **Autofit the columns** (same process as used in Word tables).
   k. You decide you don't like the pink color. Click to the **Design** tab, click the **Colors down arrow** Colors and click **Concourse.**
   l. Click the **First slide**, click **Home** tab, click the **title placeholder**, and the **down arrow** for the font color A. Click **Light Turquoise, Text 2, Darker 50%** (fourth column, fourth row).
2. Create a pie chart.
   a. Click the **New Slide** New Slide icon on the Home tab, Slides group. The Title and Contents layout appears as this is the default layout after the title slide.
   b. Click the **title placeholder** and type **Pie—Parts to a Whole.**

c. In the content placeholder, click the **Chart** icon. Click **Pie** in the left pane, **Pie in 3D** in Pie group. Depending on your monitor, you may be able to go directly to Pie in 3D.

d. Type the following data in the right-hand screen. When finished close the data sheet.

Race	Number
White	34294
Black	3391
Indian	232
Asian	1340
Native Hawaiian/Pacific Island	38
Two or more races	117

e. With the Pie chart selected, click **Layout** tab under Chart Tools to alter the look of the pie. Click the **title placeholder** and type **Population Race for 65 and older in the US*.**

f. Click **Insert** tab, **insert text box**, and draw a **text box** at the bottom of the slide. Type ***Thousands representing millions; data source http://www.census.gov/compendia/statab/2012/tables/12s0010.pdf.**

g. With the Pie selected, click **Layout** tab, **Data Labels** Data Labels icon, and then **More Data Label Options** at the bottom of the menu. Place a **check mark** in the **Category Name** box and keep the check marks in Value and Show Leader Lines boxes. Click **Close.**

h. Click the **Legend** Legend icon in the Layout tab and click **None.**

i. Click the **3D Rotation** 3-D Rotation icon. Type **100** for the *x*-axis, **50** for the *y*-axis. Click **Close.**

j. Click **each pie wedge data label** and drag it away from the pie wedge. Click the **White pie wedge** and drag away from the pit. Your pie should now look like the pie in **Figure 6-29.**

k. Now you want to see a trend with the population from this age group to those under 5 years old to see what is happening with regard to race in the US and how that might impact our planning for delivering health care. Which chart type is best suited to comparing the two? Why?

l. Using the following data, create your **chart type** comparing the two. This is for children under 5 years of age.

m. Save the presentation—**Chap6-Exercise3-LastName.**

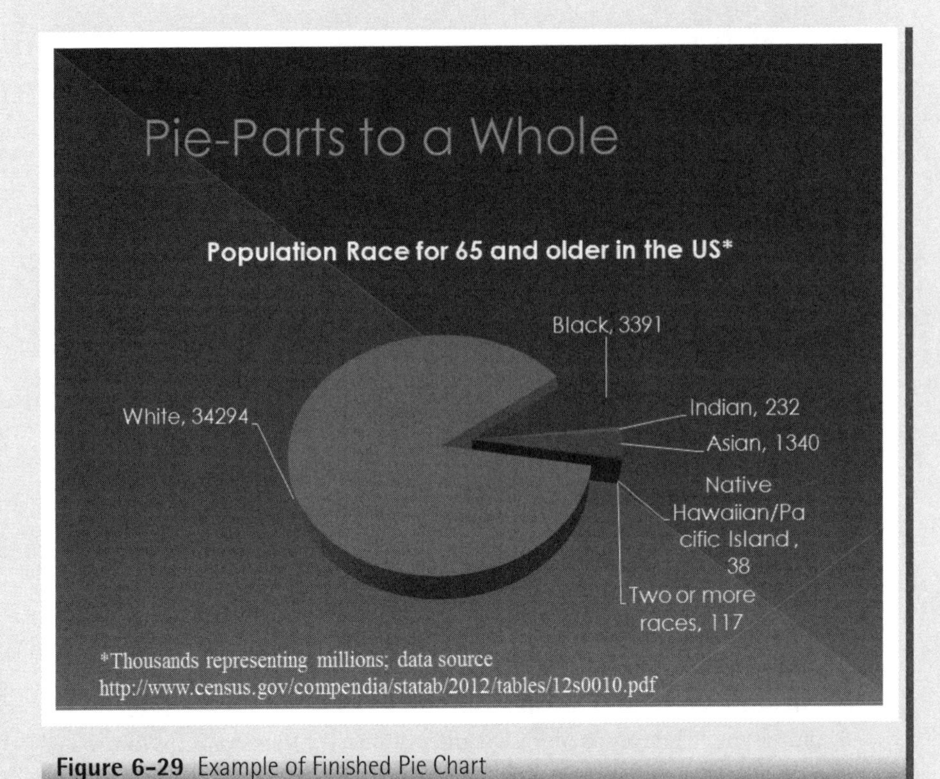

Figure 6-29 Example of Finished Pie Chart

Race*	Number
White	15575
Black	3230
Indian	298
Asian	1006
Native Hawaiian/Pacific Island	53
Two or more races	838

*Race as classified by http://quickfacts.census.gov/qfd/meta/long_RHI525211.htm

3. Create a column chart.

   a. Click the **New Slide** icon on the Home tab, Slides group. The Title and Contents layout appears as this is the default layout after the title slide.

b. Click the **title placeholder** and type **Column-Comparison Over Time.**

c. In the content placeholder, click the **Chart** icon. Click **3-D Clustered Column** chart and **OK**. In the worksheet enter the following data:

Category	Nurse Practitioner	Physician Assistant
2005	74812	81129
2007	84397	86214
2009	89579	93105
2010	90770	96876
2011	90583	94870

d. With the chart selected, click **Layout** tab under Chart Tools and then the **Axis Titles** option. Click **Primary Horizontal Axis Title** and type **Year**. Repeat the process for the Vertical axis selecting **Rotated Title** option and type **Yearly Salary**.

e. Right-click the *y*-**axis**, click **Format Axis Title**, **Number**, **Currency,** and set it to **0** decimal points. Save the presentation (see **Figure 6-30**).

f. Give credit to the source with a footnote at the bottom http://nurse-practitioners-and-physician-assistants.advanceweb.com/Features/Articles/National-Salary-Report-2011.aspx.

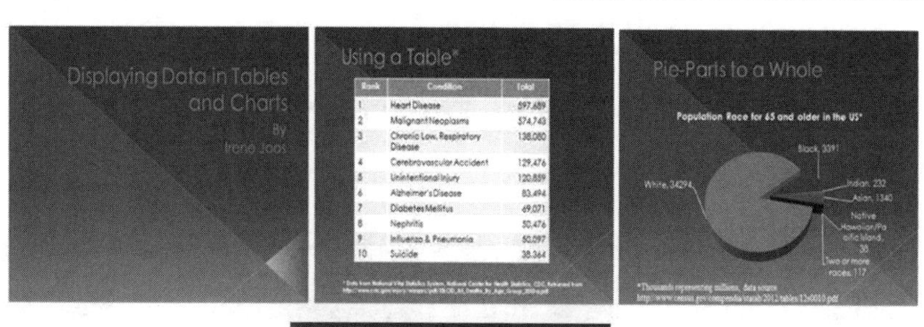

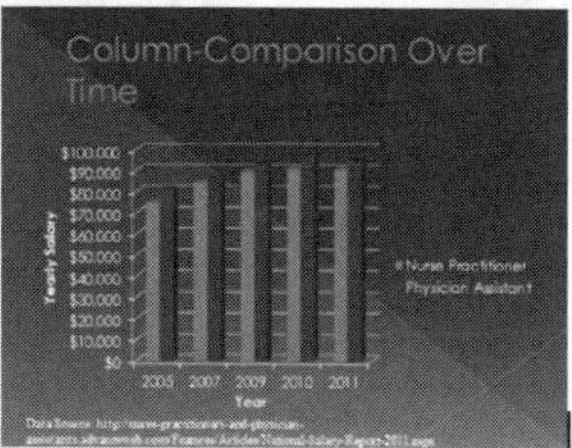

Figure 6-30 Finished Presentation Exercise 3

g. What does this chart tell you about the salaries of nurse practitioners and physician assistants?

EXERCISE 4 Is This a Good Design? How Can It Be Improved?

Objectives

1. Review selected slides for how they can be improved.
2. Use selected features of PowerPoint to redesign slides to better represent the concepts visually.

Activty

1. Open the PowerPoint presentation titled **Chap6-Exercise4-Revised.**
2. Look at Slide 1. Go to **Slide 2** and add the content from **Slide 1**. This means to **add a title** to the slide, **add a design**, **ungroup the shape** and **recolor** it, and **add the text** to the shape in the correct hierarchy. This is an example of enhancing a slide with visuals and making sure there are no more than three text slides in a row.
3. Now go to **Slide 3**. Review the text. Go to **Slide 4** and enhance the slide by using shapes (rectangles and arrows) to show flow of process, and text boxes to contain information from Slide 3.
4. Go to **Slide 5** and review the text. Using the information from Slide 5 create an enhanced **Slide 6** using rectangles, curved arrows, and WordArt to show how each concept builds on the previous concept.
5. Go to **Slide 7** and review the text. Using the information in Slide 7 create enhanced slides (**Slides 8** and **9**).
6. Save the presentation as **Chap6-Exercise4-LastName**.

Assisgnments

ASSIGNMENT 1 Converting a Boring Presentation into a Wow Presentation

Directions

1. Select one of the chapter PowerPoints from one of your courses or one that the faculty provides to you. Most of these PowerPoints are talking points or a summary of the chapter key points and don't adhere to the acceptable guidelines for professional presentations.
2. Following the guidelines presented in this chapter, revise selected slides (at least eight) to enhance the presentation.
3. Make sure you use a table, clip art, picture, chart, SmartArt, and bulleted lists (not complete sentences).

4. Discuss what you learned from this assignment. (Alternatively, you can write a short paragraph about your learning from this assignment or add it to your weekly journal.)
5. Save the file as **Chap6-Assign1-LastName** and submit following the directions of the professor.

ASSIGNMENT 2 Showing Off What I Learned!

Directions

Prepare a PowerPoint presentation on a topic related to technology in health care that you will present to the class using a computer and data projector. Use your creativity and the knowledge gained from this chapter to produce quality slides; follow the good design tips given in the chapter.

1. Include a minimum of 10 slides, with at least one of each of the following: Title slide, Bulleted list slide, Mixed-format slide with a bulleted list and clip art that is integral to the slide, Altered clip art on a slide, Table slide, Graph slide, SmartArt slide, Recolored shape slide, Imported clip art slide, Imported picture slide (generally .jpg files).
2. Introduce some variety into the layout of the slides. For example, avoid more than three bulleted list slides in a row. Use some of the shapes to enhance the slides.
3. Create a transition between slides. **Save** the presentation as **Chap6-Assign2-LastName**.
4. **Print** an outline of the presentation and a handout displaying three slides to a page. Prepare at least one notes page. Turn in the printouts or an electronic version of the presentation if instructed to do so.
5. Make sure you add a footer to the slides alerting the audience to the altered clip art, sources of the imported clip art and picture, and altered shape.

ASSIGNMENT 3 Where Do I Go from Here?

Directions

Software programs are always being updated to add new features. It's important to keep up with new and advanced features once you have the basics mastered. The focus of this assignment is to learn a new feature in PowerPoint.

1. Select one of the features listed here to learn how to use that feature:
   - Insert Action buttons.
   - Publish a slide show to the Internet.
   - Turn your presentation into a video.

- Add narration to the presentation.
- Design a research poster presentation.
- Link spreadsheet or Word table data to your presentation.
- Add quality transitions and animations to your presentations.
- Another of your choice approved by your professor.

2. Use the Help feature in PowerPoint and/or the Internet to find two quality resources that explain how to use the selected feature.
3. Develop a PowerPoint presentation that teaches your classmates how to use that feature as well as the conditions under which you might use it. Save the file as **Chap6-Assign3-Lastname** and submit as directed by the professor.

chapter 7

Introduction to Spreadsheets

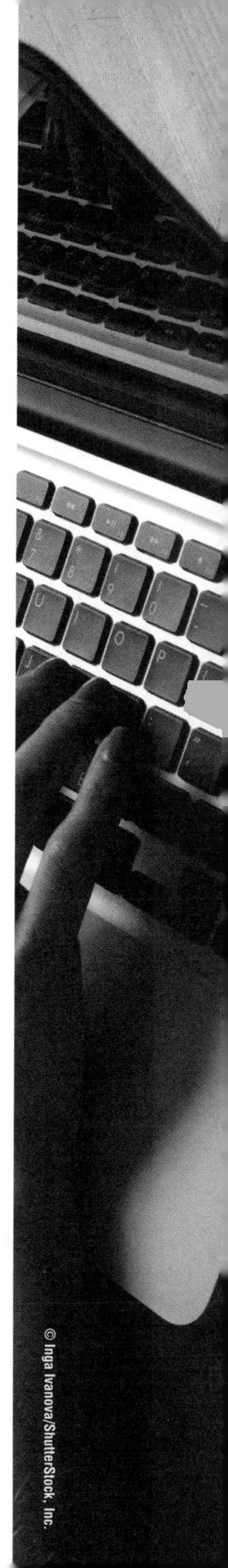

Objectives 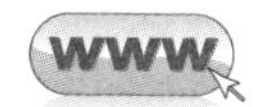

1. Identify uses of the spreadsheet in general as well as for healthcare applications.
2. Define basic terminology related to spreadsheets.
3. Review selected functions for using Excel 2010.

Common Spreadsheet Terms

Spreadsheets do for numbers and charts what word processors do for writing. Although their strength is their function as numeric calculators, most spreadsheets also have a database management component for organizing, sorting, and retrieving data and a chart component for creating and printing graphs. This chapter explains how you can use a spreadsheet to process and display numerical information. See Chapter 8 for additional Excel database functions.

The advantages of computerized spreadsheets include their accuracy and speed. Spreadsheets also have the capacity to recalculate formulas automatically when you change any numbers in the calculation. Spreadsheets have many uses; for example, they can manage inventories, tax returns, statistical procedures, grade records, personnel files, budgets, and quality assurance information.

Figure 7-1a shows Excel 2010 for Windows with the Home tab selected and below that some details showing the formula bar with data

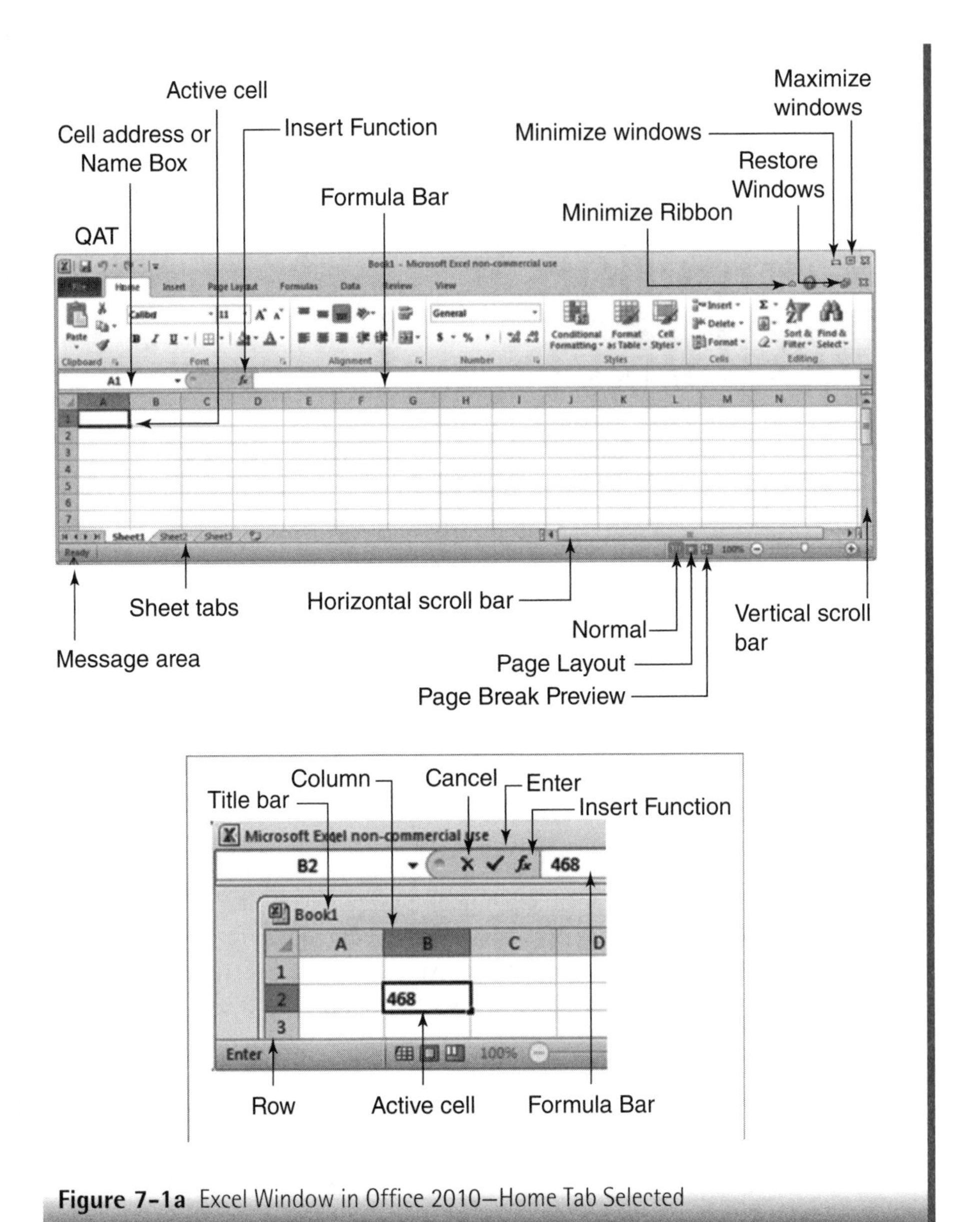

Figure 7-1a Excel Window in Office 2010—Home Tab Selected

in a cell; **Figure 7-1b** shows Excel 2011 for the Mac. Note the differences in the two interfaces. No matter which version you use, however, the basic concepts are the same.

The various parts of a **worksheet** are described next.

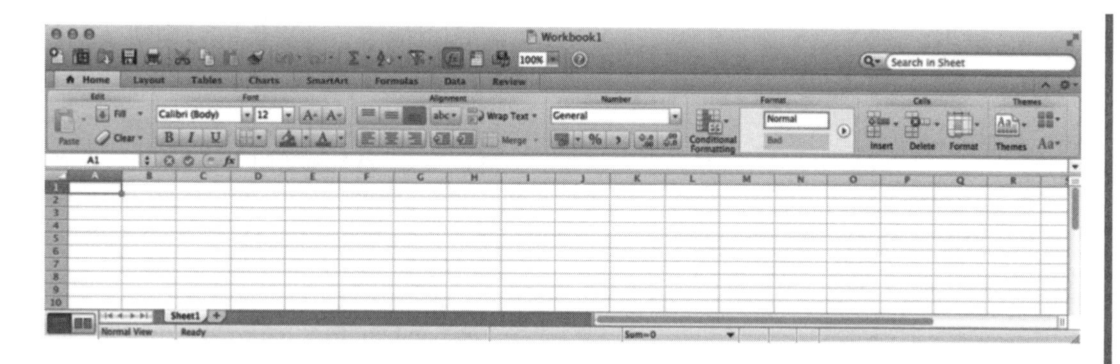

Figure 7-1b Excel Window in Office 2011 for Mac OS X

Parts of a Worksheet

Row — **Rows** run horizontally across the spreadsheet. Beginning with 1, they are numbered down the left side of the worksheet. Although the maximum number of rows varies with different spreadsheets, more than 1 million rows are available in an Excel worksheet.

Columns — **Columns** run vertically down the worksheet. They are labeled from A to Z, going from left to right. After Z, labeling continues with AA to AZ, BA to BZ, and so on. More than 16,000 columns are available in Excel 2010.

Cell — A **cell** is a placeholder for data. Each cell occurs at a specific intersection of a row and a column. The program labels cells with the column letter and then the row number (e.g., A1 or T112).

Cell Address (Cell Reference) — The **cell address** is the label for each cell. Use it to reference the cell when creating formulas or using functions.

Active Cell — The **active cell** is the cell in use; the program outlines or highlights it so that you can locate it quickly on the worksheet. In Figure 7-1a, the column letter and row number for the active cell is outlined. The row and column headers for the active cell is marked by a different color—yellow. The address of the active cell appears in the **Name Box** on the spreadsheet screen.

Range (Block) A group of cells defined by the upper-left and lower-right corners is called a **range** or block of cells. For example, the range of cells from A1 to E6 would include the cells in columns A, B, C, D, and E in rows 1, 2, 3, 4, 5, and 6. A block of cells on a worksheet is outlined and all but the first cell is shaded blue. Blocks of cells may be contiguous (next to each other) or non-contiguous (rows and columns of cells not next to each other).

Workbook (Notebook) A **workbook** or notebook is a collection of worksheet pages. Excel workbook pages are called worksheets once they contain data. In Excel they are called Sheet1, Sheet2, etc, until otherwise renamed. All the worksheets are saved together in one file and referred to as a workbook. In some programs, when the workbook is blank, it is called a sheet. When they contain data, they are called worksheets. In Figure 7-1a, the worksheets are labeled Sheet1, Sheet2, and Sheet3. You can change worksheet names to more effectively reflect the worksheet content and type of data on the worksheet. For example, if the worksheet contains charts, the worksheet could be labeled Chart-Freshmen Expenses, Chart-Nursing Shortage, and so forth. Spreadsheet programs have a default number of worksheets in each workbook is three; you can add more worksheets to a workbook or delete the unused ones if desired. You can also set the default number of worksheets if you consistently use more.

Worksheet A **worksheet** contains labels (letters), values (numbers), formulas and functions, lines or borders, and images. It can also contain charts, illustrations, tables, links, and special graphics like SmartArt and text boxes.

Template A **template** is a formatted workbook with labels and formulas but no specific data; templates are helpful when multiple uses of the same spreadsheet are necessary. You might use a template for a yearly

B1 [Company Name]

Inpatient encounter form1 [Compatibility Mode]

[Company Name]
Inpatient Encounter Form
[Date]

		Patient Name	Patient 1	Patient 2	Patient 3	Patient 4	Patient 5	Pati
		Patient MRN Number	1111	1112	1113	1114	1115	1116
		Patient Room Number	111	112	113	114	115	116
		Patient Diagnosis	xxx	xxx	xxx	xxx	xxx	xxx
Service Category	Service	Service Code						
Admit	Low Complexity MDM: 30 min.	99221						
	Mod. Complexity MDM: 50 min.	99222						
	High Complexity MDM: 70 min.	99223						
Follow-up Visit	Low Complexity MDM: 15 min.	99231						
	Mod. Complexity MDM: 25 min.	99232						
	High Complexity MDM: 35 min.	99233						
Admit D/C Same Day	Low Complexity MDM	99234						
	Mod. Complexity MDM	99235						
	High Complexity MDM	99236						
D/C	Discharge Day Mgmt.: < 30 min	99238						
	Discharge Day Mgmt.: > 30 min.	99239						
...ical ...re	Constant Attention: 1st hour	99291						

Figure 7-2 Inpatient Encounter Form Template

personal budget or for the budget of a healthcare unit, for example. In this kind of application, the labels and the calculations that you use remain stable over time; only the values change. A variety of interesting healthcare-related templates are available on Office.com. (See **Figure 7-2**.)

Spreadsheet Screen Display

The screen displays for most spreadsheets are similar. Spreadsheets look like pages from an accountant's ledger (or columnar pad), containing many rows and columns. A series of letters, denoting columns, go horizontally across the screen; a series of numbers, denoting rows, run vertically down the left side of the screen. Like other Office 2010 applications (previously discussed in Chapters 4, 5, and 6), Excel has a **ribbon** consisting of **tabs**, **groups**, and command buttons (See Figure 7-1a). **Scroll bars** appear along the right and bottom sides of the screen, along with the View buttons and the Zoom slider. Features specific to the spreadsheet screen display include the current cell address, the active cell (indicated by a black border), the formula bar or input line, sheet tabs, and the message area.

Current Cell Address

The current cell address indicates the *active cell* and is displayed on the left side of the formula toolbar.

Formula Bar	The **Formula Bar** is the toolbar at the top of the spreadsheet. The entered data or formula appears in this location on the screen for the active cell.
Message Area	The **message area** shows which actions will occur when a function or button is activated. It may also show error messages. It is usually in the bottom left corner of the status bar.

Getting Ready to Use a Spreadsheet

Before you open a spreadsheet, it is important to consider carefully the goals of the project so that you develop an optimally useful spreadsheet. Consider the following questions:

1. What is the purpose/goal of creating this spreadsheet?
2. Which type of data is necessary in the spreadsheet (e.g., inventory supply information, infection control, home medication tracking, or numbers for income or expenses)?
3. Are monthly, quarterly, or yearly time intervals needed?
4. Is there a need to make comparisons of data between units or across time periods?
5. How many data elements or time intervals are there? Is one worksheet adequate or would it be better to divide the data elements or time intervals among several sheets? For example, if you were doing an inventory of computer equipment in an organization, you might put all the computers by type or location on one page and all of the printers by type or location on another page. However, if the same inventory was for your personal computer-related equipment, one worksheet might be fine. If this were a budget, you might divide the budget into monthly or quarterly worksheets.

It is often most logical to place categories of data in columns because the width of columns can be customized easily to fit the data. You can then enter the specific data for each record, situation, or individual in each row under the appropriate column.

Once you have determined the goals of the project, the general process for creating the worksheet includes the following steps:

1. Create a file name that reflects the type of data in the worksheet. For example, UNIT 93 Budget 2014–2015 or Smith-CollegeExpenses.

2. Enter worksheet-identifying information on the first few rows. This information includes data such as name of the organization, department or division, the project (quarterly budget, inventory), and spreadsheet originator. Alternatively, this data may be entered in a separate worksheet called documentation where you may enter items like company name, workbook title, date, revision dates, purpose, name of developer, and so forth. This would be the first sheet in the workbook.
3. Enter labels that identify the columns and rows.
4. Enter the data.
5. Enter formulas and functions.
6. Format the data and labels (e.g., fonts, size, justification, number format).
7. Format the worksheet (e.g., borders, shading, color).
8. Create charts or graphs.
9. Print worksheets and/or charts.

Accomplishing Tasks in the Worksheet

This section will cover some common tasks for working with worksheets and the workbook.

Entering Data and Formulas

Spreadsheets allow you to enter two types of data: constants and formulas. Constants include dates, numbers, text, logical values, and error values. Formulas perform mathematical operations on values such as subtracting one value from another, comparing which is larger, and so forth. Formulas remain when you change values, and they recalculate the results keeping the spreadsheet up to date.

To enter data:

1. Click the **cell** for the data entry. For example, cell B10. The cell address will display, and the cell will be highlighted or outlined.
2. Type the **data**. If entering values it is generally faster to use the numeric keypad found on full sized keyboards.
3. Press the **Enter** key to go to the cell below the active cell, press the **Tab** key to go to the cell to the right, or press an **arrow** key to go to the cell in the direction of the arrow key.

Which key you use depends on the location of the next cell for data entry. If entering numbers from the numeric keypad, you may select the range of cells for data entry, and then use the Enter key on the numeric keypad. For example, select B10–F10, type the number, and press the enter key. This is generally faster since there is no tab key on the numeric keypad.

When you type data, the data appear in the formula bar. For example, in Figure 7-1a, 468 has been typed into cell B2, the active cell. If you enter new data into a cell that already holds data, the new data will overwrite the original data. In Excel, continuous data such as a column of dates are entered using the AutoFill feature—enter the first date, use the AutoFill feature (black plus sign at bottom right corner of cell or range of cells) and drag to the range of cells, and it will count by 1 day.

Typically, in spreadsheets, text is aligned to the left, and numeric values are aligned to the right. However, you can change this alignment. Unless otherwise indicated for data such as a social security number, phone number, or street number, the digits 0 to 9 and certain characters are treated as numbers in Excel. Other characters that are commonly treated as numbers include these symbols: – + . ( ) $ % / *. The program treats numbers as positive (+) unless you place a negative sign (–) in front of it. Unless the user changes the format, the spreadsheet will use a standard default approach to displaying numerical data. When you place a percent sign (%) after a number, the number may appear as a decimal. For example, 45% may appear as .45. Some spreadsheet programs automatically convert any numbers beginning with a dollar sign ($) to include two decimal spaces. For example, $12 would be displayed as $12.00. While all spreadsheet programs use default approaches to displaying data, you can alter how percentages, currencies, and other data types display.

Entering Formulas

Use the following numeric operators in formulas:

Symbol	Meaning	Symbol	Meaning
^	exponentiation	=	equals
*	multiplication	+	addition
/	division	–	subtraction
<	less than	>	greater than

When multiple numeric operators appear in a formula, the program calculates the formula using certain ordering rules called order of precedence. The first operator evaluated is parentheses, then exponentiation, followed by multiplication and division, and finally addition and subtraction; if there is a tie, calculation proceeds from left to right. Calculations enclosed in parentheses will always be calculated before other operations. For example:

5 * 5 + 3 would be calculated as 25 + 3, or 28
5 * (5 + 3) would be calculated as 5 * 8, or 40

A symbol (=) precedes a formula or function to let the spreadsheet know a formula or function follows. For example, = B2+B3.

Saving Worksheets

Each spreadsheet program has specific conventions for saving workbooks. Similar to word processing programs, spreadsheets replace newer versions of a workbook by overwriting older versions. The cautionary warnings in regard to saving word processing documents are equally important with workbooks.

To save a workbook:

1. With the workbook open, select **File**, **Save**, or press **Ctrl+S**.
2. Select a **location** and type a **name**.
3. Click **Save**.

Save your work often and before you try something new! Excel 2010 saves files in the .xlsx format, which is XML based. This format ensures the possible integration of Excel data with outside data sources and keeps the sizes of the files relatively small. Files containing macros are saved in the .xlsm format. You can also save Excel files in other formats including *.html or older versions of Excel (.xlt or .xls). A file name can contain letters, numbers, and spaces but not any of the following characters: / \ : * ? " < >. Excel automatically adds a file extension (usually .xlsx) to the file name when you save it. As in Word 2010, you can save Excel workbooks as Excel 97–2003 workbooks.

Using Charts

Charts are often effective for displaying spreadsheet data and illustrating trends. Many viewers find it easier to understand data in graphic form; spreadsheets make it easy to convert data into graphic forms. A good chart lets the reader instantly see the point of the data; it graphically compares and contrasts data. Some terms related to charts are defined here:

Axis — The **axis** is the horizontal (*x*) and vertical (*y*) plane or line on which the data are plotted. It provides a comparison or measurement point.

Categories — Categories are labels for the ***x*-axis** and ***y*-axis**.

Chart Type — The **chart type** refers to the way the chart will display the data. Examples include pie and bar charts.

Data Series — A **data series** is a group of related data points on a chart that originates from rows and columns in the worksheet. These values are used to plot the chart.

Legend — The **legend** is the information that identifies the pattern or color of a specific data series or category.

The best choice for the type of chart depends on the data to be displayed. For example, when comparing parts to a whole, such as a department's budget to the total budget for the organization, a pie chart might be useful. The following questions will help you make design decisions when creating a chart:

1. Is this the right chart to convey the data in the worksheet?
2. How would a viewer expect to see these data displayed?
3. Does the chart add to the understanding of the data and help the audience to make decisions?
4. Which questions or solutions does the chart suggest?

The process of creating a chart is discussed later in this chapter.

Introduction to Excel 2010—Basics

This chapter focuses on Excel 2010. It provides specific information about the Office 2010 version of Excel for Windows 7, which is similar to Office 2007 and Office 2011 for the Macintosh operating system. As in other Office 2010 applications, the **Backstage view** is a new feature in Excel (See Figure 4-11). The basic functions remain the same, as in older versions. Chapter 4 described the basics of applications running in a Windows 7 environment; those basics apply to Excel as well. Thus many of the skills learned in Chapters 4 and 5 will carry over into Excel.

Starting Excel is just like starting other Windows programs. Click the **Start** button at the lower-left corner of the screen, select **All Programs**, click **Microsoft Office**, and then **Microsoft Excel**. Figure 7-1a shows the Excel window. Alternatively, if an Excel icon appears in the Quick Launch area to the right of the Start button, click it to open Excel immediately. There may also be a shortcut on the desktop.

The Ribbon in Excel: Microsoft's "Fluent User Interface"

The ribbon consists of task-oriented tabs and groups of related tasks. (See Figure 4-4.) Each tab contains a different group of commands or tasks that help you use Excel. The File tab in Excel contains the same commands as it does in Word. (See Figure 4-2a.) It is helpful to compare the ribbons in Word and Excel on your computer screen to see the similarities and differences between them.

A brief description of each tab and its groups in Excel 2010 appears next.

Home — The most commonly used commands and features in Excel are on the **Home tab** (**Figure 7-3**). The Cut, Copy, and Paste commands appear in the Clipboard group. The Font group looks very similar to that in

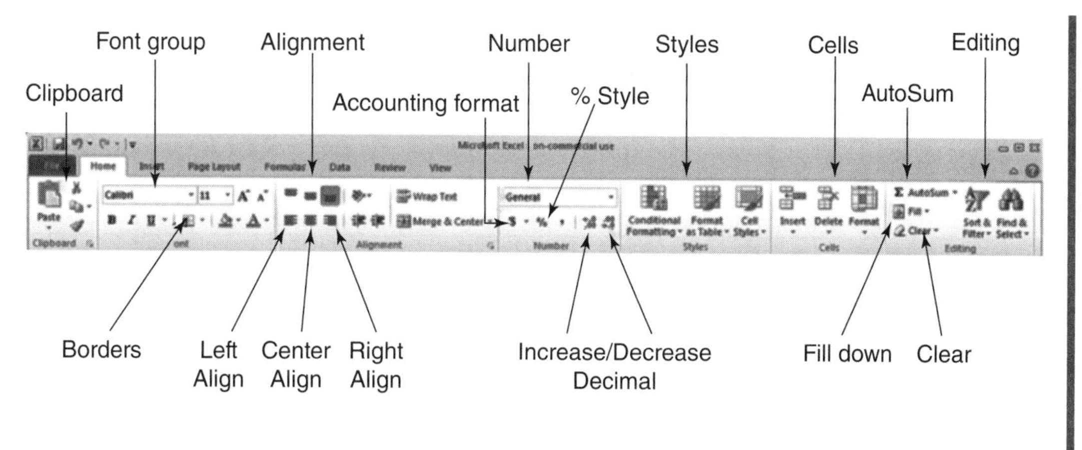

Figure 7-3 Home Tab and Groups in Excel 2010

Word; it also has a Borders icon. The Alignment and Number groups appear next, followed by the Styles, Cells, and Editing groups. Clicking the dialog launcher arrow box opens a dialog box. The Quick Access Toolbar appears above the ribbon in the Title bar; you can move it below the tabs and customize it to suit your preferences.

Insert

The **Insert tab** (**Figure 7-4**) provides quick access to groups related to tables, illustrations, charts, hyperlinks, and text objects. Seven large icons represent the various chart types. The Insert Chart dialog box (**Figure 7-5**) appears when you insert a chart type in the worksheet and provides access to Design, Layout, and Format contextual tabs for customizing charts. As long as a chart is selected in a worksheet, the Chart Tools tab appears on the right side of the ribbon.

Page Layout

Groups on the **Page Layout tab** (**Figure 7-6**) are Themes, Page Setup, Scale to Fit, Sheet Options, and Arrange. Here you can quickly change a document's theme to match a similar theme available in Word and PowerPoint. The Page Layout commands help you arrange items on the worksheet and prepare it for printing.

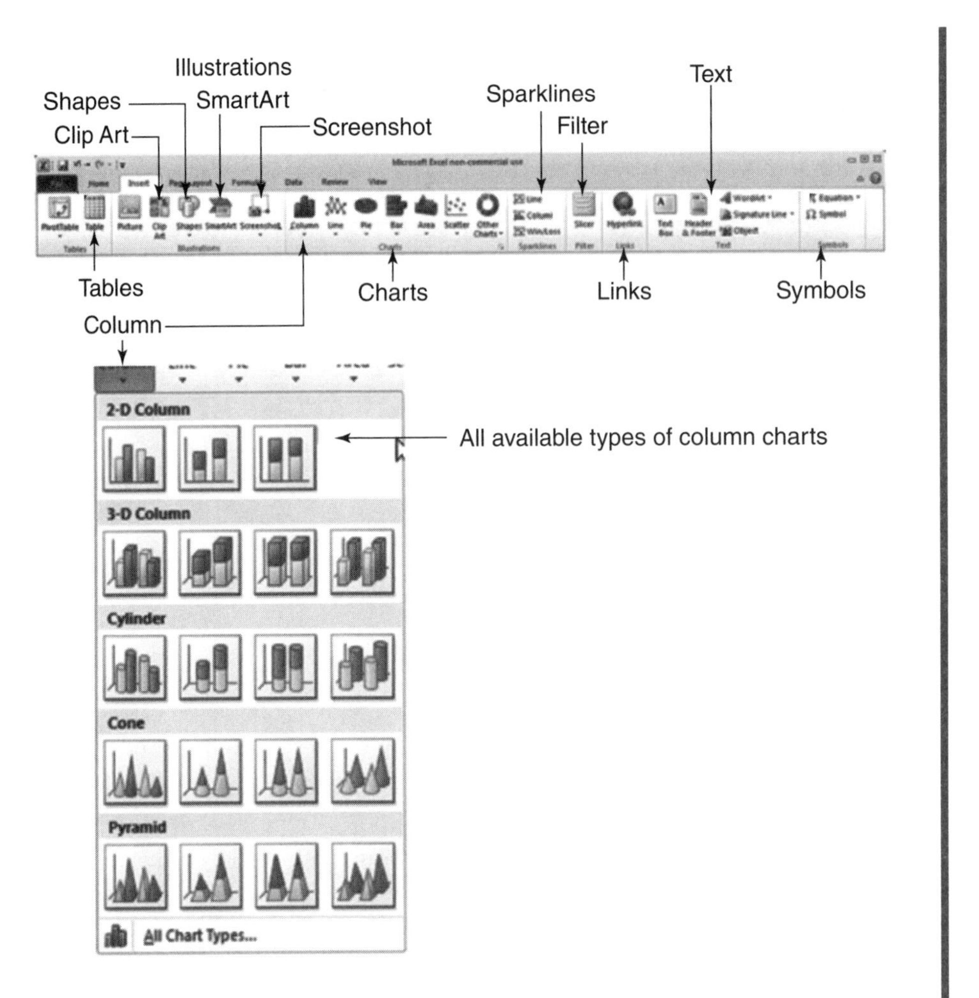

Figure 7-4 Insert Tab and Groups in Excel 2010

Formulas	Use the **Formulas** tab (**Figure 7-7**) to build formulas, check formulas, and create names for cells and tables. Groups are Function Library, Defined Names, Formula Auditing, and Calculation.
Data	The **Data tab** and groups (**Figure 7-8**) allow you to import external data, view linked spreadsheets (Connections group), sort and filter data, outline data, and use data tools. Some of the same icons for sorting and filtering appear in drop-down menus on the Home ribbon.

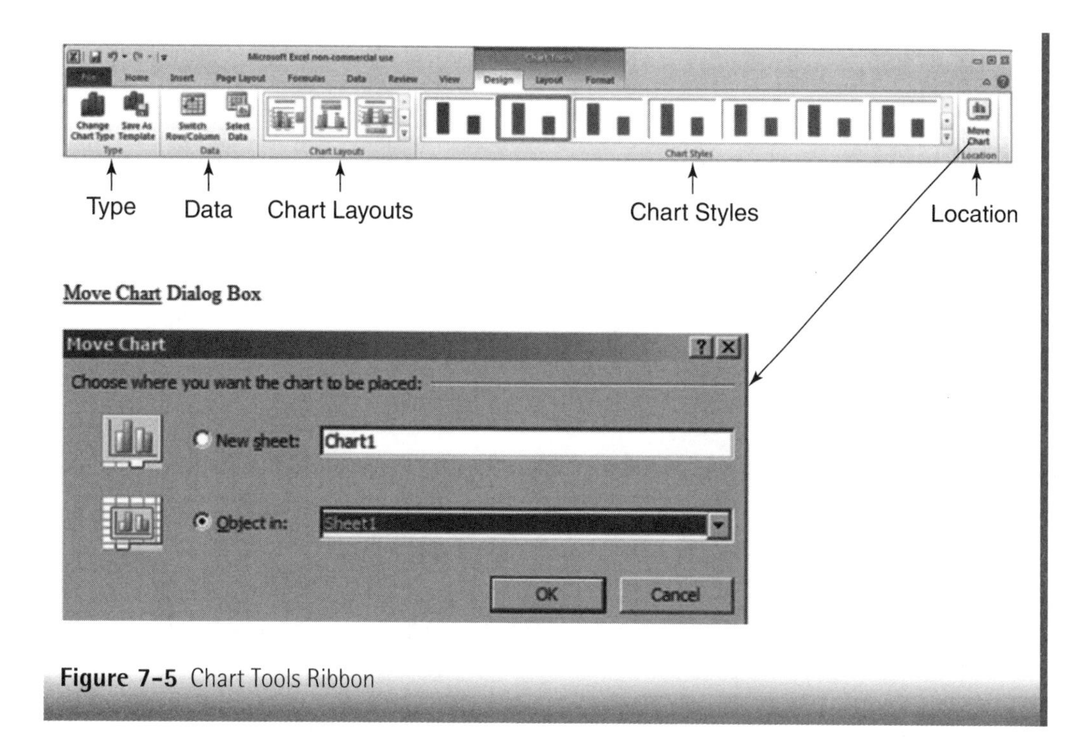

Figure 7-5 Chart Tools Ribbon

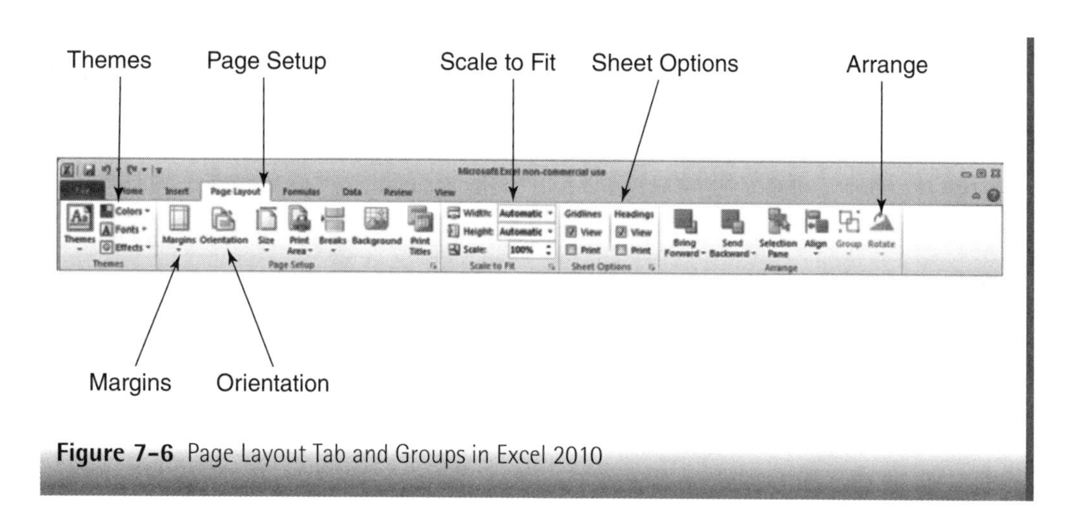

Figure 7-6 Page Layout Tab and Groups in Excel 2010

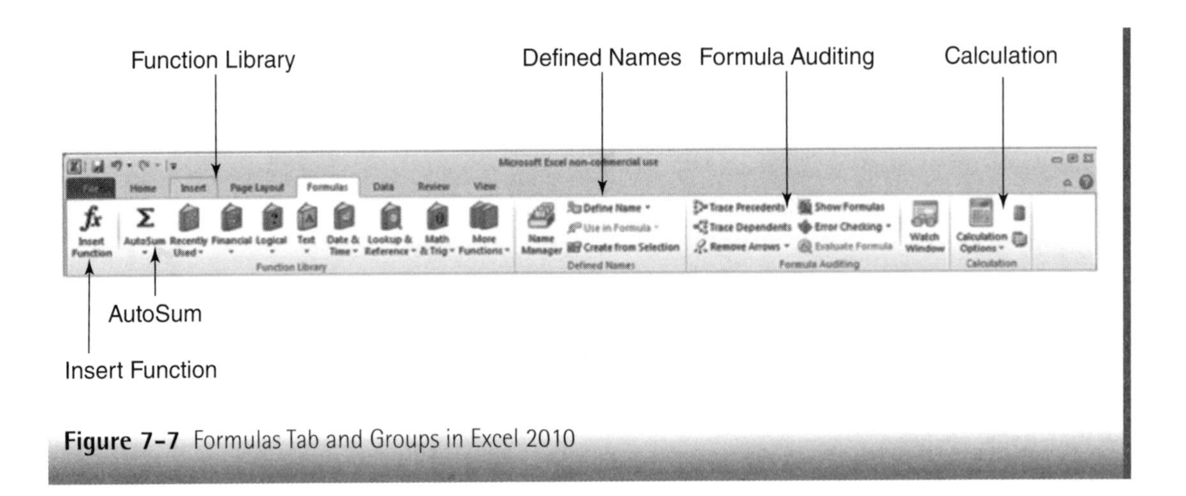

Figure 7-7 Formulas Tab and Groups in Excel 2010

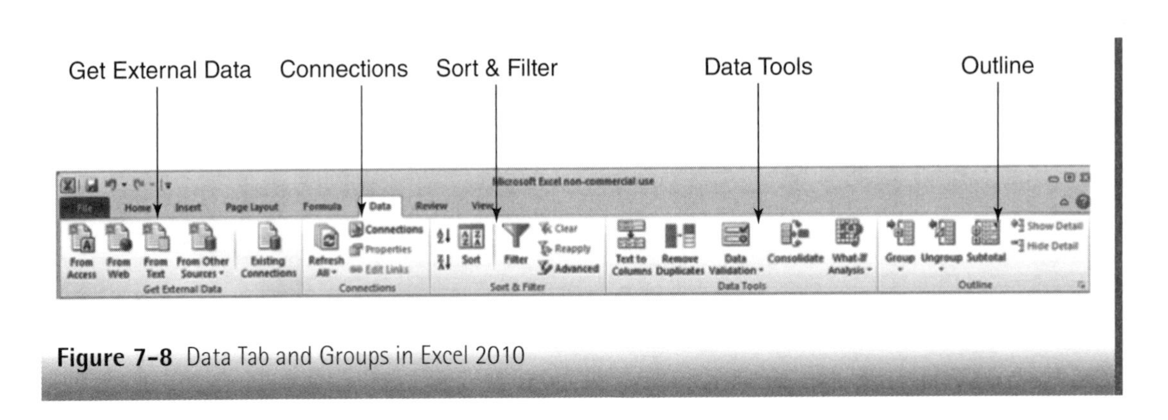

Figure 7-8 Data Tab and Groups in Excel 2010

Review	Functions relating to proofing, commenting, and protecting or sharing the contents of the active Excel sheet appear on the **Review tab** and its groups (**Figure 7-9**). Spelling, Research, Thesaurus, and the new Translate feature are part of the Proofing group.
View	The groups on the **View tab** are similar to those in Word, with some exceptions. Many refer to how spreadsheets are viewed in preparation for printing, as drafts, or arranged in the window. (See **Figure 7-10**.)

Excel also has **contextual tabs** that appear when necessary. Editing a header or footer will display the Header & Footer Tools tab, for example. Other context-sensitive tabs include Chart Tools, Drawing Tools, Picture Tools, Pivot Chart Tools, SmartArt Tools, and Print Preview Tools.

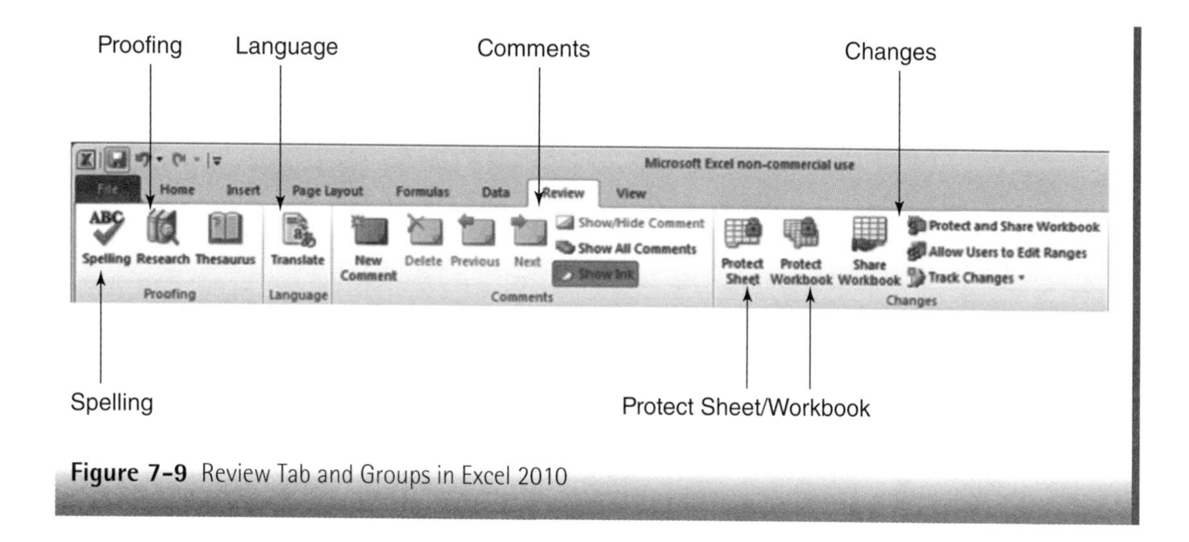

Figure 7-9 Review Tab and Groups in Excel 2010

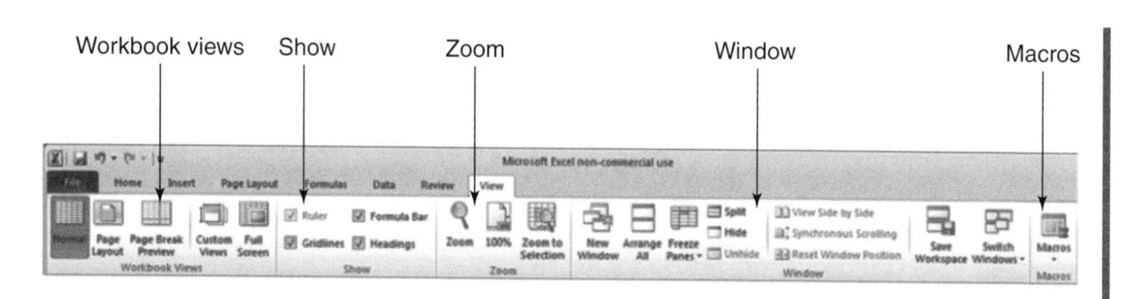

Figure 7-10 View Tab and Groups in Excel 2010

Moving Around in the Worksheet

You can navigate in a worksheet with the mouse, arrow keys, or key combinations. The simplest way to move is to place the mouse in the desired cell and click. However, if your hands are on the keyboard, the quickest way is to use the keyboard keys. Here are some of the keyboard strokes for moving around:

Arrow Keys	Move one cell in the direction of the arrow key. For example, the up arrow key moves you up one cell.
Tab Key	Move one cell to the right.
Shift+Tab	Move one cell to the left.
Ctrl+Home	Move to the beginning of the worksheet (cell A1).

Page Up/Page Down	Move to the cell one screen up/down in the same column.
Alt+Page Up/Page Down	Move left/right one screen in the same row.
Ctrl+End	Move to the intersection of last row and column containing data.
Home	Move to the beginning of the row.

To go to a specific cell:

1. Type the **address** in the cell address area, and press **Enter**.
2. Alternatively, **press F5** or **Ctrl+G** for the **Go To** dialog box.
3. Type the desired **cell address** in the reference box.
4. Press **Enter** or click **OK**.

Entering Data and Correcting Errors

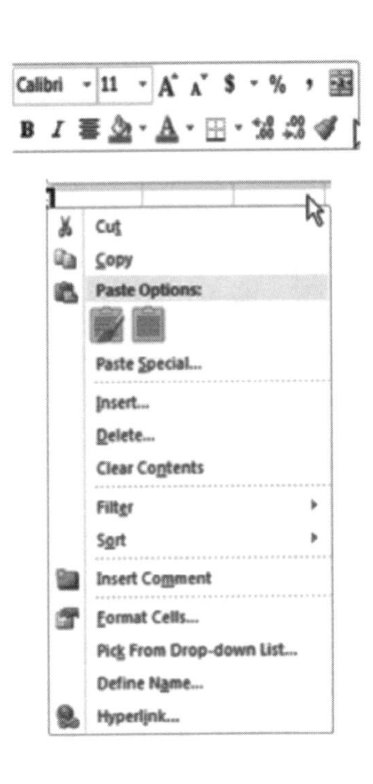

Figure 7-11 Menu that Appears When a Selected Cell or Section in the Worksheet Is Right-Clicked

In Figure 7-1a, the message area appears at the lower-left corner of the screen. It says "Ready" when you can enter data. After typing the data and before doing anything else, the message area says "Enter." You can accomplish data entry in several ways, including the following:

1. Press **Enter**.
2. Use the **mouse**, **Tab** key, or an **arrow** key to move to another cell.
3. Click **Enter** ✓ on the formula bar when entering formulas.

When you notice an error after entering data, you may change it in one of three ways:

1. Retype the data and press **Enter**. This will automatically overwrite the error.
2. Place the cursor in the cell where the error occurred and right-click. **Figure 7-11** shows the dialog box that appears. Choose **Delete** to

simply remove the data; choose **Cut** if you want to place the contents somewhere else in the spreadsheet.
3. Place the cursor back in the cell to be changed. Double-click and then make appropriate changes to the cell contents.

The Mouse Pointer

Inside the spreadsheet the mouse pointer takes on different appearances. Described here are a few of them and their meaning.

- When you see the "wide white plus sign" , use it to select cells that you want to work with in the spreadsheet. For example, use it to select a range of cells.
- Use the "four-headed arrow" to move cells or groups of cells from one place to another.
- Use the "two-headed arrow with vertical bar" to widen rows or columns. This pointer shape appears when you are between rows and columns (numbers and letters). For example, it appears when you are on the border between columns A and B or rows 1 and 2.
- Use the "little black plus sign" to AutoFill contents of a cell to another cell or range of cells. You will see this pointer shape in the lower-right corner of a cell when you are over the little square.

Using AutoFill

AutoFill is a built-in, time-saving feature in which Excel automatically inserts data by following a pattern you have begun in a worksheet. For example, when the column headings are months, follow these steps:

1. Type **January** or the first needed month.
2. Press **Enter**.
3. Place the cursor at the lower-right corner of the cell containing January; a black plus sign appear. (See **Figure 7-12a**.)
4. **Hold down** the mouse button and **drag** the cursor along the row until you have all 12 months. **Release** the button.
5. You can also **click** the right mouse button over the symbol below the last selected cell; a menu box will appear, as shown in **Figure 7-12b**. More choices then become available.

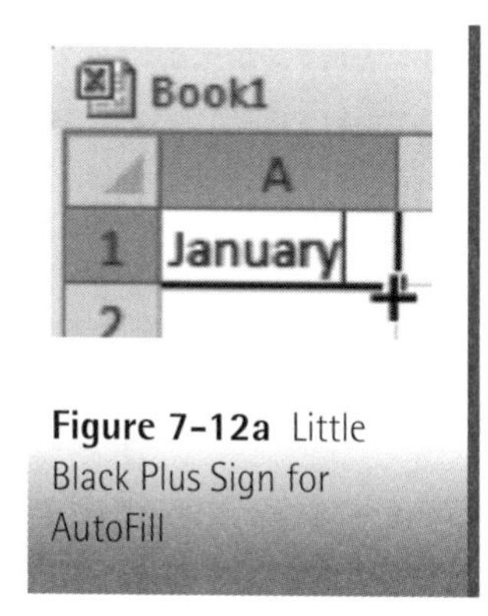

Figure 7-12a Little Black Plus Sign for AutoFill

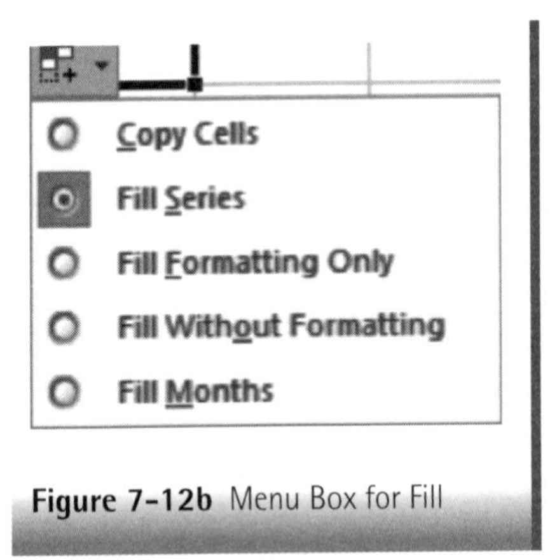

Figure 7-12b Menu Box for Fill

As you drag the black plus sign across the cells, the month will appear below the cell so you can see what Excel will insert there when you release the mouse button. To AutoFill a series of numbers, type the first two values in adjacent cells, such as 1 and 2 in cells A10 and A11 or 5 and 10 in cells A10 and A11. Select both cells (A10 and A11), and drag over the cells to place the data. For example, drag over cells A12 and A13. The AutoFill function will count by 1 or 5 as you AutoFill to cells A12, A13, and so forth.

Viewing the Worksheet

The View tab (Figure 7-10) provides options for changing how you view the workbook on the screen, such as normal page layout or full screen view. You can turn off and on the gridlines, the formula bar, and headings. Other choices relate to the Zoom feature, adjusting windows, and macros.

When working in the worksheet you can view parts of the worksheet by clicking the arrow keys on the scroll bars. The arrow keys on the scroll bar will move the worksheet one row or column at a time in the direction of the arrow. For example, clicking the down arrow on the vertical scroll bar moves one row down in the worksheet; clicking the right arrow moves one column to the right. Clicking in the blue area between the scroll bar and the arrow moves the display by an entire screen either vertically or horizontally, depending on the scroll bar selected. Note that this does not change the active cell; it just changes the view of the worksheet.

Common Commands

This section includes some common features you will use when working with spreadsheets.

To create a new worksheet:

1. Click the **File** File tab.
2. Click **New** and click Create or double-click **Blank Workbook**.

Alternatively, if the **New** button appears on the Quick Access Toolbar simply click it. Selecting the New button opens a new blank worksheet. Pressing **Ctrl+N** also opens a new workbook.

Existing templates or ones available on Office.com appear to the right of and below the Blank Workbook icon.

To access an existing worksheet:

1. Click the **File** tab. Click **Recent**. Note that a list of Recent Documents appears in the middle pane and Recent Locations in the right pane. Choose the desired workbook.
2. If the workbook is not there, click **Open** and look for the workbook in the file/folder in Documents library or wherever you saved the file.
3. Click the desired **file**.

To select cells:

To Select	Do This
A single cell	Click the **cell**.
A range of cells	Click a **cell** at one end of the series and **drag** the mouse to highlight the desired range of cells. Make sure the pointer is the white plus sign when you are holding down the mouse button to drag. If it is a four-headed arrow or a black plus sign, the data will be moving or autofilling, respectively.
Entire rows/columns	Click the **row or column heading** (the shaded horizontal or vertical area containing row numbers or column letters); the black arrow appears (**Figure 7-13**). **Drag** to include more than one row or column and to delimit the area selected.
Multiple cells, columns, or rows that are not contiguous	**Hold down** the **Ctrl** key while **clicking** all desired cells, columns or rows; then release the **Ctrl** key.
Entire worksheet	Click the **rectangle** at the left of the columns just under the formula bar.

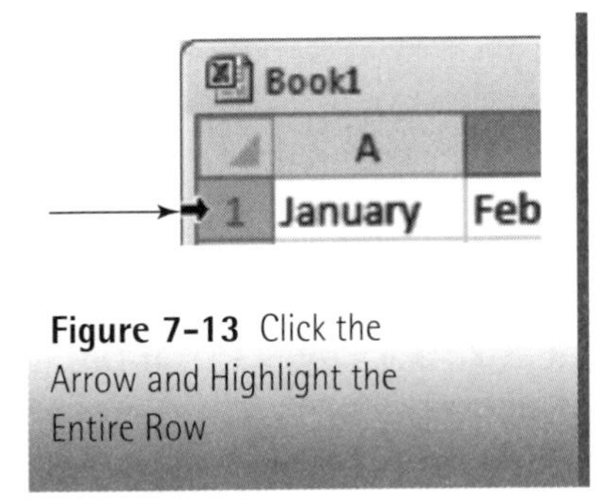

Figure 7-13 Click the Arrow and Highlight the Entire Row

If you need to clear cells, cut, copy, and change cell formats, or to apply formulas to a series of cells, first select the cells. The Clear command acts as an eraser and eliminates information or formats from a worksheet. You may clear one or more cells at one time. The cells remain on the worksheet and retain a value of zero.

To clear cell contents:

1. Select the **cell** or **range of cells** to clear.
2. On the **Home** tab, in the **Editing** group, select the **Clear** button.
3. Choose the appropriate command—clear all, formats, contents, or comments.

Here is another way to clear the contents of a cell:

1. Select the **cell** or **range of cells.**
2. Right-click the **selection.**
3. Choose **Clear Contents.**

To delete the contents of a cell:

1. Select the **cell** or range of cells.
2. Press the **Del** key to erase the cell contents.

NOTE: Delete is most commonly used to delete cell contents, whereas the Clear Contents is most commonly used to delete comments and formatting.

To change the size of a column:

1. At the top of the worksheet in the column letters, place the cursor on the **vertical line** (called a separator) to the right of the column to resize. The cursor will appear as a vertical line with arrows pointing left and right.
2. Drag the **column lines** to the size desired *or* double-click to use the "size to fit" option.

If you enter more numbers in a cell than the program can show after you press Enter, the cell will look similar to this: 2.34681+879 . Excel displays dates that can't fit in a column as pound signs (#####).

To insert a cell, row, or column:

Cell — Place the cursor where you want the new cell; right-click. Figure 7-11 shows the menu that appears. Choose **Insert**; then select the appropriate option in the dialog box (**Figure 7-14**).

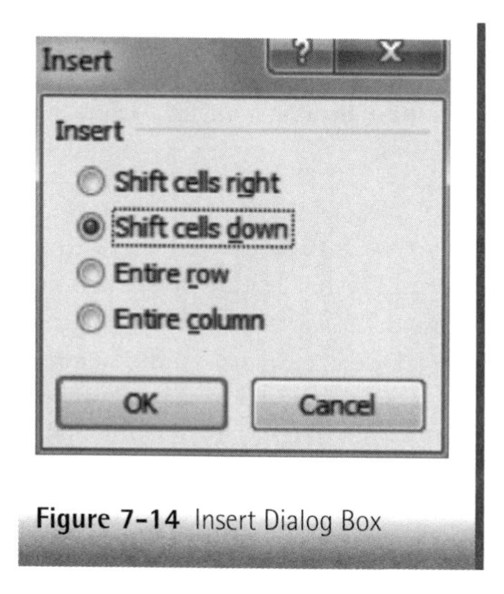

Figure 7-14 Insert Dialog Box

Column	Right-click the **column heading** (such as C or E), and choose **Insert** from the pop-up menu.
Row	Right-click the **row number** (such as 5 or 8) and choose **Insert**.

Using this technique, Excel inserts rows *above* the current row and columns to the *left* of the current column. You may insert more than one row or column by highlighting a number of row or column headers equal to the number to be inserted and following the steps above.

The Insert, Delete, and Format commands appear on the Home tab in the Cells group. To use them, place the cursor in a cell or a column or row heading. If you click once on Insert, for example, Excel inserts a cell, column, or row depending on what you have selected. If you click the drop-down arrow ▾ below Insert, a menu appears (See **Figure 7-15**.) A similar menu appears if you click the drop-down arrow below Delete.

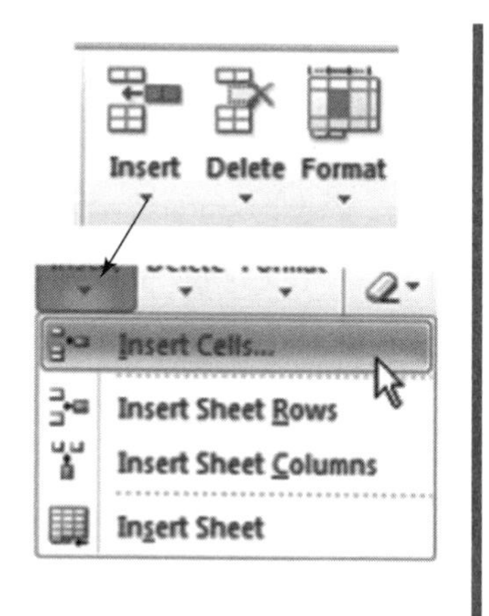

Figure 7-15 Home Tab, Insert Drop-Down Menu

To delete a row/column:

Here are several options.

1. Place the cursor on the **heading** for the row or column to be deleted, and click to **highlight** it. Press **Delete**.

2. **Right-click** the row or column header, and select **Delete** from the menu that appears.
3. Select the **row** or **column header**, and click **Delete** in the Cells group on the Home tab.

The save, save as, print, cut, copy, and paste functions work the same way in all Office 2010 applications; we have reviewed them in other chapters. It is always a good idea to use the Print Preview feature before printing a worksheet. There are many options for presenting data in an appropriate print format by adjusting headings, color, alignment, type size, SmartArt, and so forth.

Working with Excel—Multiple Worksheets

In the work world many spreadsheet applications require working with multiple worksheets containing a larger amount of data. Excel, by default, includes three worksheets in a workbook file. (See the sheet tabs in Figure 7-1a.) Here are some common features when working with larger worksheets.

To move between worksheets:

1. Click the **appropriate sheet** tab at the lower-left corner of the worksheet.
2. If there are many sheets and all aren't displaying, use the navigation buttons to navigate to additional sheets. For example, click the **last sheet** button to see the last sheet in the workbook.

To change the default number of worksheets:

1. Click the **File** tab.
2. Click **Options** at the bottom of the File menu.
3. In the **When creating new workbooks** area, choose the desired number of worksheets in **Include this many sheets** area (See **Figure 7-16**.)

To add a worksheet to this workbook only:

Here are several options.

1. Click the arrow next to **Insert** in the Cells group on the **Home** tab and choose **Insert Sheet**. A new worksheet is added to the left of the selected worksheet.
2. Click the **rectangle** next to Sheet 3. Pressing **Shift+F11** will have the same effect.
3. Right-click the **sheet tab** and choose **Insert** from the pop-up menu. Select **Worksheet** in the Insert dialog box, and then click **OK**.

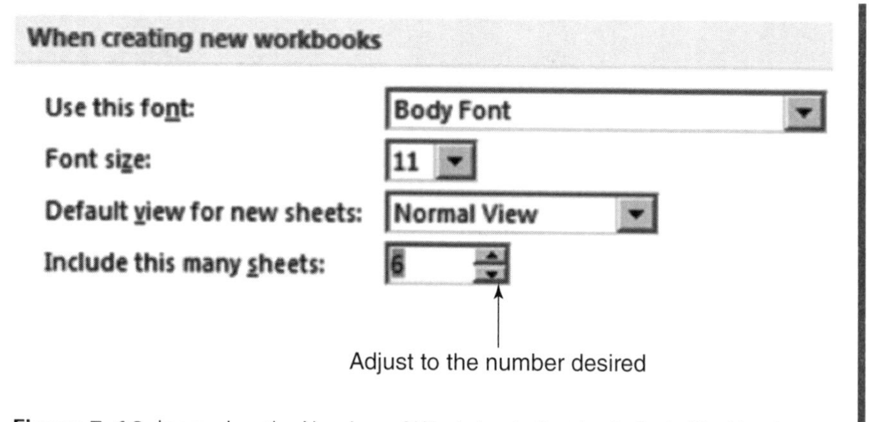

Figure 7-16 Increasing the Number of Worksheets for the Default Workbook

To reorder worksheets:

1. Right-click the **worksheet tab**.
2. Select **Move** or **Copy**; then select the order desired from the dialog box and click **OK**.

Most people use the easier drag-and-drop method to reorder sheets.

To delete a worksheet:

1. Click the **arrow** below **Delete** in the **Cells** group on the **Home** tab and choose **Delete Sheet** .
2. Right-click the **sheet label** and choose **Delete** from the pop-up menu that appears.

You may copy and paste data between the sheets in a workbook. Any formulas based on data in one worksheet that are not copied to another will result in the error message #REF, because the formula will be looking for the reference data in the cells of the new worksheet.

Working with Excel—Multiple Workbooks

Just as in Word, where it is possible to have multiple documents open, multiple workbooks may also be open in Excel at the same time; you may copy data and paste data between workbooks as well. Open workbooks are shown in the taskbar at the bottom of the screen and can be selected from there.

To view two worksheets from the same workbook:

1. On the **View** tab in the **Window** group, click the **New Window** button .
2. On the **View** tab in the **Window** group, click **View Side by Side** .
3. In the Workbook window, click the **worksheets** that you want to compare.
4. To scroll both worksheets at the same time, click **Synchronous Scrolling** in the **Window** group on the **View** tab. This option acts like a toggle switch and can be turned off and on as necessary.

To view two worksheets from different workbooks:

1. **Close** other documents.
2. Open the **first workbook**, and then open the **second workbook**.
3. Click **View** in the **Window** group; choose **Arrange All**.
4. Select **Tile**, **Horizontal**, **Vertical**, or **Cascade** from the dialog box.
5. Click **OK**.

The tile option will arrange the windows side by side in small, even rectangles to fill the screen; the horizontal option arranges windows one above the other; the vertical option arranges windows side by side; and the cascade option creates a stack of windows with only the title bar of the inactive windows showing.

The save, save as, print, cut, copy, and paste functions work the same way in Excel as they do in all Office 2010 programs (See Chapters 4 and 5 for a review of these functions.

Formatting Cells—Numbers

Cell entries are considered to be either labels or values. Values can be numbers or formulas. The first character typed determines the type of cell entry. In addition to the numbers 0–9, Excel treats the following characters as values: – + / *. E e ( ) $ %. An equal sign signals that a formula or function follows.

The default format for numbers is general. Any numbers entered into Excel appear exactly as typed. You can change number formatting to signal that the values are decimals, percentages, currency, time, or other types of numbers. As you make different selections, Excel presents examples in the dialog window to allow a view of the effects of the format.

To format cells:

1. Select the **cells** to format.
2. On the **Home** tab, go to the **Number** group.
3. Select the **desired format** from the shortcut icons in the Number group.

See Figure 7-3 for examples of formatting types. If you click the down arrow beside **General**, a Number Format menu appears that provides more choices (See **Figure 7-17**.)

To see more cell format options:

1. Click the **dialog launcher arrow** in the **Number** group.
2. Click **More Number Formats** in the Number Format menu. **Figure 7-18** shows the Format Cells dialog box that appears.

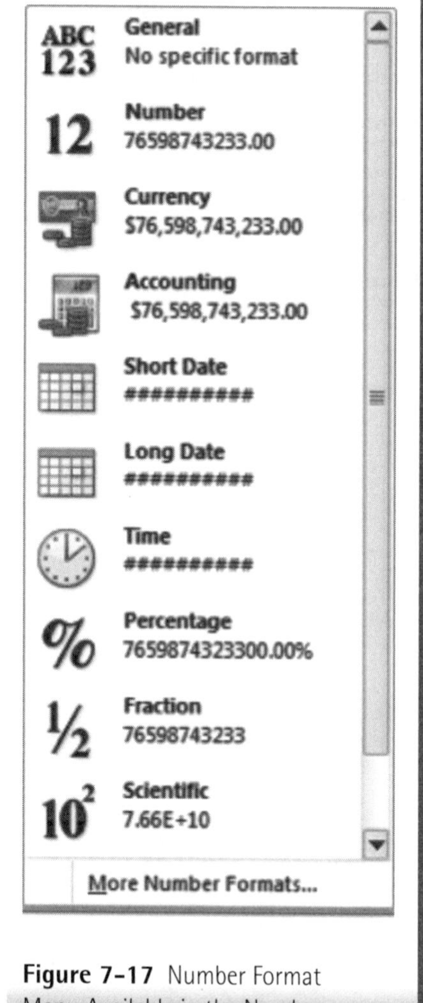

Figure 7-17 Number Format Menu Available in the Number Group, General

The changes you can make to a worksheet, particularly after it is complete, are nearly endless. For example, you can modify the font type and size, color, spacing, alignment, and styles. **Figure 7-19** shows the Cell Styles menu that appears after you select the drop-down arrow in the **Styles** group of the **Home** tab.

Using Formulas and Functions

Formulas help you analyze the data on a worksheet. With formulas, it is possible to perform operations such as addition, multiplication, and comparison and to enter the calculated value on the worksheet. A **function** is a more complex preprogrammed formula. An Excel formula or function always begins with an equal sign (=). Entering a formula is just like typing an equation on a calculator.

To build a formula:

1. Type an = **sign** in the cell where you want to place the formula.
2. Type the **formula** by typing cell addresses or by selecting cells with the mouse.
3. Press **Enter** or click the **Enter** button in the formula bar.

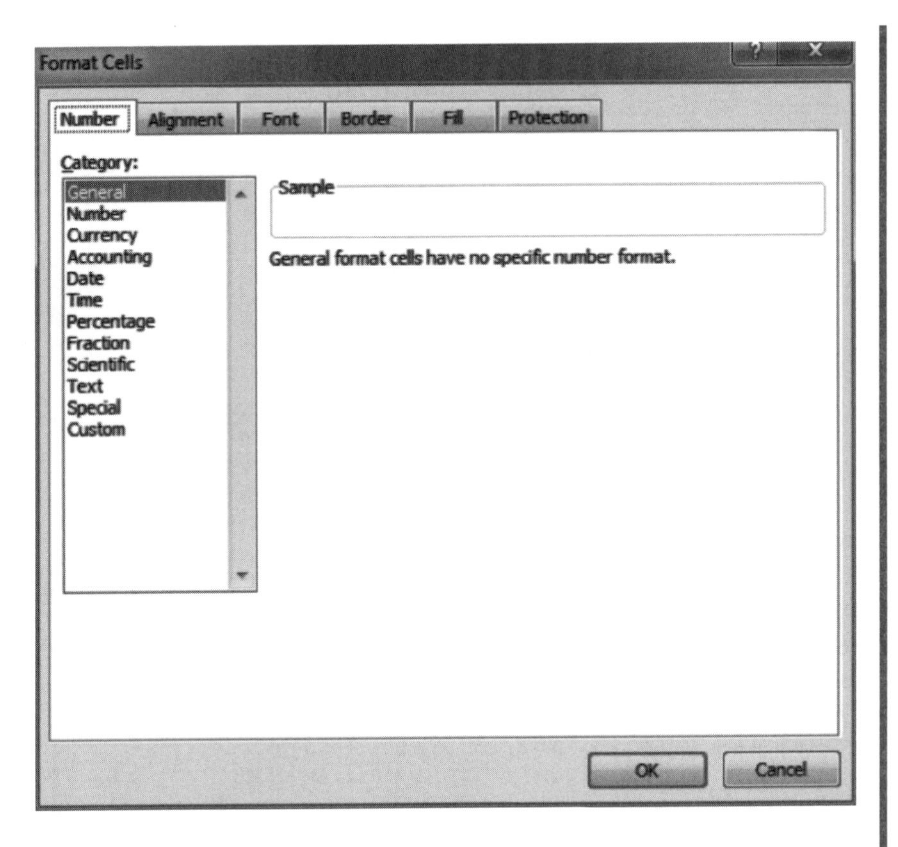

Figure 7-18 Format Cells Dialog Box

In **Figure 7-20**, we added two cells by typing = and then clicking on cells D2 and D3. Note that the formula appears in the cell and formula bar in the top example. After you enter the formula and press the Enter key, the total appears and the formula shows only in the formula bar. When using formulas in Excel, the standard rules of precedence listed earlier in this chapter dictate how the mathematic calculation proceeds.

The AutoSum function **Σ AutoSum ▾** is the most commonly used function; it automatically adds a series of numbers in either rows, columns, or both. This function is found on the Home tab in the Editing group and in the Function Library on the Formulas tab.

To use the AutoSum function:

1. Highlight the **cells** for summation and include a blank space at one end of the series.
2. Click the **AutoSum** button **Σ;** the sum displays once you press **Enter**.

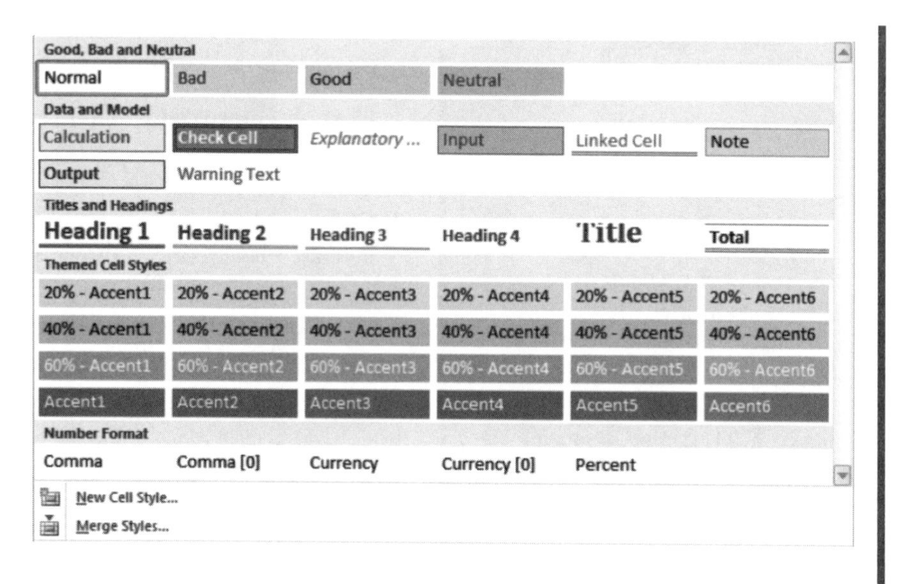

Figure 7-19 Cell Styles Menu

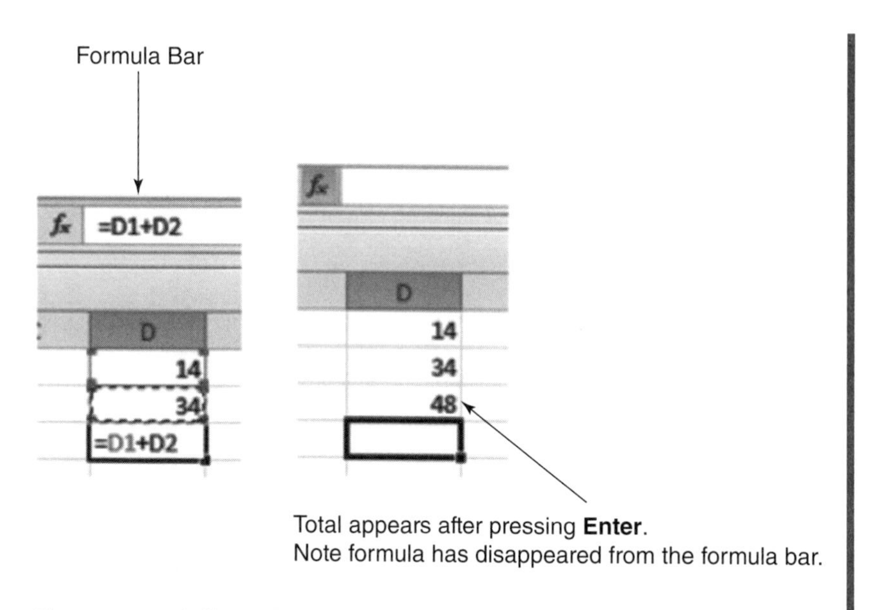

Figure 7-20 A Simple Formula for Adding Cells

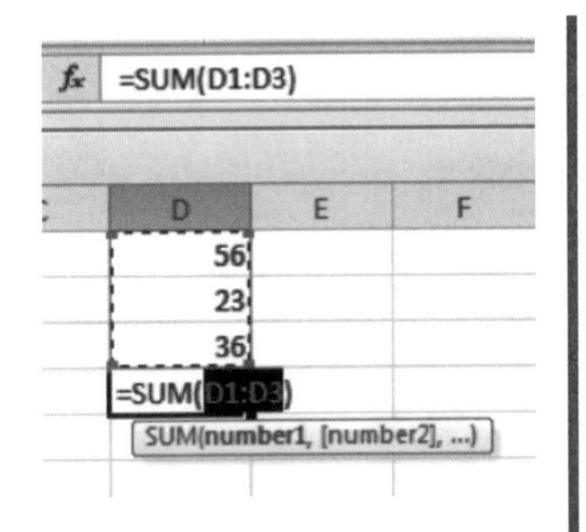

Figure 7-21 Confirm Range of Cells with the AutoSum Feature

Another way to use this function is by following these steps:

1. Click an **empty cell** where Excel will display the sum.
2. Click the **AutoSum** icon.
3. Confirm that the range of cells to be added is correct, as shown in **Figure 7-21**.
4. Press **Enter** or click the **Enter** button ✓.

Excel includes commonly used formulas in numeric functions; this eliminates some of the required steps for writing a formula. Excel 2010 includes 356 built-in functions that are useful in finance, mathematics and statistics, and engineering.

To access these functions:

1. Click the **Formulas** tab.
2. Choose the **appropriate function** from **Function Library** group.

To see more statistical functions:

1. Click the **Formula** tab.
2. Click **More Functions** and then **Statistical**. **Figure 7-22** shows the Statistical Functions menu found in the Function Library.

Commonly used functions include the following:

Function Name (Attribute)	Purpose
=SUM(range)	Sums the indicated values.
=AVERAGE (range)	Averages the indicated values.
=COUNT(range)	Counts the number of cells within a range that contains numbers.
=MAX(range)	Returns the largest value within a range.
=MIN(range)	Returns the smallest value within a range.
=STDEV(range)	Computes the standard deviation for the range.
=VAR(range)	Determines the variance for the range.
=IF(condition, true, false)	Returns a true value if condition is met; returns a false value if the condition is not met.

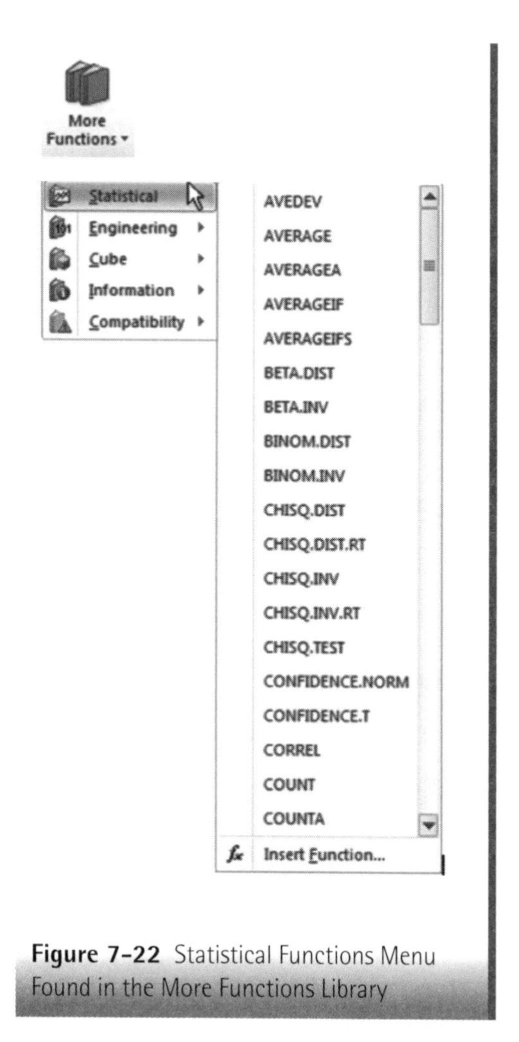

Figure 7-22 Statistical Functions Menu Found in the More Functions Library

If any values change in a function, the result also changes. The parts of a function include the following components:

= sign + function name + parentheses ( ) + arguments within the parentheses

Examples

=SUM(B3:B5)
=AVERAGE(F1,F4,G1,G3,G5)

If the cell addresses to be included in the function or formula are adjacent to each other, a colon is used to separate them (B3:B5). The colon (:) can be thought of as a vertical ellipsis; in other words, you have left something out—in this case, cell B4. If the cell addresses are not adjacent, then a comma is used between them. You can combine both adjacent and nonadjacent cells in the same function. The result of the calculation appears in the selected cell, but the function appears in the formula line, as shown in **Figure 7-23**.

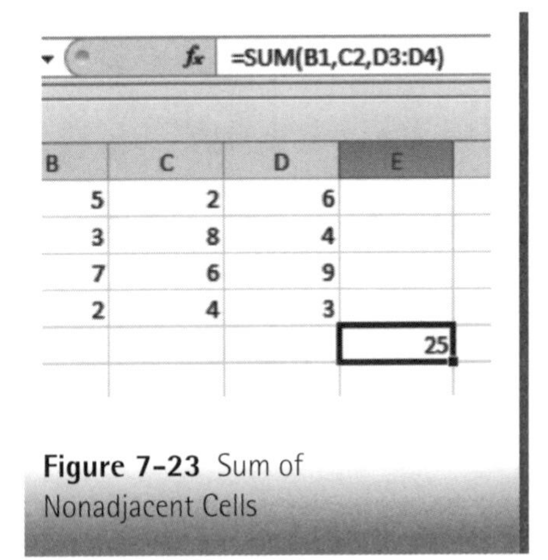

Figure 7-23 Sum of Nonadjacent Cells

To sum cells:

1. Click the **cell below** or to **the right** of the values you want to total.
2. Choose **Home**, **Editing**, and then **AutoSum** Σ AutoSum ▾ . Alternatively, choose **Formulas** and **AutoSum** Σ AutoSum .
3. Press **Enter** or click **Enter** button on the formula toolbar.

If you want to select different cells from those Excel defaults to select them with the mouse or type them in. Be sure your cursor is within the parentheses ( ). Click the first cell you want to include. You will need to add a comma between nonadjacent cells or a colon if the cells are adjacent to each other as shown in Figure 7-23.

Absolute Cell Addresses

Relative addresses are cell addresses in formulas that are designed to change when the formula is copied to other cells. **Absolute addresses** are cell addresses in formulas that remain the same despite other changes in the worksheet; they are fixed. Excel indicates absolute addresses by a dollar sign ($) preceding the part of the address that is to remain absolute. For example, if the number in C5 is to be the divisor in a formula no matter where the formula is moved, that address should appear in the formula as C5.

The following combinations are used to keep certain parts of an address constant:

CR	Both the row and column addresses always remain the same.
$CR	The row changes, and the column address always remains the same.

C$R	The column changes, and the row address always remains the same.

Database Functions–Sort and Filter

Sorting Data

Excel allows you to sort data on the worksheet. **Sorting** enables you to specify the order of the data in the columns. It is possible to sort data alphabetically or numerically. All data relevant to the sort must be included in the sort area.

To sort data:

1. Using the mouse, select all involved **data**.
2. Click **Sort & Filter** in the **Editing** group on the **Home** tab (**Figure 7-24**), and designate whether to sort data in ascending (1, 2, 3 or A, B, C) or descending order (10, 9, 8 or Z, Y, X). Choose **Custom Sort** to see other sorting options.

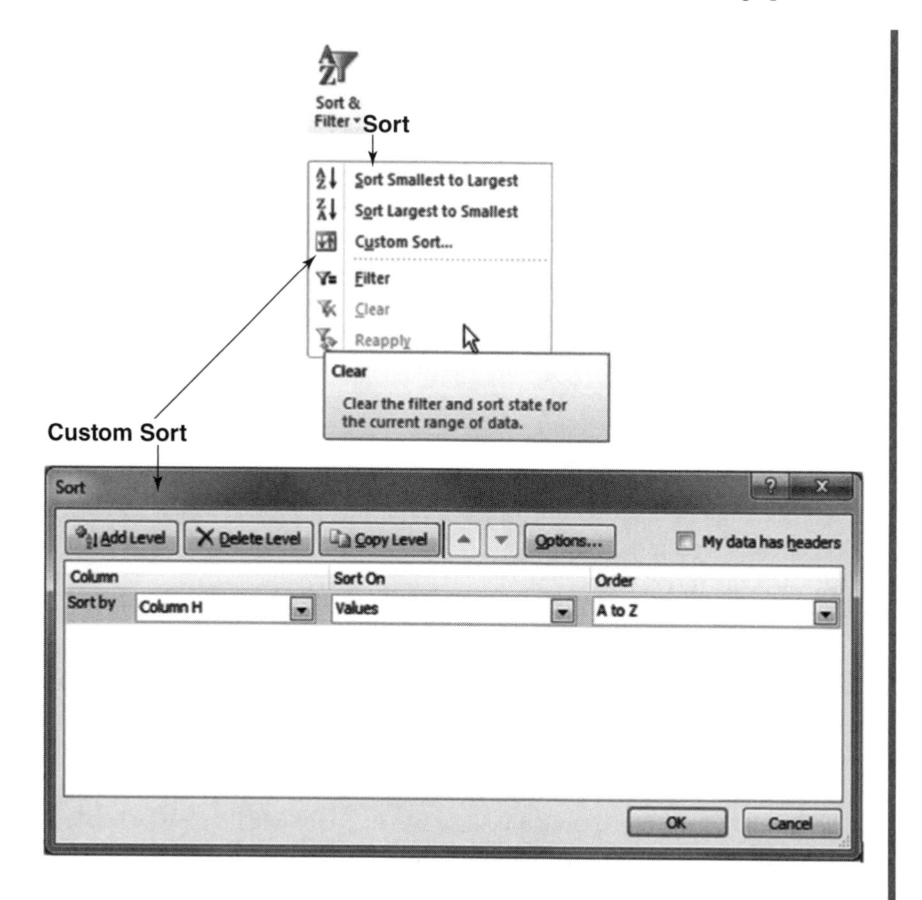

Figure 7-24 Sort & Filter Option on the Home Tab, Editing Group

If the data have a header, exclude it from the data range so Excel does not sort it. Or you can include the header and then use custom sort. Select **My data has headers** option. When you use the Sort By option, you will see the headers and will not have to remember what they were. Figure 7-24 shows the Sort & Filter group on the Data tab and the Advanced Filter dialog box.

Filtering Data

Filtering allows you to select specific records for review. It does not rearrange data, but rather hides data you do not want to display. This feature makes it easier

to manage large lists. When you select **Filter** on the Data tab, a drop-down arrow appears in the selected column(s). **Figure 7-25** shows a list of options in the Sort & Filter group on the Data tab. If you click the **Advanced** option, the advanced filter dialog box appears as shown in this figure. You could first **filter** the data desired, and then sort the filtered data by smallest or largest order. In the example shown in **Figure 7-26**, we first selected the range of cells to filter, then clicked **Sort & Filter**, and then **Filter** to place the arrow on the hours cell. In the dialog box, we then selected **Number Filters** to show the number filter choices available.

Graphing Data

To represent the data in graphic form, use the charting feature in Excel. Excel has many chart options several of which were explained in Chapter 6. The important point when selecting charts is to select the correct type for the data it represents.

To create a chart:

1. Select the **data** on the worksheet graph. Include the appropriate column and row headings.
2. Click the **Insert** tab.
3. Choose a **chart type** from the **Chart** group—Column, Line, Pie, Bar, Area, and so forth.
4. Choose one of the options available in that group. (Figure 7-4 shows the options when Column is selected.) Once you have selected a chart type, the graph appears in the worksheet and the contextual Chart Tools tab appears with its Design, Layout, and Format tabs (See Figure 7-5).
5. On the Chart Tools, Design tab, choose a **Chart Style** if graph style adjustments are necessary. If you want to see how the data will look in another

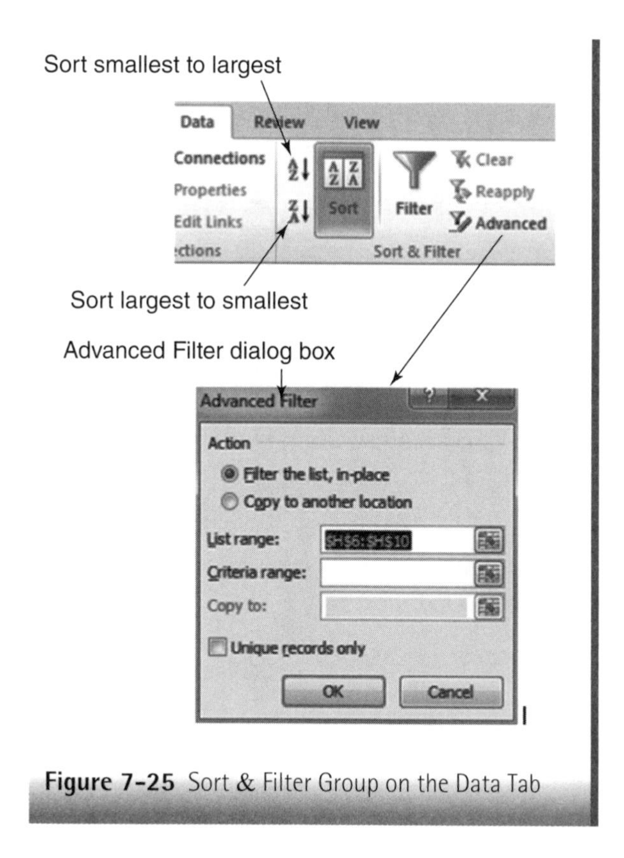

Figure 7-25 Sort & Filter Group on the Data Tab

chart type, click **Change Chart Type** in the Type group. Choose another **chart type**. When you have a chart type you like, click one of the options in the **Chart Layout** group. See which one works best with the graph.

6. Click the **Chart Title** icon on the **Chart Tools Layout tab**.
7. Type the **title**. It will appear in the Formula bar as you type.
8. Press **Enter**. Alternatively you may click the Title placeholder in the Chart and type the title.
9. Choose a **location** for the chart—the open worksheet or a new one. By default the chart will appear on the open worksheet.

To move the chart within the current worksheet, click the **border of the chart** (four-headed arrow) and drag to its **new location**. You can also resize the chart by using the double-headed arrow on the chart border (this works in the same way as sizing a window).

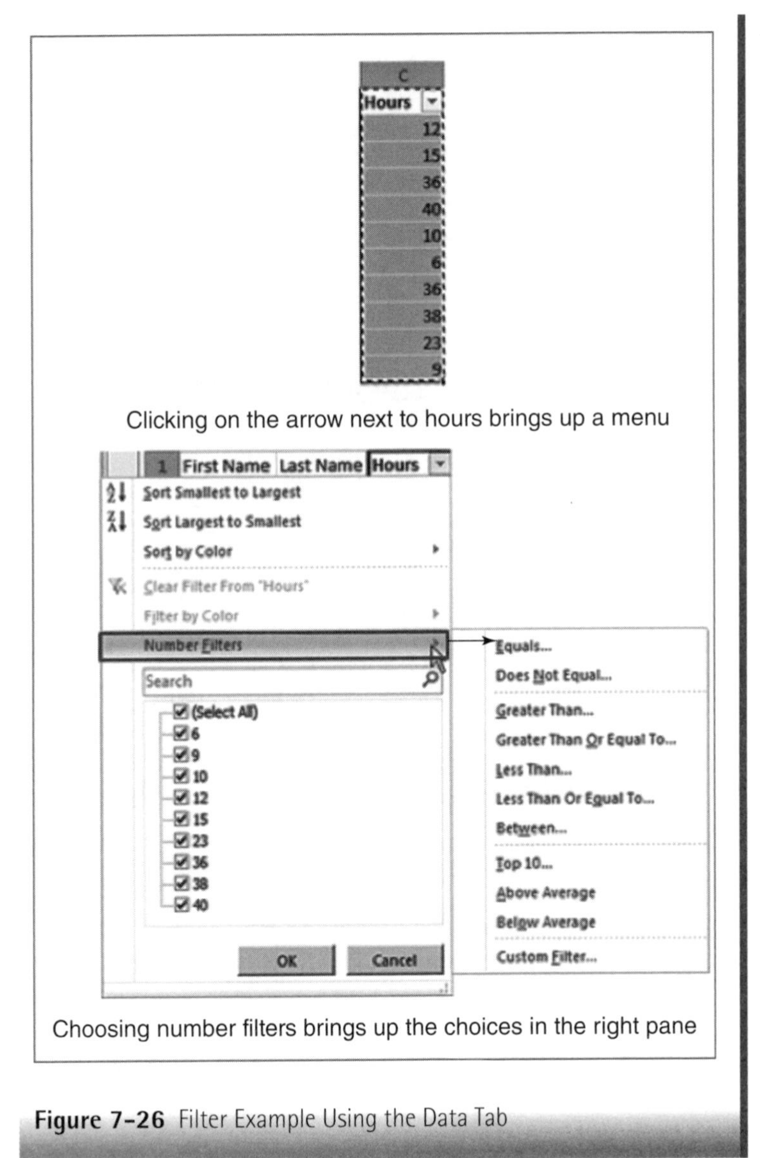

Figure 7-26 Filter Example Using the Data Tab

To move the chart to another worksheet, click **Chart Tools, Design Tab**. Now click the **Move Chart** icon at the right end of the Chart Tools, Design Tab ribbon, select **New Sheet**, type a **name** for the sheet, and click **OK.** (See Figure 7-5.) This option automatically enlarges the chart.

10. Use the layout and format tabs to make any necessary adjustments to the chart.

Scenarios

Scenarios are a type of what-if analysis tool. A scenario is a set of values that Excel saves and can substitute automatically in the worksheet. Use scenarios to forecast the outcome of a worksheet model. You can create and save different groups of values in a worksheet; you can then switch to any of these new scenarios to view their results. For example, when creating a budget with uncertain revenues, you can define scenarios with different values for the revenue. It is then possible to switch between the scenarios to perform what-if analyses.

The What-If Analysis button appears in the Data Tools group on the Data tab. When using the Scenario Manager, it is possible to have as many as 32 variables that change from scenario to scenario.

Summary

Spreadsheets can simplify tasks requiring calculations, such as budgeting, inventory tracking, and quality assurance. This chapter provided basic information about using spreadsheets—specifically, building simple formulas, using common functions, and developing charts to represent data visually in Excel 2010.

Exercises 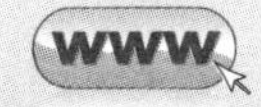

EXERCISE 1 Create a Simple Salary Worksheet

■ **Objectives**

1. Create a simple spreadsheet.
2. Use simple formulas and functions.
3. Format a worksheet.
4. Print, save, and retrieve a spreadsheet.

■ **Activity**

1. Open **Excel**.
   a. Click **Start**, **All Programs**, **Microsoft Office**, and **Microsoft Excel**. An **Excel** button may also appear in the Quick Launch area of your taskbar or in another area of the Start menu.
   b. Once you see the spreadsheet on the screen with "Ready" in the message area, you can begin. Be certain that you are in the correct cell for performing the remaining actions in this exercise.
2. Practice moving the cursor.
   a. Practice moving from one cell to another using the mouse and the arrow keys.
   b. Move from cell **A1** to cell **C5**.
   c. What happens to cell C5?
   ____
   d. What shape does the pointer assume when it is inside the worksheet?
   ____
   e. Look for the current cell address in the Name box on the Formula toolbar. What do you see? ______________________________
3. Practice entering data.
   a. Type your **first name** in cell **C5** using lowercase letters and press **Enter**.
   b. Type your **last name** using lower case letters and press **Enter**.
   c. Go to cell **C6**, press the **spacebar**, and then press **Enter**.
   d. What happens? ______________________________
   e. Erase the **name** from cell **C5**.
4. Save the worksheet.
   a. Click the **File** button then **Save,** or press **Ctrl+S,** or click the **Save** button on the Quick Access Toolbar.
   b. Select the correct **storage location** for the file.
   c. In the File name box at the bottom of the screen, type **Chap7-Exercise1-LastName**; click the **Save** button or press **Enter**. Remember that the computer stores the workbook as an Excel file.
5. Enter spreadsheet ID information.

a. Click cell **A1**.
b. Type **UNIT BUDGET**, and press **Enter**.

6. Use the process in this step to enter the labels on your spreadsheet. Do not waste your time making the data look nice at this point. Formatting comes after the labels and data are entered.
   a. Click cell **A3**.
   b. Press the **Caps Lock** key.
   c. Type **LAST** in cell **A3**. Press **Alt+Enter**. Type **NAME** and press the **Tab Key**.
   d. Type **FIRST**. Press **Alt+Enter**. Type **NAME** and press the **Tab Key**.
   e. Type **SOCIAL**. Press **Alt+Enter**. Type **SECURITY**. Press **Alt+Enter**. Type **NUMBER** and press the **Tab Key**.
   f. Type **CARE**. Press **Alt+Enter**. Type **LEVEL** and press the **Tab Key**.
   g. Continue typing the labels as shown in **Figure 7-27**. Be sure to press **Alt+Enter** after entering each word and press the **Tab Key** for the last word to move to the next cell.
7. Enter the data.

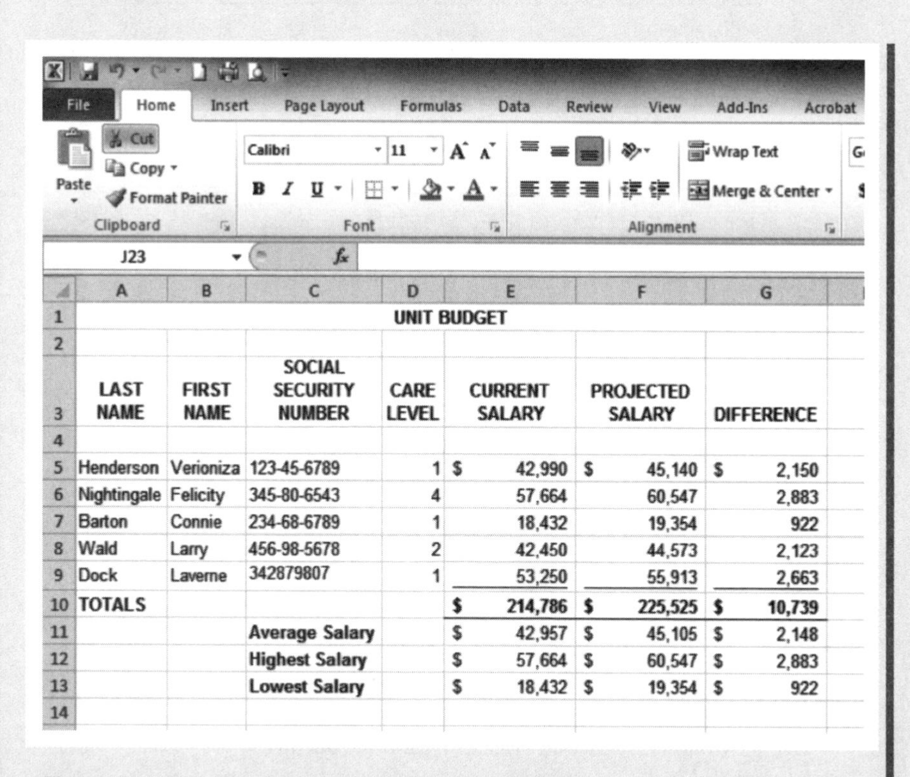

	A	B	C	D	E	F	G
1				UNIT BUDGET			
2							
3	LAST NAME	FIRST NAME	SOCIAL SECURITY NUMBER	CARE LEVEL	CURRENT SALARY	PROJECTED SALARY	DIFFERENCE
4							
5	Henderson	Verioniza	123-45-6789	1	$ 42,990	$ 45,140	$ 2,150
6	Nightingale	Felicity	345-80-6543	4	57,664	60,547	2,883
7	Barton	Connie	234-68-6789	1	18,432	19,354	922
8	Wald	Larry	456-98-5678	2	42,450	44,573	2,123
9	Dock	Laverne	342879807	1	53,250	55,913	2,663
10	TOTALS				$ 214,786	$ 225,525	$ 10,739
11			Average Salary		$ 42,957	$ 45,105	$ 2,148
12			Highest Salary		$ 57,664	$ 60,547	$ 2,883
13			Lowest Salary		$ 18,432	$ 19,354	$ 922
14							

Figure 7-27 Exercise 1: Labels and Data Unit Budget

a. Press the **Caps Lock** key to turn off the caps lock function. Click cell **A5**.
b. Type the following data in the cell as indicated and press **Enter** after each name:

Row	Column A
5	Henderson
6	Nightingale
7	Barton
8	Wald
9	Dock
10	TOTALS

c. Fill in the rest of the data as shown here. Remember, if you turn on the **Num Lock Key** you can use the numeric keypad and its **Enter** key to enter all these data items. Select the range **B5:E9**.

Row	B	C	D	E
5	Veronica	123-45-6789	1	42290
6	Felicity	345-80-6543	4	57664
7	Connie	234-68-6789	1	18432
8	Larry	456-98-5678	2	42450
9	Laverne	342-87-9807	1	53250

8. Create formulas. Project a salary increase of 5% for each healthcare worker.
   a. Click cell **F5**. Type **=(E5*1.05)** and press **Enter**.
   b. Click cell **F5**.
   c. Place the pointer at lower-right corner of the cell until it turns to a **black plus sign** PROJECTED SALARY E 44404.5 .
   d. Drag through cell **F9** and release the **mouse button**.
   e. Which formula appears in cell F7? ______________________
   f. Click cell **G5**. Type =. **Click** cell **F5**. Type –. Click cell **E5**.
   g. Click the **check mark** ✓ on the formula toolbar or press the **Enter** key.
   h. Place the pointer at lower-right corner of the cell until it turns to a black plus ✚ sign.
   i. Drag through cell **G9** and release the **mouse button**.

9. Use functions. Use the Sum function to total the salaries and differences in the budget.
   a. Select cell range **E10:G10**.
   b. Click the **AutoSum** button. What totals do you get?

      ____

   c. Add the following labels in the designated cells:
      Cell C11: **Average Salary**
      Cell C12: **Highest Salary**
      Cell C13: **Lowest Salary**
   d. In cell **E11**, type =**average(E5:E9)**. Press **Enter**.
   e. In cell **E12**, type =**max(E5:E9)**. Press **Enter**.
   f. In cell **E13**, type =**min(E5:E9)**, Press **Enter**.
   g. Select range **E11:E13**. Use AutoFill to drag through **column G**.
   h. Change Henderson's salary to 43,000 by typing **43000** in cell **E5**.
   i. What total do you see now in cell E12? ______________________
   j. Change Henderson's salary back to the original value.
10. Format labels, numbers, and the worksheet as a whole.
    a. Click **column header A** and drag the **mouse** over all the columns through **G**. Select the **Format** button in the Cells group and then choose **AutoFit Column Width** from the drop-down menu. (See **Figure 7-28**.)

       Did it adjust all the column widths to fit the content? If not, click the column header A and drag the mouse over all the columns through G. Place the cursor on the vertical line between G and H and double-click. Is that better?
    b. If necessary, click the **Home** tab. Click the **Font down arrow** Calibri 11 and select **Arial**.

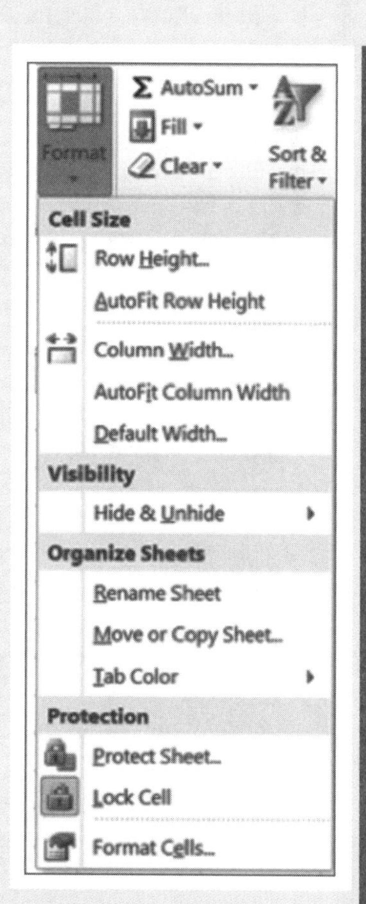

Figure 7-28 Format Dialog Box

c. Click the **Size down arrow**, and select **10**.
d. Select cells **A1:G3**. Click the **Bold** **B** button.
e. Select cells **A3:G3**.
f. Click the **Merge & Center** Merge & Center button.
g. Select the range **E5:G5**. Hold down the **Ctrl** key and **select** the range **E10:G10** to **E11:G13**.
h. Click the **Currency** $ button on the formatting toolbar.
i. Click the **Decrease decimal** button twice.
j. Select the range **E6:G9** and click the **Comma** , button.
k. Click **Decrease decimal** button twice.
l. Select cell **A10**. Click the **Bold** **B** button.
m. Select the range **E9:G9**. Click the **Underline** **U** button.
n. Select the range **E10:G10**. Click the **Underline** **U** button.
o. Click the **Bold** **B** button.
p. Select **Average**, **Highest**, and **Lowest Salary**. Click the **Bold** **B** button.
q. If you still need to make adjustments in how the data fit into cells, place the pointer on the vertical line between the columns and adjust their width.
r. The last formatting that you need to do is to center the labels. Think about how you would accomplish this task using Word. What should you do in Excel? Do it now.

   If all of these steps have been completed correctly, the spreadsheet should look like the one in Figure 7-27.

11. Save the **worksheet**.
12. Sort the information by last name.
    a. Select cells **A3** to **G9**. **Click** the **down arrow** on the **Sort & Filter** icon in the **Editing** group on the **Home** tab. (See **Figure 7-29**.) Click **Sort A to Z**.
    b. What do you notice about the column letters and the row numbers? Click the **Undo** button.
    c. Sort the information by **first name**.

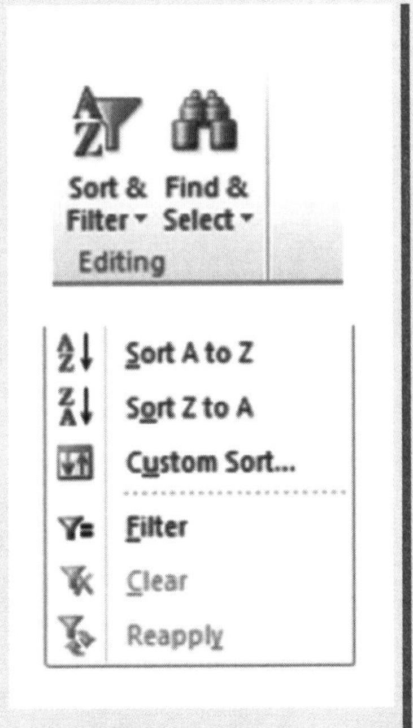

Figure 7-29 Sort & Filter Menu

d. Select range **A5:G9**. If you use A3:G9, you will need to click the square in the sort dialog window that says My data has headers or it will sort the headers along with the data.
e. Select **Custom Sort** from the **Sort & Filter** menu options.
f. From the Sort dialog box that appears choose **Column B** under **Column**.
g. Click **OK**. Now the worksheet is sorted by first name.
h. Click the **Undo** button.

13. Sort the worksheet by **last name** and then save the **worksheet**, as you did in Step 11, but change the name to **Chap-7Exercise1Sort-LastName**. Notice what happened to the underline in the data. How could you avoid that?
14. Exit **Excel.**
    a. Click the **File** tab, and then **Close**.
    b. Click the **Close** button in the upper-right corner of the screen to close **Excel**.
15. Reopen **Excel** and find the sorted file.
    a. Which steps will you use to see where you stored the budget file? ______________________________
    b. What is the full file name of the sorted budget file? ______________
    c. Open **Excel** and click the **File** button.
    d. Click the **sorted file** from the **Recent** option on the file menu.
    e. Click the **File** tab and **Print** option to see the print options for your worksheet. You can also access this command from the Quick Access Toolbar if the Print Preview icon appears there.
    f. Exit **Excel** and any other open applications. Be sure to exit Windows fully, and turn off the equipment as instructed.

EXERCISE 2 Create a 6-Month Budget

Objectives

1. Create a 6-month budget using selected spreadsheet commands.
2. Use selected functions and simple formulas.
3. Add color to highlight selected information.

Activity

1. Create the identifying information.
    a. Open **Excel** and save the worksheet as **Chap7-Exercise2-LastName**.
    b. In cell A1, type the heading for the spreadsheet: **6-MONTH BUDGET**.
    c. In cell B2, type **BUDGET**. In cell C2, type **ACTUAL**. In cell D2, type **DIFFERENCE**.

2. Add the labels.
   a. Type **JAN** in cell **A3**.
   b. Use the AutoFill function to fill the labels through cell **A8**. Place the cursor in the lower-right corner of cell **A3**. Using the black plus sign 3 JAN, drag through cell **A8**. Cell A8 will have **JUN** in it.
3. Enter the data.
   a. Select the range of cells **B3:C8**.
   b. Using the numeric keypad type the **data,** beginning with the budget for January and pressing the Enter key after use entry.

Month	Budget	Actual
JAN	1450	1390
FEB	1450	1425
MAR	1475	1410
APR	1500	1430
MAY	1450	1380
JUN	1500	1450

4. Add functions. Use the AutoSum function for finding sums in row 9, columns B and C. In column A type **TOTALS**, select **B9:C9,** and click the **AutoSum** button.
5. Which formulas would you use to compute the differences between the budgeted amounts and the actual amounts for JAN? Enter this **formula in column D3**.
6. Which feature would you use to copy the formula to compute differences for each month? Copy the **formulas** to the **appropriate cells**.
7. How would you write the function to determine the average for the 6-month BUDGET and ACTUAL amounts? In cell A11, type **Averages**, and then enter that function to determine those averages in cells **B11** and **C11**. (Click cell **B11** and click the **Sum function down arrow** Σ ▾. Select **Average**. Make sure the correct range is selected. If not, select the correct range.)

HINT: The range should not include the total for either column. Press **Enter** or click the **Enter** button on the formula toolbar once the correct range is selected. Drag to cell **C11**.

8. Format the numbers.
   a. Select **range B3:D9.**
   b. Go to the **General** option in the **Number** group on the **Home** tab.

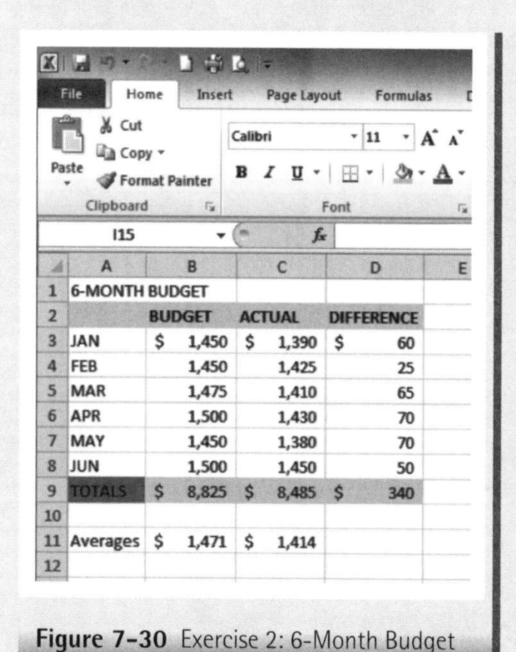

	A	B	C	D	E
1	6-MONTH BUDGET				
2		BUDGET	ACTUAL	DIFFERENCE	
3	JAN	$ 1,450	$ 1,390	$ 60	
4	FEB	1,450	1,425	25	
5	MAR	1,475	1,410	65	
6	APR	1,500	1,430	70	
7	MAY	1,450	1,380	70	
8	JUN	1,500	1,450	50	
9	TOTALS	$ 8,825	$ 8,485	$ 340	
10					
11	Averages	$ 1,471	$ 1,414		
12					

Figure 7-30 Exercise 2: 6-Month Budget

c. Click the **down arrow** and choose **Number**.

d. Format the **first** and **last row** as **Currency**, no **Decimal places**. Format the remaining numbers as **comma**, no **Decimal places.**

9. Click cell **B9**, click the **down arrow** beside the **Fill Color** button, and select **yellow**. Select cell **C9**, and add a color fill of your choice. When would you use color in formatting the worksheet? When would using gray shading be a better option?
10. **Save** the workbook. Submit it as directed by your professor. See **Figure 7-30** for the finished product.

EXERCISE 3 Create a Chart

Objectives

1. Use the Chart Wizard to create several chart types.
2. Print several chart types.

Activity

1. Create a spreadsheet.

a. Create a spreadsheet representing the expenses for three months.
b. Save the file as **Chap7-Exercise3-LastName.**
c. Include the following categories in the spreadsheet: utilities, rent, food, car expenses, and personal expenses. Either use the figures below or fill in your own. Use Column A for Expenses, B for January, C for February, and so forth.

A	C	D	B
Expenses	JAN	FEB	MAR
Utilities	225	195	175
Rent	850	850	850
Food	325	315	335
Car Expenses	35	25	175
Personal Expenses	250	175	185

2. Select the range of cells **A3:B8.**
   a. Click the **Insert** tab.
   b. Click the **arrow under Pie** Pie in the **Chart** group.
   c. Choose the **3-D pie** 3-D Pie.
   d. Go to **Chart Tools** and click **Layout** Chart Tools Design Layout Format.
   e. Click the **Chart Title** Chart Title **arrow**. Select **Above Chart** from the menu items that appear.
   f. Click the **Chart title** in the chart and type **January Expenses.**
   g. With Chart selected, click **Layout** tab under **Chart** tools.
   h. In the Labels group, click the **Legend** icon and click **Show legend at the top**. Place the legends in the pie wedges.
   i. With the chart selected, click the **Legend** icon and click **None**. Click **Data labels** icon in the Labels group and click **More Data Labels** option.
   j. Check **Percentage** and **category** to select and **value** to deselect. Click **close.**
   k. Click each **category** and drag out to better arrange them on the chart.
   l. Click the **rent wedge** and drag it out about ½ inch to explode it. See **Figure 7-31** for a finished pie chart.
   m. Experiment with different chart types. Is there one that presents all of the data in a better way?

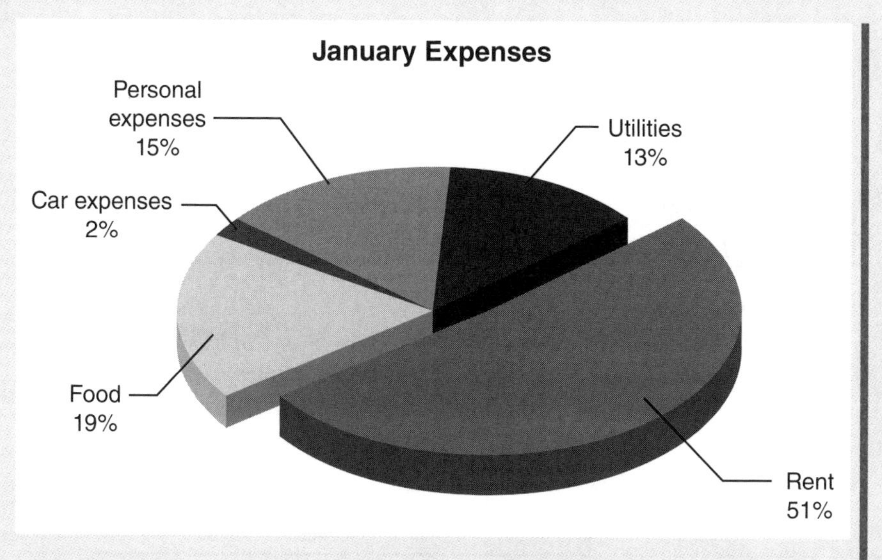

Figure 7-31 Exercise 3: Pie Chart for January Expenses

3. Using the steps learned here, create and save a column chart (any subtype) that compares all of the expenses for the 3-month period. Place it next to the pie chart. Save the work and submit per the directions of the professor.

Assignments

ASSIGNMENT 1 Create a Simple Spreadsheet

Directions

1. Create a spreadsheet for any of the following:
   a. A unit budget that includes last year's costs, this year's costs to date, and cost projections for next year if costs increase 5%.
   b. A drug worksheet that lists the dose by weight for a class of drugs (e.g., emergency drugs for premature babies or for cardiac arrest, a comparison sheet giving safe doses of narcotics) and formulas for calculating the drugs for persons weighing different amounts.
   c. A personal budget of your living costs for the past year, the current year, and projected for next year if all costs increase by 3%.
   d. A special topic approved by your instructor.
2. Use the appropriate formulas and functions.

3. Create a new sheet, copy the original worksheet to the new sheet, and conduct one "what-if" question.
4. Save your work and name it **Chap7-Assign1-LastName.**
5. Submit your work as directed by your professor.

ASSIGNMENT 2 Create a Grade Sheet

Directions

1. Use a spreadsheet to create a grade sheet that includes headings for students' first and last names, ID numbers (Student ID number), and the test scores for a midterm exam, a project, a final exam, and the final grade.
2. Enter the data under the headings as they appear here:

ID	Last Name	First Name	MIDT	PROJ	FINAL EXAM	Final Grade
6789	Titmouse	Martha	95	98	87	
4534	Finch	Jerry	87	75	90	
9084	Cardinal	Sam	65	70	67	
9087	Robins	Sally	85	80	90	
1234	Nuthatch	Jamie	85	90	95	
1234	Wren	Timothy	90	95	90	

3. The midterm exam and project are each weighted to be 30% of the final grade, and the final exam is weighted to be 40% of the final grade. Enter a formula to calculate the final grade for each student in Final Grade column.
4. Using the appropriate functions, enter the function to calculate the highest and lowest grades and the average for the midterm, project, and final exam grades.
5. Give each grade a percentage weighting so that all three grades total 100%. Place those percentages in a row you add between the headings and the first row of data.
6. Using the percentages and grades, determine the final numerical grade for each student.
7. Adjust the columns so that the spreadsheet is visually pleasing.
8. Practice creating a scenario showing how Martha's grade would change if she earned a 95 on the final exam.

9. Sort the spreadsheet in alphabetical order by the last names of the students.
10. Save the spreadsheet as **Chap7-Assign2-LastName**.
11. Submit the work as directed by your professor.

ASSIGNMENT 3 Create a Chart

Directions

1. Use the data from Assignment 2 to create a chart that compares all five students' grades on each of the three different parts that determine the grade for the course.
2. Print the graph. On the back of the paper, indicate why you selected the chart that you did. Alternatively, place the explanation about choice of chart on another worksheet as many people are no longer printing work.
3. Save the workbook as **Chap7-Assign3-LastName**.
4. Follow the directions provided by the professor for submitting your work.

chapter

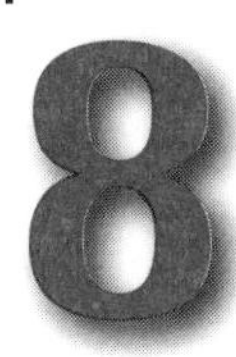

Introduction to Databases

Objectives 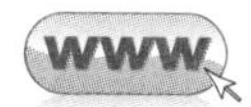

1. Identify the data types that are best managed through databases.
2. Identify the advantages and uses of databases.
3. Describe the characteristics of databases and their associated features.
4. Define terms related to database applications.
5. Describe the database design process.
6. Interpret basic directions for using Excel's database functions for simple databases.
7. Perform selected queries and filters on Excel's data table.
8. Examine selected issues related to database use in health care.

Introduction

When you are born, the State Vital Statistics office enters you into a database of vital statistics. Shortly thereafter the Social Security Administration issues you a Social Security number and places you in yet another database. The U.S. Census Bureau records you in the census every 10 years. When you obtain your driver's license the state places you in yet another database. Government agencies and other public and private entities use electronic databases in all aspects of modern society. Libraries catalog their collections in databases. Businesses track inventory, manage customer information, and maintain accounting data in databases. Educational institutions track applications and enrollments, drop and add students to courses, and produce class lists using databases. Healthcare institutions use a variety of database programs to manage and track patient information, employee data, research data, and trends. These databases reside on all types of computers, from large mainframes to personal computers. This chapter introduces basic database concepts and terms, with an emphasis on how they are them in health care. The chapter then introduces basic database skills, with several sample database exercises to reinforce these skills.

Database management systems help people organize, store, and retrieve data. These programs permit the user to create table structures, modify these structures, store data, and retrieve data in a variety of ways. They act as efficient file systems; they are, however, only as effective and efficient as the accuracy of the data and the structure of the tables within them. Most end users do not create the data structures; rather they use previously designed database input and query forms and reports. A basic understanding of these data structures is critical to assist in the development of the database that meets the end user's needs.

Electronic databases offer the following advantages for managing data:

- They reduce data redundancy (duplicate data in a variety of places).
- They reduce in data inconsistency (data stored differently in the same file, such as the format used to store a person's name—full name, including first and middle names, or first name, middle initial, and last name).
- They increase data access.

Some professionals believe that automated databases offer a data security advantage. They believe that with centralized data, control over access is much easier. Others believe that automated databases create a data security disadvantage because the increased access to data results in increased security concerns. The increased use of mobile devices to access patient records makes the database more vulnerable. The interest in mHealth (mobile health care) adds to the security and privacy concerns for mHealth databases (He and Pan, 2012, p. 8). Healthcare administrators need to make and communicate decisions about what healthcare professionals can and can't do with their own mobile devices when they use them in healthcare environments. In addition, healthcare providers must make the traditional decisions about who has access to which data and at what level. Should everyone have the ability to correct and add data or do some users warrant viewing rights only with no revision rights? In the healthcare arena, should receptionists at the information desk have access to a patient's diagnosis and physician's name or do they need access to only the patient's name and room number? Should executive administrators have the ability to chart all patient medications, or should only the nurses on the unit have that ability? These are the types of questions that healthcare providers must answer and then work with the IT department to implement the decisions.

Effective information systems produce accurate (free of errors), timely (available when needed), and relevant (useful and appropriate for the decisions to be made or the task at hand) information that healthcare providers can use for effective decision making.

Database and Database Management Characteristics

A **database** is a collection of stable stored data that you can access to provide a total picture of an entity, as well as to answer questions and make decisions. In this definition, "entity" means the focal point of the database. It can be a person (a patient or a healthcare worker), a thing (medications, vital signs), a place (hospital), or an event (admission). "Stable" means the data elements do not change. Healthcare providers use the stored data to calculate values that do change, such as a patient bill. Each time a healthcare provider produces a bill, it relies on the stable data elements to make its calculations of the total cost of care.

As mentioned earlier, a key characteristic of the data in a database is that it shared with users who need information for decision making. This requirement means that many healthcare providers must be able to access this database at the same time. However, only one user at a time will be able to edit data elements.

Finally, the data in the database are interrelated by connections to the various entities in the database and the relationship of those entities. For example, patients are prescribed treatments ordered by providers based on their diagnoses, which in turn are based on symptoms monitored by staff.

Database Models

A **database model** or schema refers to the structure of a database, which includes how the schema stores, organizes, and uses that data. Data dictionaries generally store these structures and depict them in a graphical way. The database model defines a set of operations that you can perform on the stored data in the database; as a consequence, each model structures, organizes, and uses data differently. For example, hierarchical and network models are commonly used on mainframes and minicomputers, whereas personal computer database programs almost always use a relational model. **Table 8-1** describes these models in more detail. No matter which structure you select, the model underlying the design of the database program influences or limits the permitted searching options. It also influences the maintenance of the database.

The first generation of database models (from the 1960s) was a single flat table. **Table 8-2** presents a simple flat model insurance based example. Of course in actual practice there would be more fields in this table. Note that each user has a unique ID number but may have the same insurance company.

TABLE 8-1 DATABASE MODELS

Model	Description
Flat table*	A flat model consists of a single table with columns and rows of data elements. Columns identify the data that will be entered into the cell in each row. Most of the time the type of data (e.g., numbers, text, date) expected in the column is also identified.
Hierarchical*	A hierarchical model is like a tree or organizational chart. During searching, the program searches each root and branch in sequence, checking for a match. This process is commonly called traversing the tree. Some terms commonly associated with this model include "root," "parent," "child," and "siblings." When designing the database, each child in the hierarchical model can have only one parent. This will show one-to-many relationships common in the real world.
Network*	The network model was developed to solve problems caused by the hierarchical model's inability to store certain types of data easily. The network model permits more than one parent per child. However, it requires multiple links to the various fields, making it much more difficult to revise or edit. Two constructs are important here: records and sets. A record contains fields and sets that define the one-to-many relationships between records. As a consequence, lower levels of a branch can be connected to multiple upper branches or nodes.
Relational	A relational model relies on flat tables for its structure. These tables are called relations. The columns in the table are called attributes with domains as the set of values attributes can take. Designers use only one data element per field, which means tables must be reduced to their simplest form. The term used for this process of reduction is "normalizing the table." For example, a parent with two children would become two tables that are linked based on a common field. Each table has rows (records) and columns (fields). Each entity is its own table, and columns describe this entity. For example, a patient table might include the patient's name, address, phone number, age, sex, insurance number, and so forth. All columns describe the entity—the patient—in some way. Each database consists of multiple linked tables.
Entity-relationship	An entity-relationship model defines entities (a thing or object in the real world) and relationships (how these entities relate to each other).
Object-oriented	The object-oriented model defines and manipulates objects. Traditional databases are not structured to handle drawings, images, photographs, and recordings well. In contrast, the object-oriented structure stores data and procedures that act on those data as objects. This approach has been of special interest in health care where images such as X rays or pictures of wounds also need to be accessed through a database.

TABLE 8-1 (CONTINUED)

Model	Description
Dimensional	The dimensional model represents data in a data warehouse so that it can be easily summarized. It is a task-specific database model.
Semi-structured	This model permits the specification of data where data items of the same type have different sets of attributes.
Hypertext	One task-specific model is the hypertext model encountered on the Internet. This design relies on objects linked to other related objects. The object may be text, pictures, data files, or sound files. This structure is particularly useful for organizing large amounts of diversified data as seen in an electronic health record (EHR). The disadvantage to this setup is that it is not possible to perform numerical analysis on the data, nor can it be certain how people will access each part of the database.

* These models are rarely seen today except in older legacy systems.

Designers developed the second generation of data models in the 1970s; two examples are the hierarchical and network models described in Table 8-1. The third generation of database models is the relational database, which is based on tables that link the various entities around which the tables are designed. The fourth generation of database models, as seen in the examples in Table 8-1, deal with task-specific data. These structures include the entity-relationship or Entity-Attribute-Value (EAV), object-oriented, and Internet models. The EAV model helps manage the large volume of heterogeneous data that a patient may acquire over time (Collen, 2012, p. 39). In such areas as artificial intelligence, CAD/CAM, and health care, developers are using object-relational databases models. They overcome the shortcomings of object and relational models.

TABLE 8-2 FLAT MODEL EXAMPLE–INSURANCE

IDNo	L_Name	F_Name	Primary Insurance	Secondary Insurance
345123	Jones	Joseph	BC/BS	None
098456	White	Pat	BC/BS	Medicare
000456	Makarosky	Mildred	Aetna	None
888054	Cross	Chris	Medicare	None
678923	Nelly	Florence	Cigna	Medicare

Data Relationships

Another important concept in understanding databases is relationships—that is, how the data in the database are related.

The simplest of these forms is the one-to-one relationship. For example, in **Figure 8-1** there is one healthcare provider in Table B with one security entry in Table A. No two healthcare providers have the same ID, password, security answer, and so forth. However, most **data relationships** are not this simple.

The next relationship type is one-to-many. In Figure 8-1, at 8 a.m. one patient in Table A receives multiple medications from Table B (the medication table). Thus an entity from one table (Patient A) has multiple entries in a second table (Medications).

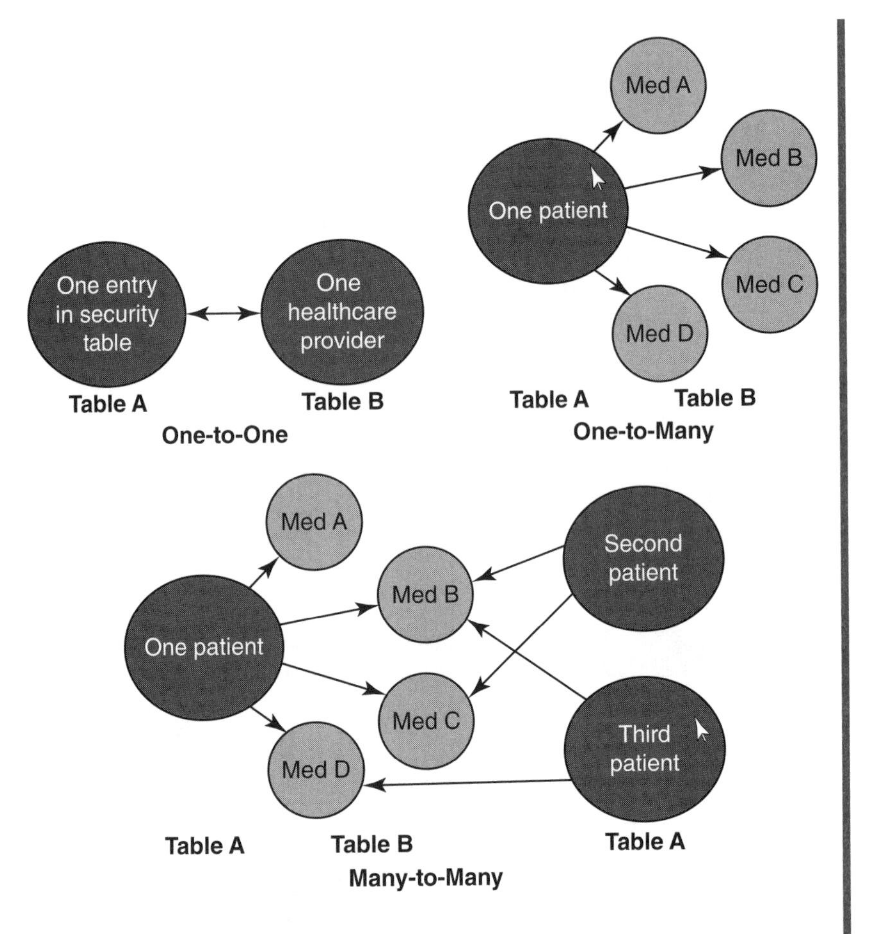

Figure 8-1 Database Relationships

There are also times when the relationship between entities is a many-to-many relationship. This means that many entities (patients) from one table may have many relationships with entities from the second table (medications). For example, an individual patient may be receiving several different medications. At the same time, several other patients may also be treated with many of these same medications.

When healthcare professionals work with database designers, it is the healthcare professional's responsibility to help the designer identify how the entity in one table relates to the entities in other tables.

Database Languages

A database system provides for two types of languages. The **data-definition language (DDL)** defines the properties of the data. This is where you define data integrity constraints. For example, the range of values for this field is 0 to 10 and the database will accept nothing outside that range. The **data-manipulation language (DML)** sets the procedures for how users retrieve, insert, delete, and modify the data. An example of this is the DML SQL (structured query language).

Database Terms and Structure

The following terms describe the structure of a database from smallest unit to largest. Recall from Chapter 2 that a computer stores data as bits. Bits are organized into bytes, which represent a character or symbol. When discussing databases, the bytes are further organized into fields, records, files, and databases (See **Figure 8-2**).

Bit — A **bit** is a zero (0) or one (1).

Byte — A **byte** is a combination of 0s and 1s that represents a character or symbol. For example, H may be given by the byte sequence 0100 1000 and I the byte sequence 0100 1001, together making the word "HI."

Data — **Data** are raw facts consisting of numbers, letters, characters, and dates. They are the content within each field. Other names for data include "data items" and "elements." Examples of data include Jones, 210-11-1234, and Chicago.

Field — A **field** (also called an attribute) is a space within a file that has a predefined location and length. Only one data item is in each field, a concept referred to as the use of atomic data. For example, a patient's temperature, pulse, and respiration data should be stored in separate fields,

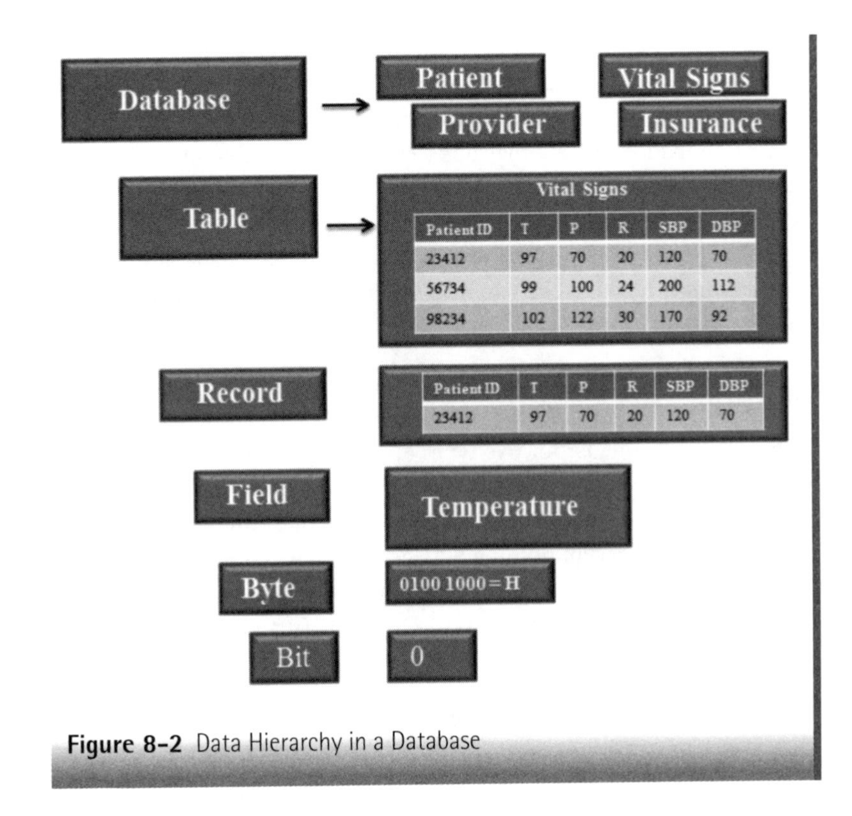

Figure 8-2 Data Hierarchy in a Database

not together in one field, such as a "vital signs" field. Examples of field names include last name, first name, city, state, diagnosis, systolic blood pressure, diastolic blood pressure, pulse, and height. A field name should reflect the data to be stored in that location.

Data Types

Data types refer to the description of which data should be expected to appear in a field. These types are software dependent; each program defines them. Most programs support alphanumeric (characters and numbers), numeric (numbers), short numeric (short, whole numbers), currency (money), character (letters), date and time, logical (equal to, greater than, or less than), memo (comment), and object (pictures or objects) data types. In object-oriented databases, the developer can define new data types (classes) and an object begins an instance of a class.

Record — A **record** is a collection of related fields or associated fields organized around a focal point. For example, a patient is a focal point around which certain data are collected and stored. A patient chart is a record. A college transcript is a record. In a relational database each row in a table is referred to as a record.

File — **Files** are collections of related records. For example, all of the patients in St. Luke's Hospital make up a file. A printed telephone book is an example of a paper file. It holds all the records of people with listed numbers, including their name, address, and phone number.

Database — A **database** is a collection of files that is analogous to a file cabinet; it holds related drawers of records. It is organized in such a way that a computer program called a database management system can quickly retrieve the desired data.

Database Management Systems — **Database management systems (DBMSs)** are the programs that enable users to work with electronic databases. They permit data to be stored, modified, and retrieved from the database.

The following definitions describe some additional database concepts that are important when working with databases:

Key Field — One or more fields with a unique identifier constitute **key fields**. Using key fields ensures that no duplicate records will appear in this database because a key field accepts only one record with that combination of text and/or numbers. An example of a key field used by Medicare is a Social Security number. Social Security numbers are not permitted to be used as a key field by institutions such as healthcare and educational institutions. They are required to use some other unique number such as JO345987.

Calculated Fields — **Calculated fields** are generated by performing mathematical operations on other fields. For example, use a calculated field to sum the total cost of five different medications based on their associated prices.

Hypertext — **Hypertext** is a growing database concept for use with large amounts of disparate information such as text, pictures, film, and sounds, where any object can be linked to any other object.

Link — A **link** is a logical association between tables based on the values in corresponding fields; it is a connection between two tables in a relational database program. The existence of a link permits you to query or ask questions of multiple tables and extract only the desired data from these tables. The linked field must be of the same data type and the linked field must appear in both tables.

Table — The **table** is the structure that is used to store the data. It consists of vertical columns, which are fields, and horizontal rows, which are records. A relational database consists of multiple tables linked together in some logical way for easy data retrieval.

Database Functions

Commonly available **database functions** allow for table structure creation, data or record editing, database searching, record sorting, and report generation. In the healthcare arena most databases are large and require a database professional to actually create and maintain them using large DBMSs like Oracle. Healthcare providers will provide input into the type of information needed to provide care and manage healthcare resources. In some cases, the need may be for a smaller database to manage a smaller project. In that case, a desktop database like Access or a spreadsheet like Excel with some database functions may be very useful. Providers may enter data directly into the database or import it from a larger database available to the healthcare provider.

Once these databases are designed and populated, healthcare providers and other healthcare employees may or may not be able to edit clinical patient data or records. If they can see records but not change them, the type of permission is called read-only access. If they are able to edit and view these data, it is called read-write access. Regardless of access type, if the edits involve patient data the system should maintain an audit trail of access and changes. While healthcare providers and other employees may not be able to edit or change entered patient data, they may be able to search, sort, and generate reports from the databases.

Creating the Database

There are two steps to creating the database: designing the structure (sometimes called the schema) and entering the data. Entering the data will populate the data fields in the database. For the most part, the expert in database design will create the database per input from the end user.

Designing the Structure

Designing the structure of the database requires identifying the field names, field types, and field widths plus relationships. What fields are required to provide the answers to the questions and generate the necessary reports? This structure design is generally stored in a **data dictionary**, which is a file that defines the basic organization of a database. The data dictionary lists all of the associated tables in the database as well as the names and data types for each field. In addition, it often includes comments about the range of acceptable data. For example, it may require that state names be entered as a two-letter abbreviation such as "PA" or "OH."

According to Shah (2012) future data models for health care will focus on producing a database that meets or addresses the following:

- Flexible patient-centric "person" models.
- Flexible multifacility "organization" models.
- Support for robot patient identification and deduplication.
- Support for separation of personal health information from clinical and transactional attributes.
- Support for multiple simultaneous entity roles.
- Support for long-term storage and change management of all entity attributes.
- Support for multiple applications and devices within the same structures (2012, para 5).

Editing Data or Adding Records

Editing data or records involves adding records, deleting old records, or changing data in active records. Healthcare institutions usually establish policies and procedures that govern what you can change in a patient record. These guidelines may not apply to nonclinical databases, however. For example, you may need to change an employee record to reflect a new phone number, name, or address; a patient registration form must reflect any changes in insurance, place of residence, or next of kin since the last admission.

While most databases will let you replace or override the previous data with new data, this practice is much less common in health care. Frequently these databases retain all data with a time stamp, thereby preserving an audit trail of what was modified, when it was modified, and who modified the data.

Searching the Database

Searching is the process of creating data subsets or locating specific records in the database. Terms used to describe this process include "search," "**query**," "find," and "ask." The power of a database derives from this search function and the ability to extract data. Additional terms related to searching are described next.

Answer Table

In some databases, the **answer table** is a temporary table in which the program stores search results. The program overwrites the first search when you conduct a new search or deletes the results when you exit the program. In other databases, the program automatically saves the answer tables or results in a Queries object.

Boolean Searching

Boolean searches are among the most commonly used features for searching any database; they provide the ability to narrow or expand a search as well as to eliminate some records. The following describes the basic uses of three of the most often used Boolean operators—AND, OR, and NOT. Chapter 12 presents additional discussion on Boolean operators.

AND — **AND** searches provide records that include both terms on either side of the AND. For example, a search for "computer AND health" elicits only records that include both terms. If one term is missing, that record does not show in the search results. The match must be exact. If a record includes the terms "computers" and "health," the search results will not include that record. The singular term "computer" is not considered the same as the plural term "computers."

OR — **OR** searches provide records that have either term. For example, a search for "hepatic OR liver" finds records that include either the term "hepatic" or the term "liver."

NOT — **NOT** searches provide records that exclude the term following NOT. For example, a search for "computer NOT bedside" elicits records containing the word "computer" and eliminates records that include the word "bedside."

Other operations, such as **NEAR** and **ADJACENT**, are also available, although they are not as common as AND, OR, and NOT. What is important is that you refine the search strategy to make it as efficient as possible for eliciting the desired information.

The following search options may or may not be available in the database you might use. When available, they make searching more efficient.

Exact Match An **exact match** search finds only entries that are an exact match for a specified word. Any minor difference results in exclusion of that entry from the results. For example, when searching for "child," the query finds only "child" and not "children," "infants," or "teenagers."

Pattern A **pattern** search permits the use of wild cards in place of a character. For example, "nur*" would match the string "nur" and any word with "nur" as the beginning string. Thus, this query would find "nurse," "nurses," "nursing," "nursery," "nurture," and "nurturing."

Range Operators such as greater than, less than, equal to, or some combination of them are logical operators. **Range** searches using these operators return records that fit the operator, such as "all patients with a pulse greater than 110."

Select Fields In a **select fields** search the user selects the fields to display in the search results. You may select all the fields or only certain select ones. For example, a healthcare worker may choose to display only the patient name and room number in the results or may choose to display additional fields such as diagnosis, doctor, primary nurse, and laboratory test results.

Sorting and Filtering the Database

The sorting function permits you to arrange records in a variety of ways and filtering permits you to work with some subset of the records. For example, you may sort a list of patients on a clinical unit in alphabetic order and then sort by the names of the assigned primary nurse, thereby rearranging the order in the database. This feature allows you to arrange the data in the order that makes sense for the desired result. Two other terms that we use when sorting are "ascending" and "descending." An ascending sort puts the items in alphabetic or numeric order from A to Z or 1 to NN (the highest number). A descending sort puts the items in the reverse order, going from the highest value to the lowest.

Filtering permits you to create some subset of records. For example, you might want to make rounds on all of Dr. White's patients. You would filter on the field

Physician to see all of those patients. You may filter on one or several fields. You might also want to see all the patients with the diagnosis of cancer who are scheduled for chemotherapy this morning.

Generating Reports

Another powerful feature of databases is the ability to generate multiple reports from the same database or data subset. Most programs permit multiple report formats for displaying the same data. This is a significant advantage in health care, where you may include data such as the patient's weight in several different reports; with a database, providers do not need to record the same measurement on each of these reports.

Other Terms Related to Databases

As automation makes it easy to collect a wide range of data, it has driven additional strategies to deal with the wealth of generated data, such as the following.

Data Mining

This concept refers to database applications that look for patterns in already-created databases. Do not confuse **data mining** with the use of software that presents data in new ways. Data mining software actually discovers new relationships between the data items that providers did not previously recognize. Kob and Tan (2005) identify these applications for healthcare data mining: treatment effectiveness, healthcare management, customer relationship management, and fraud and abuse detection (pp. 66–67).

Data Warehouse

A **data warehouse** is a collection of data designed to support decision making. Its purpose is to present a picture of the general conditions of the entity both at a particular time and historically. With this type of structure, software extracts data from other systems and places them in the warehouse database system. Along the way it collectively scans many different databases from the institution for the data relevant to or supportive of decision making. Generally, a warehouse supports summary data, not detailed data; it does not deal with the day-to-day operations of an institution. Use of the data warehouse's contents supports analysis of trends over time.

Data Mart

A subset or smaller-focus database designed to help managers make strategic decisions is a data mart. Sometimes it comprises a subset of a data warehouse.

Like a data warehouse, a **data mart** combines aspects of many databases within the institution, but with a focus on a particular subject, department, or unit. In health care, many individual clinical departments will maintain a data mart specific to that department while sending the same data forward to the institution's data warehouse.

Distributed Database

A **distributed database** is stored in more than one physical place instead of in a single, central location. This is done in one of two ways: either parts of the database are stored in different locations, or the data are replicated in multiple locations. This practice of deploying the database speeds up service to local users while simultaneously reducing the vulnerability of the database. The downside has to do with increased security issues and the potential for noncompliance with standards. Distributed databases are one of the approaches designers use to build an electronic health record (EHR), where providers pull the latest reports (such as lab or radiology results) into the patient's record from the departmental system (lab or radiology) as necessary.

Knowledge Generation and Management

"In the next 10 years, data and the ability to analyze them will do for doctors' minds what X-ray and medical imaging have done for their vision." (Grundy, 2012, para 1). Knowledge generation and management depend on data capture at the source and then the processing of that data to extract new meanings (understanding patterns) and to disseminate that knowledge to aid in quality decision making at the point where it is needed. Key to this development is a set of tools, techniques, and technologies (Bali, Wickramasinghe, & Lehaney, 2009, pp. 1–7). The quality of the stored data in the databases is crucial.

Big Data

Big Data is an emerging concept that describes the use of analytics to analyze aggregated data (Ortiz, 2013). Big Data means "a large amount of data ... that meets three criteria: volume, variety [type of data], and velocity [real or near real time]" (Hamilton, 2012, p. 1,). Many are predicting that Big Data will be the future of healthcare as it is currently changing how businesses make decision. In healthcare Big Data will be used to cost-effectively grow the volume of data to find out what happened, why it happened, and what might happen in the future. The potential to improve the quality of health care and patient outcomes by using external data from all healthcare systems, organizations, and agencies provides enormous opportunities to identify local knowledge and best practices.

A Few Database Design Tips

The most difficult task in developing any database is to create the database structure. This time-consuming task requires the designer to pay attention to detail. As a healthcare professional, it will be your responsibility to effectively convey your database needs to the professionals designing the database. What information do you need? In what form? These are two key questions that the team needs to answer. Remember the purpose of the database is to help you provide efficient, quality care.

Here are some questions to answer before creating table structures:

1. What output do you need? Which reports or screen outputs are necessary? For example, which information needs to be on the daily plan of care?
2. What queries do you anticipate? What questions will you ask the database? What questions do you have when caring for patients?
3. Which fields are necessary to produce the desired output and to answer the search questions? When asking these questions, what are the details you need to know?
4. What is necessary to define the record accurately?
5. Which field names are desirable? What are the common terms that the standards use to identify these data? For example, what is the difference between "list of diagnoses" and "problem list"?
6. Which data type will be placed in each field? For example, blood pressure (BP) is a number or numeric data, so you would never record text data or a letter in the BP field.
7. What serves as the unique identifier for each record? How do you ensure that patient records are never mixed, even if patients have the same name? The administrative simplification provisions of the Health Insurance Portability and Accountability Act of 1996 (HIPAA) mandate the adoption of standard unique identifiers for all healthcare providers and health plans that accept Medicare.
8. How will this table or file relate to other tables or files? What are the relationships?
9. Are there any redundant (duplicate) data in this table? Are healthcare providers charting the same data twice because of problems in the database design?

Here are some tips for improving the data in the database:

1. Collect meaningful data.
2. Enter data into the system at point of capture. The further you are from the point of capture in time and space, the greater the chances of data entry errors.

3. Design data collection to allow entry of accurate information. Where possible specify data ranges or use data masks, such as XXX-XX-XXXX for how to correctly enter the Social Security number.
4. Provide infrastructure that supports timely data collection. For example, mobile devices that are taken into the room or clinic.
5. Establish standard definitions for data items and concepts. This makes for easy comparisons and data retrieval.

Common Uses of Databases in Health Care

Databases have many uses in health care. For example, healthcare administrators who deal with staffing, scheduling, personnel records, and inventory control issues frequently use multiple databases. Clinical databases hold patient records, such as lab, radiology, and pharmacy data, that you use to provide patient care. Some clinical databases may be specialized, dealing with one specific disease or procedure, such robotic-assisted surgery. Educators use databases for test banks, student experiences, and student records. The FDA uses biosurveillance databases for monitoring, identifying, and tracking biological events of national concern. Medicare uses a claims database. Research-related databases are utilized for literature access, data collection, data storage, and data retrieval. Chapter 12 discusses additional databases specific to accessing healthcare literature.

Examples of databases that may be of assistance in your practice are listed below. Chapters 12 and 14 present additional examples of databases you will likely utilize within health care.

International Databases

Below are a few international examples. As with all databases, some are easy to use while others take some time to learn. Some focus on actual statistics (WHO and OECD) while others (ISPOR) are like a literature database with a specific focus.

WHO	World Health Organization, Data and Statistics tab. This index provides access to data and analysis for monitoring the global health situation. It contains data as well as analysis links on such topics as mortality and burden of disease, health systems, noncommunicable diseases, millennium development goals, infectious diseases, and so forth. URL: http://www.who.int/research/en/index.html.
ISPOR	The International Society for Pharmacoeconomics and Outcomes Research database. Includes over

325 databases from 45 countries. Notice the tabs across the top; three of them are of note—Research Tools, Decision Makers Tools, and Patients Tools. This database permits key word searches and returns information about presentations at their conferences. Many of these studies contain a wealth of data. URL: http://www.ispor.org.

OECD — The Organisation for Economic Co-operation and Development (OECD). One of the data subsets deals with health status. It is a little more complex to use than the WHO database. URL: http://stats.oecd.org/index.aspx.

National Databases

These are some examples of databases and statistics focused at a national level. They vary in who has access to them and whether there is a fee for the data and related reports. Some are government and state sponsored (CDC, U.S. Census Bureau, OSHPD, NPDB, and HIPDB) while others are affiliated with a professional organization (NDNQI and Partners).

CDC — The Centers for Disease Control and Prevention (CDC) maintain a large database of statistics about aging, alcohol use, diseases, deaths, life expectancy, and so forth. This URL takes you to an index for data available at this site—http://www.cdc.gov/DataStatistics/. Also note the many datasets accessible from this site. For example, the CDC's WISQARS™ (Web-based Injury Statistics Query and Reporting System) provides fatal and nonfatal injury, violent death, and cost of injury data from a variety of trusted sources. URL: http://www.cdc.gov.

U.S. Census Bureau — The U.S. Census Bureau contains several interactive screens for locating quick facts and simple stats. These data cover topics, such as finance, jobs, housing, people, and education, which can impact healthcare planning and trends. URL: http://www.census.gov/.

NDNQI — The National Database of Nursing Quality Indicators® (NDNQI®) provides hospitals with unit-level performance reports. This is a program of the American Nurses Association National Center for Nursing

Quality. There is a fee to access the data and reports and is only open to acute care in-patient hospitals. URL: https://www.nursingquality.org/default.aspx.

OSHPD — California's Office of Statewide Health Planning and Development (OSHPD). The Data tab provides access to a wealth of topics, such as various hospital utilization and financial data. URL: http://www.oshpd.ca.gov/.

Partners — Partners in Information Access for the Public Health Workforce is a collaboration of United States government agencies, public health organizations, and health science libraries. They have a wealth of data and statistics regarding public health issues. URL: http://phpartners.org/.

NPDB and HIPDB — This site contains two databases—the National Practitioner Data Bank (NPDB) and the Healthcare Integrity and Protection Data Bank (HIPDB). These databases are part of a confidential information clearinghouse that Congress created to improve healthcare quality, protect the public, and reduce healthcare fraud and abuse in the United States. URL: http://www.npdb-hipdb.hrsa.gov/.

Introduction to Using Excel for Limited Database Functions

Because many of you will not develop a database using a program such as Access or larger program such as Oracle, but you do have access to Excel, the remainder of this chapter describes using Excel for some database functions. Learning about Excel's database functions will provide you with a basic understanding of the process of working with databases. If you need to develop additional database skills, consider taking a database course or two.

If needed refer to Chapter 7 for an explanation of the basic Excel interface and features.

Large Datasets

When working with large datasets in Excel, the rows and columns may scroll off the screen making it difficult to accurately enter the correct data in the correct cell. The freeze pane command keeps the columns, rows, or both on the screen. With the freeze pane turned on, you can scroll through the spreadsheet keeping the rows, columns, or both visible. See **Figure 8-3** for results of the freeze pane command.

To freeze pane (row and column):

1. Make the active cell **one row below** and **one column to the right** of the header information you need to keep on the screen.
2. Click **View** tab and then **Freeze Panes** Freeze Panes.
3. Click **Freeze Panes** option from the menu. You will now see a line showing the rows and columns that are frozen.

To freeze the first column only:

1. Click **View** tab and then **Freeze Panes** Freeze Panes.
2. Click **Freeze First Column** option from the menu. You will now see a line showing the first column frozen.

To freeze the first row only:

1. Click **View** tab and then **Freeze Panes** Freeze Panes.
2. Click **Freeze Top Row** option from the menu. You will now see a line showing the first row frozen.

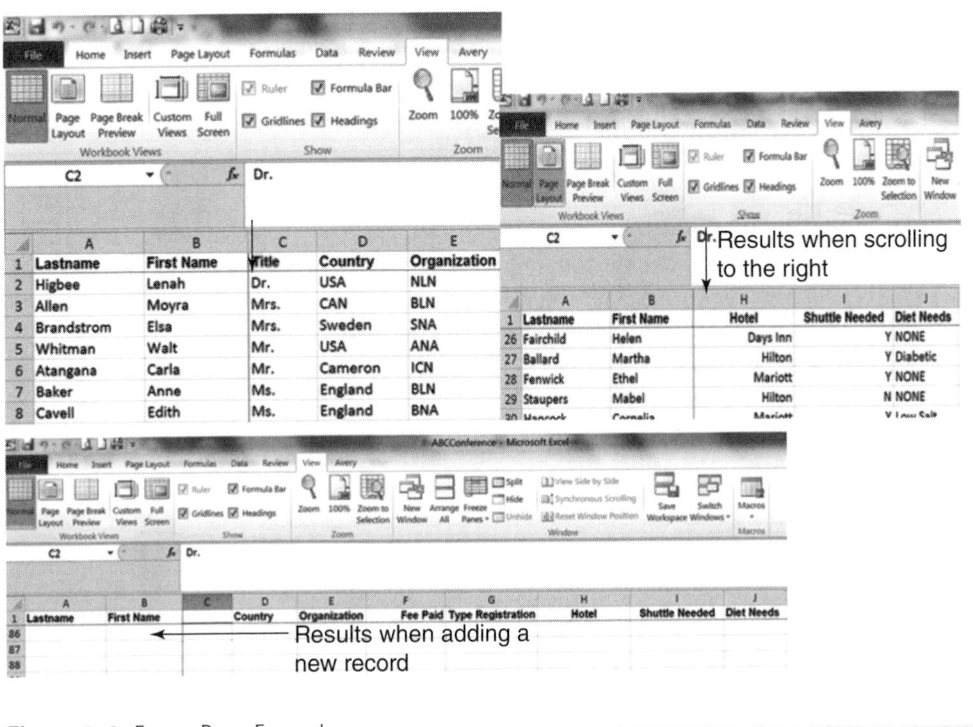

Figure 8-3 Freeze Pane Example

To unfreeze the pane(s):

1. Click **View** tab and then **Freeze Panes** .
2. Click **Unfreeze Panes.**

Creating a Table

Tables are the basic form for storing data in Excel. A table in Excel is an area on a worksheet that contains rows and columns that enable data analysis and management. First you will want to convert the selected data to a table and then conduct the analysis. Remember, a database table has fields (columns) and records (rows). You should leave no blank rows when using tables in Excel.

Converting data into a table:

1. Select the **range of data** to include in the table. Include the row and column headers.
2. Click **Insert** tab, and then **Table** in the Tables group. Make sure there is a check mark in the square to the left of **My table has headers**.
3. Click **OK.**

Adding a record (row) to the table:

1. Click the **last cell** in the table and then press the **Tab** key. Alternatively, you can add a new row (record) above or below the current record. Click the **cell below** where you want to insert the new record, click **Home** tab, click **Insert down arrow** in the Cells group, and click **Insert Table Rows Above**. If the current row is the last one, click **Insert Table Rows Below**. In addition, you can place your mouse pointer over the small square on the bottom right of the table and drag down one or multiple rows.
2. Type the **data** for the new record.

Adding a field (column) to a table:

1. Click any **data cell** to the right of the new field. Don't select a cell with the field name.
2. Click **Home** tab and then **Insert down arrow** in the Cells group.
3. Click **Insert Table Column to the Left.**
   You can also insert a column to the right when you select the last field on the right.

Editing a record in a table:

Do this the same way you would edit cells on the worksheet as described in Chapter 7. You can also search for a record using the data entry form and then edit it in the dialog box. See the next section for details on how to do this.

Deleting a record (row) in a table:

1. Click a **cell** in the record you want to delete.
2. Click **Home** tab, and the **Delete down arrow** Delete in the Cells group.
3. Click **Delete Table Rows.**

Deleting a field (column) in a table:

1. Click a **cell in the field** you want to delete.
2. Click **Home** tab, and the **Delete down arrow** Delete in the Cells group.
3. Click **Delete Table Columns.**

Creating a Data Entry Form

When working with an Excel database, you may want to consider creating a data entry form to create a new database table or add records to an existing one. This form permits scrolling through the records one record at a time, searching for specific records, and editing or deleting individual records when necessary.

Adding a data entry form:

1. Click a **cell** in the Table.
2. Add the Form button to the Quick Access Toolbar (click the **down arrow** next to the Quick Access Toolbar, click **More Commands**.) In Choose Commands from box, click **All Commands**. Scroll to the **Form button**, click **Add** and then **OK**.
3. Click the **Form** button on the Quick Access Toolbar. See **Figure 8-4** for data form example that the program generates automatically from the fields in the table.

Adding a record with a form:

1. In the data form, click **New**.
2. Type the **data** for the new record (row). Press the **Tab** key to move to the next field.
3. When you have entered all data, press **Enter** to add the record to the table.

Moving through the records:

1. Use the **scroll bar arrows** in the data form to move one record at a time in the direction of the arrow.
2. Use the **Find Next** or **Find Prev** options to move to the next record or previous record.

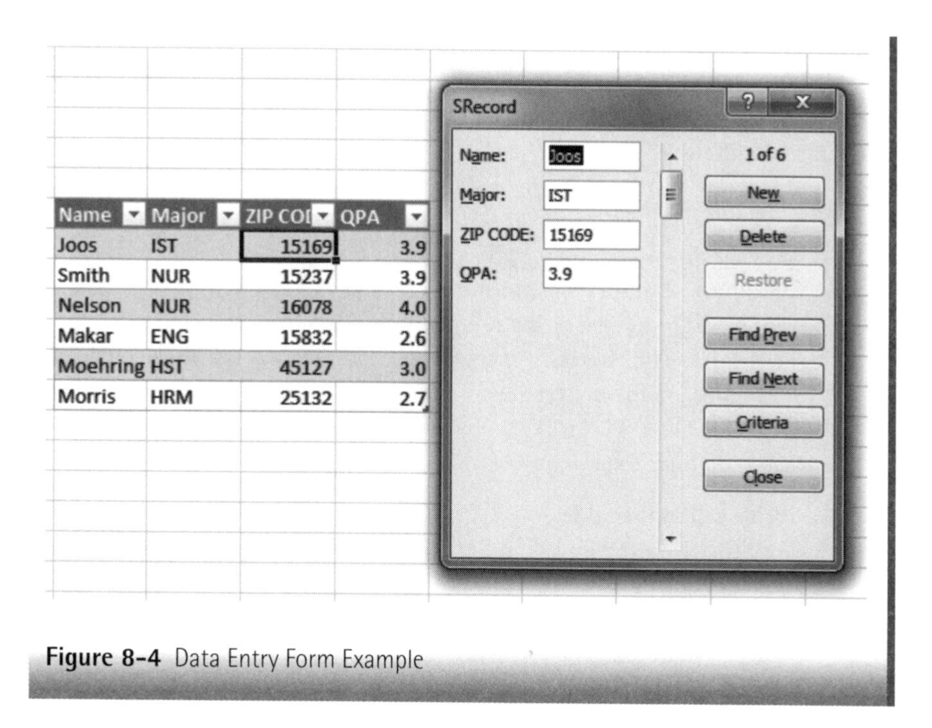

Figure 8-4 Data Entry Form Example

Finding a specific record:

1. Click the **Criteria** [Criteria] button on the data entry form. You can add multiple criteria. For example, two or three fields. This is an AND search.
2. Type the **search criteria** in the correct field and click **Find Next** or **Find Prev**.
3. Click in the form field to make changes to a specific record.

Deleting a record:

1. In the data form, find the **specific record**.
2. Click the **Delete** [Delete] button.

Sorting and Filtering Data

Sorting and **filtering** data in a table provides you with many options for manipulating the data, such as rearranging the data and creating data subsets in addition to a few aggregation functions. Sorting arranges data in an order specified for the data in the sort field. You can sort one or multiple columns using text, dates, and values sorts. Filtering creates data subsets that match the criteria that you specify.

You can filter on text, date, and values data types. You can search for a specific record using the filter option. In addition, you can also create custom sorts and filters as well as sort by cell color, font color, or icon. Chapter 7 covered nontable sorting and filtering.

To sort data (one column or field):

1. Click the **down arrow** Name City Rank next to the field to sort.
2. Click the **type of sort** to perform. You may sort text in A to Z or Z to A, dates from oldest to newest or the reverse, and values from smallest to largest or the reverse. The choices you see depend on the data in the selected field. See **Figure 8-5** for an example of choices for a number sort field.

To sort data (multiple columns or fields):

1. Click a **cell in the table.**
2. Click the **Data tab** and then **Sort** in the Sort & Filter group. (See Figure 7-24.)
3. Click the **Sort by down arrow** and click a **field**. Choices available depend on the content of the field.
4. Select one of the **Sort On** options and then **Order**. Choices available depend on the content of the field.
5. Click **Add level** and repeat the steps from 3 and 4.
6. Click **OK**.

To filter data:

1. Click the **down arrow of the field** to filter.
2. Remove the **check mark** from any of the items that should not display in the filtered subset and click **OK** or click the **date, number, or text filter option** to see the options for filtering and pick one. See **Figure 8-6** for filtering options for a date field. These options vary depending on the field data.

To remove the filter:

1. Click the **down arrow** for the field to which the filter applies. This icon tells you the field is a filtered field.
2. Click **Clear filter from name of field** to clear.

Some Advanced Features

Excel contains additional database features as discribed below. These are more complex functions and are beyond the scope of this textbook except to let you know they exist. Office.com provides training on these tools.

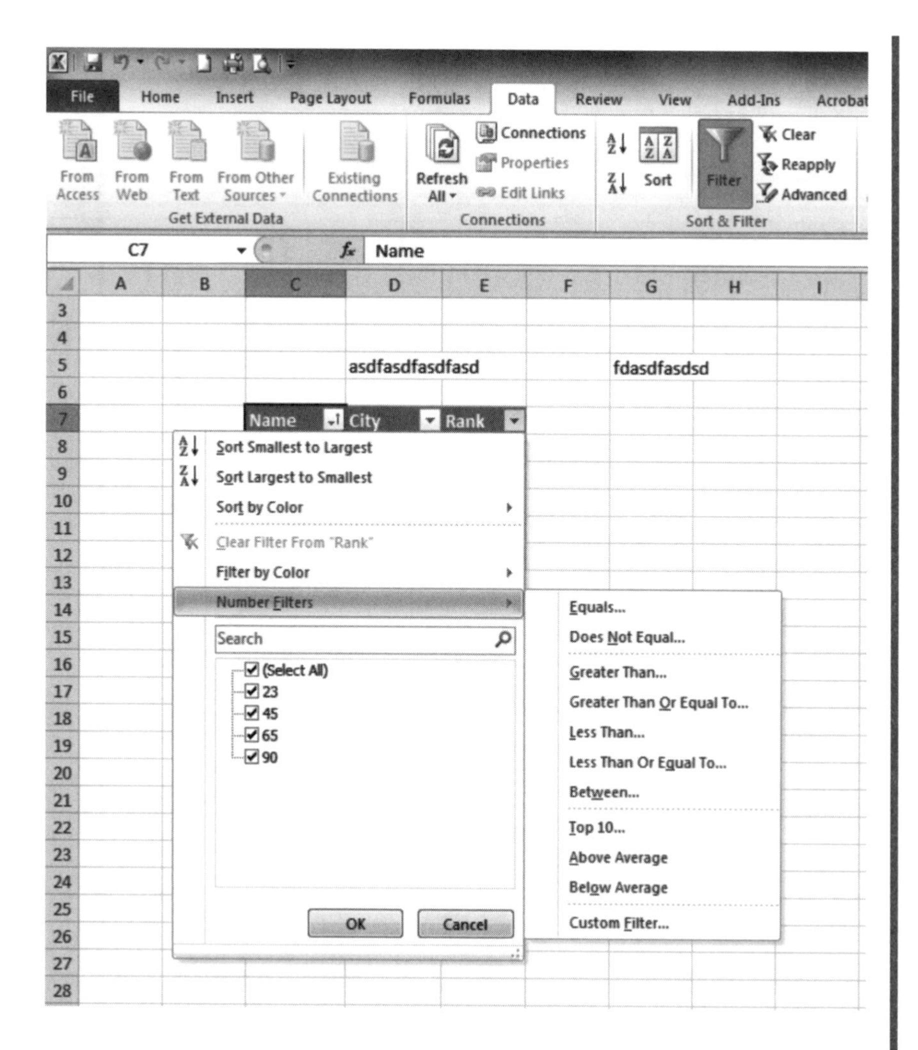

Figure 8-5 Sort & Filter Choices from a Table Using a Number Field

What-If Analysis The **What-if Analysis** is a set of tools that permits you to predict or test future results by manipulating some variables. For example, what would happen to my budget if tuition increases by 10% next year?

Goal Seek **Goal seek** permits you to identify the target or goals and then manipulate current arguments or values to achieve the goals set.

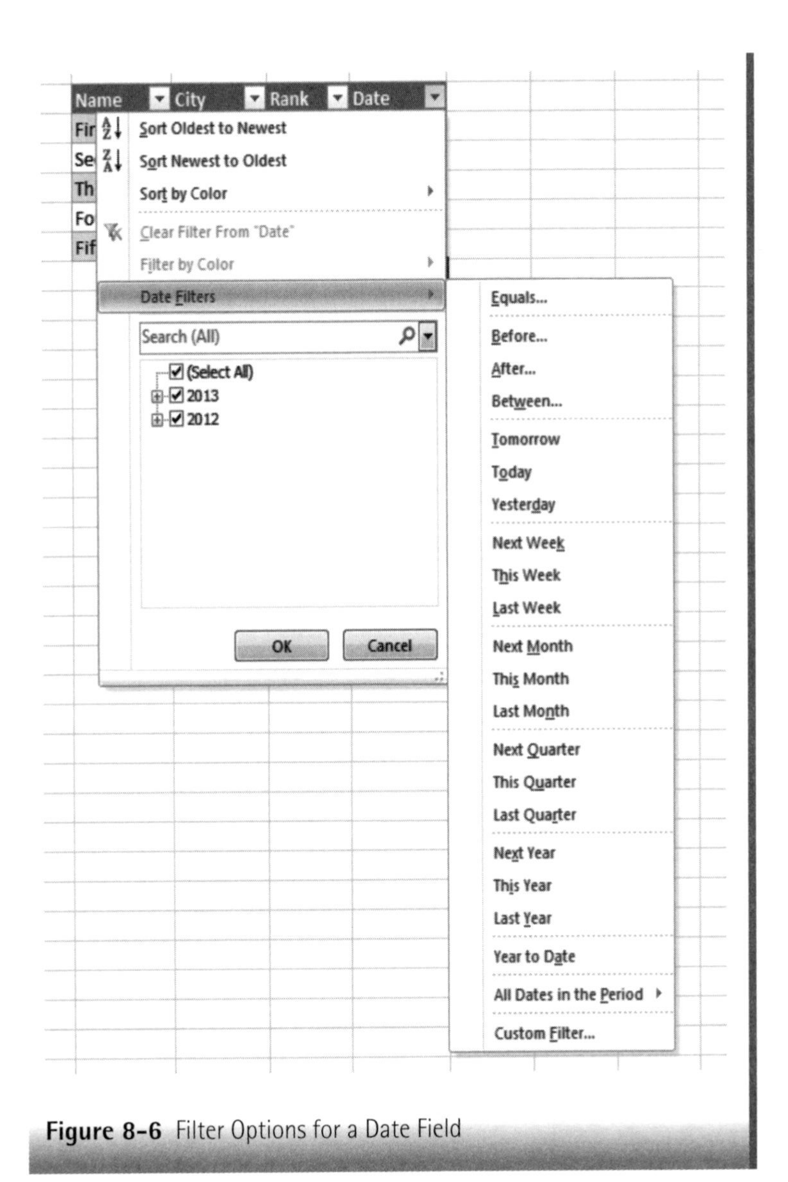

Figure 8-6 Filter Options for a Date Field

Scenarios — **Scenarios** are a set of values created from the What-if Analysis tool button that permit you to display new values based on selected cells. This requires you to work with current data.

PivotTables — A **PivotTable** provides a summary report that allows you to quickly compare long lists of values and look at data in ways not normally apparent from a regular worksheet or table. A PivotTable pivots one column against another column.

Data Validation — The **Data Validation** tool permits a restriction on entering data outside the validation rule. For example, zip codes would be restricted to five numbers only. A message appears if you try to enter data outside that range. Access the Data Validation tool on the Data tab.

Structured References and Total Row

A **structured reference** is another tool to use in formulas and functions, much like the range name feature. It uses a table element, such as the column name (field), as a reference in a formula. Use of a structured reference in formulas requires brackets. For example, =[registration fee]-[amount paid]. Once you complete the formula, Excel automatically copies the formula down the column.

A **total row** is an aggregate of data that appears as the last row of a table to display summary data, such as Sum and Count Numbers. The Subtotal function calculates values for a range of data in the table.

Summary

This chapter presented basic database concepts necessary for understanding the world of databases, including information about the database structure and related terms. We introduced specific directions for using Excel to demonstrate some of these concepts. Learning how to use databases increases your ability to retrieve and use information contained in them, for example, to assess the results of searches, sorts, reports, and data collection activities that can facilitate the decision-making process.

References

Bali, R., Wickramasinghe, N. and Lehaney, B. (2009). *Knowledge management primer*. New York: Routledge.

Collen, M. F. (2012). *Computer medical databases: The first six decades (1950–2010)*. New York: Springer Publishing.

Grundy, P. (2012). Bringing Knowledge Home. Washington, DC: Institute of Medicine of the National Academies. Retrieved from http://www.iom.edu/Global/Perspectives/2012/BringingKnowledgeHome.aspx

Hamilton, B. (2012). Big data is the future of healthcare. Cognizant 20-20 Insights. Retreieved from http://www.cognizant.com/InsightsWhitepapers/Big-Data-is-the-Future-of-Healthcare.pdf

He, D. and Pan, L. (2012). Database security for mHealth. Chicago, University of Illinois. Retrieved from https://wiki.engr.illinois.edu/download/attachments/200481540/final.pdf

Kob, H. and Tan, G. (2005). Data mining applications in healthcare. *Journal of Healthcare Information Management*, *19*(2), 64–72.

Ortiz, T. (2013). Drowning in data, but starving for knowledge? How to define big data for healthcare. Big Data Healthcare Forum 2013. Retrieved from http://www.bigdatahealthcaresummit.com/media/7442/2926.pdf

Shah, S. (2012). How to design next-generation HER data models. Retrieved from http://www.healthcareguy.com/2012/06/04/how-to-design-next-generation-ehr-data-models/

Exercises 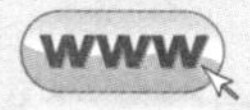

EXERCISE 1 Where Do We Begin?

Objectives

1. Define the fields necessary to create a simple database.
2. Create a data dictionary for an Excel table.
3. Relate data dictionary design concepts to the structure and design of EHRs.

Activity

1. You are involved in opening a small free-standing clinic in the basement of a senior citizen's center. This center serves over 500 people a day in a variety of activities. The director of the center wants this clinic to provide a convenient way for their clients to obtain health monitoring, updated vaccines, wellness literature, quick answers to questions, and so forth. It will be staffed with three RNs, one nurse practitioner, and two assistants. There will be backup support from two local physicians. One of the center employees is skilled in databases, but knows nothing of database needs in a clinic. Your task is to identify what data might be needed.
2. Review Creating the Data Dictionary at the Centers for Disease Control and Prevention at http://www.cdc.gov/rdc/B3Prosal/PP323.htm.
3. Create a data dictionary that identifies the data, data type, and data description.
   a. Open **Excel**.
   b. On **Sheet 1** enter the following **data**:

      Cell A1 = Company and/or Project Name: Data Dictionary
      Cell A2 = Created on: Cell B2 = Date
      Cell A3 = Created by: Cell B3 = Your name
      Cell A6 = Version Cell B6 = Description
      Cell C6 = Changed by: Cell D6 = Date

   c. Click **Sheet 1** tab and rename it **Documentation**. (See **Figure 8-7**.)
   d. Bold **appropriate cells**, adjust **column widths** as necessary.
   e. Click **Sheet 2**. Create the **data dictionary template** on this sheet. This is the template you will use to create the data dictionary for the scenario in 1. For an example, see **Figure 8-8**. You can also find or create your own. Name this sheet **Template.**

	A	B	C	D
1	Company Name - Project Name - Data Dictionary			
2	Created on:	2/7/2013		
3	Created by:	Irene Joos		
4				
5				
6	Version	Description	Changed By	Date
7	1	First draft	Irene Joos	2/7/2013
8				

Figure 8-7 Data Dictionary Documentation

	A	B	C	D	E	F	G
1	<Entity Name>	<what is this entity? For example, client, nurse, insurance, and so forth>					
2	Field Names	Description	Type	Additional Type Information	Default Value	Required Field?	Unique Value?
3	<data element name>	<what is this data element? A person's social security number, name, etc.>	Character, Integer, Currecny, Date, etc.	<what is the max and min length or any notes you want to make on the data>	<what defaul values if any?>	Yes/No	Yes/No
4	<data element name>	<what is this data element? A person's social security number, name, etc.>	Character, Integer, Currecny, Date, etc.	<what is the max and min length or any notes you want to make on the data>	<what defaul values if any?>	Yes/No	Yes/No
5							
6							
7							
8							
9							
10							
11							

Figure 8-8 Sample Data Dictionary Template

f. Click the **Template sheet** if necessary and select the **worksheet** (click the **Select All button** in the top right of the worksheet). Copy this worksheet to **Sheet 3.** (On Sheet 2, press **Ctrl+C,** click **Sheet 3,** click cell **A1** and press **Ctrl+V** to paste it in **Sheet 3.**)

g. Decide on an **entity** and enter the **data elements** for that entity. See **Figure 8-9** for the start of the data dictionary. You can then add additional sheets to describe different entities like insurance, diagnosis,

	A	B	C	D	E	F	G	H
1	Client	The focus of this data table is the client seen in the client						
2	Field Names	Description	Type	Additional Type Information	Default Value	Required Field?	Unique Values?	
3	ID Num	Unique number will will assign to each client.	Number	can have no negative numbers, and will be 4 digits in length	None	Yes	Yes	
4	Lname	Client's last name	Character	maximum length = 20	None	No	No	
5								
6								
7								
8								
9								
10								

Figure 8-9 Sample Data Element in Data Dictionary

visits, and provider. This data dictionary can now be used when working with the database administrator/designer to make sure those elements required by health professionals are in the database.

h. Make a note on the documentation sheet about what you learned from this exercise.
i. Name this workbook **Chap8-Exercise1-LastName**. Submit it as directed by the professor.

EXERCISE 2 What Excel Features Let Me Work with It as a Database?

We are using Excel to demonstrate selected database functions available in Excel. Most databases used in health care are large and developed by database administrators. This will, however, give you a feel for querying a minimal database to find information and will introduce you to some database functions in Excel.

Objectives:

1. Create a simple table in Excel.
2. Manipulate the data in the table with sort and filter features.
3. Apply a Subtotal and Total row.

Activity

1. Open Excel file **Chap8-Exercise2** and rename it **Chap8-Exercise2-LastName.**
2. Click the **Documentation** sheet, add **your name** in B2 and the function **=today()** in B3.

3. In A1 replace the **[Date] text** with the **current year**.
4. Click the **Registrations** sheet tab.
5. Scroll down to the **last row of data**. What happens to the field names? What problem do you see with that?
6. Click cell **C2**, **View** tab, **Freeze Panes** icon, and **Freeze Panes** option. Now what happens when you scroll down the worksheet?
7. Now go to cell **A71** and add **your name**, your **country**, **title**, **organization**, **fee paid**, **type of registration**, **hotel**, **shuttle needed**, and **diet needs**.
8. Remove the freeze panes (**View** tab, **Freeze Panes** icon, **Unfreeze Panes**).

Create a Table

1. Select range of cells **A1:J71.**
2. Click **Insert** tab and then **Table** icon. Make sure the My table has headers, is checked and click **OK**.

Sort the Table

1. Click any cell in **Column A**. We are sorting on last name, in alphabetical order.
2. Click **Home** tab, **Sort** icon in Editing group, and **A-Z sort** icon. The table is now sorted by last names going from A to Z.

Filter Table and Count the Records

1. Click the **down arrow** next to the **Country** field Country ▾.
2. Check Select All ☑ (Select All) to remove checks from all the countries.
3. Check England ☑ England and click **OK**. You should now see only records of persons from England.
4. You now want to see how many participants are from England without physically counting them. Click cell **D72** to make it the active cell (this is the first blank row below the table). Type **=subtotal(103,[country])**. Press the **Enter** key. You should now see a subtotal of the number of records for this data subset (HINT: 14). The 103 is the function number code for COUNTA which counts all records that are not blank and the [fieldname] tells it what field of records to count. Use function number codes when working with a table in Excel. (See **Figure 8-10**.)
5. Select the **total worksheet**, click **Copy**, click the **Sheet 3** tab, and click **Paste keeping formulas and formatting**.
6. Rename the sheet **FilterResults**.

	A	B	C	D	E	F	G	H	I	J
1	Lastname	First Name	Title	Country	Organization	Fee Pa	Type Registratio	Hotel	Shuttle Neede	Diet Needs
4	Asbridge	Jonathan	Mr.	England	BNA	$300	Full	Hilton	N	NONE
6	Baker	Anne	Ms.	England	BLN	$300	Full	Days Inn	N	NONE
9	Beasley	Christine	Dr.	England	BNA		Full	Hilton	Y	NONE
18	Carter	Peter	Mr.	England	BNA	$200	Day	Hilton	N	NONE
20	Cavell	Edith	Ms.	England	BNA	$200	Day	Best Western	N	NONE
31	Farmborough	Florence	Dr.	England	BNA	$300	Day	Mariott	Y	Vegitarian
32	Fenwick	Ethel	Ms.	England	BLN	$300	Full	Mariott	Y	NONE
39	Hunt	Agnes	Ms.	England	BNA	$300	Full	Days Inn	Y	NONE
47	McLaughline	Louisa	Ms.	England	BNA	$300	Full	Days Inn	Y	NONE
49	Nightingale	Florence	Ms.	England	BNA	$300	Full	Days Inn	Y	Vegitarian
51	Pattison	Dora	Ms.	England	BNA	$300	Full	Best Western	Y	Low Fat
52	Pearson	Emma	Dr.	England	BNA	$300	Day	Hilton	N	NONE
54	Quinn	Tome	Mr.	England	BNA	$300	Full	Mariott	y	NONE
61	Saunders	Cicely	Ms.	England	BNA	$200	Day	Days Inn	N	NONE
72				14						

Figure 8-10 Filtered Table with Subtotal Results

Clear the Filter

1. Click a **cell** in the table on the Registrations sheet and then click **Data** tab.
2. Click the **Clear** Clear button in the Sort & Filter group. Notice that the number of records increased to 70. Notice on the sheet FilterResults the number also changed from 14 to 70.

Add a Total Row

1. Check to make sure the Total Row is selected in the Table Style options. (Click **Design** tab, check to make sure there is a check mark in Total Row option.)
2. Make the active cell **F72 Fee Paid Column.**
3. Click the **down arrow** in F72 and click **Sum**. The results should be $14,000. Because we are working with a table, notice that the formula in the formula bar (=subtotal(109,[Fee Paid]) – 109 is the table number for SUM and [Fee Paid] is the column or field name.

On Your Own

1. Determine how many people need a ride from their hotel to the conference.

HINT: Check out the COUNTIF function.

2. You notice that Canada is both CANADA and CAN. Search and replace CANADA with CAN.

EXERCISE 3 Which Databases Are Available Online and Can I Import Them into Excel?

Objectives

1. Import data from another source.
2. Identify knowledge required to find the data.
3. Use data from online databases to answer selected questions.
4. Identify knowledge required to find the data.
5. Use the data to create an Excel chart.

Activity

As part of your community service project, you are giving a talk to a group of teenagers on safety issues and want to provide data on the leading causes of death for 15- to 19-year-olds. You believe this data will emphasize the key points in your presentation.

1. Obtain data from the Centers for Disease Control and Prevention.
   a. Go to **http://wonder.cdc.gov/Welcome.html**.
   b. Click **Detailed Mortality** under Mortality and agree to the terms at the bottom of the page.
   c. In #1 select **ICD-10 113 Cause List**.
   d. In #2 select **YOUR STATE**.
   e. In #3 click **Five-Year Age Groups**, **15-19 years**, and leave the rest at default setting.
   f. In #4, select **2010**.
   g. Leave the #5 to #8 default settings and click **Send**. Depending on the time of day and connection speed this could take a few minutes.
   h. Once the results appear, click the **Export** Export button on the far right.
   i. Save the file to **your storage** device.
   j. Start **Excel**, and click **File, Open**. Change the type of file to **Text Files or All files** so you can see the downloaded .txt file. Click the **file** you just downloaded and click **Open**. The Text Import Wizard will open.
   k. In Step 1 select **Delimited** in the Original data type. Click **Next**.
   l. In Step 2, Click **Tab** in the Delimiters option and in the Text qualifier drop-down list. Click **Next**.
   m. Click the **Notes** column in data preview and the **circle** in Do not import column (skip). Click **Finish**. You should now see the data in Excel.

n. Create a **Table** for the imported data. **Sort** the Death field from **largest to smallest**. What are the leading causes of death for 15- to 19-year-olds in your state? Does this support what you want to say about safety and prevention?

o. Using what you learned in chapters 6 and 7, create an appropriate Excel chart of the top 10 causes of death. Place the chart on its own worksheet.

p. Save the Excel spreadsheet as **Chap8-Exercise3-1-LastName** and submit as directed by your professor.

2. Obtain U.S. Census data.
   a. Go to **http://www.census.gov/**.
   b. Click **Statistical Abstract** at the bottom of the page in Special Topics.
   c. Click **Health & Nutrition** on the left-side pane.
   d. Click **Health Insurance** on the pop-up window.
   e. Click **Excel** format for **People With and Without Health Insurance Coverage By State**.
   f. Save the file to your storage device and call it **Chap8-Exercise3-2-LastName**.
   g. Go back and look around this site. What do you need to know to use it? See if you can answer these questions from the data at this site: What is the population and rank of your state? How many people per square mile in your state? What is the average income of your state?
   h. How does this site compare to the CDC site visited in activity 1?
   i. Place the **answers** to questions g and h on a **new sheet** in Excel. Call the sheet **AnsGH** and resave this file.
3. Create two Excel charts.
   a. Open the **Excel file** from activity 2 if necessary.
   b. Select the appropriate data to **create a column** chart of **all states** and the **percentage** (%) of people who don't have health insurance. Place the chart on its own chart sheet in Excel. Do NOT sort the data first. Make sure you only select cells needed to produce the chart.

HINT: You might need to hide the total row. Press and hold down the Ctrl key while selecting noncontiguous cells. Adjust the chart to make it more presentable—add a title, vertical and horizontal axis titles, and remove the legend. See **Figure 8-11a** for an example.

c. Create a **second chart** of the **total number** of children in each state without insurance. Place those data on their own chart sheet in Excel and adjust as in B. See **Figure 8-11b**.

d. Which three states have the highest percentage of people without health insurance and the largest number of children without health insurance? Why might this be of interest to you as a healthcare provider?

4. Place the answers to the questions from this activity in the Excel spreadsheet on its own sheet named **ans**. You should have four worksheets–ALL, children, ans, and 2009. ALL Children ans 2009

5. Save the work as **Chap8-Exercise3-3-LastName**.

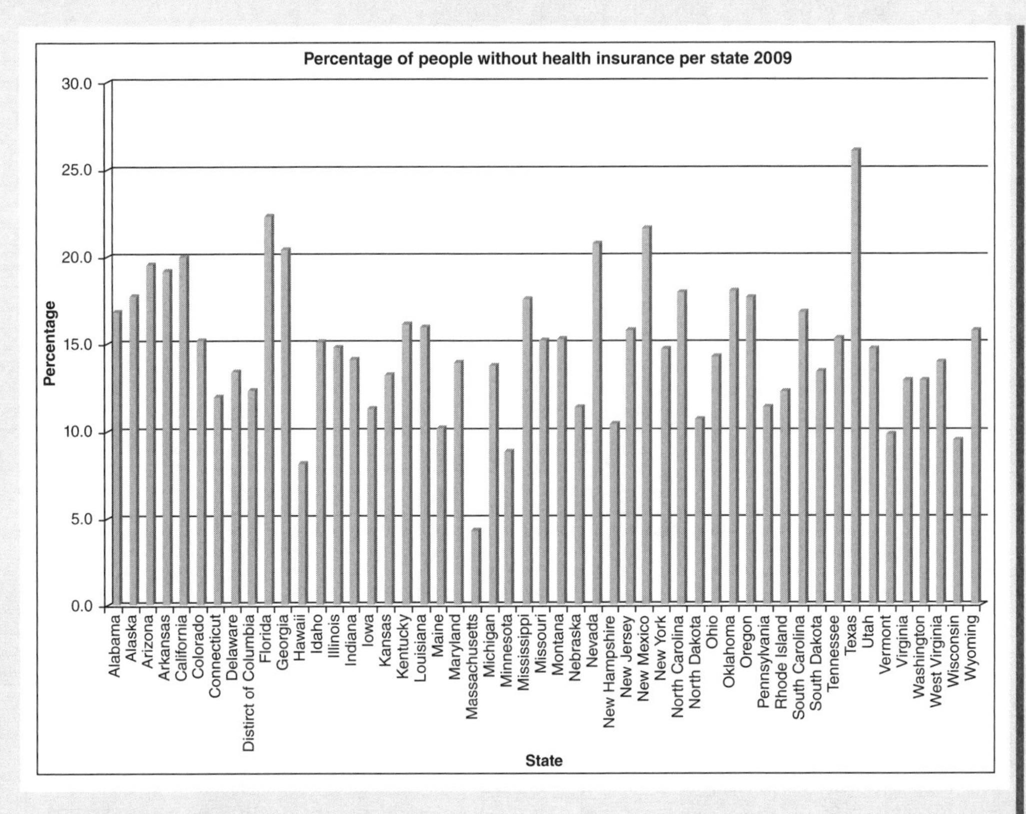

Figure 8-11a Exercise 3: Column Chart Results Chart A

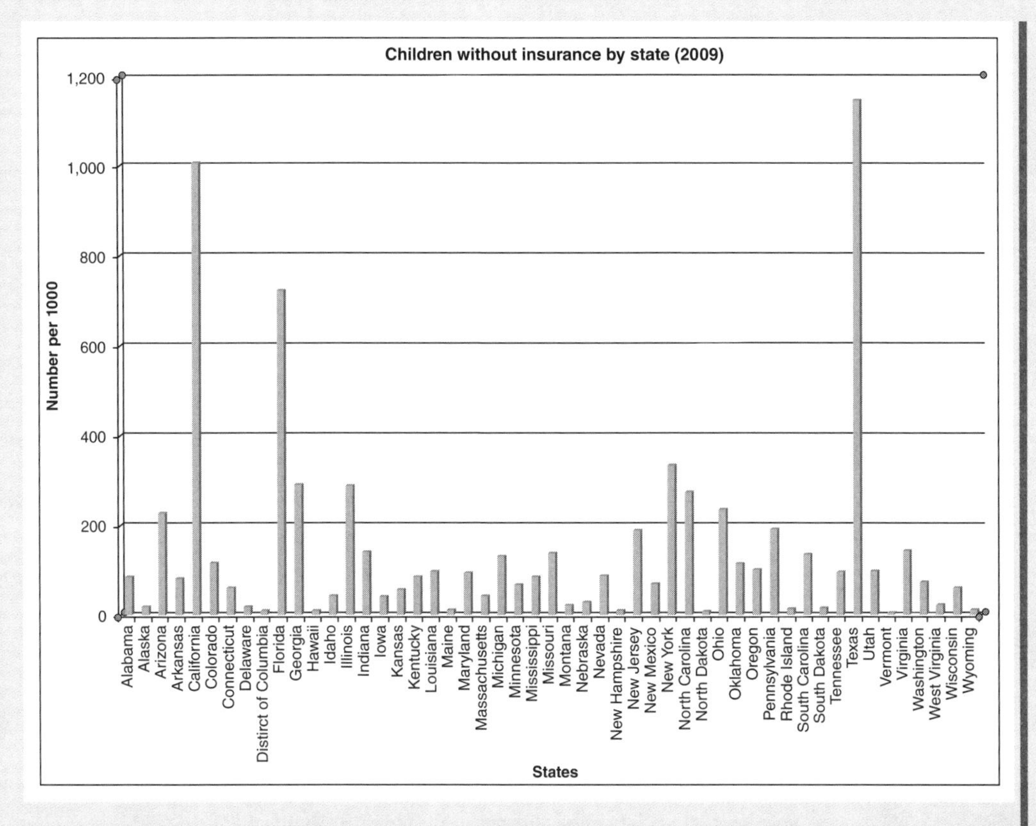

Figure 8-11b Column Chart Results Chart B

EXERCISE 4 Can I Create a Simple Excel Database?

Objectives

1. Design a record structure to use in some aspect of health care.
2. Enter records.
3. Generate an interesting chart.
4. Print a report.
5. Save the file.

Activity

Some activities can include patient registration database, a work list for caring for a group of patients, a tracking clinical experiences database, or some other topic of interest to you that is approved by the professor.

1. Generate a **few questions** you will ask of the database. This dictates fields needed in the database.
2. Create the **Table structure** in Excel.
3. Add at least **10 records**.
4. Make at least one **calculation**, one **sort**, and one **filter**.
5. Create **one chart** on its own sheet.
6. Save the work as **Chap8-Exercise4-LastName** and submit as directed by the professor.

Assignments

ASSIGNMENT 1 What Do I Need? How Can a Database Help?

Directions

1. Interview five to ten nurses regarding what databases are in use in their facility and what information is provided to them. Include what is helpful and what needs to be improved. You can include what databases you have access to in the process of providing patient care. What is helpful and what needs to be improved in those databases?
2. Select one database and identify the fields in the database and expected data types for each field.
3. Identify the additional data that would be helpful—data not currently available and what data types you would expect in that field.
4. Find one article that provides evidence that databases are improving patient outcomes.
5. Create a paper describing your findings. Use appropriate word processing features in your paper. For example, include tables and charts.
6. Save the paper as **Chap8-Assign1-LastName**. Submit according to the directions provided by the professor.

ASSIGNMENT 2 Will Standard Languages Help?

Directions

1. Go to http://www.nursingworld.org/OJIN. In the search box type **standard languages**. Select the article Rutherford, M., (Jan. 31, 2008) "Standardized Nursing Language: What Does It Mean for Nursing Practice?" *OJIN: The Online Journal of Issues in Nursing*. Vol. 13 No. 1.

2. Read the article, keeping in mind it was written in 2008.
3. What impact have standardized languages had on the databases used in nursing and the research on outcomes? Support statements with resources.
4. Does your clinical database use any standardized languages? If so, which one(s)?
5. Prepare a blog or short paper on what you found. Name your blog or paper **Chap8-Assign2-LastName**.

chapter

9

The Internet

Objectives 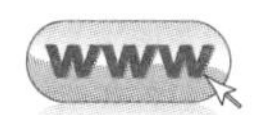

1. Describe the Internet.
2. Define related Internet terms.
3. Explain the components of an Internet address.
4. Identify the hardware and software that are needed to connect to the Internet.
5. Use browsers to explore the Internet.
6. Download files from the Internet.
7. Describe the Web page creation process and the healthcare professional's role in that process.

Introduction

According to the International World Stats (2012), 2,405,518,376 people worldwide accessed the Internet. Asia (44.8%) makes up the largest percentage of users with Europe (21.5%) and North America (11.4%) second and third, respectively. If you compare the number of users to the total population for that region, North American use comes in at 78.6% followed by Oceania/Australia (67.6%) and Europe (63.2%), respectively. In 2000, 5.8% of the world population used the Internet; in December 2012 that percentage grew to 34.3% (Internet World Stats, 2013). But what is the Internet and what should you know about it?

This chapter focuses on the Internet. People access the Internet for the purpose of communicating with others, obtaining information and files, and accessing Web servers to purchase products or services, watch movies, play games, and so forth. This chapter begins with a brief definition and description of the Internet and World Wide Web. Following this information is a discussion of Internet services; means of connecting to the Internet; addressing, browsing and locating information; use of search engines; and downloading files. We also include in this book a brief description of the process of creating Web pages. Additional information on Internet communication (e.g., email, newsgroups, list services, video chats) and informational resources (searching and search strategies) appears in chapters 10 and 12, respectively.

The Internet

Most of us think of the **World Wide Web (WWW)** as the Internet. In fact, the Internet is more encompassing than the WWW. Any function such as communications (email, listservs) and file downloading that uses the Internet networking protocols is part of the Internet, even when you do not use the **Hypertext Transfer Protocol (HTTP).** For example, downloading a file from an FTP (file transfer protocol) server over the Internet becomes part of Internet services.

The **Internet**, sometimes referred to as the information or global superhighway, is a loose association of millions of networks and computers around the world, all of which work together to share information. It is a truly global network that provides people with quick access to information and services from all over the world. WWW is the universe of hypertext servers that serve up web pages to web browers.

Structure

No one source foots the bill for the Internet; everyone pays for his or her part. For example, colleges and universities pay for their connections to some regional network. This regional network, in turn, pays a national provider for access.

Many institutions and companies donate their computer resources in the form of servers and computer technicians to hold up some part of the Internet. Other companies own and operate components of the Internet in the form of communication lines and related switching equipment. The main lines that carry the bulk of the traffic are collectively known as the Internet backbone and; network service providers (NSPs) maintain the backbone. In the United States, the NSPs maintain the network access points (NAPs) and metropolitan access exchanges (MAEs). These designations are changing, such that in many parts of the world they are now referred to as Internet eXchange Points (IXPs).

Some of the major players in this system are Verizon Business (formerly UUNET), AT&T, CenturyLink (formerly QUEST and Savvis), and Sprint. These companies sell access to **Internet service providers (ISPs)** and other large businesses (sometimes called **commerce service providers [CSPs]**). The ISPs and CSPs, in turn, sell access to the Internet to other large businesses, organizations, and smaller ISPs. The smaller ISPs then sell access to smaller businesses, organizations, and finally individuals. Through their interconnection, these networks create high-speed communication lines that crisscross the United States. These high-speed communication lines extend communication to the United Kingdom, Europe, Australia, Japan, Asia, and the rest of the world. Some of these countries provide Internet speeds much higher than those found in the United States. It is important to note that not all points along the route are well developed or have the extensive backbone found in some countries. In the United States, the backbone has many intersecting points. If one point fails or slows, the system quickly reroutes data over another part. This redundancy was one of the key points in the Internet's development. In some parts of the world, the network may have less redundancy, making it more vulnerable to slowdowns or breakdowns. In addition, governments in some countries control the backbone in their country, which means they dictate who gets access to the rest of the world.

Control

No one organization governs the Internet. Instead, this massive network relies on a group of organizations to affect a system of checks and balances to make sure things work. A few key players include:

ISOC	The Internet Society (ISOC) is a supervisory organization composed of individuals, corporations, nonprofit organizations, and government agencies from the Internet community. It holds the ultimate authority for the direction of the Internet and provides a home for several organizations that deal with Internet issues and standards (http://www.isoc.org).
IAB	The Internet Architecture Board (IAB) is responsible for defining the overall architecture of the Internet (the backbone) and all the networks that attach to it. It approves standards and the allocation of resources such as Internet addresses (http://www.iab.org).
IETF	The Internet Engineering Task Force (IETF) focuses on the operational and technical issues for keeping the Internet running smoothly as a whole (http://www.ietf.org).
W3C	The World Wide Web Consortium (W3C) manages the Hypertext Mark-up Language (HTML) standard, other

	Web-related standards (e.g., SHTML, SML, and CSS), and other specifics as they relate to the Web part of the Internet. This organization promotes interoperability for the various Web components (http://www.w3.org).
ISPs	Backbone ISPs, cable and satellite companies, regional and long-distance phone companies, and various agencies of the United States and other countries' governments contribute to the Internet telecommunications infrastructure.
IANA and InterNIC	The Internet Assigned Numbers Authority (IANA) and the Internet Network Information Center (InterNIC) are the two organizations responsible for assigning IP addresses and domain names, respectively (http://www.iana.org and http://www.internic.org).

Protocols

Communicating with other computers, many of which don't share the same structure or operating systems, requires a means for computers to "talk" to each other. That is, computers must speak the same language. For the Internet, this base protocol (set of rules) is called **Transmission Control Protocol/Internet Protocol (TCP/IP)**. Every computer on the Internet must use and understand this protocol for sending and receiving data. TCP/IP uses a "packet-switched network" that minimizes the chance that data will be lost when it sends the packets over the transmission medium.

The TCP part of the protocol breaks every piece of data into small chunks called packets. An electronic envelope encases each packet and each packet contains the Web addresses for both the sender and the recipient. Once the protocol creates packets, the IP part of the protocol determines the best route for sending the packet from one point to another point. Each packet may arrive at its destination by a different route. Routers examine the destination address and then send the packet to one router after another, until it reaches its final destination. Each router sends the packet by the best route available at that time. When the packet arrives at its destination, TCP takes over. Its function is to identify each packet, make sure that it is intact, and then reassemble the packets to reconstruct the original data.

In addition to these protocols, you may encounter others—for example, FTP for transferring files, telnet for remote logging in, and mail protocols such as POP3 (Post Office Protocol 3), SMTP (Simple Mail Transfer Protocol), and IMAP (Internet Message Access Protocol). Most of the time, these protocols operate seamlessly from the perspective of the typical Internet user.

The World Wide Web

Some consider the World Wide Web (WWW, also known more simply as the Web) the easiest of the Internet services to use. This part of the Internet is the graphical portion that stores electronic files, called Web pages, on servers that users access from their computers. Web pages may contain highlighted keywords (hypertext). Selecting a keyword takes the reader to another part of that document related to that word, to another document at that site, or to another site that provides additional information. In addition, some graphics and buttons may be hyperlinks, permitting the user to go to different sites or to obtain more information at the current site. The Web uses the HTTP protocol to communicate.

The following terms relate to the World Wide Web.

Client–Server — **Client–server** computing is the de facto model for network-oriented computing. Servers and clients interact with one another while exchanging information. Servers provide the information—in this case, Web pages—and clients consume it. The client is the computer or mobile device that knows how to communicate with a Web server.

Hyperlinks — **Hyperlinks** are words or images linked to other parts of a file or to other files at the same site or other sites. When the pointer of a mouse moves over a hyperlink, it turns into a hand.

Hypertext — **Hypertext** is linked text that provides additional information to the user. For example, a hypertext term might open a window with the definition of that term.

HTML — **Hypertext Markup Language** is the tagging used to code Web page files so that a browser can display them regardless of the user's computer or mobile device. The tags include commands for linking text and graphics and displaying the page in a browser.

HTTP — **Hypertext Transfer Protocol** is the communications protocol for accessing and working with the World Wide Web. Do not confuse it with HTML, which is the tagging language of the Web.

Web Browser — **Web browser** software interprets HTML code and displays that Web page or information on a local computer or mobile device in readable form. A few of the major browsers are Internet Explorer (IE), Firefox, Chrome, Opera, and Safari.

Web Servers **Web servers** are computers that hold information users request. Web servers recognize the requests, process them, and then make them available to the end user.

Services on the Internet

Many services are available on the Internet. Basically, the services available on the Internet fall under several categories: electronic communications, information services, information retrieval, storage, and entertainment.

Electronic Communications These services permit you to communicate with other people on the Internet via electronic mail, bulletin boards, chat rooms, instant messages, blogs, list or discussion services (such as listservs), news groups, and social networks such as Facebook and LinkedIn. In addition, electronic communications media include video sharing services such as YouTube, photo sharing services such as Flickr and Photobucket, and theme-based image collection sites like Pinterest. Chapter 10 describes these services.

Information Services Information services include remote login and other means of information access. These services permit you to log in to other computers from your computer for the purpose of obtaining information. The two main services in this area are telnet, which many librarians use, and the Web, which we all use. Growing in use are streaming applications, which permit users to view videos and podcasts of educational materials and to interact with one another in real time. The focus in this book however, is information access.

Information Retrieval These services permit users to obtain files from other sites and bring them to their own computers, a process commonly referred to as file transfer. **File Transfer Protocol (FTP)** is the most commonly used protocol for transferring files from one computer to another. Since the development of the Web, the interface for transferring files has become more user friendly and is not command driven.

Cloud Storage — **Cloud computing** refers to delivery of hosted services over the Internet or a proprietary network. With the advent of mobile devices many users store and access their data over the Internet via a cloud storage service.

Entertainment — These services consist of listening to the radio, watching TV programs and movies, and playing games interactively over the Internet.

These services are now easier to use than they were a few years ago. For example, when transferring a file, you do not need to know all of the commands for downloading files or for activating FTP—knowledge that was essential for completing these operations in the past. Most of the time today, file transfer is a matter of clicking on a download hyperlink and responding to prompts. You can even download graphics by right-clicking the image and selecting "Save picture as" from the shortcut menu. In this way, this service isolates the user from the background commands necessary to use these services.

Connecting to the Internet

This section outlines the equipment and software necessary to access the Internet. The desired services determine the necessary equipment for accessing the Internet. For example, using the Web to access and play multimedia files requires a higher-level computer than accessing a text-based email program on a UNIX computer. In addition, software programs are necessary for each type of accessed service; most ISPs and browsers now come with many features bundled into one easy-to-install program.

Computer or Mobile Device

Although the equipment requirements for accessing the Internet are not very demanding, the level of processing power necessary depends on what the user intends to do on the Internet and the requirements of the ISP. Each provider lists the minimum hardware and operating system requirements necessary to use its services. If you expect full multimedia information to appear on the computer instantly, you may need a more powerful computer with higher-speed connections and full multimedia capabilities—sound cards, speakers, and good graphics—or a mobile device with sound and a camera for using video chats and conferencing.

Network Connection

From home, the computer needs to have a network connection to the Internet. Generally ISPs provide this connection through a phone line or cellular service, digital subscriber line (DSL), satellite dish, cable, or fiber-optic connection. On campus, the connection is through campus network connections, which are either wired or wireless. **Broadband** connections such as **DSL**, cable, and fiber, are faster than dial-up access and provide an ongoing connection to the Internet. Unfortunately, this nonstop access also means that the end user is more vulnerable to hackers. To protect against hacker incursion into their computers, broadband users should install a personal firewall as well as antivirus and antispam software. Chapter 13 provides additional information about Internet related security.

Modems

A **modem** provides an interface between the computer and the transmission channel for converting the data into a form that the ISP can transmit via the selected transmission line. At home, this can be a dial-up modem, a DSL modem, a cable modem, a satellite modem, or a wireless router/modem.

Dial-up modems are still in use in many parts of the United States because of the high cost and lack of availability of other types of connectivity. They are the slowest means of connecting and they tie up the phone line; however, they are readily available and are relatively inexpensive. Because cellular services may be more widespread in some areas, access may be through the cellular service.

DSL modems provide connectivity by using the digital portion of the regular copper telephone line. This type of access is faster than a dial-up connection, does not tie up the phone line, is a little more expensive, and is always "connected" unless you turn it off, which most people do not do. The downside is the lack of availability in some areas and the inherent security issues that arise because the computer, when on, is always connected to the Internet.

Cable modems work with a cable TV line. The cable provider may rent these modems to the user or individuals may get their own from the ISP or other sources. They provide faster access to the Internet than traditional phone and DSL modems. A cable modem typically has two connections, one to the cable wall outlet and the other to the computer via an Ethernet card. Costs vary greatly depending on location and cable provider; speed fluctuates dependent on how many people are sharing the bandwidth at the same time. Security issues exist with cable as well.

A **satellite Internet connection** uses a satellite dish antenna and a transceiver (transmitter/receiver) that operates in the microwave portion of the radio spectrum. The installer generally provides and configures the modem, sets up the dish, and brings the system to a wall jack. These connections are subjected to weather interference and latency, but provide an option for fast Internet connections in rural areas not reachable by DSL or cable.

Fiber-optic connections (such as the Verizon FiOS service) rely on a wireless router to provide the connectivity between the computer, phone wire, and fiber-optic panel. This option provides for faster connection speeds than DSL or cable, but is more expensive. It also sets up a wireless connection so all devices in the home may access the Internet at the same time. Many ISPs now bundle this option with TV and phone service.

Cards and Adapters

A special device is necessary to move the data from the computer or mobile device through the transmission media (e.g., phone lines, cables, radio waves) to the access provider. Some computers (i.e., laptops) have built-in wireless and network cards instead of using modems (aircards) that plug into your computer and provide cellular access to the Internet.

A **wireless card** provides connectivity to mobile computers. It converts the data into radio signals. This type of connection can be very fast and might be available in areas that other mediums do not service. The downside is that the device must be within a 10- to 20-mile radius of a hot spot or access point. The number of wireless access points is increasing daily with free Wi-Fi (Wireless Fidelity) available to customers in many cafes, airports, and bookstores.

A **network card** in a computer enables a direct connection to a network. It is the typical connection found in college dormitories, laboratories, and offices. This type of access does not need a modem but does require a special cable and an active network port.

A **USB cellular adapter** is also called a wireless broadband adapter or air card that connects a laptop to a network for data access and transfer. The adapter plugs into a USB port, although some models use the PC card slot. You can also use some cell phones as the wireless access point for access and transmission of data.

Software

The software necessary to access the Internet depends on how you are accessing it and who provides the connection service. Communication protocols that coordinate data transfer to and from the local computer or device and the Internet (e.g., TCP/IP) and protocols for the various services (such as email, Web, and FTP) are necessary. Service providers generally install these during the setup process when making the connection.

Internet front-end software is the software with which the user interacts (the browser). It might be a comprehensive program, such as Internet Explorer, Chrome, or Firefox, or a program the service provider offers. At the very least, a browser is required to display the Web pages. Beyond that you might also install antivirus, antispam, and email software.

You might also install a variety of **plug-ins**, which are additional pieces of software that process specific types of content. For example, you might need

Adobe Reader for viewing PDF files, Macromedia's Flash for viewing Flash files, or Apple's QuickTime for watching QuickTime movies.

There are also **apps** (short for applications), which are nimble programs for use within the browser. For example, Google Maps provides helpful maps and directions and LastPass provides password management.

Access Providers

Access providers are organizations that provide access to an Internet host computer. They often supply the software necessary to connect to the Internet as well as the appropriate connection equipment. Because several types of access providers exist, users need to choose the type of access that is appropriate for them.

Internet Service Providers

ISPs provide access to the Internet and email. Many also provide special services such as news, data storage, Web hosting, and specialized databases. Examples include America Online (AOL), Verizon, Comcast, DirectTV, and a host of others depending on your geographic location. There is considerable competition among ISP providers.

Here are some considerations for selecting an ISP:

- What do the costs cover? Are there data limits? Do they offer bundles?
- Do you have any contract options?
- What are their connection medium and speeds?
- Is the connectivity fast and reliable at *all* times of the day? In other words, what is the ratio of subscribers to bandwidth?
- Is there reliable and responsive technical support on a 24/7 basis?
- Is there space on the server for personal home pages?
- Are all of the desirable services available, such as email, instant messaging, Web and related multimedia files, FTP, newsreader, and telnet?
- What is the maximum size for file attachments and for the email account?
- What tools are available for privacy and security? Does the ISP offer a firewall? Parental controls? Free virus protection?
- Do you get to choose your account logins and passwords? How many users can you have on one account?
- Does the ISP provide secure backup services so that you can store your personal data?

Free Internet Access

Some community-based computer networks are designed to help local citizens access and share information and resources at no cost; others are free ISPs that make their money from paid sponsors or advertisers. Funding to support community-based access is generally made available through local libraries, government agencies, or interested local businesses such as airports, bookstores, and malls. This type of service generally restricts use to people who live in or are visiting the community. Many of these networks rely on a group of volunteers to assist in developing and maintaining the system. In many cases these free services have limited security, so users should use caution accessing personal information such as financial data over these networks.

Temporary Access for a Fee

Local businesses such as hotels, coffee shops, or delis, might provide Internet access. Sometimes these locations are called cybercafes. Some of these providers have time restrictions; others charge varying fees for temporary access. Some hotels provide free access in the lobby or bar area, but charge for access from guests' rooms. Sometimes the access is limited to the hotel-provided computers. Other times the access is offered by Wi-Fi. In all cases, security is an issue.

Company or Institutional Access

An employee or student in an institution might have Internet access through the organization's computer and connection facilities. Once you connect to the network, you have access to all of the capabilities the organization provides, including Internet access and email. Some companies provide mobile users with cards to plug into their laptops that give them access to the corporation's network through a cellular connection; others require a physical presence at the facility or allow users to connect remotely from a home connection. The user must remain an employee or student to continue to use the access, and he or she is subject to the policies of that organization or institution (acceptable use policies).

User IDs and Passwords

Except for free Internet access options you must have a **user ID** (name) and **password** to use the services of the ISP. You may choose the user ID or the institution may assign one using its naming standards. For example, some institutions use the user's last name, first letter of first name, and middle initial; others use the last name, first letter of first name, and a number; thus a user ID might be Abraham.Lincoln, lincolnax, or lincolna1. Many ISPs let users choose their own IDs; the ID could then be ngtcrawler, nurseJane, or hojo. If you are selecting an ID on your own, it is wise to select a neutral rather than provocative ID. For example, sexyme, drugpusher, and partyanimal are not appropriate ID names for a professional healthcare worker.

It is important that each user on that system be uniquely identified. No two system users can have the same user ID on that system. Some ISPs and institutions handle duplicate IDs by assigning numbers to the end; thus ngtcrawler becomes ngtcrawler2 and nurseJane becomes nurseJane2.

Although the user ID is public knowledge, the password is private. In some cases you create the password when you create your account; in others the granting service provider provides a temporary password. The first time you login, you will be required to create a new password. You should safeguard passwords just like you do your personal identification number (PIN) for a bank account (ATM). Do not give the password to anyone or write it down where others can see it. In addition, each system has its own criteria for acceptable passwords. For example, many systems require a minimum number of characters and a combination of letters and numbers; thus the password bri8ll might be acceptable or may be rejected as too short or not containing a symbol. Avoid using dictionary words and common-knowledge words such as a spouse's name or a pet's name as passwords; they are too easy for someone to break. Use nonsense combinations that make sense to you. An example might be gcle2009, where g = green, cle = Camry LE, and 2009 = year of the car. Additional information on forming strong passwords and protecting your accounts appears in Chapter 13.

The Cloud

Cloud computing refers to delivery of hosted services (third-party) over the Internet or a proprietary network. The official definition from the National Institute of Standards and Technology reads: "Cloud computing is a model for enabling convenient, on-demand network access to a shared pool of configurable computing resources (e.g., networks, servers, storage, applications, and services) that can be rapidly provisioned and released with minimal management effort or service provider interaction. This cloud model is composed of five essential characteristics, three service models, and four deployment models" (Mell and Grance, 2011, p. 2).

According to Mell and Grance (2011, p. 2), the five essential characteristics of a cloud hosting service are:

1. On-Demand Self-Service. The provider sells its services as part of a package on demand without interaction with the service provider. The provider manages the service—the consumer needs only a personal computer/mobile device and Internet access.
2. Elasticity and Scalability. Clients use what service they need to the extent that they need it (scalability), when they need it (elasticity).
3. Measured Service. Users generally but not always pay for cloud computing services by the minute or the hour, or some other metric (i.e., on a pay-as-you-go or pay-for-what-you-use basis). This pay-for-what-you-use model is similar to the way you pay for electricity, fuel, and water and some refer to it as utility computing.

4. Broad Network Access. The service is available any time and, anywhere over the Internet or proprietary network on mobile devices (smart phones, tablets, laptops, or other handheld devices), desktops, and workstations.
5. Resource Pooling. The provider pools its dynamic computing resources to serve multiple users according to user demand. Examples of resources include software, storage, processing, memory, and bandwidth.

Regardless of the service or selected deployment model, the goal of cloud computing is to provide easy, scalable access to computing resources and IT services. In our mobile society, access to your documents, photos, files, and so forth, from any place and at any time is a must. Before you use a cloud service you must sign some form of service-level agreement (SLA). Certain SLAs for free cloud storage (such as SkyDrive, iCloud, Dropbox, and GoogleApps) require that you agree to Terms and Conditions. When users check the "I agree" box they have signed a legal contract giving them access to and use of the service. At the organizational/company level, SLAs are far more formal and complex.

When selecting a cloud service, keep these items in mind:

- What features does the service provide?
- Does it permit mobile access?
- How easy is it to use?
- Does it provide for synchronization with the data on my local computer or mobile device?
- What does it cost and how much storage does it provide?
- What help and support does it provide?
- How well is my personal data protected?
- What can they do with my data?
- What is the SLA agreement?

Understanding Addressing

While you must have a user ID to access many of the services on the Internet, your computer must have a unique address when connecting to the Internet. This address allows the computer to obtain information from a Web server and, in turn, to receive information from other computers. Although humans use words and graphics to communicate, computers prefer to use numbers. This section discusses IP addresses, domain names, and URLs—all terms that we use to locate and differentiate one computer and its files from all other computers and files on the Internet.

IP Addresses

An **Internet Protocol (IP)** address is a unique identification number that distinguishes each computer on the Internet. The university or service provider assigns this number to the computer. To communicate effectively, no two computers can have the same number at the same time. A computer may use a fixed (static) address or a dynamic address that changes each time the user accesses the Internet.

The IP address uses a number from 0 to 255 for each part of its four-part number. For example, this number may be something like 208.34.242.17 (IPv4, 32-bit). Because of the explosion of computers connected to the Internet a new IP scheme (IPv6, 128-bit) is now in use. This IP address looks like this 2001:db68:0:0:3421:0:453:8:1. What is important for you to understand is that your computer needs an IP address when connecting to the Internet in order for things to work. Most of the time assigning an IP address is a behind the scenes function. Your ISP provides an IP address during system setup and configuration.

Domain Names

A **domain name** is an address, similar to that used by the postal service, that points to a computer with a specific IP address. It is a description of a computer's location on the Internet. Domain names create a single identity for a series of computers that a company uses. A special Domain Name System (DNS) computer looks up the name and matches it with its assigned IP address. Examples of domain names are www.adobe.com and intranet.school.edu.

A period separates components of the domain name (**Figure 9-1**). On the left is the more specific name for the computer; to the right is the category that describes the nature of the organization. The first item is the name of the host server (www or online). The host registers with an organization or entity like the Internet Network Information Center (InterNIC) for the second-level domain name. This second domain name represents the organization and so takes on names representing that organization. For example, Google uses google.com while a college would use its name unless otherwise taken. The last item (e.g., com or edu) is the top-level domain name and describes the purpose of the organization or entity that owns the second-level name. The type or nature of the organization dictates its name.

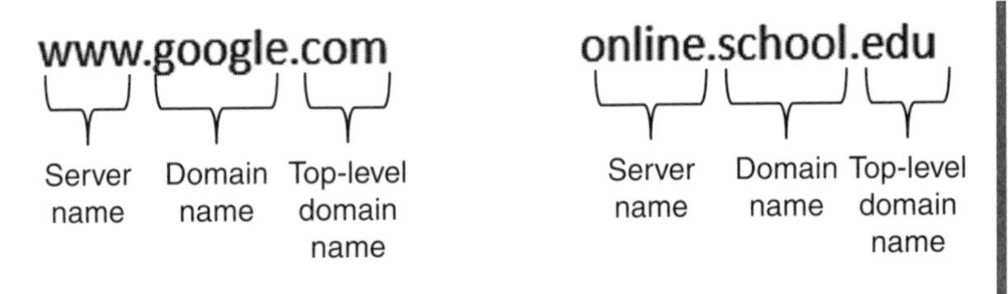

Figure 9-1 Domain Name Scheme

Here are a few of the common top-level domain names. Various users are always proposing additional top-level domain names.

aero	Air transportation industry
biz	Business
com	Business or other commercial enterprises
edu	Postsecondary institutions
gov	Government agencies or departments
int	International organizations
k12	K-12 public schools with state.county (k12.pa.us; some use .org)
mil	Military
net	Network service providers or resources
org	Organizations, usually nonprofit or charitable
pro	Professionals or other licensed people

All these top-level domain names are in use in the United States. There are also country top-level domain names such as "ca" for Canada and "nz" for New Zealand.

A domain may also contain other components between the host (Web server) and the second-level domain; these are called subdomains. Large organizations use subdomain names that support many Internet servers. For example, the U.S. government and its many agencies differentiate one agency from another through use of the subdomains. An educational institution may have subdomains for each school or department. For example, in the address www.nursing.school.edu, "nursing" might represent the nursing school's or department's Web server (www). Also, countries sometimes use a similar naming system; for example, co.uk, "co" is the equivalent of .com and "uk" represents the United Kingdom.

Anyone can register with the InterNIC to obtain a second-level domain name or use a service like GoDaddy.com, which is the leading site for domain name registrations. To see who owns specific domain names, go to www.networksolutions.com/whois/index.jsp. Some enterprising people have registered a variety of names of big corporations and now make money selling the rights to these second-level domain names to those organizations.

Understanding domain names will help you identify the type of information that you can obtain from a certain site. Knowing that the site is a government agency, such as the IRS (http://www.irs.gov), means that the forms and instructions there are legitimate. Sites such as those that the U.S. National Library of Medicine (http://www.nlm.nih.gov) and the Centers for Disease Control and Prevention (http://www.cdc.gov) operate are very likely to provide current and reliable information. However, information from someone's personal home page may or may not be accurate or reliable. Note the difference between the Web sites for http://www.irs.gov and http://www.irs.com or http://www.cdc.gov and http://www.cdc.org where the only difference is the top-level domain name. The same thing happens with slight variations in second-level domain names. Note the difference between http://www.webmd.com and http://www.mdweb.com.

URLs

URLs help a computer locate a Web page's exact location on the Web server. Although IP addresses and domain names locate the computer, they do not locate the Web documents on the server. The URL helps the computer find the actual Web pages. See **Figure 9-2** for an example.

Consider the following URL http://www.nursing.pst.edu/foundations/courses/nsg412.html (this is not a real URL). The first part, http://, identifies the communications protocol that the computers are using to communicate with one another. Other examples are FTP and telnet. Most URLs today start with http:// because most users are accessing the World Wide Web. Some will start with https:// because it is a secure server connection.

The second part of the URL, www.nursing.pst.edu, identifies the Web server or host computer that contains the page. Recall that the first part of this address describes the local host site, and the second part describes the domain name that is registered to that institution. The institution can decide how it wants to set up its local host. For example, the institution may name its local host or Web server www, or www.healthschools, or www.dept.

The third part, /foundations/courses/, tells the server where it can find the file to display. The slashes represent folders, just like those on your computer. This part of the URL provides the computer with the information about the location of a Web page file. If there is no path but a / after the top-level domain name, it looks for an index or default HTML file.

The last part, nsg412.html, is the actual file name for the browser to display. Most of the time it will be an HTML or HTM file. HTML files are static Web pages in which the content is created at the time the page is created. Web pages

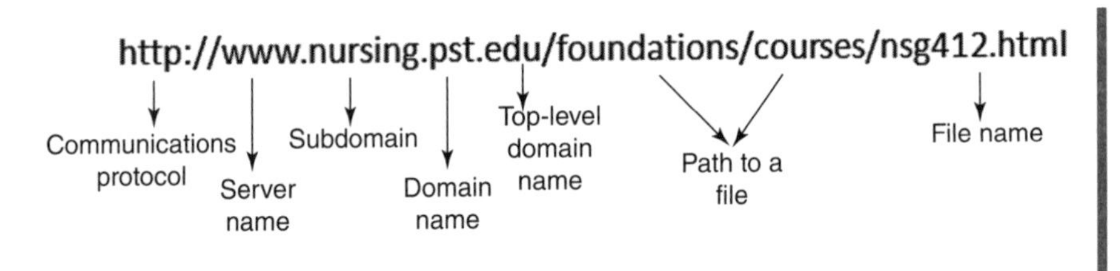

Figure 9-2 URL Explained

today tend to be dynamic, meaning that they are interactive. Such a Web page can accept and retrieve information from and for a user. These Web pages generally require some form of HTML and either a program or script. Programs and scripts are instructions that tell the computer how to perform a task; examples include CGI (Common Gateway Interface), ASP (Active Server Pages), DHTML (Dynamic Hypertext Markup Language), and Java applets.

When you type URLs in the location or address box in a Web browser, no spaces can appear between their parts; the URLs must have forward slashes and be typed exactly as given. If you type the numeral one (1) for the lowercase letter "L", the computer will not be able to find the site and will return an error message. If the URL appears in an electronic form, you can highlight it and use the copy and paste feature to place the URL in the address text box to avoid typing errors. Note that most current browsers do not require you to type the "http" part of the URL as it is the default. If you access a secure site such as the one ADP (Automatic Data Processing) operates, which is a business that processes payroll data, you need to type https://. Alternatively, you may be able to click on a hyperlink to go to that URL.

Web Browsers

A **Web browser** is the software program that displays Web pages on the World Wide Web. Although many different browsers are available, currently the top five browsers are Chrome, Internet Explorer, Firefox, Safari, and Opera. See **Figure 9-3** for a comparison of browser usage in the World versus the United States. This information changes over time. A site located at http://gs.statcounter.com/ maintains these current statistics. For example, Chrome overtook Internet Explorer on the world scene and may soon overtake Internet Explorer in the United States. Internet Explorer is bundled with Windows computers, and Safari is bundled with Apple computers. Many users download and use Chrome or Firefox on either a Mac or a PC. In the professional world, the IT department is more likely to install Internet Explorer and Firefox while many users install Chrome on their personal computers.

Although these browsers are in competition with one another, they are very similar in how you interact with them. Other browsers are also available that allow you to surf the Internet without leaving traces on the computer of where you have been. Browzar (http://www.browzar.com) is one such example. Some people prefer to use these types of browsers on public computers, while at home they may use an anonymous proxy server (a server that acts as an intermediary for requests keeping the user anonymous). Some Web sites are browser-specific and do not display their pages well if not using the correct browser. In those cases, there will be a notice on the Web page, such as "best viewed with" and the name and version of the browser.

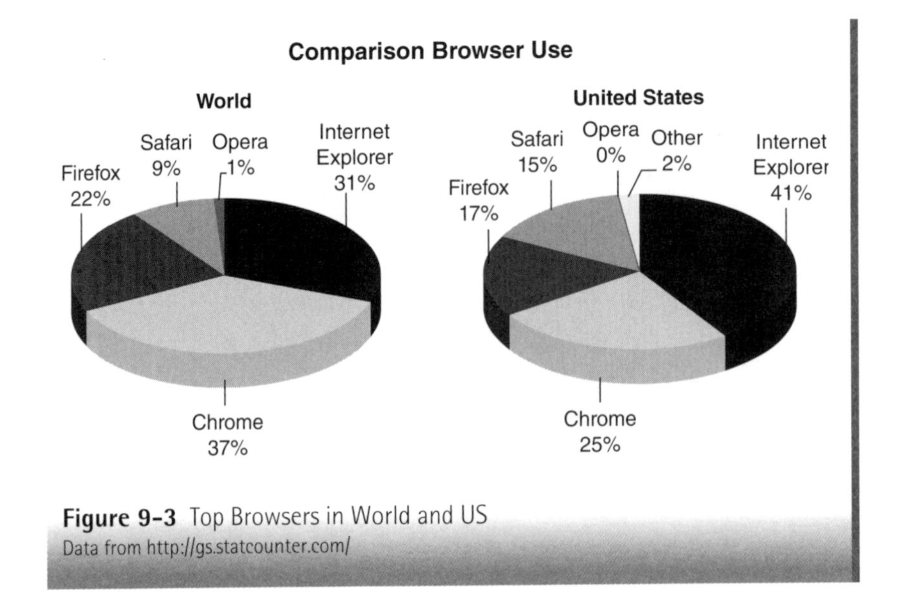

Figure 9-3 Top Browsers in World and US
Data from http://gs.statcounter.com/

Because developers are constantly revising browsers, like most software, you need to check and install the updated version of your browser on a regular basis. Frequently the IT department will update computers at work and in school labs, but you are responsible for performing this task on your own personal computer. Today, many browsers have an option to automatically update the browser. All browsers have a way to check for the version and update numbers. Note also that mobile devices also need to be set to regularly update software.

To check for the version of Internet Explorer on the computer:

1. Open the **browser**.
2. Click the **down arrow** on the Command bar or click the **Help** on the Menu bar. (See **Figure 9-4**.)
3. Click **About Internet Explorer**. A window appears with the version number.

To check for the version of Chrome on the computer:

1. Click the **browser**.
2. Click the **Customize and control** button on the Address bar. (See Figure 9-4.)
3. Click **About Google Chrome** on the menu. A window appears with the version number.

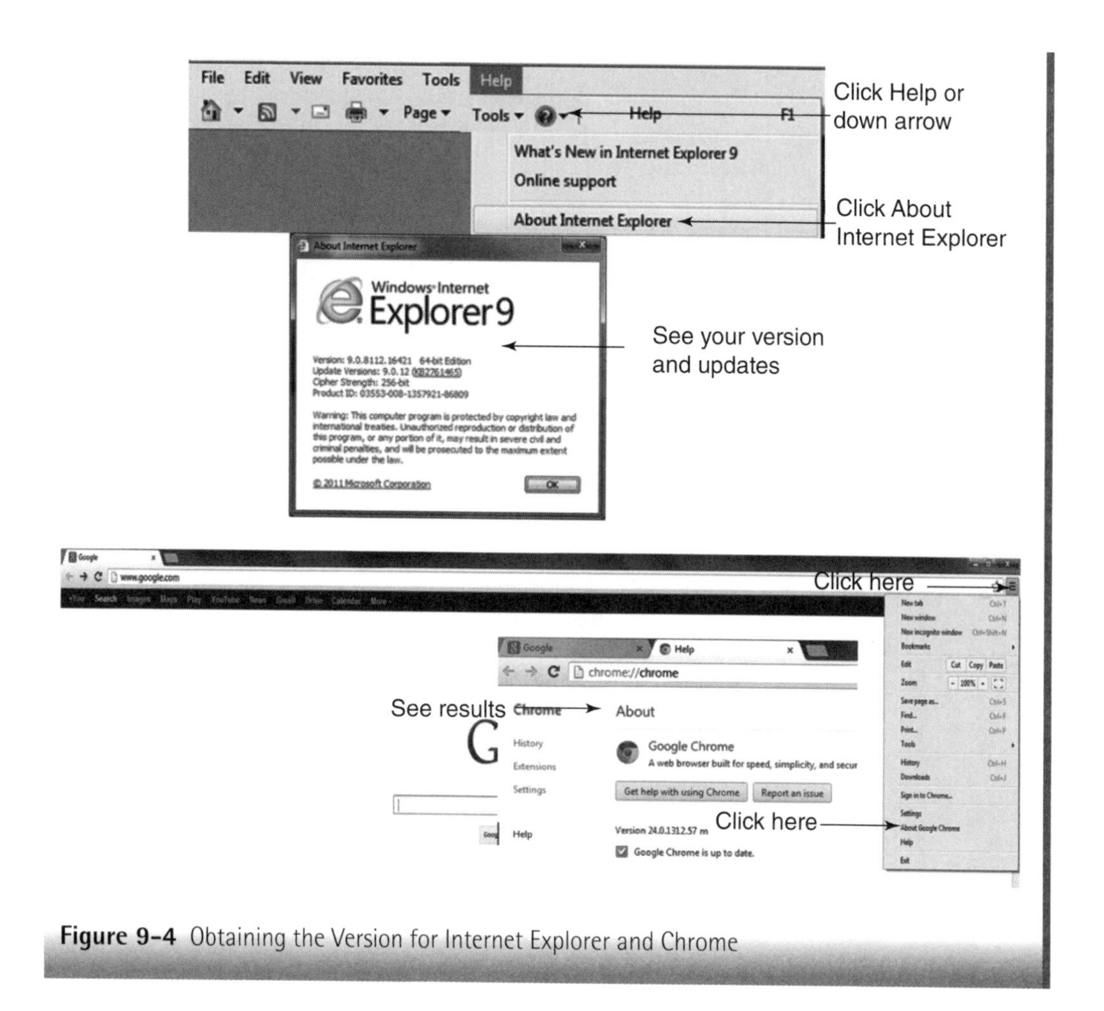

Figure 9-4 Obtaining the Version for Internet Explorer and Chrome

To check for updates for Internet Explorer:

1. Open the **browser**.
2. Click **Tools** on the Menu bar and then **Windows Update**. Because Internet Explorer is part of the operating system, the screen will show updates that are necessary.
3. Windows will now check for and display the neccessary updates. (Make sure you have a live Internet connection.)
4. A window displays the updates necessary.
5. Follow the provided directions to get the updates.

6. Internet Explorer will update automatically if you set the operating system to perform this task. All the user has to do is say "yes" to the message that appears asking if it is okay to do this. If the system set up does not call for automatic updates, you can change that setting.

To check for updates for Chrome:

NOTE: Google Chrome automatically updates the browser when it detects that a new version is available. This update happens in the background with no action necessary by you. If updates are available but not installed, you will see the Chrome icon on the browser toolbar.

1. Open the **browser**.
2. Click **Update Google Chrome** icon.
3. In the confirmation dialog that appears, click **Restart** to save your browser settings including open tabs. Once the update is complete, the browser reopens to the saved settings. Alternatively, you can select **Not now** and system updates will apply the next time you use the browser.

With each new version, developers add capabilities to the browser. However, the basic functions—the ability to use the back, forward, stop, search, print, and home buttons—remain constant. Newer versions will build in your current settings and retain items such as your bookmarks or favorites.

Main Elements of a Browser

Like the applications in the Microsoft Office suite, Web browsers have similar main elements—title, menu bars, toolbars, scroll bars, status information, and page tabs. Here are some features of the browser window. See **Figure 9-5**.

Menu and Toolbar — The Menu and Toolbar provide access to a series of commands like File, Edit, View, Favorites, Tools, and Help. Most browsers permit you to customize these toolbars for how you work.

Page Tabs — Page tabs, sometimes referred to as tabbed browsing, permit you to open a new Web site in a separate tab for quick access when you are working in multiple Web sites.

Address or Navigation Bar — This is where you enter the site URL for accessing a Web page use the Back and Forward buttons to go back to the previous resource and forward, respectively,

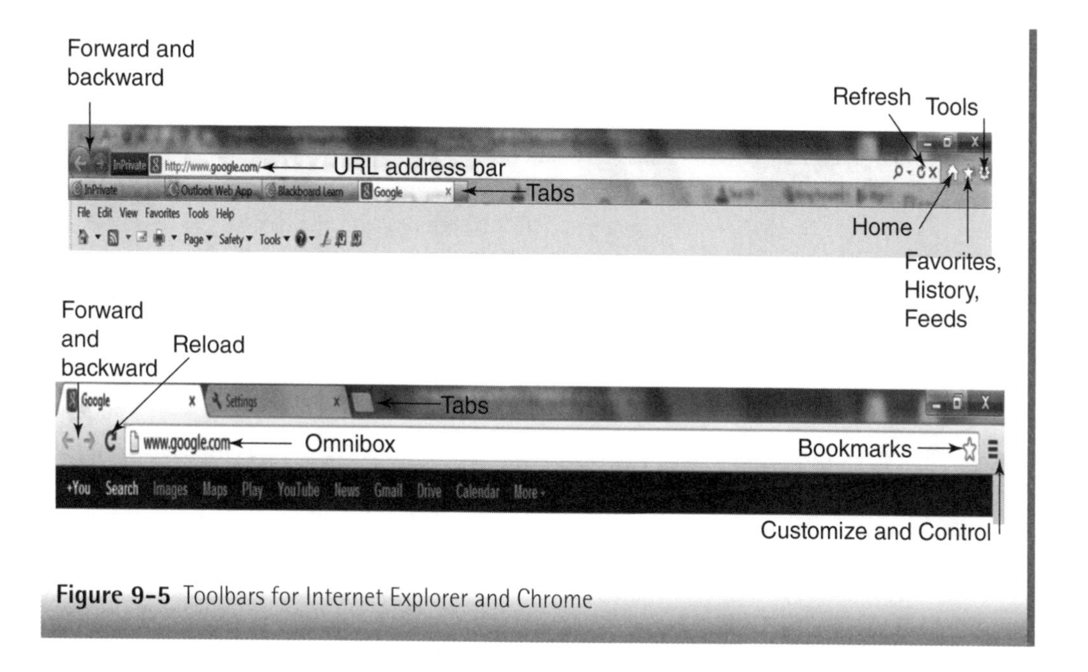

Figure 9-5 Toolbars for Internet Explorer and Chrome

use the refresh or reload button to reload the current resource, use the stop button to cancel loading the resource, and use the home button to access the user's home page, use the favorites (bookmarks) button, and use the tools button to customize the browser. Chrome calls this button Customize and Control.

Browsing Window This is the main window that displays when viewing Web pages. In most browsers it also contains the search box or place for you to type your keyword search. Some browsers merge the search box with the address bar.

Orientation to Internet Explorer and Chrome

While all browsers have similar functions, there are also some differences. In this edition we will look at both Internet Explorer and Chrome because they are the top two browsers. Firefox and Safari are close in functionality to Internet Explorer; once you learn one browser you can easily function in the other. Chrome takes a slightly different approach in providing not only searching but a portal to other Google programs like gmail, blogger, YouTube, and so forth. You can consider it a portal with browser functionality. Chrome features more of a minimalist approach with lots of keyboard shortcuts.

Internet Explorer	Chrome	Functions of Browser Buttons
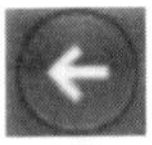	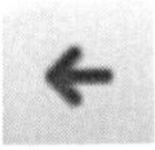	The **Back** button retrieves the last page viewed in this session. It permits you to retrace your steps backward, one Web page at a time. This button becomes active only after you have visited another site.
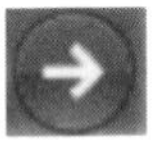	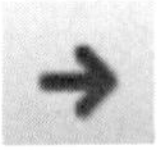	The **Forward** button retrieves the previous page viewed this session. It allows you to retrace your steps forward, one Web page at a time. This button becomes active only after the Back button has been used.
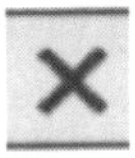	Press **ESC**	The **Stop** button interrupts the browser from loading a requested page. Use this function if it is taking too long to connect to a page. Clicking the Stop button stops loading of the Web page and permits you to continue doing something else or to go to another site.
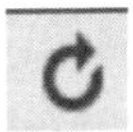	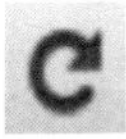	The **Refresh** or **Reload** button updates the current page displayed in the browser. Use it to view a site visited earlier whose content changes frequently, such as a stock market, sports event, or weather site.
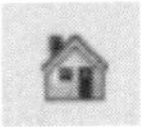	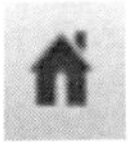	The **Home** button retrieves your home page—that is, the page displayed when the browser opens. Do not confuse it with the term "home page"—that is, the main page of a host's site. In Chrome you may have to click the Customize and control button, Settings, and under Appearance click the box to Show Home button because it does not display by default.
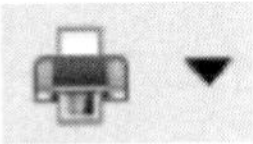	Ctrl+P	The **Print** button prints the current Web page or frame. In Internet Explorer, one copy of the current page is sent to the default printer. Additional options are available by clicking the down arrow to the right of the Print button. In IE or Chrome, press Ctrl+P to access open print options.

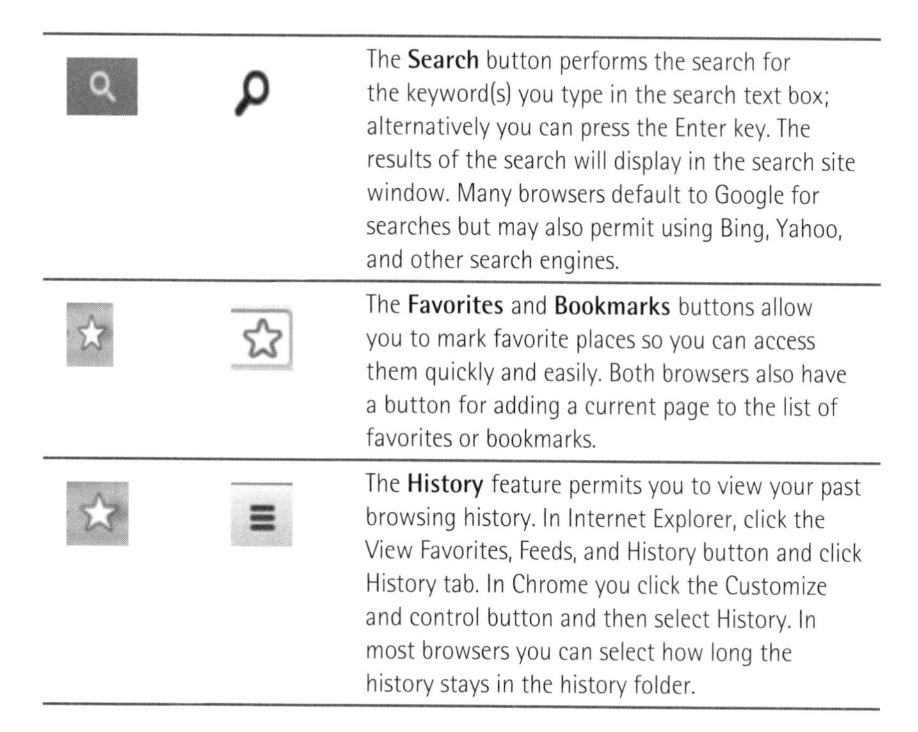

		The **Search** button performs the search for the keyword(s) you type in the search text box; alternatively you can press the Enter key. The results of the search will display in the search site window. Many browsers default to Google for searches but may also permit using Bing, Yahoo, and other search engines.
		The **Favorites** and **Bookmarks** buttons allow you to mark favorite places so you can access them quickly and easily. Both browsers also have a button for adding a current page to the list of favorites or bookmarks.
		The **History** feature permits you to view your past browsing history. In Internet Explorer, click the View Favorites, Feeds, and History button and click History tab. In Chrome you click the Customize and control button and then select History. In most browsers you can select how long the history stays in the history folder.

Note that you can customize many of these features. For example, in Internet Explorer you can set the number of days a URL will stay in the history folder. To do this, click Tools, Internet Options, Setting button in browser history, and then adjust the number of days to keep the page in history.

Starting the Browser

Chapter 4 described several ways to start programs. To start the browser, double-click the **browser icon**. If the browser is not on the desktop, click the **Internet Explorer** or **Chrome** option on the Quick Launch area of the taskbar. If that option is not available, use the **Start** button and **All Programs** to find the browser.

When the browser starts, a specific home page opens. This page may be the institution's or browser's Web page. You can change your home page in both browsers.

To change the home page in Internet Explorer:

1. Select **Tools**, **Internet options** from the toolbar.
2. Make sure that the **General** tab is selected.
3. If you did not open the desired home page, select the **text** in the **Address** text box of the current page.

4. Type the new **URL**, and click **Apply** button. If you currently display the desired home page, click the **Use Current** button and click **Apply** button.
5. Click **OK** to close the Internet Options dialog box.

To change the home page in Chrome (See **Figure 9-6**):

1. Select **Customize and control** ≡ button.
2. Under On startup, click **Open a specific page or set of pages**.
3. Type the **URL**
4. Click **OK**.

Now when the browser starts, it will point to the new home page. Use this same process to change how long sites stay in the history folder. For Internet Explorer, follow these steps: **Tools**, **Internet Options**, **General** tab, and adjust the **Setting** button under the Browsing history section. Chrome stores history for 10 weeks or until you delete it. There is no option for changing the length of time it stays.

Browsing or Surfing the Net

Browsing or "surfing the net" refers to the process of clicking hyperlinks to go to another part of a document, to a different document, or to another site. To use a hyperlink, click it. Most Web pages identify text hyperlinks by placing them a

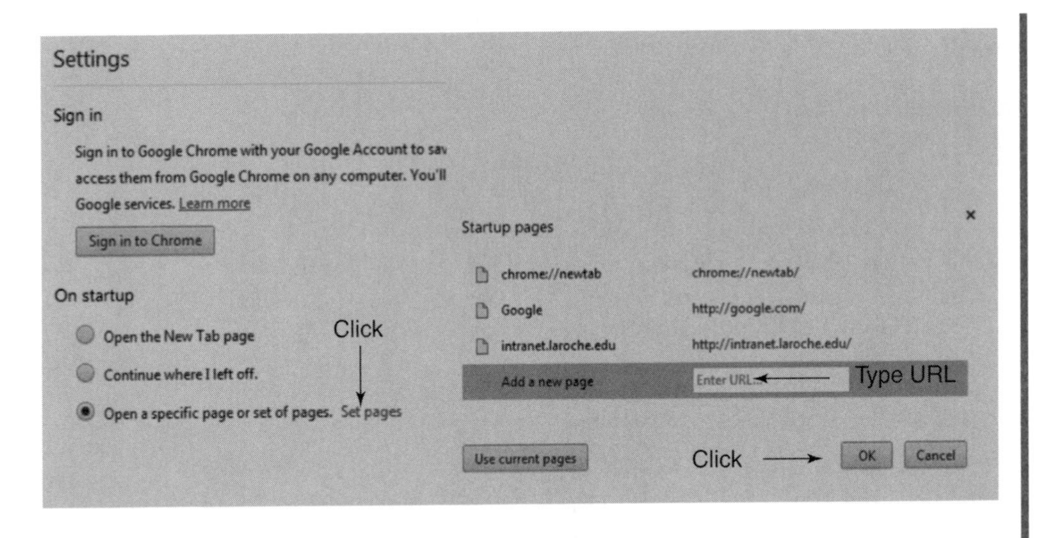

Figure 9-6 Setting Default Homepage in Chrome

different color and often by underlining them. The pointer changes to a hand when placed over a hyperlink. Be patient: Sometimes it takes considerable time to load a Web page. Graphic-intensive Web pages may come in faster through a broadband connection. Heavy traffic on the Internet slows the loading time.

If you have the URL for a site, you can simply type it in the URL address text box or in the Omnibox in Chrome to access the site. Most current browsers do not require typing the http:// part of the address; the browser automatically inserts that part. If you are going to a secure site, type https:// followed by the address. The computer requires the user to be exact; thus, you must make sure that the address is correct.

To go to a site by typing the URL:

1. Click the **text** in the Address box or Omnibox to select the text.
2. Type the **URL** and press **Enter**.
3. Click any **hyperlinked** objects or text to surf.

Using the History List

The **history list** keeps track of sites that you visited over the past several days and offers a convenient means of redisplaying those pages. Unlike favorites or bookmark lists, which store page locations that you specifically designate as candidates to revisit, the browser saves history items automatically when visiting a site. Most browsers store all visited sites in this folder regardless of how you arrived at the site. Some locator or address drop-down lists store sites only where you explicitly typed the URL. You can use the InPrivate browsing feature in Internet Explorer or Incognito feature in Chrome to keep your browsing private. These features disable cookies, temporary Internet files, history, and other data. The browser generally disables toolbars and extensions by default.

To use the history list in Internet Explorer:

1. Click the **View Favorites, feeds, and history** button and then the **History** tab.
2. Select how to view date, site, most visited, and so forth.
3. Click the **site** and/or related **actual pages** at the site.

To use the history list in Chrome:

1. Click **Customize and control** button.
2. Click **History** option. You will now see URLs by date and time.
3. Click the **site** to revisit. Note that you can also search using the search option.

Printing a Web Page

There are some subtle differences between Internet Explorer and Chrome when it comes to printing. When you click the printer icon, Internet Explorer sends one copy of the current document to the default printer. When you click the printer down arrow, the user has the option to select what to print after selecting Print (see **Figure 9-7**). Chrome has no printer icon to click. It does however provide for printing similar to the print command down arrow in Internet Explorer.

To print a Web page from Internet Explorer:

1. Go to the **Web page** to be printed.
2. Click the **Printer** button. If you are printing a site with frames, the active frame will be printed.

To access print options from Internet Explorer:

1. Click the **down arrow** next to the printer icon on the toolbar and then click **Print**.
2. Make the appropriate selections from the Print dialog box—Number of **copies** and **Pages**. You may also have the option of selecting a printer.
3. Click the **Options** tab and make appropriate selections from there.
4. Click the **Print** button.

To access print options from Chrome:

1. Go to the **Web page** to be printed.
2. Click the **Customize and control** button.
3. Click the **Print** Command.
4. Make the appropriate selections as to number of copies, printer, and so forth.
5. Click the **Print** button.

Both browsers give you the option to preview the material before printing and to change the print setup. The print preview function can be very useful in helping you determine how many pages will print before you actually click the Print button.

Saving a Web Page

Sometimes you may want to save a Web page to capture the content or the tagging (the inserted codes in the file that tell the browser how to display the page). When saving a Web page, several options may be available:

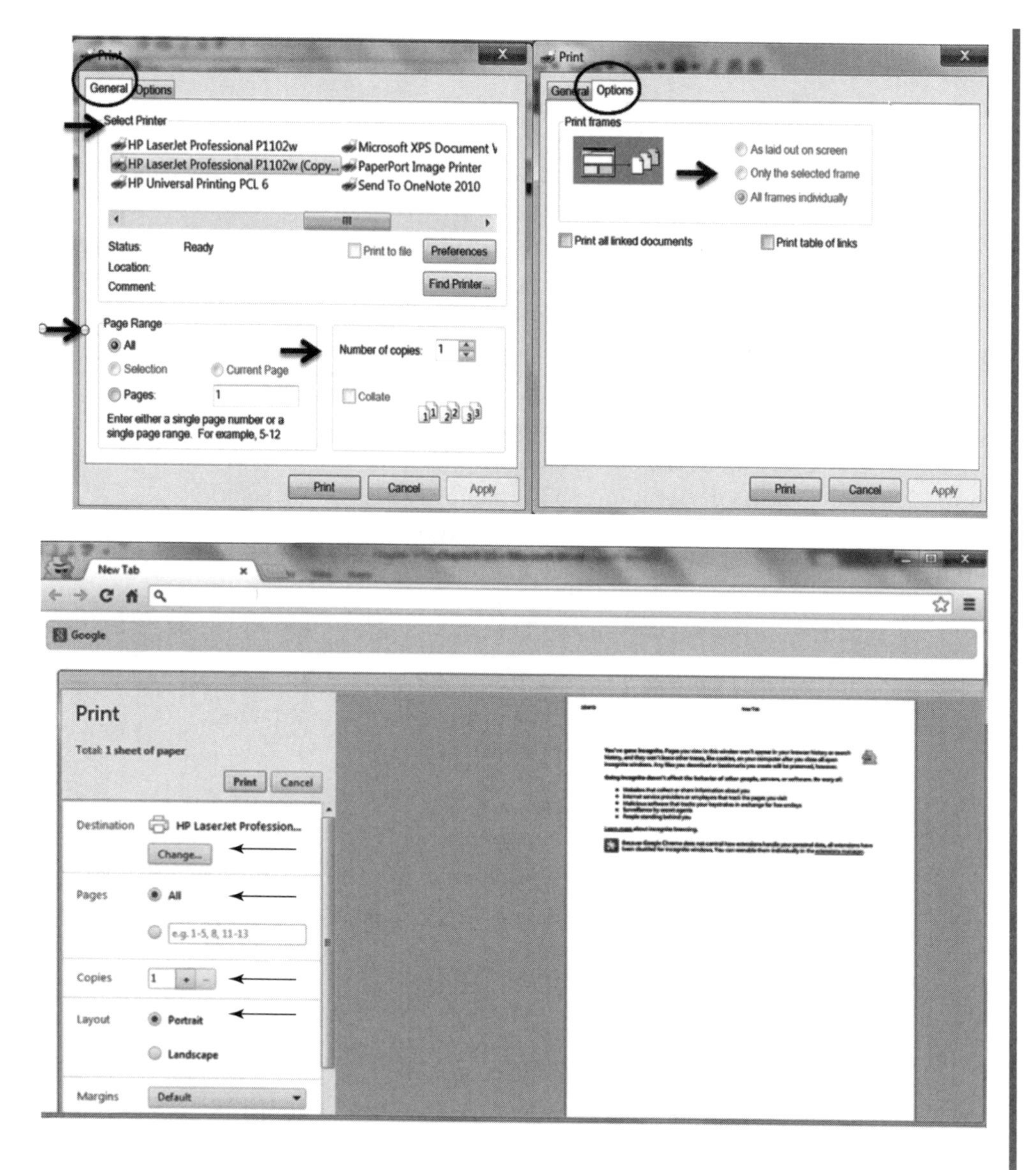

Figure 9-7 Print Options for Internet Explorer and Chrome

- **Web Archive** saves a snapshot of the current page in a single archive-encoded file. This option is not available in earlier versions of Internet Explorer and some current browsers like Chrome.
- **Web Page, HTML Only** saves only the code (tags) and text on the Web page; it does not save the graphics, sounds, or any other files displayed on the page but not embedded in the page.
- **Text Only** saves just the text from the current Web page in straight text format, permitting it to be imported into any word processor. It does not save the code and is not available in all browsers.

To save a Web page in Internet Explorer (See **Figure 9-8**):

1. Select **page you want to print.**
2. Click **File** and **Save as**. The Save Webpage dialog box appears.
3. Select the **location** and **file name** or accept the **defaults**.
4. Select one of the options for **file type**.
5. Click the **Save** button.

To save a Web page in Chrome (See Figure 9-8):

1. Select **Customize and control** and **Save page as**.
2. Select the **location** and **file name** or accept the **defaults**.
3. Select one of the options for **file type**.
4. Click the **Save** button.

On occasion you might want to save just a graphic from the Web site. Make sure you are not violating copyright rules or plagiarizing when you do this.

To save just an image from a Web page:

1. Right-click the **picture or image**.
2. Select **Save picture as** or **image as** or **target as**.
3. Select the **location** to which to download the graphic.
4. Type a **file name** or accept the **default**.
5. Under **Save as type**, select a **graphic file format** such as .jpg or .gif if provided that option.
6. Click the **Save** button.

To copy information from a Web page into a document without saving:

1. Select the **information** to be copied.
2. Click the **Page** button in Internet Explorer or right-click the **selection** and then **Copy**. In Chrome click the **Customize and control** button and then **Copy** in the Edit section.
3. Go to the document, and click **Paste** when the cursor is at the appropriate spot.

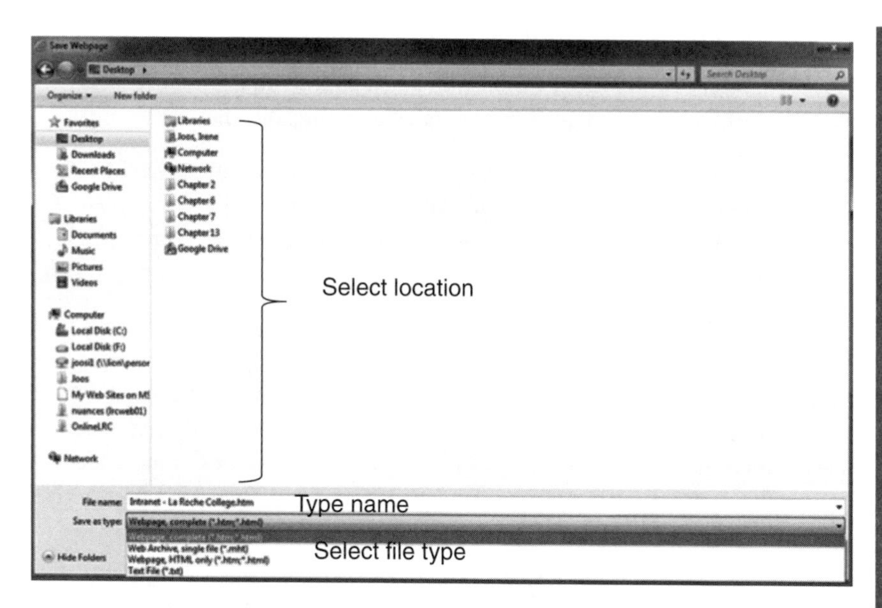

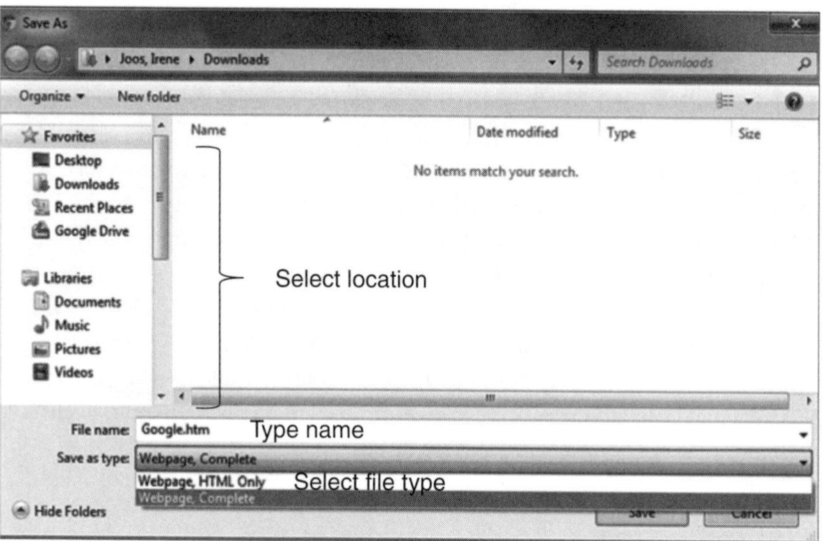

Figure 9-8 Save Web Page in Internet Explorer and Chrome

To create a desktop shortcut to a frequently accessed Web page:

1. Right-click somewhere in the **Web page**, but not on a graphic.
2. Select **Create shortcut** from the shortcut menu, and click **OK**.

You can use two other saving features for Web pages. First, you can save the file as a desktop background. Second, you can send a Web page to someone else through email. You can find these features on the shortcut menu once you are on the appropriate page.

Creating a Bookmark or Favorite

Bookmarks or **favorites** save the URLs of frequently visited sites. Use this feature to help organize a list of Web pages so that you can easily find them later. The basic functions necessary to use this feature are in all versions of most browsers, although the exact procedure for saving bookmarks or favorites varies between browsers.

The basic functions are as follows:

- Adding and removing bookmarks or favorites from your list.
- Organizing the list of URLs into categories or folders.
- Editing and arranging the bookmarks or favorites.

A number of factors make it difficult to create bookmarks. For example, many computer facilities provide a prescribed set of bookmarks or favorites, such as those that a library or computer lab may designate. The facility may place limitations on what you may change or add to this set. In addition, you may not have access to your bookmarks and favorites when you use a different computer. For these reasons, we recommend that you create a folder to hold these items on a removable storage device, rather than a folder on the hard drive. Exercises 1 and 2 at the end of this chapter describe the procedure for doing this. If you are using a personal computer, the process of creating and managing bookmarks and favorites is similar to the procedure that we discuss in Chapter 3.

Managing Internet Files

Each visited Internet site sends temporary files to the computer. These files include cookies, temporary Internet files, and surfing history.

Cookies

Cookie files are designed to enhance the online experience by recognizing the visitor when he or she returns to a Web site and recording what the visitor did at that site. For example, a cookie might remember what reservations a visitor made the last time the visitor accessed www.hotels.com or which credit card number the visitor used to order something from an online store. Although cookies should be harmless when you use a personal computer, they may pose a problem when you use laboratory or work computers. Sites can only read cookie files they place on the hard disk; they cannot read files that other sites place or other files on that computer. See Chapter 13 for more information on cookies.

Temporary Internet Files

Sites send **temporary Internet files** to the computer for the purpose of speeding the loading of graphics files when you visit a Web site multiple times. The problem with these files (and with cookie files) is that they take up space on the hard drive and remain there. Therefore, you must periodically delete these files. How often you should perform this depends on how frequently you use the Internet. Failure to purge these files periodically could lead to a full hard drive. These files also serve as a record of visited places on the Internet that you may not want others to know. You can delete these files through the browser interface or directly from the hard drive.

History Files

A history file keeps track of what sites you visit on the Web. If anyone else uses that computer, it may be wise to delete the history folder contents. For example, an abused client might search the Internet for resources about abuse. If the client doesn't know about deleting the history files, the abuser might become aware of this research. For this reason, the healthcare professional should make the client aware that he/she should delete the history files before leaving the computer. Some laboratories configure their computers to automatically delete the content of this folder when the user logs off. You may also set your browser to automatically delete these files upon exit from the browser.

To delete cookie, temporary Internet, and history files through Internet Explorer:

1. Open **Internet Explorer**.
2. Select **Tools** from the Menu bar, then **Delete browsing history** (See **Figure 9-9**).
3. Click the **Delete Temporary Internet files**, **Delete Cookies**, and **History** options. There are also other options to delete form data, passwords, and so forth.
4. Click the **Delete** button.

To delete cookies and history files through Chrome:

1. Open **Chrome**.
2. Select **Customize and control** then **Tools**, and then **Clear browsing data**.
3. Place checks in **History**, **Cache**, and **Cookies**. You also have a few other options.
4. Click the **Clear browsing data** button.

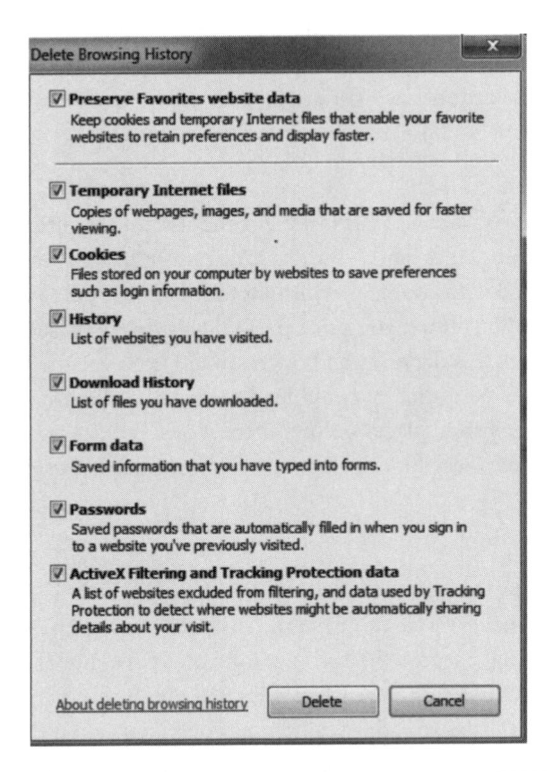

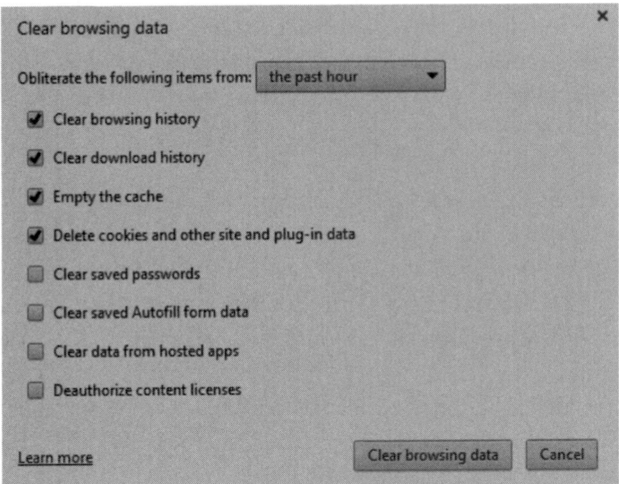

Figure 9-9 Delete Files in Internet Explorer and Chrome

Internet browsers offer a number of additional features beyond those described in this chapter. Both Internet Explorer (http://support.microsoft.com/ph/807) and Chrome (http://support.google.com/chrome/?hl=en-GB) have help systems on their Web sites where you can learn more about the features offered by these browsers. In addition you should take the time to explore several other browsers.

Search Sites (Engines) and Searching

The Internet contains a vast amount of information. Unfortunately, there is no single source to index the Internet that is analogous to the Library of Congress, which indexes books. Instead, you must search to find the information wanted. You should design your search of the Internet to find relevant information in an effective and efficient manner (more on this topic in Chapter 12).

Search sites are places on the Internet where you go to find information. **Search engines** are software programs that you use to find and index information. Several hundred different search sites and engines are available on the Internet. Generally, they are in three main categories, although the differences between these categories are disappearing as each site increases its functionality.

Directory

A directory is a hierarchical grouping of WWW links by subject and related concepts. People who search the Web and then group the links by subject create such directories. Therefore, they preselect the information appearing in the directory. The amount of irrelevant information in directories is far less than that from keyword search sites or meta search engines. Not all search sites include directories.

Directory sites are great choices for finding information quickly when you know little about the topic and the topic is broad. They are not good for ferreting out obscure facts. Links to outdated or moved Web pages also pose another problem. Yahoo, Open Directory, and About are three popular directory sites.

Keyword Search

A **keyword search** site comprises a server or a collection of servers dedicated to indexing Internet pages, storing the results, and returning lists of links that match particular queries. They provide access to the largest portion of information on the Internet, but often return a lot of irrelevant information. Spiders or bots normally generate the indexes. The terms "search site" and "search engine" are not synonymous; they are different.

Most keyword search sites have advanced search features for narrowing the search, but the results set they return may still be very large. Google and Ask are two popular keyword search sites. Mahalo is a human-powered search site unlike Google and Ask. This means you receive fewer results but higher quality results, much like a directory.

Meta Search Engines

Meta search engines are not really search engines. Rather, they work by taking the user's query and searching the Web using several different keyword search sites at one time. These tools are gaining in popularity because they permit one-stop searching.

Meta search engine sites provide a good picture of what is available because they use several different search engine sites and they do not preselect information as do directory sites. They may restrict some of the advanced search features, however. A few examples of these tools are Mamma, Yippy, and Dogpile.

Each of these search tools has a different interface or appearance, but all share several common features. Understanding how to use search sites begins by understanding a few key terms:

- **Hits** are a list of links that the search site returns as search results.
- **Query** refers to the combination of terms that you enter into a search engine to conduct a search.
- **Ranking** is a process of indicating how relevant a hit may be. Many times a search engine will organize the search results by their ranking. Because the methods that search engines use to rank pages vary, ranks may not always be useful.
- **Robots** are programs that create a database of links that they access when you conduct a search. These computer programs search the Web, locate links, and then index the links to create the results database. The program usually uses the words in the URL and title of the HTML file and counts the frequency of these words at the Internet site. Some robots search the full text, whereas others review only a portion of the site. Robots are also called *spiders* and *crawlers*. The problem with this approach is that programmers can fool the robots by using tricks in the coding; also, robots cannot access any pages that do not have links to them or that require a login.

Search Site Issues and the Invisible Web

The Internet is publishing information faster than search sites can index it; that is, search sites cannot keep pace with the sheer volume of information being produced. Adding to the problem is the issue of *who* is publishing to the Internet. Government agencies, nonprofit institutions, and educational institutions published early Web pages. Today, however, more Web sites that market or sell products and services are publishing to the Internet. With the advent of social media sites, individuals are also producing information through blogs, social networking sites, and so forth.

Current search engines have limits as to what they can index. This is creating an area of the Web referred to as the "Invisible Web" or "Deep Web" (Cohen, 2013). In addition to the sheer volume of information to be indexed, other factors influence what a search site can index. Examples include the editorial policies of family-friendly and news sites; database sites that require users to type search strings, as in the scheme that CDC databases use; requirements that visitors log in to visit certain parts of a site, as is the case with the *Chronicle of Higher Education* site; pages that contain only images; certain file types such as pdf and exe; dynamically generated pages; placement of documents behind firewalls; and some social media postings and comments. Some search sites acknowledge these difficulties by providing for links to current news sites such as CNN's sites or by having links to databases that index only images, videos, and so forth.

According to Basu (2010) advances in search engine technologies is ongoing. For example, we can now search and index pdf and Flash content. Basu provides a list of 10 Invisible Web search engines designed to index this "hidden" information. Examples include Infomine (http://infomine.ucr.edu/) and the WWW Virtual Library (http://vlib.org/).

Accessing Search Sites

Using a search engine begins by accessing the search engine site on the Internet. Open the browser and type the URL for the search site. Some users' default home page is a specific search site such as Google. To see other search sites available, type "search sites" or "search engines" in the Search text box and press Enter.

Portal-type directory structures (such as the Librarians' Internet Index) and clearinghouses or reference sites (such as Search Engine Watch, Search Engine Showdown, HowStuffWorks, and ReferenceDesk) also provide links to the most popular search sites as well as a wealth of other reference sites. Likewise, many ISPs and college/university libraries provide links to search sites on their main pages. A good place to start when conducting an Internet search is to confirm what your library recommends as quality search sites. Chapter 12 presents more on specifics for searching related to health care.

Transferring Files

One of the functions that most Internet users want is the ability to transfer files from a server on the Internet to their own computers. Before the advent of the Web, using the FTP (File Transfer Protocol) communications protocol and program was the only way to transfer files from one computer to another over the Internet. To do this, the user had to access FTP and then type commands such as "fetch" and "put" to tell the computer what to do. With today's Web browsers, transferring files is as simple as clicking a download button and telling the computer where to place the file. The FTP protocol functions behind the scenes of the Web browser.

Because of the file limitations of certain email programs, some organizations give their employees access to the organization's own FTP server so that they can move files around from one place to another. This process is generally faster and considered more secure than working over the Internet. There are no graphics on the FTP server—just the files. There are also no file size limitations, so this approach is the preferred choice when transferring large files. If you need to transfer a variety of other types of files, such as compressed (zip), program (exe), and database (mdbx) files, use of FTP may be necessary because some firewalls block files with these extensions. In contrast, if you need to save the current Web page in HTML format or capture a graphic, follow the directions given earlier in this chapter. The browser works well for transferring these files.

To use FTP, the following items are needed:

- A local computer that is capable of running FTP with an Internet connection.
- A remote computer running FTP with an Internet connection.
- The Internet address for the remote server. This is usually ftp.same-second-domain.same-high-level-domain.
- An account on the remote server (perhaps). Some FTP sites are run as anonymous sites, which means a login is not necessary or, if a login is necessary, the user ID is something like "anonymous" and the password consists of the user's email address or even nothing.

To access FTP through a Web browser:

1. Start the **Web browser**.
2. In the Address or Location text box, type **ftp://ftp.domain.topdomain**.
3. Log in if required.

4. Browse to find the **file** to transfer and **right-click** it, click **Save Target As**, or click the **Download** button if there is one.
5. Select a **location** in which to place the file and a **file name** if needed, and then click **Save**. The file will be transferred.

Two commonly used terms regarding transferring files are **download** and **upload.** Downloading is moving a file from one computer (generally a server) to another (generally a local PC). This generic term does not specify how you should accomplish this task, just that you transferred the files. Uploading is transferring a file from a local computer to a remote server (the reverse direction from downloading); use this process when moving local HTML files to a Web server for publishing on the Internet.

Here are some points to consider when retrieving files from the Internet:

- *Know what you want to download.* Some FTP sites are cryptic and assume that the user knows the file name and understands the site's organization. When at an FTP site, look for a file that describes the site and its organization; this file is usually a text file with the title "index," "read.me," or "files .lst." Select it, and read how things work at that site.
- *Keep security in mind.* Downloading files from the Internet can introduce a virus or malware into your system. Most sites take precautions to prevent viruses from entering their files, so the files will likely be clean. However, to be on the safe side, it does not hurt to check the downloaded files (especially files with an .exe or .com extension) with an antivirus program before installing them on the computer. Many experts believe that there is a greater chance of getting a virus from email files than from FTP sites.
- *Know the system requirements for the file.* Many sites assume that users know which operating system—Windows 7 or 8, Linux, or Mac OS X—they are using, as the site typically provides different versions of files for different systems. Many sites will also tell the downloader how large the file is, how much space is necessary on the hard drive to run the program, and how much memory the program requires. Make sure that the file is the correct one for the system you are using.
- *Obey copyright laws.* Several types of files are available for download. Freeware files are available without cost. For example, many free graphics files are available for use when you are creating Web pages. Although some are totally free for use, others have restrictions such as "free for use at nonprofit Web sites." If you use the file, some sites require acknowledgment of the developer or originating site on the Web site that uses the file. You can try Shareware files for free; if you like the program, you pay a small fee to

register it. Many times the registered version is a later, better version than the shareware one. Finally, you can download program or application files. Some of these programs provide a trial (limited) version; others require the user to buy the full program before downloading it. Trial versions usually last 30 days and then become unusable.

Failure to follow copyright laws can create serious legal problems for people who violate these laws.

Creating and Evaluating Web Pages

This section of the chapter provides an overview of creating Web pages and evaluating their design. It is not intended to make you a full-fledged Web designer, but focuses on providing some helpful information for design and evaluation. Chapter 12 presents material on evaluating the quality of the content of a Web site. After visiting various Web sites, most users begin to appreciate well-designed sites and develop criteria for what they find most appealing in a site's design. In addition, while many healthcare professionals may not do the actual coding for Web pages, they may provide input into the content and layout as well as the means by which users move around the site. This sort of assessment becomes easier when the professional has some basic background in Web design issues.

Creating Web Pages

Many Web page creators want to start the process by tagging the documents; that is a mistake. There is a structured process for designing Web pages. This process serves as a guide for things to consider when creating Web pages. Some of these guidelines might not apply when creating virtual health-related communities or using social media where users actively create content. Paying attention to these items at the beginning of the Web page development process will save time and energy in the long term.

- *Decide what the site is to accomplish.* Answer these questions: What is the intent of this site? What do I want to accomplish with this? What are the purposes and goals of this site? Create a statement that reflects the answers to these questions to serve as a guide during the development and maintenance of the Web site.
- *Identify the target audience to help focus the design and content.* Many Web sites are created without identifying the *who* — that is, the intended users of the site. A design that appeals to teenagers, for example, might not be appropriate for professional audiences.
- *Develop a site map showing the relationship between the parts.* Which pages will comprise the site? How will they link or relate to other pages? Keep in mind that users can access these pages in various ways and may not always land on the site's home page.

- *Develop criteria for inclusion of content.* How will developers make decisions about which content to include? What are the criteria for inclusion? Keep in mind the intent of the site and the target audience.
- *Decide who will be responsible for maintaining each part of the site.* Consider how often they will need to update the site pages, and then determine a schedule for reviewing and updating the parts. While the Webmaster is responsible for the design and coding of the Web site, others are generally responsible for creating the content.
- *Decide on the design that best presents the content.* A consistent look to the site helps keep the user oriented as to place. It is helpful to place navigational aids consistently in the same place on each page that identify the *who, what, when,* and *where* of the content. Make these navigational aids, such as buttons, easy to follow. Develop these standards at the beginning, and then use them consistently.

Once you address these guidelines, you should consider some specific things regarding design and layout. Although these points serve as a guide, good design is a matter of a person's own personal taste and style. Good design is mindful of the intent of the site and the target audience. Decide whether it is more important to have a flashy site, albeit one where some people may not be able to access all its features, or if it is more important that all people who use the site can access its features.

- *Consider differences in user resources.* Remember that some people still access the Internet through dial-up modems and not the faster Ethernet, cable, DSL, or fiber-optic connections. Graphics take longer to load than text, and the audience will be lost if they have to wait too long for the graphics. Use the 10-second rule: The page should load from many different types of connections in 10 seconds. Also, consider that not everyone uses the latest technology, so some users may not have the latest version of a browser or the same size monitor the developer used during the design of the Web site. When in doubt about design, keep it simple.
- *Design a template or layout to use with most of the pages.* Make sure that there is a descriptive title in the same place on every page along with buttons and navigational aids to take the user back to the home page or to other pages at this site. Also include identifying information, such as who created the page, when they created or last revised it, and how to contact the Webmaster with questions. Many pages also include relevant copyright information.
- *Use graphics and sound as appropriate.* Graphics and sounds should add to the content, not detract from it. Although it may be possible to place many graphics on the page, do not do so unless those images help convey the message of the page. Keep in mind two key rules: "Simpler is better" and "White

space is good." Many users find graphics and sound distracting; other users may access the page in settings where sound is distracting to others. Pay attention to copyright requirements, especially when using graphics others created.

- *Keep graphics reasonable in size.* Try to maintain a balance between size, resolution, color, and look. Keep the size between 25K and 30K with a resolution of 72 dpi if possible. Use the appropriate graphic file format—gif for images and jpg for photos. Use thumbnail graphics (small, postage stamp-sized pictures), and give the user the option to look at the graphic in a larger version. Keep in mind that what most users see when the page loads is the first 4 inches of a printed page.
- *Select colors carefully.* Make sure that the colors work together and are easy to read and pleasing to the eye. If the designer lacks color sense, someone else should select the color scheme; alternatively, the designer can use an already developed color scheme. Be especially careful with colors if users will be printing the Web pages.
- *Watch the use of videos.* They take up bandwidth and therefore need to add something important to the content. Alternatively, provide a link to a multimedia server hosting videos. Give some thought to the file format—will all people be able to view the video or is specific software required?
- Consider guidelines based on Section 508 of the The Rehabilitation Act which requires that Federal agencies' electronic and information technology is accessible to people with disabilities. Additional information on these requirements can be found at http://www.section508.gov/index.cfm?fuseAction=AboutUs

HTML Files

Once you design the documents in terms of layout and content, you need to code or tag them. The **Hypertext Markup Language (HTML)** provides a mechanism for displaying text- and graphics-based documents in Web browsers. **Tagging** describes the process of indicating the appearance of contents of a Web page by specifying fonts and font-related attributes as well as location or layout of the text and graphics. HTML code consists of a series of embedded tags in the Web document that tells the browser how to display the page. The tags look like the example here:

```
<HTML>
<HEAD>
<TITLE>Welcome to Healthcare Tips Online</TITLE>
</HEAD>
<BODY>The purpose of this Web site is to provide the general public with
several tips for working with healthcare providers and becoming intelligent
consumers of healthcare services.</BODY>
</HTML>
```

In this example, the first and last tags (<HTML> and </HTML>) tell the browser that this is an HTML file. Tags placed between the HEAD tags are for informational purposes and do not display in the browser window. The TITLE tag displays the Web page title in the title bar of the Web browser. All text between the BODY tags appears in the browser window.

When a browser locates a Web document by using the URL or through a link, it interprets these tags regardless of which platform the user is using. As a consequence, the display of Web pages on Windows, UNIX, and Macintosh computers basically looks the same.

Many tools are available for creating HTML documents. We can group them into three main categories:

- ASCII or text editors require the document creator to type the tags and text directly into the document. Notepad, which comes with the Windows operating system, is an example of an ASCII editor.
- HTML converter programs take a document created in another program and convert it to an HTML file by adding the tags. The Microsoft Office suite is an example of this type of program. The user saves this file as a Web page instead of a document spreadsheet, or PowerPoint file.
- HTML editors are software programs with a graphical user interface that help the developer create HTML files without having to type the tags. Expression Web (the replacement for FrontPage) and GoLive are popular HTML editors.

Each of these tools has advantages and disadvantages. For example, using a converter program such as Word results in documents appearing differently than they do in a word processing program. The program has to interpret the formatting and convert it into HTML tags. Because this conversion is not always done cleanly, the creator may need to play with the tags to ensure that the document will display correctly. ASCII or text editors are tedious to use but provide excellent control over the Web page. HTML editors are more powerful than converters, but the creator gives up some control over the Web page design. Exercises 4 and 5 provide experience with creating a simple Web page.

Remember that HTML tags create static Web pages. The trend today is for dynamic Web pages. A dynamic Web page is one on which the content changes in accordance with parameters that the user or program provides. Terms used to describe dynamic Web relate to scripting languages such as JavaScript , dynamic HTML (DHTML), and Flash technologies for media-type pages. These are predominantly on the client's computer. Other terms relate to server-side scripting such as Active Server pages (ASP), ColdFusion, PHP (Hypertext Preprocessor), and CGI (Common Gateway Interface) to name a few.

Summary

This chapter covered Internet basics, specifically terminology and concepts such as Web, URL, searching, and hyperlinks. An introduction to connecting to the Internet and the related requirements followed. It provided a brief orientation to the two most commonly used browsers, Microsoft Internet Explorer and Google Chrome, showing both their similarities and differences. The chapter concluded with a brief discussion of the Web page development process and the evaluation of Web page design.

References

Basu, S. (2010). 10 Search engines to explore the invisible web. Essex, UK: MakeUseOf Directory. Retrieved from http://www.makeuseof.com/tag/10-search-engines-explore-deep-invisible-web/

Cohen, L. (2013). The deep web. Albany, NY: International Tutorials. Retrieved from http://www.internettutorials.net/deepweb.asp

Internet World Stats (2013). Internet usage statistics: The internet big picture. Bogota, Columbia: Miniwatts Marketing Group: Internet World Stats. Retrieved from http://www.internetworldstats.com/stats.htm

Mell, P. and Grance, T. (2011). The NIST definition of cloud computing. NIST Special Publication 800-145. Gaithersburg, MD: National Institute of Standards and Technology (NIST), US Department of Commerce. Retrieved from http://www.nist.gov/itl/cloud/index.cfm

Additional Resources

Bare Bones (http://www.sc.edu/beaufort/library/pages/bones/bones.shtml): This site is a great tutorial site for learning about searching and search sites.

Medical Information on the Invisible Web (http://websearch.about.com/od/invisibleweb/a/medical.htm): This site is a good starting point.

Search Engine Showdown (http://searchengineshowdown.com): This site has some interesting statistics about search engines. It also includes some tutorials.

Search Engine Watch (http:/searchenginewatch.com): This site has excellent descriptions of searching and search engines. It tries to keep up to date with what is happening in the world of Internet searching. It is a good reference source.

Exercises 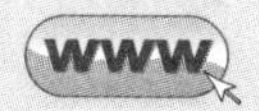

EXERCISE 1 What Can I Do with My Browser, Microsoft Internet Explorer?

■ **Objectives**

1. Define selected words related to the Internet.
2. Identify different types of Web addressing.
3. Use Internet Explorer to access the World Wide Web and to connect to different sites.
4. Organize favorites and add sites to a favorite's folder.
5. Print a document from the Internet.
6. Transfer both a home page and a graphic file from the Internet.

■ **Activity**

NOTE: If this file is provided to you in electronic format, place your answer in *italics* in this document. If no file is provided, open a blank Word document and place your answers there, along with the appropriate question number and letter

Basic Terms and Understanding

1. Use **Figure 9-10** to complete this puzzle. Submit according to directions provided by your professor; if in electronic form, use the snipping tool to paste it into your Word document.
2. Create another puzzle with at least eight terms excluding the ones used in number 1. Include such terms as 45.678.020.14 (IP address), example URL, example username, and so forth.
   a. Go to http://www.discoveryeducation.com/free-puzzlemaker/?CFID=537489&CFTOKEN=19584878 to create your puzzle.
   b. Follow the steps to **create** your puzzle.
   c. Use the snipping tool to **capture the puzzle** and copy it to a **Word** document.
   d. Submit the Word document as directed by your professor naming it **Chap9-Exercise1-1&2-LastName**. Alternatively you can post it to the discussion forum for classmates to see.
3. Do you know the host names? Place your answers in a Word document for 3 and 4.
   a. What might be the host name for a computer at the National Library of Medicine or Centers for Disease Control and Prevention?

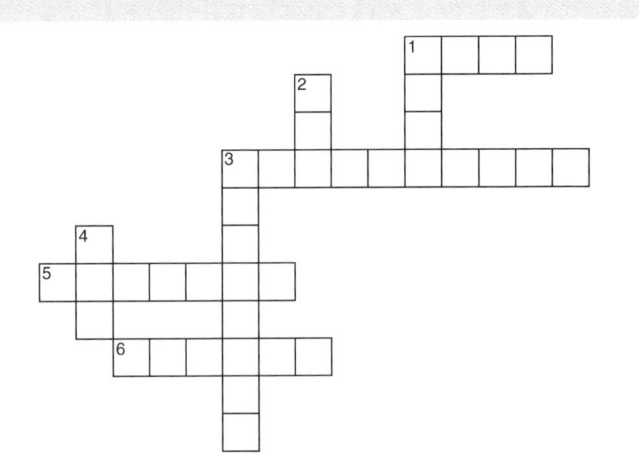

Across
1. Communications protocol for accessing and working with the Web
3. Text or graphics that provide additional information
5. Software for displaying Web pages
6. Address similar to a postal address but for the Internet

Down
1. Tagging language for displaying Web pages
2. Companies that provide access to the Internet
3. Main company page that opens when domain is typed
4. Helps to locate a Web page on a Web server

Figure 9-10 Puzzle of Internet Terms

b. Chris works part time for CVS Minute Clinic. What might be the host name for that site?
c. You are president of the local student organization chapter at your school. What might be the full Internet address of that organization?

4. Do you want to find out who owns a particular domain name?
   a. Open **Internet Explorer**.
   b. Type http://www.networksolutions.com/whois/index.jsp in the URL textbox and press **Enter**. The Network Solutions WHOIS page opens.
   c. Type **upmc.edu** in the search text box, and press **Enter**.
   d. Scroll down and answer this question: Who owns this domain name, and what is the primary IP address?
   e. Click the **Back** button on the browser toolbar. The Search window appears. Highlight the **text** in the search box.
   f. Type **WebMD.com** in the query text box, and press **Enter**. Answer this question: Who owns this domain name, and what is the primary IP address?

f. Click the **Back** button on the browser toolbar. The Search window appears.
g. **Highlight** the text in the search box.
h. Type **nursing.com** in the query box, and press **Enter**. Answer this question: Who owns this domain name, and what is the primary IP address?
i. Click the **Back** button on the browser toolbar. The Search window appears.
j. **Highlight** the text in the search box.
k. Type the **name of your local healthcare facility or school** in the query text box, and press **Enter**. Answer this question: Who owns this domain name, and what is the primary IP address? Why might this information be helpful to you as a healthcare professional?
l. Save your work as **Chap9-Exercise1-3-4-LastName**.

5. Use Internet Explorer to connect to sites.
   a. Click the **text** in the URL text box in Internet Explorer to highlight it.
   b. Type **http://www.mapquest.com** and press **Enter**.
   c. Click the **Search for** textbox, and type your **address**, **city**, **state**, and **ZIP code.**
   d. Click the **Get Map** button. A map of your location appears. How accurate is your map? Why might this information be helpful to a home healthcare professional?
   e. Click the **text** in the URL text box in Internet Explorer to highlight it.
   f. Type **weather.com** and press **Enter**.
   g. Type your **ZIP code** (your actual ZIP code, not the words) in the Zip text box and click **Search** or press **Enter**. Look around the site. What is the forecast for the next 10 days in your city? Why might this information be important to a home healthcare professional? To a patient?
6. Create and work with favorites.

NOTE: It may not be possible to complete this exercise on a public computer, as the system may prevent you from creating or customizing the system. Directions may be different for another version or operating system.

Organize Favorites and Add Sites

a. Click **View favorites, feeds, and history** button. Alternatively, you can select **Favorites** from the Menu bar. A menu appears.
b. Click **Add to Favorites down arrow** Add to favorites ▾.
c. Click **Organize favorites** option from the menu.
d. Click **New Folder** New Folder button.
e. Type **Informatics Resources** and click **Create** Create button.
f. Go to **http://www.informationweek.com/healthcare/mobile-wireless/10-medical-robots-that-could-change-heal/240143983?pgno=5** and click **View favorites, feeds, and history** button.

g. Click **Add to Favorites down arrow** Add to favorites button. Click **Add** button.
h. Repeat the process and create a second folder titled **Mobile Device Resources** in the Favorites folder. Go to **http://www.brookings.edu/~/media/research/files/papers/2012/5/22%20mobile%20health%20west/22%20mobile%20health%20west.pdf** and add that site to your **Favorites.**
i. Click **View favorites, feeds, and history** button and then **Add to Favorites down arrow** Add to favorites. Select **Organize favorites** option. You should see the two folders and two URLs as shown in **Figure 9-11**.

Add Some Sites to the Correct Folder

a. Open the **Organize favorites** dialog box.
b. Select the **10 Medical Robots URL** and click **Move** button. Select the **Informatics Resources** folder and click **OK**.

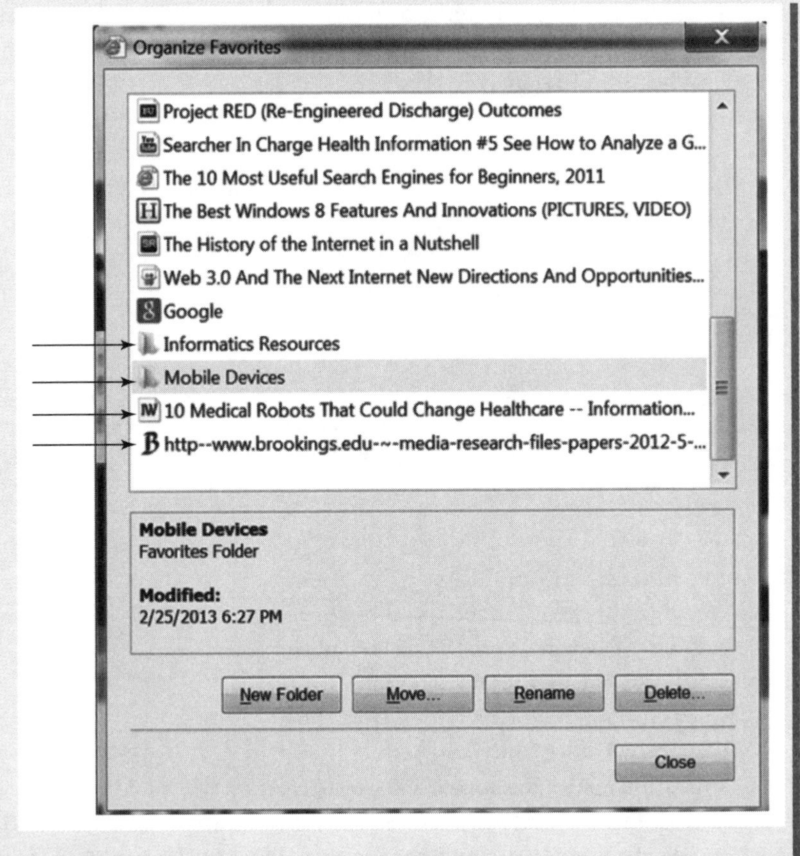

Figure 9-11 Organize Favorites Dialog Window—Internet Explorer

c. Click the **Brookings URL** and drag on top of the **Mobile Devices Resources** folder. Both files are now in their respective folders.

Note the rename and delete options in the Organize Favorites dialog box. Alternatively, you can place the favorite URL directly in the correct folder from the Add Favorite dialog window. Click **Create in down** arrow and select **Informatics Resources** folder.

7. Save Web pages.

Save Web Page as HTML Only

a. Type **www.cdc.gov** in the URL text box, and press **Enter**. The home page for the Centers for Disease Control and Prevention opens.
b. Look around the site to find the **Fast Fact** page on Pertussis (Whooping Cough).
c. Select **File**, **Save as** from the Menu bar if you are displaying the Menu bar or click the **Page Down arrow** from the toolbar and select **Save As**. Make sure to select the correct location and save it as **HTML only**. Click the **Save** button.
d. Open **Word** and the **Pertussis** file. What do you notice about this file?
e. Close **Word**.

Save a Graphic from a Web Page

a. Type **google.com** in the URL text box, and press **Enter**.
b. Click **Images** under the browser tab (found at the upper-left corner of the window).
c. Type **health care** in the search box and click the **search by image** button.
d. Look around at the images. **Right-click** on an image of your choice and select **Save picture as**.
e. Select the **location** and **file name** (if it needs to be changed). The file is now on your storage device.

8. Create a folder titled **Chap9-Exercise1-LastName**. Place all your work in that folder and then zip it (right-click the **folder**, **Send to**, **Compressed (zipped) folder**). Submit the compressed folder to the professor as directed.

EXERCISE 2 How Do I Learn More Features or Use Another Browser?

■ **Objectives**

1. Find help for learning two new features in Internet Explorer.
2. Investigate help available for learning Chrome.
3. Present the new features learned about Internet Explorer and why those features were important to you.
4. Demonstrate how to use selected features of Chrome.

■ **Activity**

New versions and new browsers appear regularly as technology grows and develops. Learning where to look for help and how to adjust to new versions are important skills for adapting to the changing Internet world.

1. Use your favorite search site and search for a help guide or tutorial on learning Internet Explorer features. Share the URL for that site with your classmates and professor. Why is it a good site?
2. List two new things you learned how to do with Internet Explorer. For example, how do you set trusted sites or permit pop-ups from certain sites?
3. Find a good help site for learning Chrome. Share the URL with your classmates and professor.
4. Now, using what you learned, repeat Exercise 1 using Chrome instead of Internet Explorer. How easy or hard was it to learn new features of a browser?

EXERCISE 3 Why Do I Need a Plug-in or Add-on?

■ **Objectives**

1. Define the terms plug-in, add-on, browser apps, and HTML5.
2. Provide an example of a plug-in, add-on, and browser app.
3. Explain why you would want to use these and what is happening with HTML5.
4. Install one of them in your browser.

■ **Activity**

1. Use a search site and search for the definitions of the words in Objective 1.
2. Open Word and place a definition for each term and the source for the definition. Provide an example of that term underneath the definition.
3. Provide a one-paragraph history of the development of those terms. Why were they needed? What functionality do they provide to a browser?
4. Select one of the plug-ins, add-ons, or apps in your browser. Look around the browser for a listing of plug-ins, add-ons, or apps installed with your browser.
5. Use the snipping tool or screen capture button to capture that screen. Paste it at the end of the Word document.
6. Save the Word document as **Chap9-Exercise3-LastName** and submit as directed by your professor.

EXERCISE 4 How Do I Select a Browser?

■ **Objectives**

1. Identify differences and similarities between browsers.
2. Review the steps for selecting a browser.
3. Using the steps provided, select one, and justify why you chose it.

■ **Activity**

1. Conduct some research and determine the most common features in browsers that are important to you.
2. Go to **http://www.wikihow.com/Choose-an-Internet-Browser** and read the steps for selecting a browser.
3. Follow those steps and select a browser that meets your needs.
4. Discuss with your classmates why you selected that browser. Why might you want to have two or three browsers installed on your computer? Under which circumstances might you use each?

EXERCISE 5 How Do I Select a Search Site?

■ **Objectives**

1. Determine the type of searching needed and the best search site for that type of searching.
2. Conduct three searches using the recommended search site.
3. Compare the results of the searches.

■ **Activity**

1. Go to this site **http://www.noodletools.com/debbie/literacies/information/5locate/adviceengine.html** and review the suggestions for different types of searching. Do you agree or disagree with the recommendations?
2. Select three types of searches you recently conducted or need to conduct this semester. Repeat them and note the results—number of hits, quality of hits, number of irrelevant returns, and so forth.
3. Try the recommendations for search sites from step 1.
4. Compare the results to those from 2 and 3. Which were better? Will this affect your future searching?
5. Create a Word document with your responses and save it as **Chap9-Exercise5-LastName**. Submit your Word document as directed by the professor.

EXERCISE 6 What Is a Vertical Search Site and Will It Access the Deep Web?

■ **Objectives**

1. Use the information from a tutorial to write a brief description of a vertical search engine.

2. Confirm that definition with another source.
3. Search a Deep Web search site.
4. Describe the results of the research.

■ **Activity**

1. Check out this tutorial at http://www.internettutorials.net/. Look around the site for **vertical search engines**.
2. Review the information provided on the vertical search engine page.
3. Click the **WedNar** link.
4. Search on **nursing informatics**.
5. Look around this site.
   - What types of materials are in its collection?

HINT: Scroll to the bottom and click the **down arrow** in the Limit to 

button.

   - Click the **Topics** tab. What information does it provide?
   - Click the **Visual** tab. What did you see?
6. Now, conduct a search relevant to your discipline.
7. Describe the results.
8. Is this site accessing the Deep Web? Explain your answer.
9. Create a Word document, PowerPoint presentation, or a Podcast to explain what you did and found in this exercise.

EXERCISE 7 Where Are We Going with Interactivity?

■ **Objectives**

1. Examine the concept of the interactivity on the Web.
2. Identify what this might mean to searching and using the Internet.

■ **Activity**

1. Go to **http://www.instagrok.com/**
2. Set the difficulty to **college level** (move to far right)
3. Type **nurse** in the search box. What concepts did it show that relates to the word nurse?
4. Click the concept **clinic**. What happens?
5. Click back on **nurse** and view the **links** on the right side of the window. What do you think of the links? Where they quality sites? Images? Videos? Can you customize the concept map?

6. Pick another word related to a concept important to you in your practice. Search using that word. What are the results?
7. How do you see this type of site helping you with the idea of concept mapping and searching? As a health professional, how do you see this helping with other professionals and your patients?

Assignments

ASSIGNMENT 1 Searching the Internet

Directions

Use a search site to answer these questions.

1. What are streaming applications?
2. What is the difference between downloaded and streaming audio and video?
3. What is the current problem with streaming audio/video on campus or from a modem connection?
4. Find a Web radio station and describe it here. What is the advantage of Web radio?

ASSIGNMENT 2 Why an E-portfolio?

Directions

1. Many schools are requiring students to prepare an e-portfolio as part of their graduation requirements given the nature of assessment in today's accrediting climate. One needs to start early to assemble this portfolio.
2. Search on portfolios and their uses. Check out whether your school has specific requirements for them.
3. Think about exercises or assignments you completed in this chapter.
4. Select two of the exercises or assignments that demonstrate your ability to find relevant information on a topic or skill in using the Internet.
5. Write a one-page summary explaining what you learned from the activity and how it might help you in your profession.
6. Add the summary and the documents to your e-portfolio as directed by your faculty member. This task may require access to Web sites or specific software that is provided by your school. If your school has no e-portfolio process, create a PowerPoint presentation highlighting the material, which follows the guidelines on creating quality presentations found in Chapter 6. You may also use OneNote to add the information and to start an e-portfolio.

chapter

10

Technology-Assisted Communication and Collaboration

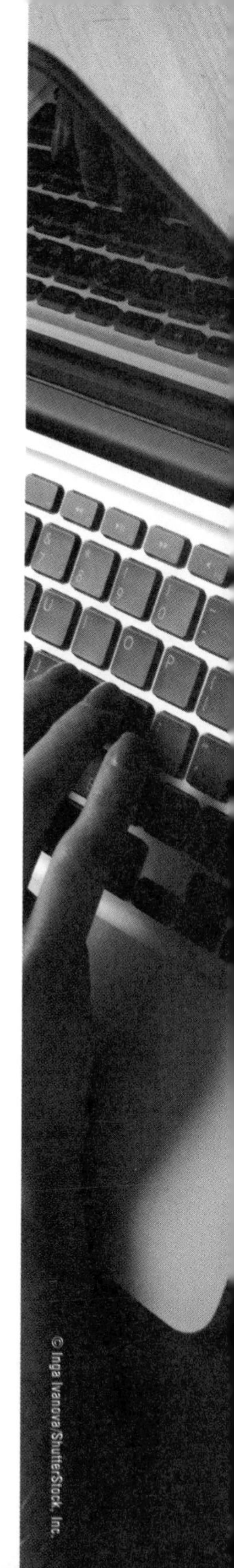

Objectives

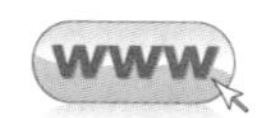

1. Compare and contrast Web 1.0 and Web 2.0.
2. Discuss general guidelines for the safe and effective use of social media.
3. Explore the purpose(s) and functioning of social media applications such as electronic discussion groups, bulletin boards, social networking sites, blogs, and wikis.
4. Identify and manage security threats when using social media sites.
5. Apply professional guidelines and resources for using social media.

Introduction

Communication and collaboration describe processes where two or more people cooperatively work together by sharing and creating new information and knowledge. In **technology-assisted communication and collaboration,** people use computer/information systems for both the communication and the collaboration processes by which they share information and create new information. This chapter focuses on Internet-based applications that you use to support the communication and collaboration process; it also explores the functionality of common Web 2.0 applications. The emphasis is on working collaboratively online for educational and professional development.

Terms Related to Computer-Assisted Communication and Collaboration

The following terms are important to understand when examining different technology/information-assisted collaboration modalities. More specific information about some of these terms appears later in the chapter.

Aggregator	An **aggregator** is a software application or program that collects information from various online sources, such as blogs, podcasts, and Web sites, for the purpose of showing that information in a single view.
Blog	A **blog** is a self-published Web site containing dated material, usually in journal format. Blogs can contain text, pictures, video, audio, and URLs of other relevant sites. Blogs generally permit readers to post their comments and reactions. Mini-blogs, or tweets, are growing in popularity. A well recognized example is Twitter which restricts posting or tweets to 140 characters.
Bulletin Board	A **bulletin board** is a public area for messages; it is similar to its counterpart that hangs on a wall. The organization of bulletin boards revolves around specific topics and might be part of an online service that you access through Internet search engines. Bulletin boards might be open to everyone, or they might be restricted to members of certain groups and accessed through passwords. Several examples of health-related bulletin boards are at http://www.healthboards.com/.
Chat	A **chat** is real-time communication between two or more users via a computer or mobile device. Most online businesses offer built-in chat features on their Web sites.
Chat Room	A **chat room** is a designated area or "room" where individuals gather simultaneously and "talk" to one another by typing messages. Everyone who is online usually sees the messages. Some students might "visit" their professor in a chat room during virtual office hours when taking online courses.
Electronic Discussion Group	An **electronic discussion group** is an email service in which individual members post messages for all group members to read.

Emoticon **Emoticon** is a way to show an emotion via text on the computer. These symbols or combinations of symbols substitute for facial expressions, body language, and voice inflections.

Instant Messaging (IM) **Instant messaging (IM)** is a communication service that permits you to send real-time messages via a private chat room to other individuals who are online. You may have several different IMs going on at the same time with different friends that you have added to your buddy list. Because there are no standards for IM systems, individuals communicating with one another must register through the same system to get an IM address. A mobile version of IM is the mobile instant messaging (MIM) technology. This permits instant messaging services accessible from a portable device like a smartphone.

Internet Conferencing **Internet conferencing** is a type of communication in which two or more people interact over the Internet in real time, receiving more or less immediate replies. This communication can involve interaction via text, audio, or video.

ListServ **ListServ** is the trade name of a software program that manages automated discussion lists. This term is commonly used to refer to all mailing lists (just as "xerox" is often used to refer to all photocopiers, not just those manufactured by Xerox). When someone posts a message to a discussion list, everyone on the mailing list receives the message via email.

Newsgroup A **newsgroup** is Internet-based discussion of informational material and articles organized around a particular topic, such as Alzheimer's disease or child abuse. Newsreaders can post a message to the newsgroup for all to read and respond to. To participate in a newsgroup, you need to have newsreader software. Microsoft Outlook provides a newsreader, but you need to add the News Command and subscribe to a newsgroup to use it.

Really Simple Syndication (RSS) **Really simple syndication (RSS)** is a scheme that makes it possible for users to subscribe to and receive information about a specific topic that others have posted to blogs, podcasts, and other social networking applications. The RSS delivers this aggregated information back through a feed and the content might then be read through a feed reader or email message.

Social Media — **Social media** consists of Web-based and mobile technologies that support social networking and microblogging activities, which turn the one-way communication of Web 1.0 into an interactive dialog, where users create online communities to share information, ideas, personal messages, and other content (Nelson, Joos, Wolf, 2013).

Social Networking — **Social networking** refers to activities, such as connecting and communicating, that you initiate through a social media site.

Spim — **Spim** is the spam of instant messaging. Part spam and part instant message, an increasing number of advertisers are using Spim.

Tags — **Tags** are terms that function as keywords associated with online content, such as blog postings, bookmarks, and Web sites. Tags make it possible for an aggregator to effectively search the Internet and group related information. Microsoft Office documents can now have tags associated with them.

Web 2.0 — **Web 2.0** is the second generation of Web utilization. This term does not refer to a change in technology, but rather a change in the creative use of Web technology and applications to enhance and expand information sharing, communication, and collaboration. Examples of Web 2.0 include the evolution of Web-culture communities, social networking sites, video-sharing sites, and blogs.

Webinar — A **webinar** is an interactive presentation, lecture, workshop, or seminar that the presenter(s) delivers over the Internet. In many cases, the participants can ask questions or offer comments via a chat or a voice application.

Wiki — A **wiki** is a Web site that permits users to collaborate in creating and editing a document using a Web browser. Users can add, edit, or delete content on the wiki.

Understanding Web 1.0 and Web 2.0

Initial Internet applications were designed for accessing information as opposed to creating information. As described in Chapter 9, starting in the early 1990s Web sites posted information and users accessed this information using a browser. In the late 1990s a number of new applications with the functionality to share and cooperatively create new information began to evolve. The new applications did not change the technical specifications that were used to build the World Wide Web, but rather represented a change in how the Web was being used. This interactive approach to how the Internet is being used is now often referred to as Web 2.0, in contrast to the previous static approach that has been labeled **Web 1.0.**

It is believed that Darcy DiNucci was the first to use the term Web 2.0 in 1999 in an English language publication; however, Tim O'Reilly is often credited with the first detailed description of the concept. **Table 10-1** lists selected characteristics associated with Web 1.0 and Web 2.0. In analyzing the differences between them it is important to appreciate that Web 2.0 does not replace Web 1.0 but rather builds on and exists in concert with Web 1.0. For example, publishing is associated with Web 1.0; however, the process of open review for online articles demonstrates Web 1.0 characteristics when a journal article is published on the Internet and demonstrates Web 2.0 characteristics when online readers post their criticisms, comments, and suggestions.

TABLE 10-1 CHARACTERISTICS OF WEB 1.0 AND WEB 2.0

Web 1.0	Web 2.0
Static—does not adapt to the user.	Interactive with the user modifying the format and creating the content.
Information created by experts. The credentials of the expert(s) determine the credibility of the site.	Information created by interaction of experts and users. The quality of the information evolves and improves over time.
Personal Web site.	Social media sites for blogging, photo sharing, and so forth.
Publishing.	Participating.
Value is in the information.	Value is in the ability to adapt and grow the information.
Standard languages.	Tagging—labels created by the user.
The Internet is the application.	The Internet is a platform for creating applications.

Just as people communicate for a variety of purposes, so too can they use these tools to support a variety of activities. Healthcare professionals should consider how they can use these tools to support their professional communication as well as how patients and healthcare consumers might use them to deal with health and other personal issues. With this goal in mind a discussion of online group communication and processes follows.

Online Group Communication

In 1964, Marshall McLuhan introduced the phrase "The medium is the message, in a book entitled *Understanding Media: The Extensions of Man*. Three years later he published a second book, *The Medium Is the Massage*. The original title planned for the book was *The Medium Is the Message* but a proofreader made an error and McLuhan preferred the error—reflected the reality that society was increasingly moving to a world of mass media and mass communication. McLuhan died in 1980 and may not have envisioned Web 1.0, let alone Web 2.0. But he understood that a message is transmitted via a channel and that the media used to create that channel can inform and embellish how that message is perceived and understood by individuals within a group and by the group as a whole (Gibson, 2008). For example, the same words that you use to say something face-to-face can take on a very different meaning if you send them by email and an even different meaning if you post them on a discussion board. As a professional working with colleagues and patients, it is important for you to appreciate how the medium of online communication can affect the message and, in turn, the communication process.

Factors Impacting Online Communication

The characteristics of social media-based communication can be described as mainly time-independent, text-based, and computer-mediated (Wilson, Nolla, and Gunawardena, 2005). The term computer-mediated indicates that the specific application will play a major role in influencing how a message is structured as well as in the meaning of the message. For example, Facebook, which tends to focus on personal relationships, uses a timeline to organize comments, activities, pictures, and events posted on an individual's site. Twitter limits messages to 140 characters and transmits bits of information. Pinterest uses a bulletin board format and messages that rely heavily on images.

The purpose of the application will also impact how and what people communicate within that application. For example, Wikipedia is "the free encyclopedia that anyone can edit" (Wikipedia, n.d.). Wikipedia as an encyclopedia does not publish original research—that is not the purpose of an encyclopedia (Wikipedia: What Wikipedia is not, n.d.). LinkedIn is designed to support the development of professional relationships while Facebook is more supportive of personal relationships. While communication styles on a social networking site tend to be informal, communication on LinkedIn is for the most part more formal than communication on Facebook. Understanding the purpose of a social media application and the networking culture can be key to achieving successful relationships and effective communication.

Many social media sites are asynchronous or time-independent. This means that people can add their comments and postings at a time that is convenient for them. It also means that when posting, individuals can take their time by carefully thinking through what they want to say, picking their words, and constructing their comments. However, that also means that as different people are commenting at different points, the flow of the conversation can be disjointed and difficult to follow. In addition, you can post a comment and no one might respond to it. Similar to a situation in which no one responds to a comment you have made in a face-to-face interaction, a lack of response in an asynchronous social media environment can produce a sense of anxiety.

Although pictures and video are used in social networking, the predominant communication is text-based. The inability to actually see the general appearance of others in the group, along with the absence of body language and intonation, make it much more likely for misunderstandings to occur. For example, a younger student in an online class who has unsuccessfully tried to "friend" a great-grandparent might post a comment suggesting that older people have problems with technology. Older students in the class might take offense and express their dissatisfaction with this generalization. While the older students might have meant to gently point out that care should be taken when generalizing, the lack of body language and intonation make it likely that their remarks will also be misinterpreted by the younger student. Text-based communication can be more effective in putting the focus on ideas rather than the personalities.

Online Tools for Collaboration

As Web 2.0 has evolved, a number of tools and applications have been developed to support online collaboration and creativity. These applications as a group are frequently referred to as social media. In this chapter, we will introduce the major types of Web 2.0 applications with an emphasis on professional use of social media. **Box 10-1** provides general guidelines for using Web 2.0 applications and for participating on social networking sites.

Box 10-1 Communication Tips for Social Media

1. When creating an account on a social media site, take the time to review the *Terms and Conditions* as well as the *Privacy Statements*. These documents are actually formal contracts. If you click *I accept this*, it is the same as signing a formal contract.
2. Begin exploring a new social media site by checking the Help section. Before you actually start to use the site, be sure your understand how to configure your settings—especially the privacy-related settings for the site. After you use the site and become comfortable with how the site actually operates, review the privacy settings again. At this point you will have a better understanding of these settings and can more effectively configure them.
3. Be honest but avoid overexposure. You should refuse to use a site if you must publicly post personally identifiable information such as your birthday, gender, address, or phone number. Begin by setting up a free email account that does not require public posting of your actual name or other identifying information.
4. Do not set up false accounts. It can actually be illegal to set up a false identity on a social media site. This is because sexual predators and other scammers like to use false identities.
5. Remember that *everything* posted on the Internet is public and permanent. Marking something private does not guarantee it will remain private. For example, both Facebook and Google have paid substantial fines to the Federal Trade Commission for failure to maintain the privacy of data they had promised to protect.

   The FTC has accepted as final a settlement with Facebook resolving charges that Facebook deceived consumers by telling them they could keep their information on Facebook private, and then repeatedly allowing it to be shared and made public (FTCa, 2012).

   Google, Inc. has agreed to pay a record $22.5 million civil penalty to settle Federal Trade Commission charges that it misrepresented to users of Apple, Inc.'s Safari Internet browser that it would not place tracking "cookies" or serve targeted ads to those users, violating an earlier privacy settlement between the company and the FTC (FTCb, 2012).
6. Social media accounts can be established for social as well as professional reasons. Maintain your professional identity by not mixing business and pleasure. When you establish an account carefully think about why you have this account and who you hope to interact with on this social media site. This means you might have a social media account for interacting with patients and consumers

such as an online support group. You might have another account in a different social media setting for interacting with professional colleagues and you might establish a third site for interacting with friends and family.

7. Remember when you collaborate on professional sites you don't have to like people to work with them. As in your face-to-face professional life, it is important to manage personal conflict so that avoidable conflict does not get in the way of the progress of the group as a whole. If you start to feel that conflict is developing, try to ask nonthreatening questions that help to explore an issue rather than be confrontational in stating your position.
8. Successful social media collaboration depends on the full participation of group members. Social media collaboration by definition relies on multiple ideas and perspectives. While you work to understand the views of others, actively share your view with tact and clear rationale.
9. Always consider online course work related to group projects and collaboration as part of your professional life. Relationships established with classmates, faculty, staff, and administrators can become an important part of your professional network throughout your career.
10. Learn how to say good-bye when leaving a social media site. Social media sites rarely involve lifelong commitments. If you have not used a specific social media site for some time, you should consider making the account inactive or canceling the account. Over time, social media sites can include a collection of contacts with whom you are no longer involved. You may need to reorganize your professional contacts and your personal contacts. A short note to professional contacts explaining that you are, for example, limiting your Facebook page to mainly family and very close friends, but would like to keep in touch via LinkedIn can be more effective than just disappearing. A short note explaining to an online support group that you have another work assignment and will no longer be part of the group is much more professional than just disappearing.

References

Federal Trade Commission (FTCa) (2012). Press Release: *FTC Approves Final Settlement With Facebook.* Retrieved from http://www.ftc.gov/opa/2012/08/facebook.shtm

Federal Trade Commission (FTCb) (2012). Press Release: *Google Will Pay $22.5 Million to Settle FTC Charges it Misrepresented Privacy Assurances to Users of Apple's Safari Internet Browser.* Retrieved from http://ftc.gov/opa/2012/08/google.shtm

Electronic Mailing Lists or Discussion Groups

People with common interests frequently join with like-minded individuals to form an organization. The types of interests and the structures of these organizations vary widely. The joining of people with common interests also occurs in the virtual world of the Internet. One of the earliest types of online discussion groups is an electronic discussion group, based on the concept of an email distribution list. These groups are often referred to in terms of the applications that are used to manage these groups. One of the most common examples of such a term is "listserv," which refers to the name of the software program used to support the functioning of the electronic discussion group. It is often used in place of the term "online discussion group." Examples of online discussion group software programs include ListProc, ListServ, and Majordomo (Hopkins, 2011). Note however that in some environments electronic discussion groups are gradually being replaced with other social media such as Twitter and blogs.

An **electronic discussion group** software application maintains the mailing list for a group of people with common interests. The membership list includes the group of people who have joined together by subscribing to the same list. The discussion group will have a computer name that reflects the interest of the group. For example, SNURSE-L is the name of an international electronic discussion group for nursing students. To communicate with other people on the list, participants send messages to the discussion group's email address. The software then sends the message to all individual member's email address. When the message is distributed to each member on the list, it is referred to as being "posted to the group."

Electronic discussion groups may be either moderated or unmoderated. On a moderated list, the list moderator reviews and approves each email message before it is posted. On an unmoderated list, no one reviews posts before they are sent to members. Most lists are unmoderated. The discussion group relies on the integrity of its members as well as online peer pressure to encourage participants to abide by the list rules. An unmoderated list will develop its own culture, so not all of the rules will necessarily be documented. For example, on some discussion groups, announcements of job opportunities are welcome. On others, these messages are considered off topic and not welcome.

To join the group (to subscribe), individuals send an email message to the application email address. This email address is different from the one you use to post messages to the discussion group. Because a computer program will read and answer the subscription request, the message must follow the specific format required by that application. If the discussion group is moderated, the moderator will read the request. In either case, you will receive a response to your email letting you know if you are subscribed. If you were successful in your request the response will include commands employed for communication with the discussion group application software and the address to use when posting a message. Be sure to save these directions for later use after subscribing. With most discussion groups, you can also access the specific procedures for joining and posting messages either through email or on the Web site that introduces the electronic discussion group.

Finding and Joining an Electronic Discussion Group

The most effective way to find a discussion list managed by ListServe is to search the CataList, which is the official catalog of ListServe lists maintained by L-Soft international, Inc. at http://www.lsoft.com/lists/list_q.html. ListServe is a commercial product and L-Soft is the vendor for this product. This service, however, does not provide the names of lists managed by the ListProc or Majordomo applications. The best way to find electronic discussion lists managed by these applications is through an Internet search engine.

Use the results in CataList to access more specific instructions for subscribing to an individual list. Procedures for joining electronic discussion groups are similar. The following steps represent the typical approach to joining a list:

1. Address the email message to the appropriate email address for subscribing. This is not the same email address that members use for posting to the discussion. For example, use listserv@lists.psu.edu to subscribe to the ListServe that Penn State University maintains. A complete list of the Penn State university discussion groups is at http://lists.psu.edu/cgi-bin/wa?HOME. Listserv@listserv.arizona.edu is the address for subscribing to an electronic discussion group that the University of Arizona maintains. A complete list of online discussion groups that the University of Arizona hosts is at http://www.lsoft.com/scripts/wl.exe?XH=LISTSERV.ARIZONA.EDU.
2. Put no other information in the header. Leave the subject line blank.
3. In the body of the message, type the following: **subscribe <list name> <firstname lastname>** (for example, subscribe nursenet Nancy Smith). Some online discussion group software programs accept the word "sub" in place of the word "subscribe," whereas others require the word "join." Some online discussion group software programs require your email address rather than the first and last names. Sometimes no names are necessary. For example, if you wish to subscribe to the Online Journal of Nursing Informatics list that Penn State maintains you would only include SUBSCRIBE OJNI-L in the body of the message.
4. Put no other information in the body of the email message. Do not sign your name, include your signature file, or thank the online discussion group. Remember that this message is *not* a communication with a person but is rather a set of commands that you are sending to a computer.

5. If the attempt to subscribe is unsuccessful, the software program will email back an error message. This message will try to indicate the type of mistake. If the message is not meaningful, get help at the local site.
6. If the attempt to subscribe is successful, a welcome message from the online discussion group will arrive. The initial email may ask that you confirm the subscription by clicking on a link or replying to the email. Once you are subscribed, you will receive an email with a great deal of information that is not entirely meaningful initially. Even so, save this message as it includes specific directions for interacting in the discussion group and other commands for managing your subscription.
7. If there is a time period when you anticipate that your participation in the online discussion group will decrease and you will not read the group's email, send a message to the online discussion group to suspend the email service. To stop receiving email from the list, send an "unsubscribe" message to the correct electronic discussion list address. The specific directions for suspending email or for unsubscribing are generally found in the list welcome message. Failure to stop online discussion group email may result in a full mailbox, with messages bouncing back to the online discussion group. This is very poor list etiquette.

Posting an Email Message to a List

It is wise to read several postings on a list before posting your own message. Each list has its own culture. It is helpful to know the list and the nature of the list before posting.

1. Send the appropriate message to the list's address. For example, DINF (dental informatics) is a forum for people interested in dental informatics. Note the difference in the list's address for posting messages (dinf@listserv.adea.org) and the address for subscribing to the list (listserv@listserv.adea.org). In both cases, the domain part of the address is the same, but the user ID part of the address is different. When posting a message to the list, users are communicating with people and not a computer.
2. Put the topic of the message in the subject line. This information is very helpful to receivers when they are reading their email directory. If the posting is a response to another person's email, use the same words to identify the subject topic as the previous sender used. Many email programs will insert the subject and address automatically if you select the reply function. If selecting the reply function with an email message from online discussion group software, confirm that the email program inserted the correct list address before posting the message. For example, if you only want to respond to the person who posted the initial message make sure you are not replying to the entire list. Posters can send a message with a request

that the response be made “offline.” This means the poster is requesting that you respond directly to them and not to the full list.

3. When typing the message, use appropriate netiquette, as discussed in Chapter 1.
4. Because some email programs clip off the header on incoming messages, always end the message with your name and email address.

Usenet Newsgroups

Usenet is a form of an online bulletin board system. With this service, users read and post messages or articles in categories called newsgroups. There is no central server but rather a large, constantly changing group of servers that store and forward messages. Use of newsgroups requires access to a newsgroup provider and a newsreader to interact with the group. Today, most Web browsers have newsreaders built into them, which has allowed more people to become involved in newsgroups. Most universities subscribe to a provider, but if you do not have access via your university a list of providers is at http://www.harley.com/usenet/newsgroup-reviews/newsgroup-reviews.html.

Newsgroups are organized by topics in a hierarchical tree structure. There are 17 topics at the root level. The first part of a newsgroup name is the hierarchy in which the group exists. Each successive part of the group name describes the group in more detail. A dot (.) is used between each part of the name. For example, the newsgroup related to nursing is named sci.med.nursing. The newsgroup for nurse practitioners is named alt.npractitioners.

Google has added another layer to the newsgroup concept. It provides a service that maintains a list of newsgroups and allows Web access using its Groups functionality. With this approach, you do not need a newsreader. Users can now search the Usenet archives back to 1981. The archives from the newsgroups can be searched in the same way that the Web is searched (Google, 2012). Additional information including tutorials with detailed directions and guidelines can be found at http://www.harley.com/usenet/index.html.

Internet or Web Conferencing

Internet or **Web conferencing** permits point-to-point (between two people) or multipoint (three or more people) conferencing using technologies and the Internet. The participants engage in real-time conversations and receive more or less immediate replies, depending on the speed of their connections. Each participant uses a video camera, microphone, and speakers, many of which are built into our devices. The participants’ voices and images transmit over the network. Web conferencing software facilitates initiating and participating in the live conference. Examples of programs used to facilitate Internet conferencing are Skype (purchased by Microsoft), ooVoo, Google video, Tango, and FaceTime to name a few.

Each has its pluses and minuses. On the higher end for multipoint conferencing are systems like WebEx, Adobe Connect, and MegaMeeting.

Some things to consider when selecting a conferencing tool are costs and features like call recording, desktop sharing, high definition video streaming, number of participants, security, and ease of use. Consider why you need a Web conference and what you hope to accomplish with the call. Answers to these questions will help you determine the features that will be necessary.

Chat, or text-based interaction, was the original form of this type of Internet communication. Now audio and video conferencing via the Internet are commonplace. With the changing demographics and the increasing need for health care, you will see more healthcare providers and consumers engaged in the use of Web conferencing. The concerns you must keep in mind when using these tools are cost, security, privacy, and infrastructure improvements.

Chat

Chat can be a function within another program or a standalone application. There are four basic uses for chat:

1. Support services on a Web site, for example, when shopping.
2. Questions and comments as part of a webinar.
3. Standalone applications for instant communication with friends or colleagues.
4. Participation in a chat session with classmates or colleagues.

Although some chat services support graphics and voice, the basic chat interface is text. In text chat, two or more people communicate by typing messages that appear in a text window, which can be visible to the other people in the same chat room. People use chat to communicate about specific topics because it offers a more rapid response than email. Many online vendors use chat to answer questions when you are shopping. Chat rooms are one of the most commonly used resources on the Internet. However, as with chatting in a crowded room, often many simultaneous conversations are taking place. In text chat, the participant will see all of the messages that are part of those different conversations in the order people have entered them into the system. Thus, following the sequence of a particular line of the conversation may be confusing.

Most chat systems allow participants to send private messages to individuals in the chat room as well as to participate with the group. If you are trying to communicate with one or two people it may be better to move into a private chat. Some chat programs, such as ICQ (http://www.icq.com) and Google chat, allow users to compile a "buddy list" of friends on the Internet. Using these programs, you can set up personal chats and/or chat rooms and chat privately with friends. Most course management applications, such as Blackboard, include a chat function for use within a specific course. These programs follow a common protocol:

1. Register as required by the chat room before you can log in. As part of that process, you will select your user name, which is the name that everyone else in the chat room will see. In public chat rooms, nicknames are recommended to ensure better privacy. As with other user IDs, each name must be unique. In Blackboard or other course management programs, there is no additional registration required; once you log in to the course management program, you have access to the chat feature. Note that many social media sites have chat capabilities built in.
2. Log in and read the messages in the current chat session. Messages from those participating in the chat session as well, as system messages and information about people entering and leaving the room, can appear in a box on the screen. Each message is preceded by the user's name to ensure that each participant can tell who said what.
3. When you are ready to participate, type your message into the text entry box, and press Enter.

Using one of the many search engines on the Internet, it is possible to find a chat room of interest. Indeed, most search engines support chat rooms and private chats. Chat rooms are usually organized around topics of interest, age, or other categories. Many Web sites also include topic-specific chat rooms.

Chat rooms can be dangerous; this is rarely a problem, however, when participating in class-related chats under the direction of a teacher or professional organization. The dangers of chat rooms usually involve dealing with strangers who have unsavory ulterior motives. This can be a danger with any Internet-related communication, but synchronous communication and the expectation of an immediate response accentuates the danger. Health professionals working with children should be especially aware of these dangers and be prepared to provide appropriate information for parents and their children. **Table 10-2** provides several resources to support this education.

Chatiquette is similar to **netiquette** in terms of the words and behavior acceptable while participating in a chat room. For more information about chatiquette, visit http://www.ker95.com/chat101/html/chatiquette.html. Information on chatiquette as it applies to an online class can be found here:

- http://www.innovateonline.info/pdf/vol2_issue5/Synchronous_Discussion_in_Online_Courses-__A_Pedagogical_Strategy_for_Taming_the_Chat_Beast.pdf
- http://ed.fnal.gov/lincon/act/intro/chatiquette.shtml

TABLE 10-2 INTERNET-RELATED RESOURCES FOR CHILDREN AND PARENT EDUCATION

Organization: Documentation	URL
California (ca.gov): Cyber Safety for Children!	http://oag.ca.gov/cybersafety
FBI: A Parent's Guide to Internet Safety	http://www.fbi.gov/stats-services/publications/parent-guide
FBI: Kids—Safety Tips	http://www.fbi.gov/fun-games/kids/kids-safety
National Criminal Justice Reference Service: Internet Safety—Internet Safety for Children	https://www.ncjrs.gov/internetsafety/children.html
The Federal Trade Commission: OnGuardOnLine: Protect Kids Online	http://www.onguardonline.gov/topics/protect-kids-online
U.S. Computer Emergency Readiness Team: Keeping Children Safe Online	http://www.us-cert.gov/cas/tips/ST05-002.html

Wikis

A **wiki** is a server application or software program that permits users to collaborate in creating and editing a document using a Web browser. In most cases you will use a wiki application that also includes wiki hosting services or the wiki might be on a server on the intranet of an organization. With wiki hosting, the document is on an Internet- or Intranet-based server and not on your personal computer. If the wiki software is on your computer, you will need to provide the group members who are working with you access to your network and/or computer.

Applications that are common in Office-type suites have been discussed in other chapters. A wiki is an application that makes it possible for people at different sites and working at different times to work together on one such application, especially a word processing application. Users who have limited technical knowledge can create a document by adding, editing, and deleting text, movies, pictures, and sounds. Wikipedia clearly demonstrates this functionality and use.

Many universities provide a wiki application for students, either as part of a course management application such as Blackboard or D2L (Desire 2 Learn) or as a free resource from the university. If available, a university-provided wiki is preferable because these wikis usually have better privacy protection. However, if this type of application is not available from the university, there are several free wiki applications available on the Internet. Some examples include:

- DokuWiki https://www.dokuwiki.org/dokuwiki
- Google Sites http://www.google.com/sites/
- MediaWiki http://www.mediawiki.org/wiki/MediaWiki
- Wikidot http://www.wikidot.com
- Wikispaces http://www.wikispaces.com/

Each of these applications provides the same general functionality; however, they each have different commands, advantages, and disadvantages. Trying out a few different wiki services will give you a feel for the services and editing approach you prefer. However, as with all other Internet-based software, whether or not you are using a university application or an application from another source, it is important to understand and use the appropriate privacy settings. First, decide if, for this project, you prefer to limit viewing access to group members. Second, you will most likely elect to limit editing access to the group members; not doing so means anyone with access can modify the content and format of a wiki document.

The functionality of a wiki makes it especially valuable for creating the required documents for group projects. The flexibility inherent in using wikis makes them an excellent tool for developing asynchronous communication and group collaboration skills. Today you can expect to find required group projects in most, if not all, educational programs for health professionals. Although many students don't like group projects, there are good reasons for these assignments.

In 2003, the Institute of Medicine (IOM) identified five required core competencies for all health professionals. Working on an interdisciplinary team is one of these five core competencies (IOM, 2003). Safe, effective patient care is not possible without cooperation and coordination between and within the various healthcare disciplines. Since this IOM report was published, each health discipline has incorporated the teaching of intraprofessional and interprofessional team skills to students in their various programs. For example, the American Association of Colleges of Nursing (AACN) developed three key documents within their Essential Series.

- The Essentials of Baccalaureate Education for Professional Nursing Practice and Tool Kit (2008)
- The Essentials of Master's Education in Nursing (2011)
- The Essentials of Doctoral Education for Advanced Nursing Practice (2006)

Each of these documents stresses the importance of interdisciplinary or interprofessional team skills and is available at http://www.aacn.nche.edu/education-resources/essential-series.

If group members are going to produce a coherent product, they must learn to work together in a non–face-to-face environment. It is the lack of such skills that make group projects so difficult and unpleasant for many students.

Learning how to cooperate and coordinate within a group is an essential leadership skill for all health professionals.

The following general rules can be helpful in establishing a culture of productivity when working with a wiki:

1. Select a group coordinator. This person will coordinate the activities of the other group members so he or she should have less responsibility for contributing content to the overall project.
2. Establish clear rules for when and how members can add, modify, and delete material, including a procedure for informing others of changes made.
3. Keep a copy of deleted materials. You may need these materials later.
4. Establish clear rules for deadlines and the consequences if members do not meet these milestones. For example, if one student does not contribute material that is needed in a timely manner, the group might remove the student from the group following the established rules.
5. Have a backup plan if something should happen to your Web site or to any of the group members.
6. Once the group members establish their working rules and procedures, be sure the professor is comfortable with these procedures.

Examples of such guidelines are at:

- http://www.udel.edu/chem/white/C342/CHEM342GrpGroundRules.pdf
- http://www.jhu.edu/virtlab/misc/Group_Rules.htm

Realizing the advantages that wiki software offers, healthcare professionals are increasingly using these applications as collaborative tools to create, synthesize, share, and disseminate knowledge in healthcare (Archambault et al., 2010). **Table 10-3** provides several example of these types of wikis.

Blog

A **blog** is a self-published Web site containing dated material, usually in a journal format. Blogs can contain text, pictures, video, audio, and URLs linking to other relevant sites. They usually include a process for readers to post their comments and reactions. Mini-blogs or tweets are growing in popularity using Twitter as a social networking service. Twitter restricts mini-blogs to 140 characters. Also growing in popularity are multi-author blogs (MABs), which are blogs that several different authors write and others often professionally edit. The difference between a MAB and a wiki is purpose and format. A wiki is organized as a hierarchical structure similar to an encyclopedia while a MAB follows the format of a journal with the latest information at the top. In health care, healthcare institutions, insurance companies, and pharmacy and medical supply companies maintain a number of such blogs.

TABLE 10-3 EXAMPLES OF WIKI APPLICATIONS IN HEALTH CARE

Name	URL
AskDrWiki	http://askdrwiki.com/mediawiki/index.php?title=Physician_Medical_Wiki
Computerized Provider Order Entry (CPOE) Wiki	https://himsscpoewiki.pbworks.com/w/page/10258531/Table%20of%20 Contents
ganfyd	http://www.ganfyd.org/index.php?title=Main_Page
Medpedia	http://www.medpedia.com/
Nursing 101	http://nursing101.wikispaces.com/
Nursing and Allied Health Resources	https://sites.google.com/site/nahrsnursingresources/
Public Health Informatics	http://clinfowiki.org/wiki/index.php/Public_Health_Informatics
WikiDoc	http://wikidoc.org/index.php/What_is_a_wiki

In a fashion similar to wikis, are a number of sites that provide an application for creating a blog and a site for hosting the blog. Examples include:

- Google: Blogger http://www.blogger.com/home
- WordPress http://wordpress.org/

Clear concise communication is always important. Because you read blogs on a screen, they require specific communication skills. **Table 10-4** presents resources that provide rules and guidelines for writing a successful blog. These are general guidelines, not specific to health care. As a professional in health care

TABLE 10-4 RESOURCES FOR SUCCESSFUL BLOGGING

Title	URL
16 Rules of Blog Writing and Layout	http://www.successfulblogging.com/16-rules-of-blog-writing -which-ones-are-you-breaking/
Problogger: How to Write Great Blog Content	http://www.problogger.net/how-to-write-great-blog-content/
7 rules of Successful Bloggers	http://www.cbsnews.com/8301-505125_162-57333218/7-rules-of -successful-bloggers/
7 Reasons Why Successful Nurse Entrepreneurs Blog or Write Articles	http://www.nurse-entrepreneur-network.com/public/749.cfm

it is important to recognize the additional ethical responsibilities in publishing a healthcare-related blog. The National Council of State Boards of Nursing published a general guide for working with social media titled White Paper: A Nurse's Guide to the Use of Social Media (NCSBN, 2011). This document contains general guidelines that also apply to blogging.

VoIP

VoIP is an acronym standing for **Voice over Internet Protocol**, which is the technology that makes it possible to transmit voice or sound via the Internet. This protocol converts your voice into a digital signal that travels over the Internet. If you are calling a regular phone number, the protocol converts the signal to a telephone signal before it reaches the destination. VoIP allows you to make a call directly from a computer, from a special VoIP phone, or from a traditional phone connected to a special adapter (Federal Communications Commission, n.d.).

Several vendors offer VoIP-based services. In some cases, you can download the software and use it for free to contact others who have also installed this same software. For example, Skype.com offers free computer-to-computer calls anywhere in the world when you use their software (http://www.skype.com/download/skype.) Calls to landlines and mobile phones do incur a charge; however, the rates are usually significantly less than those for traditional landlines or cell phones. Many computers, tablets, and smartphones now come with a webcam and microphone, which are necessary when using Skype for a video call. A broadband connection is also highly recommended.

Online Social Media and Networking

Social media are Web-based and mobile technologies that support social networking and microblogging activities whereby the one-way communication of Web 1.0 is transformed into interactive dialog in which users create online communities to share information, ideas, personal messages, and other content (Nelson, Joos, Wolf, 2013). These sites and the services that they offer allow users to construct a profile, identify a list of other users with whom they share a personal connection, and traverse that list of connections (Boyd & Ellison, 2007). Users can interact with their connections on a one-to-one basis or with all or some of their connections on a one-to-many basis. The users of social media sites can be individual users, groups within the social media site, or groups such as professional organizations or healthcare institutions. These sites offer an ever-growing variety of services that create online communities and communication. For example, they include a process for building a profile that can include text, pictures, video, and audio files that users can share with others. In addition, they provide a means of finding and connecting with others who are already in the community of users.

The nature and purpose of the connections and the interactions will vary from site to site. For example, Facebook tends to be more general purpose or personal, whereas LinkedIn focuses on building professional relationships. A list of major social networking sites, along with links to additional site information, is at http://en.wikipedia.org/wiki/List_of_social_networking_websites.

Professional Social Networking

In September 2012, *The Huffington Post* posted a slide show on their Web site entitled *The Internet Saved My Life: 10 Stories of Miraculous Survival* (Medina, 2012). In some cases, the Internet was used to connect with information, but in most cases the connection was made with other people. In January 2013 the *Court House News Service* posted a news story of a lawsuit that a family had filed against the Raphael Healthcare System in New Haven, Connecticut. The title of the article was *Hospital Worker Texted Corpse Pic, Mom Says*. The story concludes with the following statement from a hospital spokesman:

> *As a result of this incident, three employees were terminated and others have received written warnings, documented counseling, and there has been related education.* (Stuart, 2013, para 15)

While social media sites have opened up a whole new toolbox for effective and efficient communication with family, friends, colleagues, and patients, as a general rule you should consider communication on these sites both permanent and public. Such sites can empower healthcare professionals, engage patients, save lives, and ruin careers. One of the more extensive social media related resources for healthcare providers is at http://davidrothman.net/. Look around this site to get a sense of how many Web 2.0-related sites are specific to healthcare providers. Now look at the sites: http://www.doseofdigital.com/healthcare-pharma-social-media-wiki/ or http://www.healthtechnica.com/blogsphere/clinical-medical-users/ and again note the number and type of Web 2.0 applications in health care. Realizing the potential opportunities and dangers, a number of healthcare professional organizations have published social media guidelines. **Table 10-5** provides additional information on these resources and where to find them.

Patients on the Internet

The Internet has empowered many patients to take the lead in using social media sites to direct their own care. In turn, many healthcare professionals and institutions have embraced the engaged patient concept. One of the earliest supporters of the engaged patient movement was a physician named Thomas Ferguson (http://www.doctom.com/). His work led to the establishment of the Society for Participatory Medicine (http://participatorymedicine.org/). This group has seen limited participation from nursing but now a number of key physicians and

TABLE 10-5 PROFESSIONAL ASSOCIATIONS AND SOCIAL MEDIA GUIDELINES

Professional Association	Document Title	URL
American Hospital Association (AHA) and Association for Healthcare Resource & Materials Management (AHRMM)	Social Media Guidelines	http://www.ahrmm.org/ahrmm/resources_and_tools/social_media/index.jsp
American Medical Association (AMA)	Professionalism in the Use of Social Media	http://www.ama-assn.org/ama/pub/physician-resources/medical-ethics/code-medical-ethics/opinion9124.page
American Nurses Association (ANA)	ANA's Principles for Social Networking and the Nurse	http://www.nursingworld.org/MainMenuCategories/ThePracticeofProfessionalNursing/NursingStandards/ANAPrinciples.aspx
Australian Medical Association (AMA); New Zealand Medical Association; New Zealand Medical Student Associations (NZMSA); Australian Medical Student Association (AMSA)	Social Media and the Medical Profession: A Guide to Online Professionalism for Medical Practitioners and Medical Students	http://ama.com.au/socialmedia
National Council of State Boards of Nursing (NCSBN)	White Paper: A Nurse's Guide to the Use of Social Media	https://www.ncsbn.org/Social_Media.pdf
National Student Nurses' Association, Inc.	Recommendations for: Social Media Usage and Maintaining Privacy, Confidentiality and Professionalism	http://www.nsna.org/Portals/0/Skins/NSNA/pdf/NSNA_Social_Media_Recommendations.pdf
Nursing & Midwifery Council (NMC)	Social networking site guidance	http://www.nmc-uk.org/Nurses-and-midwives/Advice-by-topic/A/Advice/Social-networking-sites/
Royal College of Nursing (RCN)	Legal Advice for RCN Members Using the Internet	http://www.rcn.org.uk/__data/assets/pdf_file/0008/272195/003557.pdf

TABLE 10-6 EXAMPLES OF SOCIAL MEDIA SITES DESIGNED FOR PATIENTS

Name	Business Model and Additional Information	URL
PatientsLikeMe	Private: For-profit http://www.patientslikeme.com/help/faq/Corporate	http://www.patientslikeme.com/
23andMe	Private: For-profit https://23andme.https.internapcdn.net/res/pdf/6_2REcKn2n7ldwrslkdbrw_factsheet_v4.pdf	https://www.23andme.com/
CureTogether	Fully owned by 23andMe, Inc. https://www.23andme.com/about/press/curetogether/	http://curetogether.com/
Inspire	Private: For-profit http://corp.inspire.com/about/investment.htm	http://www.inspire.com/
Stupid Cancer	Nonprofit http://stupidcancer.org/about/index.shtml	http://stupidcancer.org/index.shtml
CaringBridge	Nonprofit http://www.caringbridge.org/finance	http://www.caringbridge.org/

patients have been using the Internet, social media, and other sources to lead this movement forward. A list of these individuals with their interesting bios is at http://participatorymedicine.org/about/board-of-directors/. In addition, a number of businesses and nonprofit organizations have developed based on the concept of the engaged/empowered patient. **Table 10-6** provides examples with links to information on their business models. Referring patients to a Web site is the same as referring patients to a healthcare provider. You want to do your homework so you can provide patients with the information necessary to make safe decisions. This includes understanding the business model of the Web site and how data related to patients may be collected and used.

Summary

The Internet is changing where, when, and how individuals, businesses, organizations, groups, and communities communicate. This chapter reviewed several of the more common tools that are driving this change. The challenge for healthcare students is to know how to use these tools to improve the effectiveness and efficiency of both their professional and personal communication.

References

Archambault, P. M., Légaré, F., Lavoie, A., Gagnon, M. P., Lapointe, J., St. Jacques, S., Poitras, J., Aubin, K., Croteau, S., and Pham-Dinh, M. (2010). Health professionals' intentions to use wiki-based reminders to promote best practices in trauma care: A survey protocol. *Implementation Science*, 5:45. Retrieved from http://www.implementationscience.com/content/pdf/1748-5908-5-45.pdf

Boyd, D. M. and Ellison, N. B. (2007). Social network sites: Definition, history, and scholarship. *Journal of Computer-Mediated Communication, 1*(1), article 11. Retrieved from http://jcmc.indiana.edu/vol13/issue1/boyd.ellison.html

DiNucci, D. (1999). Fragmented future. *Print,* 53(4): 32; 221–222. Retrieved from http://darcyd.com/fragmented_future.pdf

Educause Learning Initiative (ELI). (2006). 7 things you should know about... Wikis. Washington, DC: ELI. Retrieved from http://net.educause.edu/ir/library/pdf/ELI7004.pdf

Federal Communications Commission (FCC) (2010). Voice over Internet Protocol. Washington, DC: FCC. Retrieved from www.fcc.gov/voip/

Gibson, T. (2008) Double vision: McLuhan's contributions to media as an interdisciplinary approach to communication, culture, and technology. *Media Tropes* eJournal. Volume I: 143–166. Retrieved from www.mediatropes.com/index.php/Mediatropes/article/view/3345/1489

Google (2012). The difference between a Usenet newsgroup and a Google Group. Retrieved from http://archive.is/b98Q

Hopkins, J. (ed.) (2011) Introduction to electronic mailing lists: Listserv, Listproc, and Majordomo. Retrieved from www.uta.fi/FAST/PK5/LISTS/e-lists.html

Institute of Medicine (IOM), Committee on the Health Professions Education Summit Board of Health Care Services, Greiner, A. C. and Knebel, E. (eds.) (2003). *Health professions education: A bridge to quality*. Washington, DC: National Academies Press. Retrieved from www.iom.edu/CMS/3809/4634/5914.aspx

McLuhan, M. (1994). *Understanding media: The extensions of man.* Cambridge: MIT Press. (Original work published 1964).

McLuhan, M. and Fiore, Q., produced by Agel, J. (1967). *The medium is the massage: An inventory of effects.* New York: Random House.

Medina, S. (2012). The Internet saved my life: 10 stories of miraculous survival. *The Huffington Post.* Retrieved from www.huffingtonpost.com/2012/09/28/the-internet-saved-my-life_n_1918112.html#slide=1573743

National Council of State Boards of Nursing (NCSBN) (2011). *White paper: A nurse's guide to the use of social media.* Chicago: NCSBN. Retrieved from https://www.ncsbn.org/Social_Media.pdf

Nelson, R., Joos, I., and Wolf, D. (2013). Social media for nurses: Educating practitioners and patients in a networked world. New York: Springer Publishing Company.

O'Reilly, T. (2005). What is web 2.0. Sebastopol, CA: O'Reilly Media. Retrieved from http://oreilly.com/web2/archive/what-is-web-20.html

Stuart, C. (2013). Hospital worker texted corpse pic, Mom says. Courthouse News Service. Retrieved from www.courthousenews.com/2013/01/07/53663.htm

Wikipedia (n.d.). Welcome to Wikipedia. Retrieved from http://en.wikipedia.org/wiki/Main_Page
Wikipedia (n.d.). Wikipedia: What Wikipedia is not. Retrieved from http://en.wikipedia.org/wiki/Wikipedia:What_Wikipedia_is_not
Wilson, P.L., Nolla, A. C., and Gunawardena, C. N. (2005). A qualitative analysis of online group process in two cultural contexts. *The Electronic Journal of Communication*. Volume 15, Numbers 1 & 2. Retrieved from www.cios.org/ejcpublic/015/1/01516.html.

Exercises 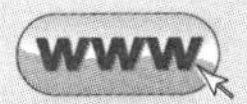

EXERCISE 1 Complete an Information Analysis of Blog Content

Objectives

1. Identify the advantages and disadvantages of different search engines in searching for blog content.
2. Systematically identify blog sites that may be of current professional interest.
3. Analyze and evaluate the format and content of information available in a blog site.

Activity

1. Select a topic that relates to your current classes or professional activities. For example, if you are writing a term paper about the role of the school nurse in preventing bullying or involved in the implementation of an electronic health record (EHR) at work you might choose one of those topics.
2. A number of search engines focus on searching blogs. Use at least two of the following search engines to search for a blog discussing your topic of interest.
   - http://technorati.com/
   - http://www.ljseek.com/
   - http://www.google.com/blogsearch
   - http://blogs.icerocket.com/
3. Begin the search process by reviewing each selected search engine; note its features or functions. For example, does the search engine offer functions such as advanced search? What is the scope of the search engine? For example, does the search engine search the Internet in general or only blogs written with a specific blog application?
4. Now try different search strategies with the selected search engines. For example, you might try the following search strings:
   - nurse bullying
   - school nurse bullying
   - "school nurse" bullying
   - school nurse role bullying
5. Next complete the same search using a selection of general search engines such as Google, Bing, Ask, and Yahoo!. This time add the term "blog" to your search string.
6. Review the results of these different approaches to finding content on a blog.
7. Using Word, write a brief summary explaining what you learned about the process of searching for content on a blog and the type of information

you were able to find. For example, did you find specific suggestions for a school nurse dealing with bullying-related problems in a school or did you find more information reflecting peoples' feelings and opinions?

8. Save the Word document as **Chap10-Exercise1-LastName** and follow your professor's directions for submitting your assignment.

EXERCISE 2 Use Skype for Face-to-Face Communication

Objectives

1. Explore the technology used in establishing a VoIP connection.
2. Analyze video-based communication.

Activity

1. Check the specifications on your computer to determine if you have a Webcam. If not you will need to obtain one to complete this activity.
2. If needed, review at least one online tutorial on using Skype. Some options include:
   - http://www.youtube.com/watch?v=X9H14EU0mEQ
   - http://www.youtube.com/watch?v=oJNvrHn6izI
   - http://www.youtube.com/watch?v=IOf2mgSsXak
   - http://www.youtube.com/watch?v=QTVElj-cg2w
3. Review the Skype site (http://www.skype.com) for a description of their services including what is free and what services you must pay for.
4. Download and configure your computer to use Skype.
5. Contact one of your classmates, a member of your family, or a friend by email and schedule a Skype call.
6. During the call, turn your video off and then turn it on again.
7. After your first call, search Skype to determine if you can find other people you know who have a Skype account.
8. On your class wiki, personal blog, or course discussion forum, share your insights and experiences in setting up your computer, scheduling the meeting, and actually using Skype for communication. Include your opinion about using Skype with a client.

EXERCISE 3 Use Social Media to Connect with Professional Organizations

Objectives

1. Establish a relationship with a professional organization within a social media site.

2. Analyze the different opportunities to interact within a professional organization on a social media site.

Activity

1. For this exercise create a PowerPoint presentation describing your experiences as you follow the steps of the activity. Use the presentation to respond to the questions included within the steps below.
2. Establish both a LinkedIn and a Facebook account.
3. Begin with LinkedIn and search for two or three professional organizations that relate to your discipline or professional interest. For example you might search for the American Nurses Association (ANA), the American Health Information Management Association (AHIMA), or the American Medical Informatics Association (AMIA).
4. Next search for the same organizations within Facebook.
5. Describe the search process used on each site, the challenges experienced, and your findings. For example, did you need to use the full name to find the organization? Did you have to search on a word such as *nursing* and then scroll through the search results to find your group?
6. Once you find an organization that is of interest to you on both LinkedIn and Facebook, determine how you can interact with this organization within the site and the type of relationship that you can establish. For example, what is the difference between joining a group or "liking" a page?
7. Once you have established a relationship with a professional organization on both LinkedIn and Facebook, determine and describe the activities that are now open to you. For example, can you join a chat or participate on a discussion board?
8. Complete your PowerPoint presentation by describing what you learned from this experience.
9. Save the PowerPoint as **Chap10-Exercise3-LastName** and submit it following the directions provided by the professor.

Assignments

ASSIGNMENT 1 Compare and Contrast a Wikipedia Article with a Textbook Chapter

Directions

1. If you are a student taking courses this term, select a chapter that is a required reading for one of your classes. If you are not a student select a chapter in a book related to your area of interest in health care.

2. Search Wikipedia and find an article on the same topic as this chapter. If you can't find an article in Wikipedia select a different chapter for this assignment.
3. Read the chapter and either highlight key points, make an outline, or create a list of the key points in the chapter.
4. Review the references at the end of the chapter and, if available, any Web page associated with the chapter. The Web page might be provided by the book publisher or by your instructor.
5. Read the Wikipedia article and highlight the key points.
6. Review the references, links, and other supporting materials for your selected article in Wikipedia.
7. Use PowerPoint to create a presentation demonstrating:
   a. The similarities and differences between a textbook chapter and a Wikipedia article.
   b. The advantages and disadvantages of each resource as well as the advantages of combining these resources.
8. Save the PowerPoint as **Chap10-Assign1-LastName** and submit per the directions of the professor.

ASSIGNMENT 2 Working with Empowered, Engaged, and Equipped Patients and Patients Groups

Directions

It has been suggested that patients working together in social networks with access to the same information as healthcare providers are increasingly functioning as peers and colleagues on the healthcare team.

1. Go to http://participatorymedicine.org/. Click the links and video on the homepage that explain the philosophy and goals of this group.
2. Watch the video at http://www.youtube.com/watch?v=2vejkD0Rl3o followed by the video at www.youtube.com/watch?v=4PObMvjvQJs.
3. Watch the video at http://www.youtube.com/watch?v=0O--uLzcQnQ followed by the video at http://www.youtube.com/watch?v=yG_H33HRPUU.
4. Write a blog defining the terms "empowered," "engaged," and "equipped" as the terms might apply to individual patients.
5. Next add a section explaining how these same terms apply to a group of patients.

6. Conclude your blog by explaining the implications for healthcare professionals of working with empowered, engaged, and equipped individual patients and groups of patients.
7. Provide your professor with a link and access to your blog if a blog function is not available in your course management program.

ASSIGNMENT 3 Creating a Social Media Resource Document

Directions

1. In this assignment, create a social media resource document that other students can use. Social media on the Internet change frequently, so check each resource before adding it to the document. In other words, make sure the address is correct, the site is still available, and that you understand the terms and conditions, the privacy statement, and the focus or purpose of the site.
2. Work in small groups (three to five people) to create the resource document. The resource document should include the following information for specific topics of interest to the discipline or course:
   a. A list of professional scheduled chats, including information on when they occur and how to access them.
   b. A list of professional association groups on Twitter and LinkedIn including the focus or tone of the discussion.
   c. A list of patient-based social media sites with a description of their mission and business model.
   d. A list of electronic discussion groups, including directions for subscribing to them.
   e. A list of newsgroups, including directions for how to access them.
3. After each small group completes its document, the class will use a wiki to create a master document identifying all resources found by the class. The wiki should be carefully organized with similar types of resources grouped together and each resource listed only once. Make sure your professor has access to the wiki if it is outside your course management program.

chapter

11

Distance Education: A Student Perspective

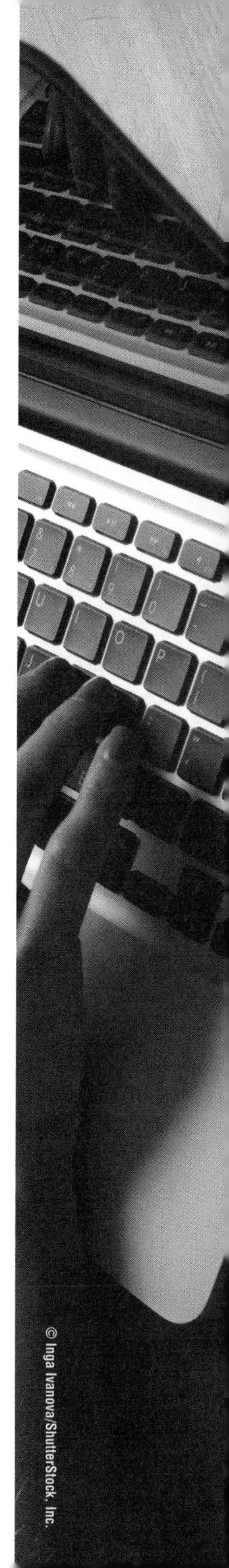

Objectives

1. Conduct a self-assessment of your readiness for learning in a distance education environment.
2. Develop appropriate learning skills for success in a distance learning course.
3. Describe how the technology used to deliver distance education can influence your learning.
4. Identify distance education courses and programs that can meet your learning and career goals.

Introduction

Most students who are 35 or younger grew up using computers in their homes and their classrooms. While these individuals vary widely in their knowledge of computers and related technology, including software programs and frequently used apps, most are comfortable using technology in their daily lives. Many K through 12 schools offer distance education course options. In many states, high schools require students to take at least one online course before they graduate. With the growth of cyber schools, a significant number of students entering college as freshman are experienced distance education learners having completed not just a number of courses, but a complete educational program online. However, other students in today's college classrooms began using computers long after they finished high school. These students may have limited or no exposure to learning in a distance education environment. Often, more experienced classmates intimidate them.

While there is significant variation in the learning experiences of the current college population, all students need to become comfortable using distance education technology. A significant proportion of their future formal and informal educational options will be delivered using these technologies. Health care is a fast-changing field in which competent healthcare providers must be lifelong learners. Increasingly, employers in healthcare settings are using distance education technologies instead of face-to-face classes to deliver required training and updates. Many states also require healthcare professionals to obtain continuing education units (CEUs) for relicensure; in most cases, you can easily obtain these CEUs through online learning.

This chapter focuses on those aspects of distance education that are important to you as a student and to your success with distance education. Whether a practicing professional, student, or prospective student, you should understand the importance of continuing your education after you complete your formal program. The content of this chapter (1) includes a self-assessment tool to help you determine what challenges you might expect to face in achieving a successful learning experience in a distance education course or program; (2) identifies the different technology options for distance education and their relationship to your successful learning; (3) outlines the study skills specific to successful learning in a Web-based distance education program; and (4) suggests techniques for finding the best-fit distance education programs for your future learning.

Definitions of Terms

We use several terms to refer to distance education including *distributed education, online education, online learning, eLearning,* and *Web-based education*; however, the definitions for these terms vary. We use the following terms and definitions related to distance education in this chapter.

Asynchronous — **Asynchronous** is a communication exchange in which the involved people are communicating at different times. For example, email and discussion boards are asynchronous because the communicants do not need to be logged in at the same time.

Blended Course or Learning — The combination of traditional classroom and online distance learning activities within a single course or group of learning activities. Some people refer to a **blended course or learning** as a **hybrid course** or hybrid learning.

Chat	Real-time text-based communication between two or more users via a computer or mobile device.
Course Management Software or System (CMS)	**Course management software or system** (CMS) is a software application an institution uses to facilitate distance education by centralizing the development, management, and distribution of instructional-related information and materials. A CMS provides faculty with a set of tools that support the development of course content such as organized learning activities and related assessments. In addition a CMS provides a portal through which learners access their course materials and activities. Two commonly used commercial CMS programs are Blackboard and Desire2Learn.
Distance Education	**Distance education** is the use of technology to deliver education when the student and the instructor are in physically different locations. In today's learning environment institutions often deliver this type of education over the Internet using a variety of technical tools such as a CMS, virtual conferences, and podcasts.
Distributive Education	Many people confuse this term with distance education. In other settings **distributive education** is the more comprehensive term that includes both distance education and hybrid learning.
eLearning	**eLearning** refers to all types of education and instruction that various entities deliver to learners via a digital medium such as a computer, tablet, or mobile phone.
Learning Management System	**Learning management system** is often used synonymously with CMS; however, this term often refers to an application used to support learning as opposed to an application that supports course development and delivery.
Massive Open Online Course (MOOC)	The meaning of **massive open online course** (MOOC) is evolving but usually refers to a model for delivering free, usually noncredit courses, via the Internet to anyone who has an interest. Some of these courses enroll over 100,000 students. While these courses can include a number of tools for students to assess their own learning, direct feedback from the instructor is

usually limited and many of these courses have a low completion rate.

Synchronous Communication

Synchronous communication is real-time communication between participants who are using their computers or mobile devices. Chat rooms and Internet meetings are examples of synchronous communication, because all of the involved individuals are on their computers or mobile devices at the same time.

Threaded Discussion

Threaded discussion is an online information exchange that is similar to a bulletin board, except that topics within each interest area are identified and organized together so that users can access and read only the discussions pertaining to a particular interest area.

Video Conferencing

Video conferencing is a conference in which participants are separated by geographic distance and communication occurs via a computer, video camera, microphone, and speakers. Along with hearing audio, the technology delivers whatever images appear in front of the video camera to the participant's monitor. A "virtual" conference can be as small as two participants or can include a large number of participants. Video conferencing is synchronous communication. However, a video conference can be recorded and accessed for review at a later time.

Virtual Classroom

A **virtual classroom** is a learning environment that exists solely online in the form of digital content and online communication. Networked computer and information systems store, access, and exchange the content. Everything in a virtual classroom occurs in a nonphysical environment, and students "go to class" by connecting to the network rather than by traveling to a physical classroom.

Webinar

A **webinar** delivers a seminar or lecture over the Internet with audio and screen components. The presenter and participants view the same screen at the same time. Depending on the software application and functionality, participants can chat by entering text, answering polls, raising their hands, and asking questions in audio format. While the webinar may be synchronous, the presenter can record and archive the presentation for later viewing.

Self-Assessment for Distance Education

Success in a distance education environment requires motivation and an interest in learning. Registering for a distance education course simply because you are late in registering for an on-campus course and it is the only course that will fit in your schedule is not usually a good idea. Students who are ambivalent about being in school and have limited interest in their classes usually do worse in a distance education environment than a traditional classroom. However, if you are a motivated and self-directed person, distance education provides great opportunities.

Some students take to distance education like ducks to water. From the beginning, they like the format and do well. Other students go through an adjustment period, but then discover how to learn in the new environment and then become successful. Unfortunately, a few students find distance education frustrating and must make an extra effort to succeed in this environment. The following questions will help you determine where you fit in this picture and where you may need to make adjustments to achieve the most successful experience.

What Are Your Literacy Skills and Background Knowledge?

Your literacy skills and background knowledge of the course content are important in ensuring a successful distance education experience. These skills include the following:

- Reading comprehension and the ability to express yourself in writing.
- Ability to follow directions.
- Basic computer literacy.
- Knowledge of and aptitude for the specific subject of study.

If you prefer to hear new information rather than to read that content, if you prefer to talk about rather than write about your ideas, or if you are uncomfortable with technology, distance education will be a major challenge for you.

Computer literacy is an important part of overall literacy. While you can succeed in a Web-based distance education course with minimal computer literacy, some comfort in working on the computer can be key to achieving success. In addition, if the course involves a field where you have little knowledge of the topic or lack the prerequisite background necessary for that topic, distance education can be difficult. For example, if you have a weak math background or struggle with mathematical concepts and are taking a statistics course online, your lack of preparation or aptitude for mathematics can be a major challenge.

What Are Your Personal Attributes?

Some students appreciate the teacher reminding them of assignment due dates. Others have already noted the key dates in each of their courses. These students might hate to hear the same information repeated and feel that the professor is nagging them. Some students like to have their work done early and do not like the sense of last-minute pressure. Other students feel they do their best work under pressure and leave barely enough time to finish the work. Some students set up a time and place to study and can resist distractions. For example, they turn off cell phones and check their email only after they finish their project. Other students do better in a traditional classroom where the professor filters out the distractions of daily life during class time. Some students believe they can "multi-task," moving back and forth from class materials to phone call, text messages and other distractions. They are usually surprised when they discover they have made errors in all these tasks. As you think about these different personal attributes, are you organized, structured, not easily distracted, and a bit compulsive about meeting deadlines? If this description fits, you should do well in a distance education course. If not, you will need to focus on creating a structured environment for your learning.

How Important Are Social Interactions?

Is social interaction and getting to know your classmates on a personal level important to your education? Distance education courses usually encourage interaction between classmates and the teacher; however, that interaction focuses on the course subject. The informal interactions that occur between classes or within student organizations are often not part of the distance education experience. For some students, the lack of informal interactions proves too isolating so that they become less interested in the course. For these students, taking a distance education course can be similar to sitting at home reading the textbook.

Because the informal social relationships that occur on campus can lead to long-term professional relationships, some schools support online student organizations. Sometimes schools will encourage a virtual coffee house or online study groups where online students go to socialize and/or learn together. This practice can be effective, but requires the student to make that extra effort to become involved in the online community.

Several universities have designed self-assessment tools to help students determine whether they should participate in distance education. **Table 11-1** provides examples of these tools. As you look over these questions and do your own self-assessment, you will discover that you are stronger in some areas than in others. While your strengths will help you and your weak areas will challenge you, your motivation is the key factor. In many cases, how much you really want to complete the course, or even the whole program, influences the final outcome.

TABLE 11-1 ONLINE SELF-ASSESSMENTS FOR DISTANCE EDUCATION

University	URL
Bellevue Community College	http://bellevuecollege.edu/distance/WebAssess/
Boise State University	http://ecampus.boisestate.edu/students/is-ecampus-right-for-me/
North Central State College	http://www.ncstatecollege.edu/academics/dl/orientation/SelfAssessment.htm
The Community College of Baltimore County	http://www.ccbcmd.edu/distance/assess.html
Western University of Health Sciences	http://wsprod.westernu.edu/wu/nursing/cgn_assess.jsp

Along with your readiness for distance education, two other factors that determine your experience are (1) how much of your total education has been delivered in this format and (2) what type of distance education technology will be used to deliver your education. Two important types of distance education technology are video conferencing and Web-based programs. The next section provides additional information about these two types of distance education technology.

The technology that delivers Web-based distance education is also an excellent tool for supplementing and supporting traditional classroom formats. The technology may be useful to deliver part of a course, a complete course, or a complete program where graduates are never on campus. Blended or hybrid learning is the name for these types of courses. The degree of immersion in distance education can have a significant effect on your adjustment to the distance education experience. Taking a Web-based distance education course during the same term you are taking traditional classes is a very different experience from taking all of your classes via Web-based distance education.

Distance Education Technology and Environment

The media and technology available to deliver distance education have moved through several generations (Bates, 2008). Initially, distance education used a print or paper format delivered by postal mail. This format is referred to as correspondence education to distinguish it from distance education, which by definition involves the use of technology. One-way broadcasting media such as television, radio, or mailed videocassettes followed correspondence education.

The next major innovation involved two-way synchronous telelearning, such as telephone-based conference calls and interactive video. The widespread acceptance of the Internet led to a fourth approach—asynchronous online learning usually delivered via course management software. The functionality of different course management software packages varies greatly:

- Each vendor has its own package with different features and functions; some of these are optional and your school may or may not select them.
- The course management software may offer a number of independent plug-in applications or modules.
- Each university will select its own configuration for integrating and/or interfacing the course management software with other university systems. The ultimate configuration will affect the functionality and, in turn, the user's experience. For example, in some universities they automatically place you in or withdraw you from an online course depending on your registration status. At other universities, the professor might be able to add or remove students at will.

These variations will influence the degree of automation, interaction, and user control.

Currently, all these generations of technology are in use, often in combination. This chapter, however, focuses on interactive video conferencing and asynchronous online learning via course management software because these are the formats in common use today.

Interactive Video Conferencing

Distance education that relies on **interactive video conferencing** is synchronous—that is, the classes occur at a set time with the students and faculty present at their classroom locations. In the Unites States, some universities use room-based video conferencing, which connects two or more traditional classrooms in real time across a network. This setup requires that students travel to the video conferencing classroom. Each classroom has a camera to capture the faculty and/or students in that classroom, a monitor to broadcast this picture to the other classroom(s), and a sound system for transmitting voice communication between the rooms. In addition to this basic setup, classrooms often include a document projector and an Internet connection for transmitting images and slides across the network. The teacher is in the originating or home classroom. The classroom(s) receiving the broadcast is/are the distance classroom(s).

In many ways, video conferencing is similar to the traditional classroom experience of both students and teachers—which is also its primary advantage.

This approach requires less adjustment for both the teacher and the student in comparison to other distance education approaches. The main disadvantages include the set time of the class, the need to travel to the classroom, the cost of equipping the classrooms with the needed technology, and sometimes the signal delay distortion. Because of these limitations, distance education is increasingly moving away from this technology for educational purposes to Internet-based course delivery options.

In many cases, the system transmits the course to one or two other classrooms; however, the number of connected classrooms can vary greatly, with as many as 15 to 20 classrooms participating in a single session. This practice is referred to as multipoint video conferencing. The functionality of the equipment in the classrooms can also vary greatly. For example, the camera may focus only on the teacher; any movement would require the teacher to adjust the camera. In this setup, students in the distance classroom(s) see only the "talking head" or the images/slides. Remembering to switch the monitor between these two options is the responsibility of the teacher. Students in the home classroom see a group shot of the students in the other classroom. In a more common setup today, the camera focuses on sound. If the teacher is talking, the camera records the teacher. If the teacher moves, the camera follows him or her. If a student in either the home classroom or the distance classroom asks a question, the camera then focuses on the student.

In this environment, time and focus or attention on task are key factors for learning. Several factors in the classroom influence the time each student remains focused on the course content. Although students can effectively manage many of these factors, doing so requires a commitment on the part of students both as individuals and as a group.

Classroom Ambiance

The traditional classroom usually has a formal environment where one recognizes protocols for behavior, such as raising your hand to talk or looking at the person who is talking. With video conferencing, students in the home classroom will experience much the same environment as students in a traditional classroom. There can be distractions from these expectations but they tend to be minor. For example, some faculty members have a tendency to talk to the distance class and forget to look at the students in the home classroom; others tend to forget the distance classroom. Some teachers have difficulty managing the technology while they teach. With experience as well as feedback, these distractions tend to fade over time.

The ambiance in the distance classroom can be quite different. Usually a student worker, technician, or one of the students in the class is responsible for making sure the classroom is open, ensuring that the equipment is turned on and working, distributing handouts, and performing other housekeeping tasks that contribute to a smoothly running class. A distance education classroom not only lacks the physical presence of the faculty member, but also the psychological presence. As a result, distance education classrooms have a tendency to become more informal and, in turn, more distracting. If the classroom sound system is muted, the faculty member may not be aware of background noise in the room, such as side conversations between students or noise from eating, cell phones ringing, or other activities. This effect can be even greater if the faculty member is focused on presenting content and has limited interaction with the students, especially the distance education classroom students.

Learning Engagement

In a traditional classroom, a teacher with strong lecturing skills can keep students' attention. Such a teacher paints a picture with words. As the picture evolves, students actively engage with the topic and the message. In contrast, watching a teacher on a monitor is very much like watching television. The student moves from active participant to passive observer; the talking head can take on a monotone quality and the mind begins to wander. To combat this effect, commercial television includes action. The action might be subtle, such as the changing camera shots with a news show, or constantly changing, as is the case with many advertisements and action shows. Many times you will hear people comment, "That was a good show—it had a lot of action." Even with this emphasis on action, however, there is a tendency to engage in other activities while watching television. Note the number of people who read, eat, knit, or find other things to do while in front of the television.

There are a number of things a teacher can do to increase the amount of interaction with students and focus the students on the topic; likewise, students can take steps to increase their individual interaction with the content. Not all of the suggestions listed here will work for every student. Review this list and select those that you believe will help you as you take distance education courses.

- Sit toward the front of the room, close to the monitor screen. This location will decrease the amount of visual distraction from others in the classroom.
- Take notes. Sometimes teachers provide students with handouts in place of notes. These handouts may include the slides used in the lecture or an overview of the lecture itself; they may be in paper form or more commonly in digital form. Use these handouts to follow the lecture and write/type

your notes on them, but do not let these handouts become a substitute for taking notes. The process of writing/typing notes will focus your attention on the content being presented.

- If the teacher lectures directly from the textbook, be sure to read the chapter before class and then highlight the points the teacher is making during the class. Many ebooks permit highlighting.
- Read the chapter before class and note key questions to ask the teacher.
- Turn off your cell phone and put it away; never engage in disruptive and inappropriate behavior in class such as text messaging.
- Do not eat during the class; some foods tend to make you sleepy.
- Drink liquids for proper hydration and to keep you awake, especially if you worked before class.
- If you are taking a late afternoon or evening class, and especially if you have been on a clinical unit before class, try to take a short nap and perform some exercise before class.
- Create classroom activities that help focus others on the content. For example, before class, ask a group of friends to pick out the key points from today's class that will be on the next test. At the break, share these ideas.

Classroom Interaction

While transmission time has improved, there may be a delay when data and voice are carried across the video conferencing network. This delay produces a trade-off between how much content the teacher can present and how much time the students can spend on interaction. To maximize time and support the learning of all students in the class, students must use appropriate classroom etiquette.

- The monitor in the room where you are located will most often show the other classroom; the monitor in the other classroom will show your classroom. Because the people there are most likely looking at you, always assume you are on camera. Avoid inappropriate gestures, positions, or behavior.
- Most classroom microphones are fairly sensitive. Keep them mute unless you are speaking.
- In most video conferencing classrooms, the teacher will ask for questions at a specific point. Be sensitive to that reality and do not ask spontaneous questions throughout the class.
- Be sensitive to time delays. Do not interrupt the teacher or other students. Keep your comments concise and your questions short. If you have a

question that is of interest only to you, send it to the teacher in an email after class.

- When speaking, look at the camera, speak in a normal tone, and do not rush through your question or comment. Do not fidget or wear jewelry that creates noise.
- Assume the equipment is working. Do not ask if others can hear you. In larger and/or multipoint classes, give your name and location when you start to speak.
- Wear colors or, if you are in a uniform, wear a sweater or jacket with color.
- If technical problems affect reception in your classroom, let the teacher know.

Web-Based Course Management Programs

By removing the limitations of time and distance, Web-based course management programs have opened a whole new world of options for students of all ages and interests. In the early 1990s, browsers were new and had very limited availability. You accessed the Internet using text-based tools with no graphics. Thus the initial courses via this medium included text-based lectures that students received by email. These initial courses demonstrated the potential of the Web-based format. One of the best-known examples is the course titled *Roadmap,* offered by Patrick Crispen beginning in 1994. The course consists of 27 classes spread over 6 weeks (Crispen, n.d.). An outline and access to the lectures are at www.webreference.com/roadmap/. At the time he offered the course, Crispen was a college student.

Roadmap is the original MOOC; however, at that time this term had not yet been coined. Over the years, more than 500,000 people have signed up for Roadmap and received their weekly email classes, learning how to use the Internet (Crispen, n.d.). Any one session of the course could have more than 10,000 students. The technical format for delivering the lecture was simple: an email message sent two or three times a week. The course and the content of each lecture were clearly presented and easy to follow. However, with 10,000 students in a class, participants could not ask questions or receive feedback. Put simply, students were on their own. While the software that institutions use today to deliver Web-based distance education provides much more functionality and even automates some feedback, such as quizzes, this same general rule still applies: Individual student support and feedback is in direct proportion to the student-teacher ratio. Larger ratios result in less feedback.

However, in a MOOC students can work together and many new opportunities for self-directed learning are in development. For example, Coursera at https://www.coursera.org/about has partnered with a number of universities to offer 370 MOOC courses as of May 2013. Duke University School of Nursing is producing one of these courses titled Health Innovation and Entrepreneurship; over 15,000 students enrolled in the first course offering (Duke University School of Nursing, 2013). **Box 11-1** lists the characteristics of a MOOC.

A number of vendors now offer software applications for delivering a Web-based course. These applications provide organization and structure with the following purposes:

- Presenting information including links to outside resources.
- Encouraging interaction between students and with teachers.
- Assessment of student involvement and learning.

Box 11-1 Characteristics of a MOOC

- There is no limit on attendance. Anyone who would like to can enroll.
- The structure of a MOOC can be identical to a standard course; however, participation is flexible and optional.
- Courses are offered by any level or type of college or university.
- To deal with the large number of students there is usually an emphasis on the use of social media to foster collaboration, participation, and peer-to-peer learning.
- The multiple conversations and learning activities with limited instructor control can make some students uneasy.
- MOOCs represent an emerging model for delivering education. They can increase the enrollment and raise the profile of the institution and/or faculty, but their full impact is not yet clear.
- The most significant contribution is the MOOC's potential to alter the relationship between the learner and the instructor and between academia and the wider community.

Source:
EDUCAUSE, (2011, Nov). 7 things you should know about MOOCs. EDUCAUSE Learning Initiative (ELI), pp. 1-2. Retrieved from http://www.educause.edu/library/resources/7-things-you-should-know-about-moocs. Reprinted by permission.

Table 11-2 lists the well-known commercial Web-based course management software vendors, with links to their Web sites. In addition, there are a number of open source Web-based course management software options; these are listed in **Table 11-3**. The cost of these applications varies greatly, and as a result universities will sometimes change their standard application to save money. This can cause stress for both faculty and students. In addition, if you transfer or take a course at a different university, be prepared for the possibility that the new school will be using different CMS.

Table 11-4 lists the common functions of most of these applications from a student perspective. A number of other functions the professor might use that

TABLE 11-2 COMMERCIAL WEB-BASED COURSE MANAGEMENT SOFTWARE VENDORS

Vendor or Package Name	URL
Blackboard/Angel/WebCT	http://www.blackboard.com
Desire2Learn	http://www.desire2learn.com/
Pearson Learning Solutions	http://www.pearsonlearningsolutions.com/pearson-learning-studio/compare-features.php
Edvance360	http://edvance360.com/
Jenzabar Learning Management System	http://www.jenzabar.com/higher-ed-solutions/learning-management-system-lms
eLearningForce SharePoint LMS	http://www.elearningforce.com/products/pages/sharepoint_lms.aspx

TABLE 11-3 OPEN SOURCE WEB-BASED COURSE MANAGEMENT SOFTWARE VENDORS

Vendor or Package Name	URL
Moodle	https://moodle.org/
Sakai	http://www.sakaiproject.org/
Canvas	http://www.instructure.com/
eFront	http://www.efrontlearning.net/open-source
OLAT (Online Learning and Training)	http://www.olat.org/
Claroline	http://www.claroline.net/?TB_iframe

TABLE 11-4 COMMON COURSE MANAGEMENT SOFTWARE FUNCTIONS

Feature	Tools
Content Delivery	• Internal Web pages • Attached files such as lectures, presentation graphics, and spreadsheets • External links • Online assessment and testing • Internal ebooks
Communication Tools	• Discussion board • Blog • Email system • Real-time chat • Home pages and portfolios • PC-based video conferencing
Group Work Tools	• Whiteboard • Wiki • Group work areas • Document sharing
Productivity Tools	• Searching within the course • Bookmarks • Calendar • Grade book and progress review

work behind the scenes; students will see them but not be able to create them. For example, the professor might send automatic messages to students who have completed a certain portion of the course or who have not signed in for a set number of days. Also note that the professor might track your progress. If the professor tracks your progress, the level of detail available to the professor concerning your participation may surprise you and other students.

Course management software makes it possible for the educational experience to be asynchronous. That is, while the course might include some synchronous activities, such as PC-based video conferencing, the majority of learning will be asynchronous; this principle sets the culture for the course. In addition, with Web-based course management software, the classroom setup no longer determines the structure of the course. The professor organizes the course content and learning experiences within the template of the software. In such an environment, key learning skills and habits can play a major role in ensuring your success.

Distance Education Learning Skills

To be successful in a distance education environment, you must approach the educational experience with an appropriate attitude and effective distance education learning skills. This section provides an overview of these attitudes and skills.

Assume You Are in Charge of Your Learning

In a traditional classroom, many students expect the teacher to orient them to the expectations and requirements for the course. In distance education, the professor makes this information available, but it is the students' responsibility to review and understand these materials. To meet this responsibility:

- Check the school's student Web site. Most schools have one that provides help guides, video clips, and so forth.
- Access the course and look over how the professor organized it; learn where things are located, and how to navigate the course. Use **Table 11-5** as a guide for the types of information you should expect to find within your course.
- Once you see how the professor structured the course, go back and carefully read the posted materials. Many students find it helpful to download these materials and to highlight key points. Put any warning and due dates on your calendar. Be specific about the details of these requirements and prepare for problems. If an assignment is due at 5:00 P.M., do not wait until 4:55 P.M. to post it. Waiting is one way to ensure your Internet service provider (ISP) will be unavailable. If you are to post an assignment in a specific place in a certain way, make sure you understand how to do that. Sending the assignment at the last minute via email to a busy teacher with many students in different classes is not a wise move.
- You should follow the file naming protocols that the course requires. Professors use these protocols to manage several different assignments from different students and become frustrated when students do not follow their directions. Expect to discover that each professor and each course will have its own format for how the professor arranges information. Different professors will use different organizational structures, different rules as to assignments, and different protocols for naming files. In fact these variations often occur between courses the same professor offers. While these variations can be frustrating, they will help you become more flexible and more knowledgeable in the end.
- Once you review the materials, make a list of your questions and post them for others in the class to see, especially if the professor creates a Q&A section in the discussion forum. You will want to review the materials first so you do not ask questions that the professor has already answered in the prepared

TABLE 11-5 CONTENT AND STRUCTURE OF A DISTANCE EDUCATION COURSE
• A list of objectives, goals, or outcomes that describes what can be achieved from the course and how this will be useful. This is frequently provided in a syllabus that includes an overview of the course content and other requirements including required textbooks.
• Clearly outlined expectations for the projects and homework as well as an explanation of how each grade is achieved and how each assignment will impact the student's final grade; some refer to this as a rubric. Due dates for all work.
• A variety of learning experiences guided through online information and resources.
• Modules that organize topics into manageable units for learning.
• Opportunity for interaction between the students and teacher as well as, in many cases, opportunities for peer interactions.
• A format with related timelines for asking different types of questions and receiving answers. For example, many faculty will not respond to questions over the weekend. However, if you were to have a significant emergency that might affect a Monday assignment deadline, send the email so it is there on Monday morning when the faculty member is back at work.
• Control, to some extent, of the learning environment so that the student can set the pace and progression through course modules.
• Examples to facilitate understanding of material being studied.
• The opportunity to practice using material and to apply material to problems or cases.
• Feedback on practice and the use of the material.
• Tools to help reflect on what is being learned and to guide the next steps in the learning process.
• Resources in the form of hyperlinks, tables, charts, summaries, and references.

materials. You want to post these questions for the class because most likely other students may have the same questions. In addition, you may get a quicker response because not only the professor, but also other students may be able to answer your question(s). The exception to this approach is those questions that deal with private issues. For example, if you have a documented learning disability and need certain accommodations, you should send questions related to these accommodations to the professor in a private email; do not post them on a course discussion board. This same principle applies if you have concerns about a grade on an assignment or your progress in the course.

Set Aside a Specific Time and Place for Learning

In a traditional class, you might read the content in the required readings, listen to the professor review this information, take notes on what the professor said, and review your notes, at least before the exam. In a traditional on-campus class, you spend a great deal of time reading, reviewing, and going to class. This consistent time spent on these tasks usually leads to effective learning. In a distance education class, these repetitive tasks of reviewing materials occur in a new environment. Reading, highlighting, and reviewing the assigned materials are important. Noting the relationship between the readings, posted lectures, and graphic presentations helps to reinforce the learning. Many times there are ungraded activities in a distance education course—but "ungraded" does not mean the activity is optional.

The learning process in a distance education course will not take any less time than the learning process in a traditional on-campus course. In fact, it usually takes more time. If a three-credit course requires 45 hours of class time and a student should spend an average of 2 to 3 hours studying for each hour of class, then a three-credit course requires at least 135 to 180 hours during the term. For a 15-week semester, that averages 9 to 12 hours *every* week. Many students will do well the first 2 to 3 weeks of the term, but then start to back off. Once you miss a week or two of an on-campus course, it can be very difficult to catch up and this is even more so in a distance education course. Plan for that letdown after the first few weeks of class and push through that period.

Use Effective Communication Skills to Build Good Relationships with Others in the Class

In a distance education environment, communication depends heavily on the written word. You make first and lasting impressions based on how well you express yourself in writing. When you post comments and questions on a discussion board, excessive spelling and grammatical errors can give the impression that you are not a capable student. If this is a problem for you, prepare your remarks in a word processing application and, after editing them, cut and paste the comments to the discussion board.

Consider alternative views when engaging in an online discussion. Always keep in mind that some of your ideas might actually be wrong. Even if you disagree, learn to understand what others are saying. If you disagree with someone, take your time and think about how best to express your ideas. Never respond when you are angry or upset. It is possible to disagree without being disagreeable. Try not to *react,* but rather to *respond.* One of the best ways to do so is to ask questions rather than to state your disagreement. If you feel a discussion is evolving into an argument, limit your comments and help move the discussion on to a more insightful approach.

When you post a comment, think about how others might interpret it. For example, "Many of the elderly have difficulty getting health information from the Internet" sounds very different from "You cannot expect older people to be able to use the computer." If half of the students in the class are over 50 and you posted the second comment, you might get a negative reaction from your classmates. When you see comments that reflect a negative attitude or bias, direct confrontation does not usually change these attitudes. For example, if a classmate in a school nursing class made the statement that many financially disadvantaged or poor parents do not bother to apply for health insurance assistance, you might suggest the class try to create a list of reasons why some of these parents do not apply for assistance. You could start the list with some of the reasons such as:

- They need help completing the paperwork due to literacy limitations.
- Agencies have hours when parents are at work and they cannot afford to miss that work.
- There is no transportation to get to the agency.

In other words, move the discussion from criticizing the parents to how you, as a healthcare provider, can find solutions.

Manage Your Stress

Taking a distance education class for the first time can be very stressful. Understanding (1) why it is stressful, (2) when you can expect the most stress, and (3) how relaxation activities can alleviate stress can be helpful in creating a successful learning experience.

The first few weeks of class are often highly stressful. During this period, you may be learning (1) the new content of the course, (2) how to learn in a distance education environment, (3) how to navigate the course management software, and (4) new computer skills. Dealing with these four overlapping learning skill sets creates a fair amount of stress for most students. Many students, for example, express concern that they will miss an important assignment and fail the course. Because they are still learning how to communicate with their classmates, they often believe they are the only ones who are anxious. If questioned, some students will say things such as: "I thought I was the only one who was worried" or "I was sure all the other students already knew everything about using the computer to take a course" or "I was afraid I was really going to look dumb." You can avoid some of this anxiety by reviewing the university's technology requirements and participating in any online orientations that the university provides before starting the course. Most students survive this period by also sharing their anxiety with other students, reviewing the materials provided by the professor, and sharing their concerns with their professors.

The next anxiety-laden moment is with the first major scheduled assignment or test. If this is an assignment, review the directions and create a checklist of items you should include. If a grading sheet or scoring rubric comes with the assignment, make sure you address each point in the grading sheet. For example, if the professor says you should document your sources, make sure you include a set of references. If the first major graded activity is a test, practice taking online tests using the orientation materials that the university provides as well as self-administered tests available on the Internet. Use the self-assessment tests in Table 11-1 as sources for practice tests. If the professor uses timed tests, use your own timer and do not depend on the course management software to alert you to the time or to stop the test if you go overtime.

The last stressful period in a course occurs during the last couple of weeks. Anxiety usually escalates if you have major assignments that you have not yet completed or if you are behind in the course. Planning ahead and leaving extra study time in your schedule during the last 2 weeks of class is the best way to manage this period. This advice works for on-campus courses as well!

Once you make the adjustments to a Web-based distance education environment, you may discover you prefer this approach and the added flexibility it provides. As we stated earlier in this chapter, we assume you will be continuing your education to obtain an additional degree, obtain certifications, or obtain continuing education units for license renewal. Distance education is certainly one of the options you should consider for these endeavors. If possible, it is usually wise to take at least one (online) course before enrolling in a full-scale distance education program. Because this may not always be possible, it may help to know that motivated students who have never taken a distance education course often do very well in a distance education program. The key is commitment and motivation.

Just as there is wide variation in the quality of traditional courses, so there is wide variation in the quality of Web-based distance education courses or programs. Selecting courses—let alone a complete program—can be an expensive process, so shop carefully.

Selecting a Distance Education Program

All distance education programs are not created equal. There are, of course, "diploma mills" that are not always easy to identify from a distance. In addition, excellent schools with well-earned reputations do not always carry that excellence forward when they turn a traditional educational program into a distance education program. To add to the complexity of the decision there are a number of online schools and universities that have placed their emphasis on recruitment rather than on student success. That being said, distance education has introduced previously unavailable learning opportunities to students who want to continue their education. Once you discover programs that are potential candidates to meet your needs, carefully assess their quality. The following questions provide an outline for that assessment.

Is the Program Accredited?

Accreditation is important from both the institutional perspective and the program perspective. Is the institution that is offering the program an accredited institution? Is the educational program being offered also an accredited program?

In the United States, one of several regional accrediting agencies accredits colleges and universities. The Council for Higher Education Accreditation (CHEA) maintains a list of these agencies (which includes links to their Web sites) at http://www.chea.org/Directories/regional.asp. The location of the university, not your location, determines the appropriate regional accrediting agency. For example, the University of Phoenix (http://www.phoenix.edu/), which has campuses in at least 40 states and an Internet presence in every state, is accredited by North Central Association of Colleges and Schools.

Specialty accrediting agencies accredit specific educational programs in health care. For example, The Accreditation Commission for Education in Nursing, Inc. (ACEN, http://www.acenursing.org/) formally the National League for Nursing Accrediting Commission (NLNAC, http://www.nlnac.org) or the Commission on Collegiate Nursing Education (CCNE, http://www.aacn.nche.edu/Accreditation/index.htm) can accredit nursing programs. In addition, in February 2013 the National League for Nursing announced that they would be creating a third accreditation agency for nursing. You can see the press release for this announcement at http://www.nln.org/newsreleases/nlnaccred_022013.htm and http://www.nln.org/aboutnln/blast/blast_accreditationupdate.htm. Each accrediting agency includes a list of the schools or programs that are currently accredited by that agency. When determining accreditation status, always check the accrediting agency Web site as opposed to the school or program Web site. Unscrupulous schools will list accreditations that they do not hold.

While it is important to determine if a program is accredited, it is also important to determine if that accreditation is meaningful. Accrediting agencies are private organizations and not subject to legal regulation. Thus, while a program might be accredited, the agency providing that recognition might be nothing more than a Web page. In other words, just as there are diploma mills selling degrees, there are also accrediting agencies selling accreditations. Two resources can help you determine the quality of the accrediting agency listed by the educational program or institution you are considering. The Council for Higher Education Accreditation (CHEA), a private organization, has developed a review process for ensuring the quality and effectiveness of accreditation agencies. Institutions of higher education have accepted the integrity of this list. CHEA's Web site (http://www.chea.org/search/default.asp) provides a list of accredited institutions, educational programs, and recognized accrediting agencies.

The U.S. Department of Education (USDE) also lists "regional and national accrediting agencies that the U.S. Secretary of Education recognizes as reliable authorities concerning the quality of education or training offered by the institutions of higher education or higher education programs they accredit" (USDE, n.d.). The USDE plays a key role in determining whether students attending an educational program are eligible for federal financial aid. USDE provides a searchable database at http://ope.ed.gov/accreditation/.

Is Every Aspect of the Program Totally Online?

Many students assume that if an institution advertises a course or program, that the course or program is wholly asynchronous Web-based distance education. However, that is not always the case. Be sure to ask if the institution offers *all* of the courses and *all* of the course content in an asynchronous Web-based format. Find out if you will need to be on campus at any point during the program. The institution may require you to come to campus for video conferences, testing, or a particular class. You may also discover that students must come to campus for a specific activity such as orientation.

Always find out if there is a clinical component to the program and how you must complete it. Many distance education programs will permit you to complete their clinical requirements in your local area. To do so, they may expect you to arrange a clinical experience that meets specific criteria. For example, a clinical course on physical assessment may require completing a set number of physical examinations under the supervision of a preceptor. Preceptors, too, must meet certain criteria. Finding a willing preceptor with the appropriate client access may be your responsibility. Facilitating communication between the preceptor and the faculty may be your responsibility as well.

If the program of interest includes course requirements outside the department, ask if they offer these courses online. For example, if the program of interest requires a statistics course taught by the math department, does the math department offer this course online? If not, what options does the university offer for meeting the requirement?

What Does the Program Cost?

Most universities will post the cost of tuition and fees on their Web sites, but it is not unusual for them to impose additional fees for courses and programs that they offer by distance education. To find the total cost, talk to personnel in the admissions office, financial aid office, and student accounts office. Ask about recurring costs, such as tuition, and about one-time costs, such as graduation fees. Ask if the institution waives any fees for distance education students. For example, if you are not on campus do you still have to pay a recreation or health fee? Also, ask whether the costs are different for out-of-state students and if they consider distance education students out-of-state attendees. Universities might apply some very unique rules in this area. For example, until August 2008, part-time out-of-state distance education students at Slippery Rock University (http://www.sru.edu) paid 2% more than in-state students. In contrast, full-time distance education students paid the full out-of-state tuition—a difference of several hundred dollars.

Also consider indirect costs. For example, if the institution requires you to be on campus for a week of orientation, what kind of housing costs might you incur? Will you have to pay shipping fees for books that you borrow from the library? The financial aid office or other students who are already in the program might help you estimate the indirect costs you might expect to pay.

Which Timelines Apply to the Program?

The best way to appreciate the timelines in a distance education program is to plan out the total program on a calendar. This plan should include the beginning and end dates of each course as well as any other requirements that are part of the program.

Begin this process by determining the number of courses and credits you must complete. Credit requirements vary among universities. For example, a nurse with an associate degree may discover that some universities accept the transfer of only 30 or 33 credits for their nursing courses. Other universities will transfer in the total number of credits that you have completed at the community college, making no distinction between nursing and non-nursing courses.

Next, determine when the institution offers the necessary courses. Distance education programs do not always follow the traditional semester or trimester schedule. Sometimes you can start courses at any time and progress through the course or program at your own pace. Other universities offer specific courses during specific terms. For example, it might offer a course related to death and dying only in the spring term, and a public health course only in the fall term. It is very important to plan your schedule for the total program by determining, if possible, when they offer the required courses.

As you develop your calendar, be realistic about the number of courses you can take at one time. Distance education courses often involve a greater time commitment than traditional courses. If you are working, going to school, and fulfilling other responsibilities, you can easily overschedule yourself. Be especially careful if this is your first experience with distance education courses.

Are the Faculty Qualified?

When considering any type of educational program, you should always assess the qualifications of the faculty. In health care, this consideration includes both the academic preparation of the faculty and their clinical expertise. For example, the authors of this book have all taught computer literacy and health informatics courses. Each of the authors has more than 20 years of experience in teaching technology. Two of the authors have master's degrees in information science in addition to their master's degrees in nursing. Two of the authors have published chapters in books and presented informatics-related papers at large national and international conferences in 2012–2013. When asking about faculty, ask about the specific faculty teaching the online courses. Part-time temporary adjunct faculty teach courses in many accredited distance education programs. Depending on the school, these faculty can vary greatly in their educational preparation as well as in their teaching and clinical experience.

In addition to these qualifications, the faculty teaching in a distance education program should be prepared to teach using this technology. While some universities do require that faculty complete an orientation program, currently, there are no specific required certifications or degrees for a faculty member who teaches distance education courses. However, you can ask questions to ascertain the university's quality in these areas:

- Does the curriculum or course approval process in place at the university include any specific criteria for distance education courses?
- Does the university offer distance education preparation courses or workshops for faculty?
- Does the university require faculty to complete any type of preparation before teaching a distance education course?
- How long or how many courses have the faculty taught using distance education?
- Is there an administrative infrastructure to support faculty who teach using distance education technology? For example, is there a director of distance education or adequate instructional technology available to support faculty?

In addition to asking these questions, it is helpful to talk to current students. How do they evaluate the faculty and their distance education experience?

Are Distance Education Student Support Services Available?

Several student support services are part of a quality distance education program. First are library services. The American Library Association: American Association of College and Research Libraries (ALA/ACRL) has established standards for distance education library services (ALA/ACRL, 2008). **Table 11-6** includes several examples of university library Web sites listing their services for distance education students. When looking at these sites consider the following: (1) what resources are available in the library collection, (2) how do distance education students get access

TABLE 11-6 EXAMPLES OF LIBRARY SERVICES FOR DISTANCE EDUCATION STUDENTS

Library	URL
Eastern Kentucky University Libraries	http://www.library.eku.edu/distance-online-learning
North Carolina State University Libraries	http://www.lib.ncsu.edu/distance/
University of Iowa Libraries	http://guides.lib.uiowa.edu/distance
University of North Carolina at Greensboro Libraries	http://library.uncg.edu/info/distance_education/
University of Wisconsin–Green Bay: Cofrin Library	http://www.uwgb.edu/library/DE/index.asp

to these resources, and (3) is a librarian available online to support student learning. Chapter 12 will help you evaluate the library collection available.

Other support services for distance education students should include the following:

- Online university and program orientation.
- Technical orientation and support (e.g., what are the hours during which technical support is available?).
- Online registration, financial aid, student account services, and university ID card.
- Academic advising and support.
- Online student organizations and government.
- Online book store access.
- Career services assistance.
- Writing assistance and/or workshops.

One of the best ways to determine whether the university is "distance education friendly" is to assess the ease of finding information about online student support services on the university's Web site.

Is the Chemistry Right?

When selecting an educational program, certain intangibles may help you decide whether you will be comfortable and successful in the program. When a university offers a program in the traditional format, you usually visit the school and talk to the people there. When selecting a distance education program, it is important to carefully assess these same elements from a distance. Talk to your previous or current faculty and ask their advice. Review the posted faculty biographical profiles and information. Telephone and/or email faculty members who teach in the program in which you are interested. How quickly and fully do they respond to your inquiries? Find out if they understand your goals and your challenges. Keep in mind that they will be not only your future professors, but also your future role models. Problems getting responses to your inquiries as a potential student are not a good sign. With distance education programs, faculty–student interaction is often a major factor in the success of students. Be concerned if all of your information is coming from the recruitment office and faculty are "too busy" to interact with potential students.

If you do not know any of the current students, ask for the names, phone numbers, and email addresses of some students who will share their experiences with you about the program. Use both telephone and email contacts to ask questions. Often you will get different kinds of information from these two modes of communication. Search the Internet using the school's name and look for comments on social media sites. Remember, if it sounds too good to be true—it probably is too good to be true.

Summary

Successful distance education experiences occur when students take an active role in their learning. This chapter identified the tools necessary to be an active learner in a distance education course. It outlined a process and tools for assessing your distance education readiness. It provided criteria for selecting a best-fit distance education program as well. It explained the impact of distance education technology on the learning process, and concluded by exploring required distance education learning skills.

References

American Library Association (ALA) and American Association of College and Research Libraries (ACRL) (2008). *Standards for distance learning library services.* Chicago, ALA/ACRL. Retrieved from http://www.ala.org/acrl/standards/guidelinesdistancelearning

Bates, T. (2008). *What is distance education?* Vancouver: Tony Bates Associates Ltd. Retrieved from http://www.tonybates.ca/2008/07/07/what-is-distance-education

Crispen, P. (n.d.). About Patrick Crispen. Retrieved from http://netsquirrel.com/crispen/about_crispen.html

Duke University School of Nursing (2013). More than 15,000 enrolled in nursing's first MOOC. *Duke Nursing Magazine, 8*(3), 6.

Indiana University Information Technology Services (2009). *Distance education student primer: Skills for being a successful online learner.* Bloomington, IN: Indiana University Information Technology Services. Retrieved from http://ittraining.iu.edu/workshops/deguide/de_student_primer.pdf

U.S. Department of Education (USDE) (n.d.). *Accreditation in the United States.* Washington, DC: U.S. Department of Education. Retrieved from http://www.ed.gov/admins/finaid/accred/index.html

Exercises

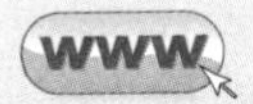

EXERCISE 1 Discovering Your Distance Education Readiness

■ **Objectives**

1. Use online self-assessments to identify your strengths and weaknesses as they relate to distance education.
2. Develop strategies for managing your distance education-related weaknesses.

■ **Activity**

1. Complete three of the self-assessment tests listed in Table 11-1.
2. Using the results of these three tests, make a list of your strengths and weaknesses as a distance education learner.
3. Using the distance education learning skills outlined in the chapter, create a list of strategies for maximizing your strengths and minimizing your weaknesses.
4. Save this file as **Chap11-Exercise1-LastName** and submit following the directions given by your professor.

Assignments

ASSIGNMENT 1 Evaluating Online Courses

■ **Directions**

1. Select an online course you are currently taking and, using a search engine, find three similar courses on the same topic. You might try the terms "distance learning," "eLearning," and "online courses."
2. Table 11-4 lists the content you should expect to find in an online distance education course. Use this information as criteria for examining the online courses you selected to review. Note that you may not be able to access all this information unless you enroll in the course, but there should be enough information in the marketing piece to give you a good idea of the course and its requirements.
3. Using PowerPoint, create a presentation outlining what you did and the results. Make sure you follow the guidelines for creating a quality presentation (remember this is a graphic presentation program so use the graphics to convey the message). Include:
   - A title slide.

- A slide outlining the process used for this assignment.
- A slide containing the criteria used for the analysis.

HINT: SmartArt works well here.

- A **table** with the **criteria** in the first column and the **three courses** in the next three columns. In the appropriate column, identify how well the course you examined meets the criteria. Give enough information to lure someone to a good course or steer them clear of one that you think has not yet been well developed. Be sure that the course title and Web address appear on the Word document. Be creative with the design, and include graphics if you wish.
- Slide with a **recommendation** and **rationale** for that recommendation.

4. Save the file as **Chap11-Assign1-LastName**.
5. Submit the file as directed by your professor.

ASSIGNMENT 2 Finding Best-Fit Distance Education Programs

Directions

1. Use the content in this chapter to create a spreadsheet with criteria for evaluating distance education programs. The criteria that you develop should be listed in column A. Later in this assignment, you will list specific distance education programs in the header row across the top of the spreadsheet.
2. Share your spreadsheet with three other classmates and add any criteria that your spreadsheet is missing.
3. Do an Internet search and select five distance education programs that are of interest to you for furthering your education. These can be baccalaureate, master's, or doctoral programs. Do not select a certificate program.
4. Complete the spreadsheet with data gathered from the Web page for each program. Create a second worksheet (tab) with the same setup.
   a. On the first worksheet, use a rating scale from 1 to 5 to fill in the cells on the spreadsheet. The lowest rating of 1 is used when the criterion has not been met; 5 is the best rating possible. In row 7, create a formula for adding the points for each program.
   b. Use the cells on the second worksheet to record your comments and collect text-type data related to these criteria for each of the programs.
5. Note where there are gaps because the information is not available on the university or program Web site. If the information related to that criterion is

not available, give the program a rating of 1. You can send an email inquiry to the admissions department and change the rating based on the response you receive.

6. Using both the qualitative and quantitative data you collected, select the program you believe is the best fit for you. Write a statement explaining why you selected this program. Be sure to refer to your criteria, including how to the criteria apply to this program.
7. Save the file as **Chap11-Assign2-LastName**. Submit as directed by the professor.

chapter

12

Information: Access, Evaluation, and Use

Objectives 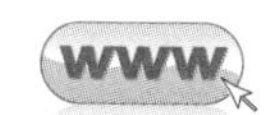

1. Define information literacy.
2. Demonstrate skills related to information literacy.
3. Define an information need, including concepts and terms that you can use to search for information.
4. Develop a variety of search strategies to locate and access information from published literature, "gray literature," and Internet resources.
5. Use a systematic approach to evaluate the quality of information from a variety of sources.
6. Identify appropriate and inappropriate uses of information.
7. Explain general principles for documenting information resources.

Introduction

Information literacy is one of the various overlapping technology-related skills required of all professional healthcare providers. **Figure 12-1** provides a model demonstrating these different skill sets and their interrelationships. The foundation of the model is basic literacy. **Basic literacy** consists of the text (reading) and numerical (math) knowledge and skills necessary to function in everyday life. This includes the ability to use information from various sources such as textbooks, newspapers, Web sites, and journals and in various formats such as maps, tables, and charts. As Figure 12-1 portrays, computer fluency and information literacy are overlapping skill sets that build on basic literacy. **Digital literacy** overlaps with and builds on computer fluency and information literacy. Digital literacy is the ability

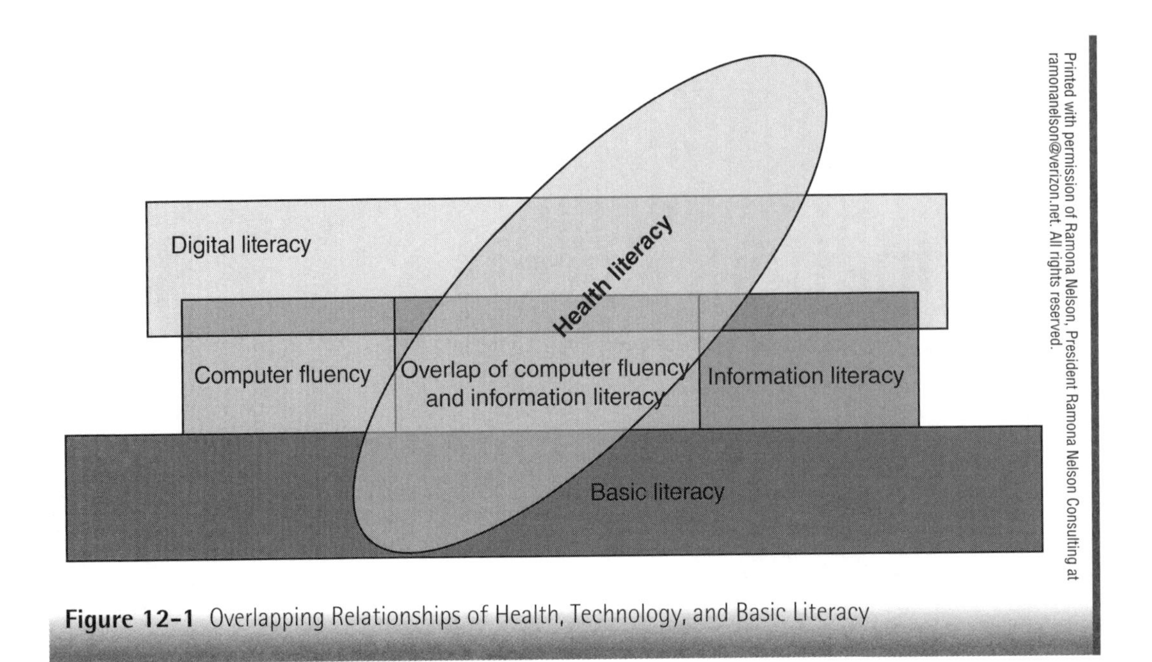

Figure 12-1 Overlapping Relationships of Health, Technology, and Basic Literacy

to understand and use digital devices of all types. In today's world, **health literacy** requires each of these literacies and therefore cuts across each of the areas of literacy within Figure 12-1. Because health literacy also includes knowledge of health and healthcare delivery, the concept of health literacy stretches beyond the technical skill areas within Figure 12-1. This chapter will focus on information literacy within this larger context including computer and health literacy.

The concept and skills that we identify today as information literacy grew out of the American Library Association's (ALA's) efforts to provide library and bibliographical instruction (BI) starting in the early 1900s. BI, which preceded the use of computers within libraries, focused on the use of book and other print materials within a library. The advent of computers, electronic information management, the information age, and the Internet changed the emphasis from "how to use the library" to information access, evaluation, and use (Gilton, n.d.).

The term information literacy was introduced in the 1980s although there is not clear documentation on who first used the term. In 2000, the American Library Association formally defined information literacy as the ability to recognize when information is needed as well as the ability to locate, evaluate, and effectively use the needed information (ALA, 2000). With this definition the ALA identified five information literacy standards for higher education. An information-literate person:

- Determines the nature and scope of an information need.
- Effectively and efficiently accesses that information.

- Evaluates information and its sources critically and incorporates selected information into his or her knowledge base and value system,
- Uses information effectively for a specific purpose.
- Understands many of the economic, legal, and social issues surrounding the use of information and accesses and uses information ethically and legally.

Starting in the late 1980s, a growing body of literature has continued to call for all healthcare professionals to be "information literate." **Table 12-1** lists a few examples of articles presenting this call. Note the concepts that these titles reflect. Critical thinking, evidence-based practice, and lifelong learning all require information literacy. In 2001, the American Nurses Association (ANA) described information literacy as a required skill for all beginning nurses

TABLE 12-1 CALLS FOR INFORMATION LITERACY

Author(s)	Title of Article and Journal	Year Published
Fox, L. M	Teaching the wise use of information—evaluation skills for nursing students in *Western Journal of Nursing Research*	1989
Weaver, S. M.	Information literacy: Educating for lifelong learning in *Nurse Educator Today*	1992
Cheek, J. and Doskatsch, I.	Information literacy: A resource for nurses as life-long learners in *Nursing Education Today*	1998
Rosenfeld, P., Salazar-Riera, N., and Vieira, D.	Piloting an information literacy program for staff nurses: Lessons learned in *Computers, Informatics, Nursing (CIN)*	2002
Innes, G.	Faculty-librarian collaboration: An online information literacy tutorial for students in *Nurse Educator*	2008
Leasure, A. R., Delise, D., Clifton, S. C., and Pascucci, M. A.	Health information literacy: Hardwiring behavior through multilevels of instruction and application in *Dimensions of Critical Care Nursing*	2009
Phillips, R. M. and Bonsteel, S. H.	The faculty and information specialist partnership: Stimulating student interest and experiential learning in *Nurse Educator*	2010
Turnbull, B., Royal, B, and Purnell, M.	Using an interdisciplinary partnership to develop nursing students' information literacy skills: An evaluation in *Contemporary Nurse*	2011

(Staggers et al., 2001). The ANA repeated this call in 2008 in *Nursing Informatics: Standard and Scope of Practice Information* (ANA, 2008).

These five standards, along with an emphasis on computer and health information literacy, provide the organizing structure for this chapter. The chapter begins with a discussion of how we can effectively access information. The ability to access information makes it possible to find all types of information from a wide variety of sources. This information may, however, be accurate or inaccurate, objective or biased, current or outdated.

Inaccurate and misleading information does not come with a label indicating that there is a problem. In fact, many times the author will assure readers that the information is credible. The reader must determine the quality of the information. Even good information can be misused. For example, the Internet includes many excellent sites with information about the importance of adequate vitamin intake during pregnancy. Referring a patient to one of these sites with no appreciation of the patient's ability to read and understand these data is a misuse of information.

Identifying an Information Need

Information needs come from a variety of sources. Common examples include a classroom assignment, a health problem in a family, or intellectual curiosity. In each case, the recommended first step is to write a statement to describe the question that will lead to an answer. Actually writing this statement helps to clarify what specific information is necessary. For example, if you were preparing to write a pamphlet on exercise for an elderly population, what information would you need? A statement of the information need might include these elements:

- Appropriate and useful exercises that are valuable for elderly clients.
- Exercises that most elderly clients should avoid.
- Guidelines on writing for the general population, especially the elderly.
- General health literacy levels of elderly clients.
- Signs and symptoms that an elderly person is exercising too much or too little.

Once the statement is written, underline the key words. Now make a list of different words that may have the same meaning or almost the same meaning as the underlined words. For example, how many different terms are there for the word "elderly"? How many of these terms might be in a pamphlet or article for the general population, and what terms are more likely to be in a document written for professionals? For example, are you more likely to find the term "senior citizen" or are you more likely to find specific age groups such as "65 to 75" in an article written for health professionals? Taking the time to carefully identify your terms and the potential location of those terms will increase both the effectiveness and the efficiency of your search.

Access

The first step in accessing information is to determine potential sources of the type of information you hope to find. Information sources used in professional and academic settings are classified as primary, secondary, and tertiary.

Primary, Secondary, or Tertiary Sources

Teachers often encourage students to consider primary sources of information over secondary sources. By definition, a **primary source** is the original source of that information. A **secondary source** uses data or information from primary sources in summarizing, describing, analyzing, or interpreting the primary source. For example, publications written by individual nursing theorists are primary sources for each of those theorists. However, a textbook about nursing theories that cites these same theorists while summarizing or describing the different theories is a secondary source. In addition, if the textbook includes other secondary sources in explaining the theory, it also becomes a **tertiary source**. While these definitions may appear to offer a clear difference, the reality is that individual publications can be a primary, secondary, and/or tertiary source depending on the context and discipline.

The context for the use of an individual source can play a major role in determining if it is a primary, secondary, or tertiary source. For example, Anton and Nelson published a research study analyzing what consumers were reading about health information on the Internet (Anton & Nelson, 2000). They conducted the research by classifying and analyzing what had been written in popular magazines about this topic. The Anton and Nelson publication is a primary source for this research and their conclusions. However, you may consider the articles cited in this research as a primary, secondary, and/or tertiary source depending on the context. For the researchers they are primary sources, but for the general population reading these same articles they are secondary and tertiary sources.

The decision about whether a source is primary, secondary, and/or tertiary also varies by discipline (User Education Services: University of Maryland Libraries, 2013). **Table 12-2** provides links to several examples of classification of information sources within the healthcare disciplines. As you look at these links you may consider sources such as journals both primary and secondary sources. These are general classifications. The final determination depends on the content within the specific source and the context in which you use it.

TABLE 12-2 HEALTH SCIENCE RESOURCES FOR IDENTIFYING PRIMARY, SECONDARY, AND TERTIARY INFORMATION SOURCES

University and Libraries	Page Title	URL
Brigham Young University Harold B. Lee Library	Terminology	http://sites.lib.byu.edu/subsutility//viewGuide.php?gid=508&nav=1
Brookdale Community College Bankier Library	Health information technology: primary versus secondary information sources	http://libguides.brookdalecc.edu/content.php?pid=116291&sid=1003445
Indiana State University Cunningham Memorial Library	Characteristics of different types of sources of information	http://libguides.indstate.edu/content.php?pid=175498&sid=1477968
University of Connecticut University Libraries	Finding nursing information: types of nursing information	http://www.lib.uconn.edu/research/bysubject/nursingtutorial/types.htm#primary
University of Minnesota Bio-Medical Library	Primary, secondary, and tertiary sources in the health sciences	http://hsl.lib.umn.edu/biomed/help/primary-secondary-and-tertiary-sources-health-sciences
Washington State University College of Veterinary Medicine	Guidelines for assessing professional information	http://www.vetmed.wsu.edu/courses-jmgay/evalguide.htm#Contents

School Library versus World Wide Web

In an academic setting the two primary sources of information include information resources available via the school library and information from the World Wide Web (WWW). You may access both of these sources via the Internet. At the college and university level, library sources are a major expense for the school and are therefore subject to careful selection by the library staff and the university faculty. The process for selecting school library resources provides a high level of assurance that these resources are of good quality and reliability. However, no library, even one with an interlibrary loan program, can provide full access to all information needed by everyone associated with the university. In addition, there are excellent resources that could not be duplicated by an individual library yet are offered free on the Internet. Excellent examples of this are the health-related resources that the federal government provides, such as Pubmed (http://www.ncbi.nlm.nih.gov/pubmed). Many times the university library Web site will suggest several excellent health science-related WWW resources.

However, research concerning sources of Internet content used by students in higher education identified six principle sources (Turnitin, 2013).

1. Social Networking and Content Sharing—answers.com; Yahoo Answers
2. Homework and Academic—Google books; Mayo Clinic
3. News and Portals—*The Huffington Post*; *The New York Times*, US.gov
4. Paper Mills and Cheat Sites—AllFreePapers; Frat Files
5. Encyclopedias—Wikipedia; Britannica, RefDesk
6. Shopping—Amazon, Barnes and Noble

Depending on how you use the site and the information on that site any of these could be appropriate. For example, a student assignment might require that students contrast and compare a paper they wrote with a paper on the same topic from a paper mill. Students doing this assignment may be surprised to discover that their own paper has more current references that are of better quality. Amazon often provides sample chapters from books listed on their site and many students use these chapters in completing their research. However, it is more likely that students will rely on the information presented in a site such as answers.com, which comes from individuals with no credentials related to the topic.

The Turnitin White Paper: The Sources in Student Writing—Higher Education (2013) lists the following key findings:

- Just over half of Internet sources in student writing come from legitimate educational resources: 57% of matches come from academic and homework sites, news, portal sites, and encyclopedias.
- Poor research practices lead students to a significant number of sites that are not authoritative: 43% of matches lead to sites that are academically suspect.
- More pointedly, 19% of content matches come from paper mills and cheat sites.
- Wikipedia remains the most popular source for unoriginal content in student writing.
- Higher education students need further instruction on proper research habits. Educators should incorporate the teaching of proper research habits upfront.

If you apply these findings to the world of evidence-based practice in health care, it would suggest that the future of quality care is dependent on the knowledge and integrity of today's health science students. Students who do not know how to identify quality information or those who elect to cheat by using resources such as paper mills will not be prepared to provide safe quality care to their patients and clients.

Searching for Quality Information

The process of accessing information begins by understanding how the computer stores data. Data are stored in an orderly and systematic structure called a **database**. As explained in Chapter 8, a database includes files that contain records. Each record refers to a specific entity and includes a set number of fields. Data related to the entity are stored in these fields. For example, if the entity is a journal article, the fields most likely include the author(s), article title, journal name and an abstract of the article, along with several other fields that hold relevant data. The process of searching for data in a database involves matching specific attributes about the entity with the field where the data element is stored. For example, if a search request is looking for a book that was written by the author Nelson, the database management system would search in the author field for the name Nelson. Each time Nelson is found in an author field, it would refer to a book written by Nelson. However, if a record includes Smith in the author field and Nelson in the title field, this book would not meet the search criteria; this source would not be a book written *by* Nelson, but rather a book *about* Nelson.

A **bibliographic database** is a specific type of database designed to store information about articles, books, and other print materials. The **fields** in a bibliographic database include the title, author, abstract, date of publication, and other details about the item being indexed in the database. Increasingly, bibliographic databases also include the full text of the article. **Table 12-3** lists some of the important health-related bibliographic databases commonly used in health care. The group or organization that produced the database may provide access to these databases or an information vendor that has leased the database may provide access to the database. Increasingly, information vendors have purchased established databases (such as CINAHL), produced their own databases, and then provide access to databases they own or lease. Vendors often combine databases along with other resources to create a discipline-specific package. **Table 12-4** lists examples of some electronic information vendors in health care; most of these vendors produce their own databases as well as lease access to databases that other groups produce.

Table 12-5 provides examples of the database offerings from selected information vendors; we collected the information in this table from the Web sites of these vendors in February 2013. Note the overlap in offered databases and the different descriptions for the same databases. In a world of exploding information

TABLE 12-3 SELECTED BIBLIOGRAPHICAL AND FULL-TEXT DATABASES IN HEALTH CARE

Database	Description
AMED	The Allied and Complementary Medicine Database is a bibliographic database produced by the British Library. It includes journals in complementary medicine, palliative care, and several professions allied with medicine, such as occupational therapy, physiotherapy, rehabilitation index, and podiatry. Additional information can be found at http://www.library.nhs.uk/help/resource/amed
CINAHL	Owned by EBSCO, the Cumulative Index to Nursing and Allied Health is available in five versions. These include (1) CINAHL Database, (2) CINAHL Plus, (3) CINAHL with Full Text (4) CINAHL Plus with Full Text, and (5) CINAHL Complete. These vary from 2999 journals that are indexed with 71 full-text journals in the CINAHL database to 4556 journals that are indexed with 772 full-text journals indexed in the CINAHL Plus with full-text version (EBSCO Industries, Inc., 2012) The CINAHL database overlaps MEDLINE; however, there are several citations in CINAHL that are not included in MEDLINE and vice versa.
ClinicalTrials.gov	Provided by the National Institutes of Health, ClinicalTrials.gov is a registry and results database of publicly and privately supported clinical studies conducted around the world. Additional information can be found at http://www.clinicaltrials.gov/
Cochrane Database of Systematic Reviews	This database, produced by the Cochrane Library, includes full-text articles that review the effects of health care. The reviews are highly structured and systematic, with evidence included or excluded to minimize bias. As of 2013 there are over 5000 reviews in the database. Additional information can be found at http://www.cochrane.org/
EMBASE	This database includes worldwide literature on biomedical and pharmaceutical sciences. Compared to MEDLINE, EMBASE is more European in focus although about one-third of medical journals are covered in both databases. Additional information can be found at http://www.embase.com/
MD Consult	This full-text database provided by Elsevier Company includes full-text articles from over 80 medical journals and clinics, 50 medical references across a wide range of specialties, clinically relevant drug information, and over 15,000 patient handouts that can be used for patient education. Additional information can be found at http://www.mdconsult.com/

(continues)

TABLE 12-3 SELECTED BIBLIOGRAPHICAL AND FULL-TEXT DATABASES IN HEALTH CARE (continued)

Database	Description
MEDLINE, PubMed, and PMC (PubMed Central)	Each of these three databases provided by the by the U.S. National Library of Medicine (NLM) overlap and are interrelated. MEDLINE (Medical Literatur, Analysis, and Retrieval System Online), includes citations from approximately 5600 scholarly journals published around the world. The MEDLINE database is a subset of the PubMed database. It can be searched directly from the National Library of Medicine (NLM) as well as through other numerous vendors who license the database. All documents maintained in MEDLINE are indexed using the NLM controlled vocabulary, Medical Subject Headings (MeSH). PubMed includes the MEDLINE database plus a number of other citations not included in MEDLINE. PubMed citations often include links to the full-text articles and chapters in books from the National Center for Biotechnology Information (NCBI) Bookshelf. PMC is a free archive for full-text biomedical and life sciences journal articles. In summary, PubMed citations come from (1) MEDLINE indexed journals, (2) journals/manuscripts deposited in PMC, and (3) the NCBI Bookshelf. MEDLINE and other PubMed citations provide links to full-text materials in PMC, the NCBI Bookshelf, and publishers' Web sites. Additional information can be found at http://www.ncbi.nlm.nih.gov/pubmed/.
MedlinePlus	Produced by the National Library of Medicine, this database of health information is designed for the general public, including patients and their families. It uses language understood by the general public to explain diseases, conditions, and wellness issues. This free, reliable, up-to-date health information resource can be used by patients and professionals. Additional information can be found at http://www.nlm.nih.gov/medlineplus/.
PsycINFO	Produced by the American Psychological Association, this database includes citations and summaries of journal articles, book chapters, books, dissertations, and technical reports in the field of psychology and mental health as well as the psychological aspects of related disciplines, such as medicine, psychiatry, and nursing. Additional information can be found at http://www.apa.org/pubs/databases/psycinfo/index.aspx.
SPORTDiscus and SPORTDiscus with full text	Owned by EBSCO, SPORTDiscus is a bibliographic database covering sport research, physical fitness, exercise, sports medicine, sports science, physical education, kinesiology, and related topics. SPORTDiscus with full-text builds on the SPORTDiscus bibliographic database and includes full-text access for more than 530 journals. Additional information can be found at www.ebscohost.com/biomedical-libraries/sportdiscus.

Source: EBSCO Industries, Inc. (2012). ***Nursing & Allied Health Literature: CINAHL via EBSCOhost***. EBSCOhost.com. Retrieved from http://www.ebscohost.com/promoMaterials/CINAHL_CHART_0512.pdf

TABLE 12-4 ELECTRONIC INFORMATION VENDORS IN HEALTH CARE

Company Name	URL
EBSCO Informational Services	http://www.ebsco.com
Elsevier	http://www.elsevier.com/
Gale Health Solutions	http://www.gale.cengage.com/Health/index.htm
OVID Technologies	http://www.ovid.com/site/index.jsp
ProQuest Company	http://www.proquest.com/
STAT!Ref	http://www.statref.com/
Thomson Reuters	http://www.thomsonreuters.com/

and competing information vendors, there are constant changes in the offered databases and the content within those databases. With this infrastructure for providing online journal access to individual libraries, an individual journal may be indexed in several different databases. You can expect the information in Table 12-4 and Table 12-5 to change within the year of publication, but the existence of different overlapping literature databases from information vendors will not change.

Although there are certainly a large number of databases and several vendors providing electronic access to healthcare information, including full-text access to many professional journals, there are some significant gaps in the online professional resources available. For example, vendors offer access to a number of online full-text medical books; however, the options for access to online books, while growing, are still limited for nursing and allied health. Examples of vendors that do offer such books appear in **Table 12-6**. Visiting the Web sites of these vendors demonstrates significant variation in the number and the currency of these ebooks. In most cases the books offered by any one vendor are limited to a select group of publishers.

The company or organization that provides the access will determine the specific database management system and, in turn, the user interface that it employs for searching that database. Many users become confused about the difference between a bibliographic database (the structure that holds the records with the content) and a bibliographical database management system. The **bibliographical database management system** is a system that provides the user interface to access the database and conduct searches. You can use several different bibliographical database management systems to access a database such as MEDLINE. In addition, the user interface for a specific bibliographical database management system will vary with the search device. For example, PubReader is a web presentation

TABLE 12-5 EXAMPLES OF DATABASES OFFERED BY SELECTED INFORMATION VENDORS

Database Name	Focus and Content of the Database
Examples of Health-Related Databases Provided by ProQuest	
Health and Medical Complete	Provides coverage from over 1,950 publications with over 1660 available in full text and of these, over 910 include MEDLINE indexing.
MEDLINE/MEDLINE with full text	Includes the entire MEDLINE database with full text and incorporates full-text journals from ProQuest Medical Library.
Nursing and Allied Health Source	Provides abstracting and indexing for more than 1070 titles, with over 890 titles in full text as well as over 12,300 full-text dissertations.
PsycINFO	Provides access to international literature in psychology and related disciplines.
Examples of Health-Related Databases Provided by Gale	
Health and Wellness Resource Center	Provides full-text medical journals, magazines, newspapers, reference works, and multimedia directed to consumers.
Nurse Resource Center	Directed to beginning students in LPN, LVN, ADN, diploma, and BSN programs, it includes encyclopedia articles, journal citations, animations, medical illustrations, disease overviews, drug monographs, and sample care plans.
Examples of Health-Related Databases Provided by EBSCO	
The CINAHL Databases	Provides access to each of the four different CINAHL databases described in Table 12-3.
International Pharmaceutical Abstracts	Provides abstracts from over 800 pharmaceutical, medical, and health-related journals.
Patient Education Reference Center (PERC)	Provides patient handouts in multiple languages that can be customized, printed, and given to a patient at the point-of-care.
MEDLINE Complete	Combines the MEDLINE database from the NLM with full text for more than 2100 journals.
PsycINFO	Note that this is the same literature database described in Table 12-3 and offered by ProQuest.

TABLE 12-6 EXAMPLES OF VENDORS OFFERING EBOOKS IN NURSING AND ALLIED HEALTH

Vendor Name	URL
EBSCOhost	http://www.ebscohost.com/ebooks/medical/subject-sets/doodys-core-titles-essential-purchases-2012/32411
McGraw-Hill eBook Library	http://www.mhebooklibrary.com/product/medical-nursing
Ovid Technologies	http://www.ovid.com/webapp/wcs/stores/servlet/content_landing_Collections_13051_-1_13151
Rittenhouse Book Distributors: R2 Digital Library	http://www.r2library.com/public/default.aspx
STAT!Ref	http://www.statref.com/titles/byResources.html

tool used to view articles in the PMC archive designed particularly for enhancing readability on tablets and other small screen devices. You can also use PubReader on desktops and laptops. Additional information about this tool is at http://www.ncbi.nlm.nih.gov/pmc/about/pubreader/.

Because vendors and information providers use different bibliographical database management systems to be used on different interfaces with different devices, this book does not give specific commands for using them. Each bibliographical database management system will provide a help section specific to that vendor. In addition, the library offering the database will offer assistance in using the databases in its collection.

General Principles for Searching

Two factors determine how much time and effort you need to exert when searching for information—your level of expertise with the topic and your knowledge of search strategies. An expert in a specific field will find it much easier to perform an efficient and focused search. For example, if you are an expert in maternity care and are looking for information about a specific complication of pregnancy, you could be expected to find the desired information very quickly because an expert knows the language and understands how knowledge is organized within the field.

If you are not an expert, then the process of searching for information is in many respects recursive. You usually begin by identifying a topic about which you want more information. For example, you may be assigned to write an article on electronic health records (EHR) and Meaningful Use (MU). As you begin the search for information on the topic you will find related information such as information on electronic medical records (EMR) and personal health records (PHR). Initially, it may be difficult to determine if this information is relevant to your assignment or not. At the same time, you may find that there is more information about this topic than you are able to effectively read and potentially use. In the process of selecting those materials that apply to your assignment and eliminating those materials that are not relevant, your search will become more focused. This initial exploration can be frustrating, but it is very important. It is during this initial stage that you become familiar with the terminology and the way in which the related information is organized. If your approach is to look for a few related articles or Internet sites and then stop your search, you will miss a significant portion of information about both the topic and the organization of information in that field. Your assigned paper will demonstrate these information gaps. To deal with this initial problem you may want to review references that you will not use as citations in your final paper. For example, encyclopedias such as Britannica or Wikipedia may be useful in developing a gist of the topic you are exploring. At this point be sure to check the cited references and note the terms as well as the sources of information sited in the encyclopedias. In other words, tertiary resources can be very useful when researching topics where your knowledge is very limited. Compare these terms with the terms you had initially written when identifying your information need. Once you have a list of terms you can start searching the appropriate databases used by health professionals. Note also that you might take advantage of the services of your school librarian to help with the initial search strategy; librarians can be very helpful in locating the best resources.

Indexing, Standard Languages, and Keywords

A record within a database will include several fields. The database management system that interfaces with the database will offer you the opportunity to search on these fields. Database management program design usually accommodates both experienced and inexperienced users. The experienced user will understand both the concept and the procedure for searching on specific fields. For example, many literature database management systems allow you to search for a specific author. In these systems, you enter a command such as "au-Nelson" or "a-Nelson." The search results from these systems would include all materials in that database that were written by an author with the last name of Nelson.

At the same time, these same literature database management systems are accessible to users who are less familiar with these concepts. These systems will compare any term that you enter in the search field to several fields. For example, you might enter the term "Nelson"; if this term is in the title, author, or even abstract field, the system would include it in the search results. **Table 12-7** shows common searchable fields used in database management systems that allow such searches.

TABLE 12-7 COMMONLY SEARCHABLE FIELDS IN BIBLIOGRAPHICAL DATABASES	
Abbreviation	Field
Au or A	Author
Ti or T	Title
Yr	Year Published
Pb	Publisher
K	Keyword
Su	Subject

The two fields that many frequently confuse are **keywords** and subject. Both fields identify the topic discussed in the reference being accessed. However, keywords and subject terms are developed very differently and using them interchangeably will often produce overlapping, yet different search results. Keywords are terms that the author, the publisher, or the developer of the literature database management system may have selected to identify the topic of the article. The design of some literature database management systems is such that any word appearing in the title, author field, and/or abstract will function as a keyword, however, there is no standardization of keyword terms. For example, an article about cirrhosis may be indexed using the keywords "liver," "hepatic disease," or "cirrhosis." The same article in different literature database management systems may have different keywords associated with it.

Subject terms, by comparison, are standardized. Individuals who are experts in understanding indexing and taxonomy concepts develop these terms in a systematic process. You may refer to standard sets of subject terms as a **controlled vocabulary**. An example of such a controlled vocabulary is MeSH (Medical Subject Headings), which is used in indexing MEDLINE. There are people who read each article in the database and then select the specific indexing terms from the controlled vocabulary.

It is also important when planning a search strategy to understand that different databases may be indexed with different subject terms. For example, **CINAHL** (Table 12-3) has its own controlled vocabulary which is different from that used by **MeSH**. As a consequence, the same article may be indexed under different terms in CINAHL than it is in **MEDLINE**. By understanding how keywords and subject terms differ, it becomes possible to maximize the advantages of both indexing approaches when developing a search strategy. By using terms and concepts that were developed when clarifying the information need, you can select a specific database or group of databases. For example, if the information need is related to the concept of nursing diagnosis, CINAHL would be a better choice of database than PsycINFO.

If you use a subject term as part of your search, you can expect to find all of the materials that relate to that term as identified by the index or taxonomy expert. In contrast, because keywords are not standardized, searching on a keyword may lead to incomplete results. For example, you may use "cancer" as a search term and miss all of the articles related to cancer that were indexed using the keyword "neoplasm." If you explore the interface of the different database management systems, you will usually find helpful tools for identifying the subject terms.

Because most library information systems permit the user to search several databases at the same time, the next step is to use the library information system to indicate which databases to include in the search. You enter the identified terms into the library information system as keywords. You then review the resulting hits from the search to find those references that fit best with the information need. Next, you examine these best-fit citations to determine the subject terms that were used to index these references. If you are searching across several databases at the same time, keep in mind that different databases may be indexing the same concept using different terms. Also, more than one subject term will be used for each article. For example, an article describing the types of injuries that occur when children are abused will be indexed on subject terms related to trauma, children, and abuse. Select the subject term that fits best with the identified information need. A new search using the subject term will result in a more comprehensive list of hits, although that list of hits may include too many or too few references.

Boolean Search Strategies

You can use several approaches to expand or exclude references from search results. These approaches are built on the concept of **Boolean search** strategies. Chapter 8 introduced the concepts of AND, OR, and NOT. **Figure 12-2** demonstrates the Boolean concepts of AND, OR, and NOT using a healthcare example. You can also use several other operators to expand or limit a search. These strategies are usually explained in the help section of the library information system or the Internet search site. Additional Boolean concepts are explained here.

Truncation

Sometimes your topic may have several words with the same base—for example, "nurse," "nursing," and "nurses." In such a case, using **truncation** may be more efficient than using the Boolean OR. With truncation, you type the beginning of the term and then use a symbol to indicate that you are searching for any citation that includes a term beginning with these letters. The specific symbol will depend on the specific database management system in use. Symbols commonly used for

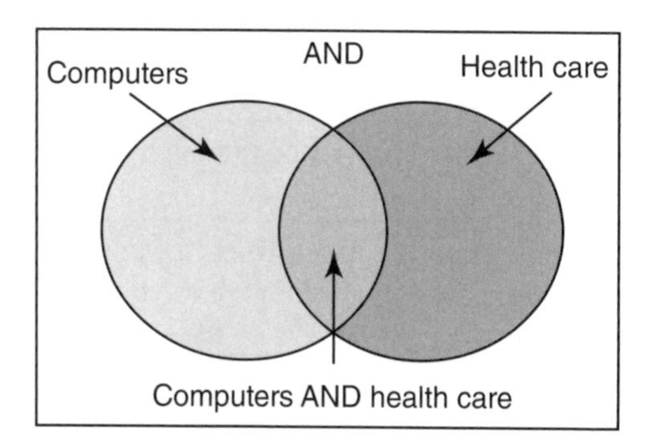

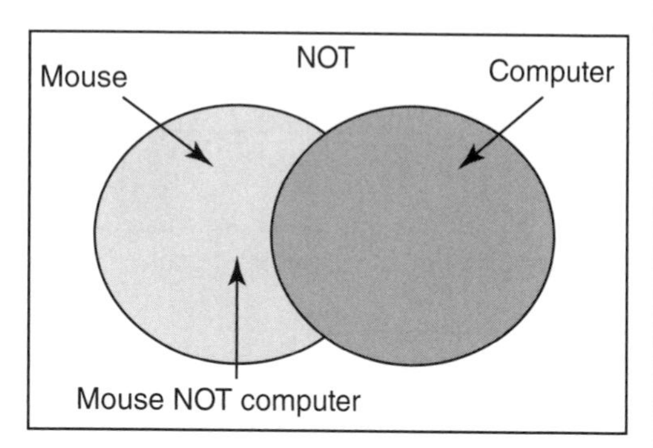

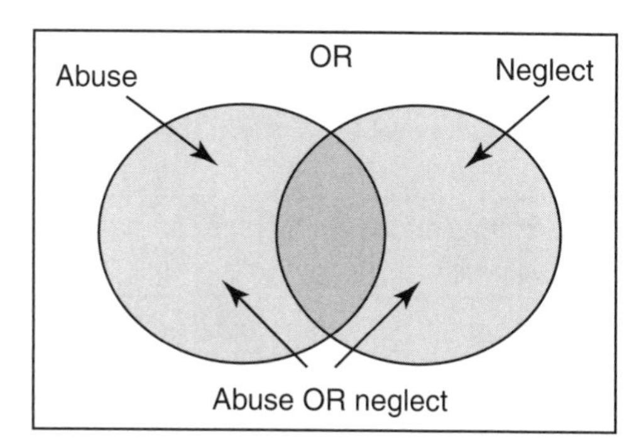

Figure 12-2 Understanding Boolean Search Strategies

this purpose include the asterisk (nurs*), question mark (nurs?), and dollar sign (nurs$). Remember that when you use truncation the search results will include every term that begins with the beginning letters. For example, when using "nurs" in addition to the terms "nurse," "nurses," and "nursing" you may also see nursery, nursemaid, and nursle.

NEAR

When the terms should be close to each other, you would use the term **NEAR**. For example, you may be looking for information on teaching people about computers. In this case, "teaching NEAR computers" might be a useful search phrase.

Web Search Sites

The Internet contains a vast amount of information. However, there are important differences between the information found on the Internet and the information resources found in an academic library even if accessed over the Internet. **Table 12-8** compares the key differences.

TABLE 12-8 KEY DIFFERENCES BETWEEN LIBRARY AND INTERNET RESOURCES

Library Resources	Resources on the Internet
Resources go through a review process.	Many resources are posted without a review process.
Resources are purchased by the library and distributed free or at a discount to those individuals or groups who have access to that library.	A wide variety of financial approaches are used to support access to the site and these may not always be obvious to the user.
Professional staff are available to assist in finding resources.	The Internet does not usually provide personal assistance.
Library resources are indexed and organized.	There is no organizational plan for the Internet.
Library resources are selected to ensure a comprehensive collection related to key topics.	The Internet provides an eclectic hodgepodge of information.
Information found in a library can usually be accessed at a later date.	Information on the Internet may or may not be available at a later date.
Because the review process and the preparation time to prepare materials for library use takes time, the information in the library may not be up-to-date.	Newer information can be found on the Internet; however, it may or may not be accurate.
Most information in the library is dated, so the user can tell how old or new the information is.	Information on the Internet may or may not be dated. If it is dated, the date may reflect the date the page was updated, rather than the date the content was updated.
The source of the information is usually clearly identified.	It may be difficult to determine the actual source of the information.

Chapter 9 introduces the concept of search sites and distinguishes between search sites and engines. **Table 12-9** provides examples of URLs for specific types of search sites—directories, keyword search sites, and metasearch sites. Although each has a different interface or appearance, all of them share certain features. Understanding how to use search sites begins by understanding relevant terms. Described here are some additional relevant terms. Chapter 9 defined other terms like hits, query, ranking, robot, search site, directory, metasearch sites, and search engine.

Stop Word

A stop word is a word that a search engine ignores in a query because the word is so common that it makes no contribution to relevancy. Examples include *and, get, the,* and *you.*

TABLE 12-9 EXAMPLES OF SPECIALTY WEB SEARCH SITES

Health-Specific Search Sites	Academic Search Sites
Healthfinder: http://www.healthfinder.gov/	Colossus: http://www.searchenginecolossus.com/Academic.html
MEDBOT: http://med.stanford.edu/medworld/medbot/	DBLP: http://dblp.uni-trier.de/
MedHunt: http://www.hon.ch/MedHunt/	Google Scholar: http://scholar.google.com/
MedNet: http://www.mednet-tech.com/	Infomine: http://infomine.ucr.edu/
PubMed: http://www.ncbi.nlm.nih.gov/entrez/query.fcgi	Qsensei Scholar: http://scholar.qsensei.com/
UCLA Information Resources: http://www.mednet.ucla.edu/	RefSeek: http://www.refseek.com/
National Institutes of Health: http://health.nih.gov/	
ISleuth: http://www.isleuth.com/heal.html	
University of Connecticut Health Center: http://library.uchc.edu/departm/hnet/inters.html	

Gray Literature

Gray literature (also called grey literature) includes works that may not have been formally peer reviewed and have not appeared in standard, recognized databases or publications. Government agencies, universities, corporations, research centers, associations and societies, and professional organizations produce this literature. Examples include some government documents, conference proceedings, online journals, and other valuable resources (CrossRef, n.d.). Because gray literature does not have wide distribution, it is difficult to locate or is not available for study. With the advent of the Internet we recognize more than ever the importance of gray literature within the domain of health information. Several libraries now provide help sheets and directions for finding gray literature within health care. Some examples include:

- New York University Libraries located at http://nyu.libguides.com/content.php?pid=27011&sid=992846
- Oregon Science and Health University located at http://libguides.ohsu.edu/content.php?pid=202165&sid=1689683
- Medical Library Association, Nursing and Allied Health Resources Section, Nursing Wiki located at https://sites.google.com/site/nahrsnursingresources/Home/grey-literature-1

Metadirectory

A **metadirectory** (sometimes called a directory of directories or directories of directories) is a directory of links to other directories. You can see an excellent example of a health-related metadirectory at http://hardinmd.lib.uiowa.edu/index.html.

Finding Search Sites and Beginning Your Search

Using a search site begins by accessing the search site on the Internet. There are several ways to find sites. For example, most academic libraries provide links to several sites. Some examples of sites with search site links and other tools include:

- http://www.noodletools.com/index.php
- http://www.searchenginecolossus.com
- http://www.internettutorials.net/engines.asp

Select any of the search sites from your university library or one of the options above. On the homepage of the search site, you will find a field or box where you enter search terms to create a **query**. Before you try your query, it is often helpful to access the help section of the Web site (it is sometimes referred to as "search tips"). Because each search site is different, you will find some variations and unique features on each one. Think of a car as an analogy: Each model is different, but all models share many common functions. The process for searching remains the same, but the tools or commands may be different.

In many cases, your first searches will result in a large list of irrelevant hits. One of the reasons for this result is that many search engines automatically assume that you intended OR between any of the words in the query. Thus, if you are looking for information about University of Virginia, many search sites return results that may include the term "university" and "Virginia"; only some of these sources will contain both terms and relate to your desired subject. The power searches, advanced search, search tips, or help at search sites can assist you to narrow your search. Boolean search strategies also help you focus your search. Many search engines use a plus sign (+) in front of the term for AND and a minus sign (–) in front of the term for NOT. A blank space between terms can be either an AND or an OR, depending on the search engine. With each search engine look at the directions and do a few searches testing how different Boolean strategies function within that specific search engine.

Evaluation of Information

Although finding information that is specific to your topic can be a challenge, finding quality information can be even more of a challenge. It is your responsibility to ensure that you use only high-quality information. The attributes of quality information provide a basis for developing criteria to evaluate that information.

Information Attributes

Information attributes apply to all information from any source. You use these attributes to develop criteria for evaluating the quality of information.

Timely

Timely information has several parts. Information that is timely is as current now as when it was written. For example, in 1992, the U.S. Agency for Health Care Policy and Research (AHCPR) released clinical practice guidelines on urinary incontinence. At that time, AHCPR had published approximately 20 clinical practice guidelines. You may be able to find a hardcopy of them in your library. You can access these guidelines at http://www.ahrq.gov/clinic/cpgarchv.htm. As noted on this Web page, the government agency has been renamed the Agency for Healthcare Research and Quality (AHRQ) and *none* of those guidelines should be used in current practice.

The concept of timely is also relative. For example, if you were writing a paper on the history of Florence Nightingale or the medical treatment of soldiers during World War II, something dated 10 years ago might still be correct and therefore still timely. In fact, materials written in the 1940s might be considered a primary source for researching medical treatment of soldiers during World War II. However, if the topic was the current treatment modalities for breast cancer, an article written 10 or even 5 years ago may no longer be timely. When you access information on the Internet or in a library, always check the date of the information at the site of the information. A word of caution applies when you do so: You should always make sure that the date reflects the date the content was updated, not the date the Web page was published or copyrighted.

The concept of timely also means having the information when it is needed. We live in a world of "just in time" information needs. For example, a clinical information system that goes down between midnight and 6 A.M. makes the information you need to provide care unavailable, or if a lab test is not entered into the PHR for 30 days, information is not available to aid in decision making when needed. Not having timely information at the point of need will affect the quality of decisions made.

Accurate

Information is accurate when it does not contain errors or misleading information that could result in an incorrect conclusion. For example, using the search phrase "HIV does not cause AIDS" will result in several hits for sites that dispute a relationship between acquired immune deficiency syndrome and the human immunodeficiency virus. Many of these sites look professional; however, the best scientific evidence indicates these sites contain inaccurate information.

Verifiable

Verifiable information can be checked at more than one source; that is, there is consensus among experts and consistency in how the data are reported. Verifiable information is usually supported by quantifiable data. As an example of verifiable information consider data about the current nursing faculty shortage. In this case, you might check government statistics, predictions from your professional organization, and health foundations, such as the Pew Foundation, to find verifiable information about this trend. While they may present slightly different numbers or predictions, each of these sites will confirm the existence of a nursing faculty shortage.

Accessible

Accessibility refers to how easy it is to obtain the information. For a number of years, MEDLINE was not generally available to the public. In the first six months that MEDLINE offered free access on the Internet, the general public conducted one-third of all searches as opposed to professional healthcare providers. With the addition of MedlinePlus (http://medlineplus.gov/), this resource has become accessible to a widely diverse audience. Information is considered accessible if you can enter a search term and the desired information is found in your search results. Four factors have a major influence on accessibility.

The first factor relates to the terms or language used to store the information. If you are using a bibliographical database, which words are in the title or in the abstract? How was the document indexed? If the information is on the Internet, access depends on which words are used on the Web page and the approach to indexing used by the Internet search engine. For example, does the Internet search engine search the whole document or just the first paragraph?

A second factor that determines accessibility is the number of references that refer to the original document. In a bibliographical database, references appear in the footnotes to an entry. Sometimes it is possible to click a footnote and be linked directly to the article. On the Internet, access is also determined by links. If several Web pages link to a document, you are more likely to find them either by browsing or by using a search engine.

The third factor that determines accessibility is your ability to focus the search. Initial searches often find either too much or too little information. One of the most effective approaches is to find one document that includes information you find useful and then use the information (words or concepts) from this document to find additional material.

A fourth factor that will determine accessibility is which functions are added to the search engine software. For example, EBSCO has added reference linking, which in turn offers three ways to link a particular article to other related resources. First, if a reference cited in the reference list of the original article is in the EBSCO database, a direct link from the cited reference to the actual reference is provided. Second, clicking on a reference link at the top of the screen will create a list of references that were cited in the original article. Finally, clicking the name of an author will create a list of other materials published by that same author.

Free of Bias

Biased information is information that someone has altered or modified in an attempt to influence the reader. Sometimes the bias is blatant and easy to identify. To confirm this point, do an Internet search using the term "abortion" or "gun control"; both topics generate strong opposing opinions. Look at several sites to determine if information is accurate and free from bias. Bias is easier to identify when you disagree with the opinion being expressed or when the information is clearly inaccurate. Sometimes, however, the information is accurate and the bias is subtle. For example, information provided by a drug company about one of its pharmaceutical products will most likely include information about side effects—but it may appear in small print near the end of the document. In contrast, the indications for which the drug is used may appear in larger print at the beginning of the document and be reinforced with a graphic. Each time the drug is referred to in the document, the trade name will be used as opposed to the generic name. These formatting choices are intended to influence you to consider the indications for the drug before its side effects and to think of the trade name before remembering the generic name.

Comprehensive

Comprehensive information is complete. Because there is always more that can be said about any topic, it can be difficult to determine if the information is comprehensive. Information is not comprehensive if missing details mislead the reader. For example, suppose there are two hospitals in your local community that do coronary artery bypass surgery, and one hospital has a higher postoperative death rate than the other. This information could lead you to conclude that one hospital provides better care than the other does. However, if the first hospital is a community hospital that takes only low-risk patients and the second hospital is a major medical center that cares for high-risk patients, the death rate data may not give a comprehensive picture of the quality of care at either hospital.

Precise

Information is comprehensive if it provides all the details. The information lacks precision, however, if the details are not specific. For example, a map on the Internet may include the specific street location for a clinic, yet fail to provide the street number for the clinic. Precision occurs when the provided details meet the specific information needs of the reader.

Appropriate

Appropriateness refers to how well the information answers your questions. Is the information on target? For example, you may be looking for information on preparing clinic nurses to use a new information system. You may be able to find a great deal of information about the new system, but nothing that helps you to prepare the new users for engaging with it. The information may be precise, timely, and accurate, and meet all the other criteria of quality information, but it does not focus on the specific needed information; that is, it does not answer the specific question that you asked. Health information is inappropriate if it fails to consider the age, culture, or health literacy level of the reader.

Clear

Information lacks clarity if you can interpret the same information in more than one way. For example, consider the following disclaimer: "There are several sites on the Internet that provide health information. Some sites provide quality information, while others do not. This is one of these sites." The reader is left to decide if this site provides good- or poor-quality information.

Criteria for Evaluating the Quality of Online Information

Knowing information attributes can help you evaluate the information you find online. Using those attributes, you can evaluate the source of the information, determine its accuracy and currency, and identify how easy it was to access and use the information online.

Source

When accessing and using information on the Internet, you should start with a reliable source. Reliable sources are usually verifiable and accurate. The source of the information on the Internet refers to both the author of the information and the location of the information on the Internet. Many times these two factors overlap. For example, you may find information about the role of weight in diabetes on an Internet site that the American Diabetic Association maintains or you might find the information on personal sites of individuals well known for their research on diabetes and weight. Many times personal sites use a ~ symbol (called a tilde) in the URL to direct you to a personal directory.

When evaluating the author as a source, it is helpful to identify the author's name, title or position, degrees or education, and professional affiliation. Remember that this may be part of the information on the Web pages, yet it may not be accurate. The author could state that he or she is the chairperson of the department of a major university and in reality be a 10-year-old child learning to design a Web page. It is up to you, as the user of the information, to validate the source. In addition, the listed author may not be the author of the document. Professional identity theft occurs when a document uses an individual's name and credentials falsely. The experience of Professor Emeritus John W. Hill, JD, PhD (http://kelley.iu.edu/facultyglobal/directory/FacultyProfile.cfm?id=8277) exemplifies this. Dr. Hill is a recognized legal expert with a distinguished academic record. If you search the Internet for his name you will find several references concerning the future of Medicare. However, as http://urbanlegends.about.com/od/government/a/Blue-Cross-On-Medicare.htm documents, these statements are fabrications. The association of Dr. Hill with these statements is an example of how someone can steal a professional's reputation and credentials and then use them on the Internet.

The URL is your major clue for the location of the information. Let's look at the following URL: http://www.widener.edu/about/campus_resources/wolfgram_library/evaluate/default.aspx. This site tells you it is a library site at Widener University. If you look around this Web site, you will see and hear a great deal of excellent information reinforcing the content in this chapter. The Wolfgram Memorial Library information literacy resource applies to all types of online information. The Western Connecticut State Libraries site provides an excellent example of how you can apply these principles in nursing and in the support of evidence-based practice (http://libguides.wcsu.edu/nurinfo).

Currency

As new information evolves, it replaces old information. With the ongoing knowledge explosion, keeping current is a major challenge in health care. In January 2009, the U.S. Department of Health and Human Services published the results of a research study dealing with relevant consumer Web sites providing guidelines for treating acute otitis media, or ear infection. The study reported that 32 months after release of the latest guidelines, only 32% of the relevant Web sites had been updated (Holland & Fagnano, 2008).

There are three important dates to consider when evaluating a Web site. The first is the original date when the information was generated. For example, if the site quotes clinical guidelines, when were those guidelines produced? Second is the last date on which the site updated its content or information. This is not the same as the last time the site modified the page, which is the third date to consider. The site may have modified design features on the page and place a new date on the page; however, the Webmaster may not have updated the content at the same time.

Another clue that the information is current is the reliability of the links. There are two ways to evaluate the links. First, do they function? Links on the Internet change constantly. If a site is poorly maintained, it will include outdated links that no longer function. Second, do the links provide current information? A well-maintained site removes links that no longer connect to quality information. If a site maintains historical data, it should identify the site as such. Note the following example at http://www.health.gov/scipich/. On April 28, 1999, the Science Panel on Interactive Communication and Health (SciPICH), an independent body convened by the U.S. Department of Health and Human Services (HHS), released its final report, *Wired for Health and Well-Being: The Emergence of Interactive Health Communication.* The panel is no longer active; HHS maintains this site for historical purposes only. However, without the historical purposes notice, the fact that the topic is very current might lead you to assume the page and related posted reports on this page are also current.

Ease of Navigation

Quality information is usually organized in a logical format. Logical technical approaches are then used to guide the user through the information. The navigation aids that a site employs may be as simple as a table of contents that provides an overview of the information in the document or as complex as the use of multiple frames. Sometimes a site map provides an overview of the information on a site. Sites may use color and graphics that help (or hinder) navigation. A site may be comprehensive, but if it is not well organized and the navigational aids do not function well, you may never find the quality information on the site.

Because a search engine may land you anywhere within a specific site, effective navigational aids are important. They provide a clear overall picture of the Web site as a whole as well as an at-the-moment location. A menu, a site map, arrows, and buttons should all flow together to provide direction. Standard terms such as "Home" and "About" are easier to understand than terms that are unique to a specific Web site.

Objective Information

Objective information is free of bias. Of course, the Internet is an excellent place for the expression of opinions as well as advertisement of ideas, products, and positions. Biases on the Internet are acceptable if they are clearly stated. For example, http://www.democrats.org is the URL for the Democratic Party; http://www.rnc.org is the URL for the Republican Party. You would naturally expect to find very different opinions on these sites. However, on some sites it can be difficult to discern the difference between an opinion, a bias, and a fact.

Errors

Several of the criteria presented will help you determine if an online resource is error free, but other clues may also be helpful in this regard. First, watch for errors in spelling and grammar. If a site is subpar as to these kinds of details, it may also be subpar with the accuracy of the provided information. Second, be cautious if the information is on only one site and no other information verifying it exists on other sites. For example, an Internet site might describe a malaria epidemic in Alaska. Malaria is caused by a parasite that is transmitted from person to person by the bite of an infected *Anopheles* mosquito. These mosquitoes can be found in almost all countries in the tropics and subtropics. Given these facts about the cause of malaria, the likelihood of a malaria epidemic in Alaska is minimal at best.

Health-Related Information on the Internet

Historically, healthcare providers have encouraged their patients to understand their health problems and to comply with the treatment protocol that they establish. Providers customize the treatment plan for the patient by taking into account the patient's goals, thereby creating a mutually agreed-upon plan of treatment. The assumption has been that healthcare providers, with their extensive education, are authorities and, therefore, must make sure the patient understands the treatment plan and will follow it. In other words, the role of healthcare providers includes responsibility for patient education.

Establishing mutual goals and providing the patient with the necessary education to achieve these goals is not always effective. Failure to follow a treatment protocol can have a significant negative effect on the patient's health status; a topic that has been widely discussed in the professional literature for a number of years. *Patient Compliance* is a MeSH heading with the following definition: "Voluntary cooperation of the patient in following a prescribed regimen" and the following caution: "Distinguish entry term *Patient Non-Compliance* from *Treatment Refusal*" (National Library of Medicine, 2013).

Failure to follow a treatment protocol or noncompliance is a recognized nursing diagnosis. **Table 12-10** provides examples of noncompliance-related diagnoses in ANA-approved standard languages.

Over the last decades access to information via the Internet has expanded and changed the focus of the healthcare provider as health educator. Patients are increasingly encouraged to move from the passive role implied by the concept of compliance and to take an active role in managing their own healthcare decisions. An example of this change appears in the *Patient Engagement Framework* (see **Figure 12-3**) that the National eHealth Collaborative (NeHC) developed. The NeHC is a public-private partnership established through a grant from the Department of Health and Human Services Office of the National Coordinator for Health IT (ONC). NeHC works "to educate, connect, and encourage healthcare

TABLE 12-10 NONCOMPLIANCE AS A NURSING DIAGNOSIS

Standard Language	Nursing Diagnosis	Definition	Source
Clinical Care Classification (CCC) System	Noncompliance of Diagnostic Test	Failure to follow therapeutic recommendations following tests to identify disease or assess health condition.	http://www.sabacare.com/Tables/Diagnoses.html?SF=DiagCode&SO=Asc
	Noncompliance of Dietary Regimen	Failure to follow the prescribed diet/food intake.	
	Noncompliance of Fluid Volume	Failure to follow fluid volume intake requirements.	
	Noncompliance of Medication Regimen	Failure to follow prescribed regulated course of medicinal substances.	
	Noncompliance of Safety Precautions	Failure to follow measures to prevent injury, danger, or loss.	
	Noncompliance of Therapeutic Regimen	Failure to follow regulated course of treatment.	
NANDA	Noncompliance (00079) Domain 10: Life Principles, Class 3: Value/Belief/Action Congruence	Behavior of person and/or caregiver that fails to coincide with a health-promoting or therapeutic plan agreed on by the person (and/or family and/or community) and healthcare professional. In the presence of an agreed-upon, health-promoting, or therapeutic plan, the person's or caregiver's behavior is fully or partially nonadherent and may lead to clinically ineffective or partially ineffective outcomes.	Herdman, T. H. (ed.) (2012) *NANDA International Nursing Diagnoses: Definitions and Classifications 2012–2014.* Oxford, UK: Wiley & Sons, Ltd.

TABLE 12-10 (CONTINUED)

Standard Language	Nursing Diagnosis	Definition	Source
SNOMED CT Core Nursing Problem List	Noncompliance with Diagnostic Testing; Noncompliance with Dietary Regimen; Noncompliance with Treatment; Noncompliance with Therapeutic Regimen; Noncompliance with Safety Precautions; Noncompliance with Medication Regimen	Core nursing diagnosis identified by cross mapping the UMLS mappings of CCC and NANDA-I concepts to SNOMED CT for use in EHRs.	http://www.nlm.nih.gov/research/umls/Snomed/nursing_problemlist_subset.html

stakeholders, who are critical to the successful deployment of health information technology and health information exchange nationwide" (NeHC, 2010a). A key activity within NeHC is the Consumer Consortium on eHealth. The goal of this program is "to spark a grassroots movement intended to empower consumers to take advantage of eHealth tools and become equal partners in their healthcare" (NeCH, 2010b).

Figure 12-3 indicates the first stage of the *Patient Engagement Framework* includes patient-specific education that focuses on topics such as the care plan, tests, prescribed medication, and procedures/treatments. But the end of Stage 5 encourages all care team members, including caregivers, family, friends, and clergy, to participate in online community support forums and resources. This would suggest that the patient is no longer a passive recipient of healthcare services, but a colleague with the ultimate responsibility for managing her or his health. It also demonstrates the need for healthcare providers to provide information and health literacy-related education for patients, families, and communities. Patients, families, and communities must be prepared to access, interpret, and utilize health information from a variety of resources including those resources on the Internet.

However, not all health information is created equal, and not everything on the Internet is correct. When knowledgeable people "surf the Web," they have

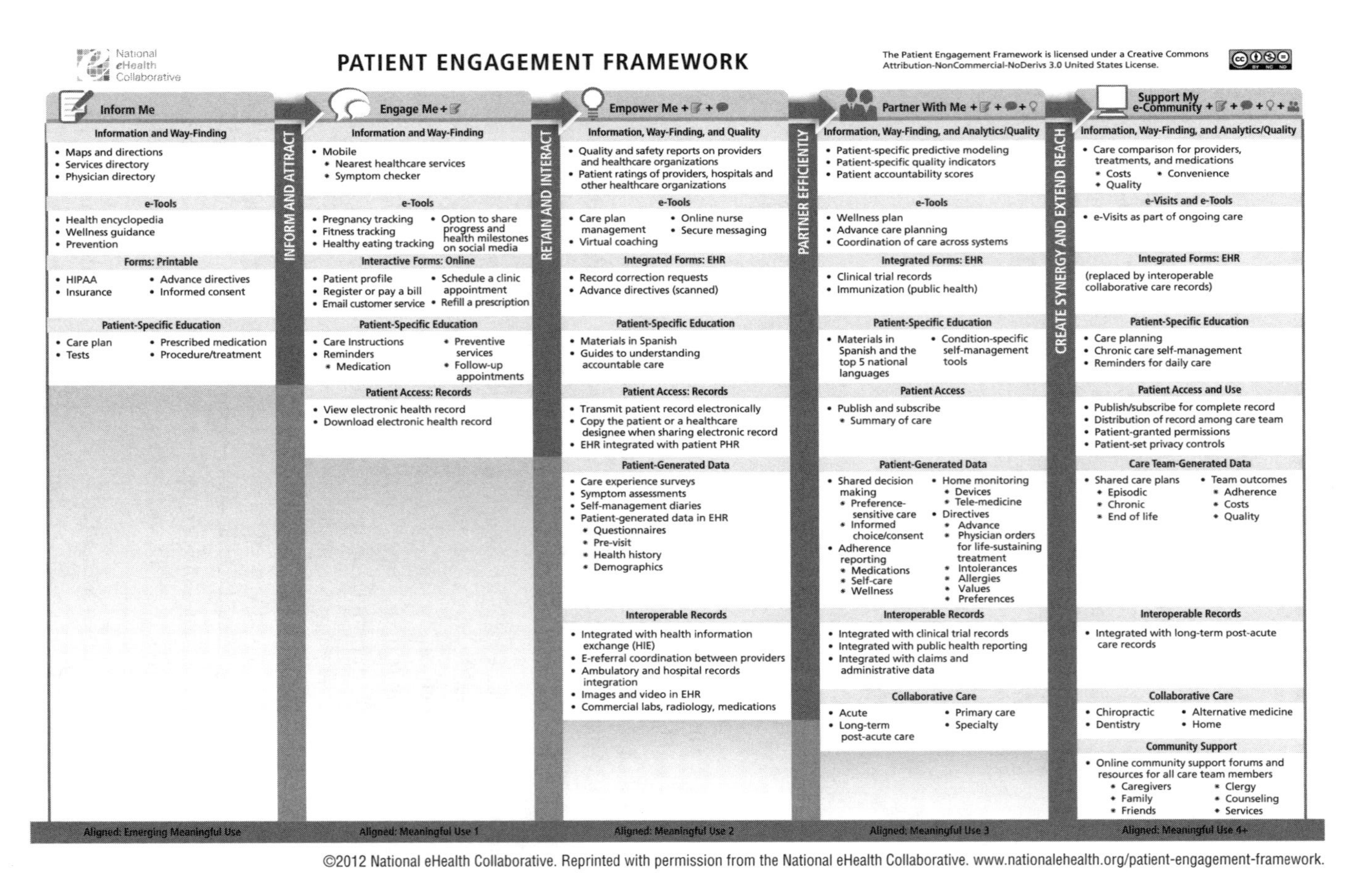

Figure 12-3 Patient Engagement Framework

found dangerously misleading or incomplete health information that looks quite legitimate on the surface. The medium itself contributes to the problem. With the right tools even a novice designer can make a Web page look legitimate. While poor design can indicate poor information, good design does not guarantee good information. Information on a Web site may be no more reliable or credible than something you heard at a party or on a talk show. While sites post much of the health information on the Internet to help people, not all of it will be useful for everyone.

Research related to this issue has concluded that as a professional or student healthcare provider you have a responsibility for educating patients and health consumers.

> ***Conclusions:*** *Google, Yahoo!, Bing, and Ask.com are by and large effective search engines for helping lay users get health and medical information. Nevertheless, the current ranking methods have some pitfalls and there is room for improvement to help users get more accurate and useful information. We suggest that search engine users explore multiple search engines to search different types of health information and medical knowledge for their own needs and get a professional consultation if necessary* (Wang, Wang, Wang, & Li, 2012).

The professional consultation referred to is a professional such as you.

Additional Criteria for Health-Related Information

The criteria discussed earlier in this chapter deal with any information found on the Internet. They also apply to healthcare information, though they are not *specific* to healthcare information. Unique criteria that do apply when the information is health related, include:

Intended Audience

Does the site clearly state who the intended audience is, including the skills and knowledge necessary to interpret the information provided by the site? This information is often included in an area titled "Mission" or "About Us." Many sites will identify information as being appropriate for the general public or for healthcare professionals.

Confidentiality of Personal Information

Many healthcare sites collect personal healthcare data. For example, many sites include self-assessment areas. A quality site will clearly state what data it collects and how it will use that data. These statements are usually in the "Privacy Notice" and/or the "Conditions of Use" area of the website. Remember that anyone can publish anything on the Web, including a statement of privacy that is incomplete or inaccurate. Be sure you know the site and the sponsors of that site before you provide personal information to an Internet site. Ask yourself, Do I trust them with my information?

Source of the Content/References

An Internet site that provides health information must be able to document the source of that information and the relationship of that source to the information. The name of the organization or institution responsible for the content should be clear. The page should clearly indicate the author's name, credentials, and personal or financial connections that could be a source of real or potential bias. In addition, the Web page should provide an easily located way to contact the author of the page. As a user, you need to evaluate the source of the information and determine whether the listed sources are, in fact, real. The references list itself may include references that do not exist.

Sensitivity to the Health Literacy of the Intended Audience

We introduced the concept of health literacy at the beginning of this chapter. Low levels of health literacy have frequently been correlated with poor health outcomes. To address this, *Healthy People 2020* incorporated health literacy into its objectives on the website: http://www.healthypeople.gov/2020/topicsobjectives2020/objectiveslist.aspx?topicid=18. "Health literacy is the degree to which individuals have the capacity to obtain, process, and understand basic health information and needed services to make appropriate health decisions" (U.S. Department of Health and Human Services, 2000). Basic to health literacy is the ability to read and comprehend information. You can use several tools to evaluate the reading level of posted materials on the Internet and utilize the technology skills identified in Figure 12-1.

In Chapter 5, we demonstrated one such tool available in Microsoft Word—readability statistics. You can learn more about this tool by using Word's help function. Comprehension is a more difficult question: It depends on the healthcare background of readers and their ability to understand and effectively use the presented information. Because anyone can access the Internet, it is important for any healthcare-oriented site to address this issue. It is also helpful if the site specifically identifies the intended audience.

Recognition by Other Authorities

Reputable sites will recognize other excellent sites that have quality information. If there are no links to a site and no references to it, you should be concerned. For example, the Consumer and Patient Health Information Section (CAPHIS) of the Medical Library Association maintains a list of the top 100 sites related to health care; this list is at http://caphis.mlanet.org/consumer/index.html.

Sites Containing Healthcare Information Criteria

The quality of healthcare information on the Internet is of great concern to many healthcare providers. A number of sites on the Internet provide guides for evaluating healthcare information. Some excellent examples include: (http://www.mlanet.org/resources/userguide.html), (http://www.ucsfhealth.org/education/evaluating_health_information/), and (http://www.spry.org/sprys_work/education/EvaluatingHealthInfo.html).

Other organizations accredit or recognize sites that meet specific criteria. One of the most respected sites is Health On the Net Foundation (HON, http://www.hon.ch/home.html), a nonprofit organization in Geneva, Switzerland. Among its many activities, HON has developed a code of conduct for providers of healthcare information. The code does not rate the quality or the information on a Web site; rather, it defines a set of rules designed to make sure the reader always knows the source and the purpose of the data accessed. You will note that Emory University's entry includes a reference to this code of conduct on its evaluation form.

In addition the federal government has attempted to educate the general population on the quality of healthcare information as indicated by these sites:

- http://healthfinder.gov/FindServices/SearchContext.aspx?topic=14310
- http://ods.od.nih.gov/Health_Information/How_To_Evaluate_Health_Information_on_the_Internet_Questions_and_Answers.aspx
- http://www.ahrq.gov/legacy/qual/hiirpt.htm
- http://www.ahrq.gov/research/data/infoqual.html
- http://www.cancer.gov/cancertopics/cancerlibrary/health-info-online
- http://www.fda.gov/Drugs/ResourcesForYou/Consumers/BuyingUsingMedicineSafely/BuyingMedicinesOvertheInternet/ucm202863.htm
- http://www.nlm.nih.gov/medlineplus/webeval/webeval.html

At this point, many of the resources for educating the general public on evaluating health information on the Internet are still based on a Web 1.0 model, where the information is posted and patients do not co-create it. However, with the advent of social media and the Web 2.0 model, many patients are now getting health-related information from these social media sites. The criteria for evaluating this information are the same but the social media environment has influenced the application of those criteria. For example, you would still consider the source of the information but on a social media site you might consider a patient, who has no professional credentials but who has consistently posted reliable information, an excellent source. **Box 12-1** provides selected patient education tips for evaluating information on a social media site.

Box 12-1 Tips for Evaluating Patient Information on Social Media Sites

1. Try to determine who established and is maintaining the site. For example, is it a moderated social support group maintained by a local hospital or is it a for-profit unmoderated site supported by advertisements? Is this a site that has been recommended by your healthcare provider(s)? The answers to these questions can help you evaluate whether information on a site may have a bias.
2. Be sure to review the Privacy Statement and Conditions of Use before establishing an account. These documents should be easy to access, understand, and print. Be concerned about sites where this is not true. Reliable sites that are well maintained want their users to understand these documents.
3. When establishing an account, provide the minimum information necessary to establish the account.
4. Spend time learning how to navigate the site and set privacy/security settings before participating.
5. Lurk on the site to learn the names and personality characteristics of individuals who frequently participate on the site. For example, do certain members tend to post information along with links to documentation or is there a formal moderator who works for the company that maintains the site? The name and credentials of professionals can usually be found on the Web. For example, most states maintain a Web site where the general public can check if someone is, in fact, a licensed physician or nurse. In other words, get to know the people in the social media group and the personality of the group from your own observations and from additional information you can find on the Internet.
6. If health information has been posted that is unclear or incomplete, ask questions or request more information. The learning that occurs is one of the primary advantages of using social media sites.
7. Avoid conflict or arguments with people on a social media site. If someone posts information you believe is wrong, ask questions and/or politely point out how this is different from your previous knowledge. The follow-up discussion can then clarify and/or correct misinformation.
8. Remind patients that information may be accurate but not applicable in all cases. For example: "Skin rash during treatment with anti-EGFR TKIs for non-small cell lung cancer (NSCLC) represents a significantly strong predictor of the efficacy in particular for patients with unknown EGFR mutation status" (Petrelli, Borgonovo, Cabiddu, Lonati, & Barni, 2012). This is a reliable conclusion from a reported research study. However, patients who experience little or no rash should not discontinue their medication.
9. Validate information posted on a social media site by looking at information on other sites or discussing information with your healthcare provider.

Using Information

The final step in becoming information literate is to make effective use of information. In this book, we limit the discussion of effective use to documenting information from the Internet.

Documenting Internet Sources

You must document information that you access on the Internet just as you would document information from any other source. Failure to document is plagiarism: Plagiarism is the act of stealing another person's ideas or work and presenting it as your own. The Internet has made it easier to plagiarize and has created additional issues regarding attribution of sources. Often, students do not even realize they are stealing. Copyright laws protect information posted on the Internet just as they do information that appears in print. These laws can even apply to posted email messages in online discussion groups. Because documentation of Internet-based information has become an increasing concern, some people have developed Web sites to help deal with this issue. One example can be seen at http://www.nwmissouri.edu/library/services/prevent.htm.

Citing Internet Information

Just as it is easy to post information on the Internet, it is also easy to remove that information, therefore, the citation for information from the Internet should include some additional data, such as the date on which the information was developed. The Internet site should provide this information; if it does not, the citation should indicate that the information source is undated. Several Internet sites give specific directions for formatting an Internet citation from their site.

The American Psychological Association (APA) is one of the most commonly used formats for citing healthcare information. The APA maintains a Web site that includes information on how to use the APA format to cite Internet resources (http://www.apastyle.org). Many university libraries and writing centers provide additional help with APA style; http://owl.english.purdue.edu/owl/resource/560/01/ is one such example.

In addition to the APA format, there are other accepted citation formats. Many libraries provide guidance on citation formats on their Web sites. The University of Texas Libraries demonstrates several of these on its site at http://www.lib.utexas.edu/refsites/style_manuals.html. Such sites often include a list of links to guidelines for citing Internet resources. Two sites that demonstrate this approach are http://nova.campusguides.com/content.php?pid=329404&sid=2707195 and http://library.lafayette.edu/help/citing/webpages; the second site includes a list of components that should be included in any Internet citation.

Summary

This chapter explored the concept of information literacy and outlined strategies necessary to identify an information need, find information, evaluate the quality of information, and cite information from the Internet. Quality health care requires good information. As a healthcare provider, it is your responsibility to search for the latest high-quality information and make appropriate use of that information in providing care to your patients. It is also your responsibility to educate patients about safe and effective approaches for becoming informed consumers of health-related information.

References

American Library Association (2000). Information literacy competency standards for higher education. Retrieved from http://www.ala.org/acrl/standards/informationliteracycompetency

American Nurses Association (2008). *Nursing Informatics: Scope and Standards of Practice.* Silver Spring, MD: Nursesbooks.org.

Anton, B. & Nelson, R. (2000). Health information on the Internet: A research approach to learning what the consumer reads in mainstream publications, in *Nursing Informatics 2000: One Step Beyond: The Evolution of Technology* (V. Saba, R. Carr, W. Sermeus, and P. Rocha, eds.). Auckland, New Zealand: Adis International, pp 746–752.

CrossRef (n.d.). CrossRef glossary. Retrieved from http://www.crossref.org/02publishers/glossary.html

Gilton, D. L. (n.d.). *Information literacy instruction: A history in context.* Retrieved from http://www.uri.edu/artsci/lsc/Faculty/gilton/InformationLiteracyInstruction-AHistoryinContext.htm

Holland, M. L. & Fagnano, B. A. (2008). Appropriate antibiotic use for acute otitis media: What consumers find using Web searches. *Clinical Pediatrics, 47*(5), 452–546.

National eHealth Collaborative (NeHC) (2010a). About National eHealth Collaborative. Retrieved from http://www.nationalehealth.org/about-national-ehealth-collaborative

National eHealth Collaborative (NeCH) (2010b). About the Consumer Consortium on eHealth. Retrieved from http://www.nationalehealth.org/consumers

National Library of Medicine (2013). Medical Subject Headings—MeSH Descriptor Data—Expanded Concept View. Washington, DC: National Institute of Health.

Staggers, N., Gassert, C., Kwai, J. L., Milholland, K., Nelson, R., Senemeier, J., Stuck, D., & Welton, J. (2001). *Scope and standards of nursing informatics practice.* Washington, DC: American Nurses Publishing.

Turnitin. (2013). White Paper: The Sources in Student Writing—Higher Education: Sources of Matched Content and Plagiarism in Student Writing. Oakland, CA: iParadigms/Turnitin.

User Education Services: University of Maryland Libraries (2013). Primary, secondary and tertiary sources. Retrieved from http://www.lib.umd.edu/ues/guides/primary-sources
Wang, L., Wang, J., Wang, M., & Li, Y. L. (2012). Using Internet search engines to obtain medical information: A comparative study. *J Med Internet Res, 14*(3). Retrieved from http://www.jmir.org/2012/3/e74/

Exercises

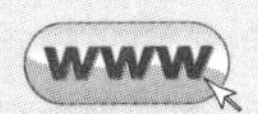

EXERCISE 1 Understanding Variations in Search Sites and Search Strategies

Objectives

1. Use the help section of an Internet search site.
2. Analyze how different Boolean search strategies are used with different search engines.
3. Evaluate the significance of the rank order of hits obtained with an Internet search.

Activity

Comparison of search sites and search strategies:

1. Select two general search sites such as Google, Bing, or Yahoo.
2. Briefly review the help section for each search site including directions for using the advanced search function.
3. Use the following list to conduct a series of searches with your first selected search site. Print the first page of hits obtained with each of the following search strategies.
   a. (Healthcare AND "social media")
   b. + healthcare + social media
   c. healthcare social media
   d. social media healthcare
   e. "social media" AND "health care"
   f. Use these search terms with the advanced search function of the search engine.
4. Develop a spreadsheet listing the six search strategies down the first column so you have created six rows on the spreadsheet.
5. Limiting your analysis to the first six hits on the printed pages, list the hits across the top cells of the spreadsheet. The hits are the column headers. As you create the column headers do not list a site (hit) more than once.
6. Put a Y in the intersecting cells indicating if a specific search strategy yielded that site and an N if it did not yield that hit.
7. Now repeat the search strategies and printing of the hits with the second search engine.
8. Add these data from the second group of searches to your spreadsheet. There are several different approaches you can use to design your spreadsheet to accept these new data. Select the one that is most effective for helping you to see the big picture.

9. Write a short paper describing how search sites and search strategies can impact the specific hits that can be obtained when searching the Internet.
10. Submit the paper as directed by the professor.

EXERCISE 2 Designing Tools for Evaluating Health Information on the Internet

Objectives

1. Using the criteria described in this chapter, develop a tool that you can use to evaluate the quality of information on a specific Internet site.
2. Evaluate the effectiveness of the tool for a user who has limited health literacy.
3. Evaluate the effectiveness of the tool for someone with a different first language and culture.

Activity

Evaluating health-related information sites:

1. Review three sites from the following list:
   http://www.virtualsalt.com/evalu8it.htm
   http://www.ala.org/alsc/greatwebsites/greatwebsitesforkids/greatwebsites
   http://www.ncbi.nlm.nih.gov/pmc/articles/PMC1446565/pdf/11236453.pdf
   http://mailer.fsu.edu/~bstvilia/papers/conHealthcareIQ.pdf
2. Using information from these sites and this chapter develop a checklist-type tool that you can use to evaluate the quality of a Web site with health-related information.
   a. Select three wellness-related Internet sites that provide information for the general public. One site should have high-quality information, another site should have inaccurate information, and the third site should be somewhere in the middle.
   b. Ask a high school student or college freshman, who would be expected to have a limited healthcare background, to review the sites using your form.
3. Answer the following questions:
   a. Did the student collect information for all sections of your form?
   b. When information was missing, did the student note this fact? For example, if the date the page was last updated was missing, did he or she note this omission?
   c. Did the student validate the data or information that was collected? For example, if the author of the information at the Internet site indicated that he or she was a college professor, did the student check the directory of the college to see if the person was listed?

d. Was the student able to differentiate the quality of the information at the three sites using your form?
e. If the student was correct, which factors influenced the student in making this decision? In other words, how was he or she able to recognize the quality of the information?
f. If he or she was incorrect, which factors misled the student? Remember the student may be correct about one page and not the other.
g. Now repeat the process with a classmate who is not taking this course or using this book.
h. If possible repeat this process with a person whose first language is not English and/or who represents a different culture.
i. From this experience, how would you revise your form? What would you stress if you were teaching patients to evaluate information on the Web? How would you revise the form for different levels of knowledge and skills?

Assignments

ASSIGNMENT 1 Evaluating Healthcare Information

Directions

1. Begin this assignment by designing two forms for evaluating health-related information at an Internet site. Design one form that can be used by a healthcare provider. The second form should be designed for use by the general public. The forms should be no longer than two pages and should include directions for use.
2. Pilot-test both forms with at least five users. Exercise 2 should be helpful to you in planning your pilot.
3. Write a paper about this project that includes the following information: Explain the rationale for the design and content of each form. Describe how you selected your users and what happened when you pilot-tested the forms with them. Outline your findings or the results of your pilot test. Redesign the forms based on your pilot and include the revised forms as an appendix to your paper. Don't forget to cite references using the appropriate format.
4. After the paper is completed, design a poster presentation based on the paper. You may find PowerPoint helpful for this part of the assignment. Present the poster presentation to your classmates. Save paper and presentation as **Chap12-Assign1-LastName.**
5. Submit both the paper and the poster presentation as directed by the professor.

ASSIGNMENT 2 Cultural Sensitivity and Health Information on the Internet

Directions

1. Please note that this assignment may be done either as an individual or group assignment.
2. For this assignment assume that you have been assigned to care for two patients who are newly diagnosed diabetics. Both patients are females. The first patient is a 57-year-old Hispanic American and the second patient is a 62-year-old African American. The initial nursing assessments indicated that English is a second language for the Hispanic American patient and that the African American patient has "low health literacy."
3. Using the library, including the reference librarian and the Internet, develop an assessment form identifying the cultural and language-related information you would find helpful in planning educational programs for these patients. For example, are there any ways to measure a patient's level of health literacy and can that information be used in selecting reading materials?
4. Prepare a list of Internet resources that either or both patients can use to understand their disease, common lab test results, their medications, their diet, and general healthcare, such as inspecting their feet. For example, can you find reliable sites for this type of information in Spanish or at a fifth-grade reading level?
5. Both patients have asked if there are any online social media sites that they might join to help them deal with this new diagnosis. Use the Internet to research this question and write a brief note on what you would recommend for these patients.
6. Save your work as **Chap12-Assign2-LastName** and submit as directed by the professor.

ASSIGNMENT 3 Standards of Care and Evidence-Based Care

Directions

1. For this assignment assume that you are assigned to a task group that is writing standards of care for pregnant women who are seen in an outpatient clinic associated with a community hospital. All patients seen in the clinic meet the "low income" requirements for such care. The clinic is staffed by midwives and physicians. Each patient is assigned her own provider for follow-up during the pregnancy. However, the schedule is designed so that each patient is delivered by whomever is on call when they go into labor. The on-call 24/7 schedule includes a midwife with physician back-up, as needed.

2. The standards of care will be used to provide a general framework for treatment and follow-up of all patients seen at the clinic. The newly developed standards of care must be evidence-based.
3. Search the following sites to identify any standards that might be useful in creating the new document.
   a. http://www.guideline.gov/index.aspx
   b. http://www.health.ny.gov/health_care/medicaid/standards/prenatal_care/
4. Find three other *reliable* sites with information about standards of care during pregnancy. Specify the criteria used to determine that these sites are reliable.
5. Use information from the five sites identified in this assignment to outline six standards of care that would guide care for all patients seen at the clinic.
6. Save this work as **Chap12-Assign3-LastName** and submit as directed by the professor.

chapter

13

Privacy, Confidentiality, Security, and Integrity of Electronic Data

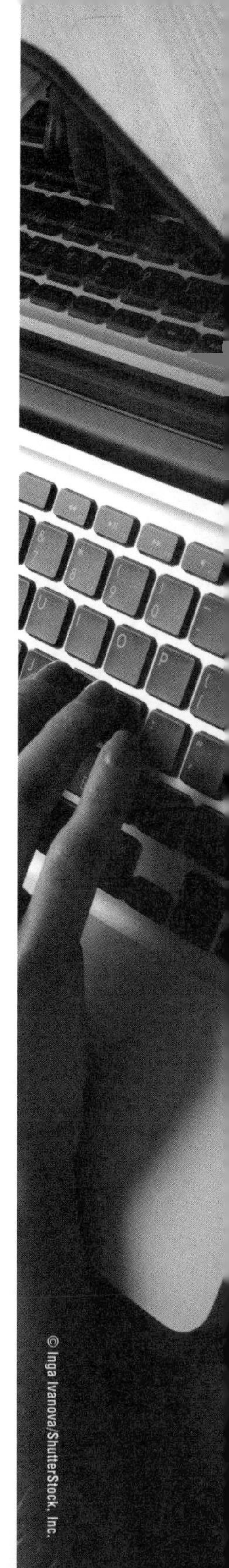

Objectives 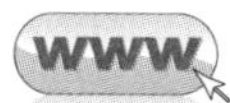

1. Discuss the concepts of privacy, confidentiality, security, and integrity as they apply to the management of electronic data.
2. Recognize common threats to the privacy, confidentiality, security, and integrity of data that electronic systems encompass and store.
3. Apply effective procedures for protecting data, software, and hardware.
4. Follow Health Insurance Portability and Accountability Act (HIPAA) principles for protecting healthcare information.
5. Discuss healthcare security issues as they relate to the Internet and the role of healthcare providers in protecting patient data.

Introduction

This chapter identifies threats to privacy and confidentiality as well as threats to integrity and security of information. **Privacy** refers to a person's desire to limit the disclosure of personal information. **Confidentiality** deals with the healthcare provider's responsibility to limit access to information so that it is shared in a controlled manner for the benefit of the patient. **Security** refers to the measures that organizations implement to protect information and systems. **Integrity** refers to the accuracy and comprehensiveness of data.

The code of ethics for healthcare professionals consistently demonstrates that ensuring the confidentiality and privacy of patient, client, and consumer information is a major responsibility of healthcare providers. Meeting that responsibility is impossible if the healthcare provider does not understand how to follow current regulations and apply effective procedures for protecting electronic data. These issues are even more of a concern with the advent of social media sites used by healthcare professionals. This chapter clarifies the regulations for protecting healthcare information. In addition, healthcare providers are responsible for ensuring the security and integrity of patient data; this chapter describes procedures for protecting data, software, and hardware.

Using Computer Systems for Storing Data

With rare exceptions, all healthcare institutions manage and store data in automated systems. These data, which relate to clients, employees, and the institution, are interrelated and interdependent. A threat to any data element in these automated systems can be a threat to the clients, the employees, and the institution. The legal and ethical implications related to storing personal health-related data are of primary concern.

Concerns with confidentiality and security are not limited to healthcare information systems. Many personal computers and mobile devices now store or access significant confidential data. Stolen data from these personal systems can be a major source of problems. **Identity theft** occurs when a person takes someone's identifying information and uses it for fraudulent purposes. There are several different types of identity theft. These are the most common:

- **Medical identity theft** occurs when someone uses another person's personal information with or without that individual's knowledge or consent to obtain healthcare and/or receive payment for such care. Victims of medical identity theft may discover that their medical records are inaccurate. This inaccuracy is not only medically dangerous for the victim, but can also affect his or her ability to obtain insurance coverage or benefits (Federal Trade Commission, 2012a).
- Child identity theft occurs when identity thieves use a child's Social Security number. For example, the child's identity may be used to apply for government benefits, open bank and credit card accounts, or rent a place to live (Federal Trade Commission, 2012b).
- Tax-related identity theft occurs when someone uses a person's Social Security number to obtain a job or to steal a tax refund.

The different types of identity theft often overlap. For example, someone may use a child's Social Security number to obtain a job, medical care, or Social Security payments. An intake history or nursing assessment may pick up warning signs of identity theft. If a patient provides a health history that includes information that is not congruent with previous medical records or comments on medical bills for services never received, the provider should investigate these types of incongruences.

Concerns with data integrity and security are not limited to healthcare or personal data. Most files on a computer represent hours of work that can be very difficult to replicate. For example, if a student spent several hours completing a term paper that a computer virus destroys, it may be difficult to convince the instructor that a virus "ate the paper."

Five major concerns arise in conjunction with electronically stored data, whether it is stored on a healthcare information system, on an Internet server, or on a personal computer:

- Providing for privacy and confidentiality of data.
- Ensuring the integrity of the data.
- Protecting hardware and devices as well as the software and apps that are used to manage and store these data.
- To the extent possible, minimizing the impact of the lost or destroyed data.
- Recognizing and prosecuting criminal abuse of computer data and equipment.

Privacy and Confidentiality

To protect privacy and confidentiality, you must address issues relevant to data storage and use. Problems of ensuring privacy and confidentiality of data include **data protection** issues and **data integrity** issues. Data protection issues include accessing data for unauthorized use and unnecessary storage of data. Data integrity issues include incomplete or inaccurate data and intentional or accidental manipulation of data.

Personal Privacy and Confidentiality

With the advent of computers, numerous companies, institutions, and government agencies maintain databases containing personal data. For example, personal information related to education, including learning disabilities and financial need data, is stored on university computers. The Department of Motor Vehicles stores personal driving record information; the Social Security Administration stores Social Security benefits information; and retail companies store personal information such as phone numbers, addresses, and items that customers have ordered as well as credit card numbers. Insurance companies maintain extensive information on their customers' personal health care. Knowing what data others are storing is an important first step in protecting individual privacy.

When individuals complete warranty or registration forms that ask for their names, addresses, and other information, companies can collect and sell these data to other companies. Simply using the Internet generates information about individuals—where they go on the Internet, who they interact with via social media sites, and which products they buy. Several organizations have evolved to respond to online privacy issues; **Table 13-1** lists several of these

TABLE 13-1 ORGANIZATIONS PROTECTING ONLINE PRIVACY

Name	URL	Description
Center for Democracy and Technology (CDT)	http://www.cdt.org/	CDT is a 501(c)(3) nonprofit public policy organization founded in 1994 to promote democratic values and constitutional liberties. Areas of focus include: preserving the open, decentralized, and user-controlled nature of the Internet; enhancing freedom of expression; protecting privacy; and limiting government surveillance.
Center for Democracy and Technology (CDT)—Health Privacy	https://www.cdt.org/issue/health-privacy	In March 2008, CDT launched an initiative to address the complex privacy issues associated with the use of health information technology.
Electronic Privacy Information Center (EPIC)	http://epic.org/	EPIC is a 501(c)(3) nonprofit public interest research center established in 1994 to focus public attention on emerging civil liberties issues and to protect privacy, the First Amendment, and constitutional values.
Privacy International (PI)	http://www.privacyinternational.org/	PI, formed in 1990, is registered in the UK as a charity focused on defending the right to privacy across the world by fighting unlawful surveillance and intrusions into private life by governments and corporations.
Electronic Frontier Foundation (EFF)	http://www.eff.org/	EFF, founded in 1990, focuses on defending free speech, privacy, innovation, and consumer digital rights. EFF's primary approach is in the courts—bringing and defending lawsuits.
Privacy Rights Clearinghouse (PRC)	http://www.privacyrights.org/	PRC is a California 501(c)(3) nonprofit established in 1992 focused on consumer information and consumer advocacy. For example, it works to raise consumers' awareness of how technology affects privacy and empowers consumers to control access to their personal information.

organizations. Notice that each of these organizations was established in the early 1990s, just as the Internet was becoming available to the general public. While each of these groups takes a different approach to protecting online privacy, all include education of the public as one of their approaches. For example, The Privacy Rights Clearinghouse (https://www.privacyrights.org/privacy-rights-fact-sheets) has more than 50 fact sheets, including a group specific to the privacy of personal health data. Each fact sheet deals with a different online privacy topic. For example, Fact Sheet 21 is a resource guide for dealing with children's online privacy (Privacy Rights Clearinghouse, 2012a).

Currently, many organizations share personal data from their databases. By sharing information across these databases, it becomes possible to create a personal profile of an individual that is more extensive than you might imagine. For example, you should read the small print privacy statements on leaflets that are mailed with credit bills or bank statements. The Medical Information Board/MIB Group, Inc. (MIB) provides another excellent example within health care. MIB is an association of approximately 475 U.S. and Canadian life and health insurance companies. By sharing information, these companies work together to ensure the consistency of health information that they collect during the insurance application process (MIB, n.d.). MIB provides free access to individuals requesting a copy of their files. Since many people do not know they have a record with MIB, few checks and balances exist to ensure the accuracy of this information. For example, a company may refuse to offer an individual life insurance and the individual may never know that the reason for the refusal was the presence of inaccurate information in the MIB file.

Patient Privacy and Confidentiality

Because many people believe that the information they share with their healthcare providers is held in confidence, they may assume a level of protection that does not exist. Once the related medical record includes that information, however, the actual confidentiality of that information is determined by who has access to those data. Healthcare information is shared not only with physicians, nurses, and other healthcare providers, but also with insurance companies and government agencies such as Medicare or Medicaid. Others obtain legal access to these records when individuals agree to let others see them, usually by signing consent forms when receiving health care.

HIPAA, which is discussed in more detail later in this chapter, establishes federal privacy standards for medical records that healthcare providers, health plans, and health clearinghouses maintain. However, a great deal of health-related information exists *outside* of healthcare facilities and their business partners and, therefore, is beyond the reach of HIPAA. This includes employee files, school records, and organizations such as MIB. Under both the HIPAA and the Patriot Act, there are certain circumstances when police may access medical records without a warrant (Burke & Weill, 2005). Although HIPAA requires that others inform you about how they may use your records without your consent, it does not require that others inform you when your records are actually shared. In addition, the Patriot Act includes provisions that prohibit notifying you if others share your medical records under the provisions of this act.

> *Under Section 215 of the Patriot Act, the Federal Government has the authority to request (i) a court order requiring a physician to produce medical records ("production order"), as well as (ii) a concurrently issued non-disclosure order ("gag order") that prohibits a physician from disclosing to any other person (except for an attorney or persons necessary for compliance with the production order) the existence of the production order* (American Medical Association, 2007).

Data Integrity Concepts

Ensuring patient privacy is necessary but not sufficient for ensuring patient safety. If the collected and processed data for providing patient care lacks integrity, the resulting care will be dangerously inadequate. Data are uninterpreted facts or observations that describe an event or phenomenon. Data integrity refers to the truthfulness and accuracy of the data. For example, one might describe a patient's weight as 130 lbs. If the patient's weight is actually 150 lbs., the data is of poor quality or inaccurate. Providers and information systems process data to produce information and are therefore the foundation for effective healthcare decisions and critical thinking. The following list of principles is the result of work by American Health Information Management Association (2007) and provides examples of appropriate data integrity maintenance in healthcare records:

- Access permissions are in accordance with clear written policies that enforce and that ensure only the appropriately educated healthcare personal can create, read, update, and delete data from any healthcare-related records.
- A data dictionary is created, maintained, and used. The data dictionary includes standardized data field definitions for each data element. For example, nursing diagnoses used in the patients' health records follow a clearly defined standardized language.
- A standardized data entry and processing format is used to ensure consistency. This includes standardized data entry screens as well as the process for entering data.
- Laws, regulations, accreditation standards, and standards of practice are reinforced and incorporated into all aspects of the data entry process.
- Data integrity policies and procedures are developed and followed. For example, different departments should not maintain a separate list of patient allergies. Rather, the patient's record should include one comprehensive list that is used by all departments.

Safety and Security

Protecting the safety and security of patient data involves identifying threats to computer systems and initiating procedures to protect the integrity of the data and system. The two main types of threats are related to the integrity of data and to the confidentiality of the data. These threats can result from accidental or intentional human actions or natural disasters. Destruction of data, hardware, and software by natural disasters include damage by water, fire, earthquakes, or chemicals; electrical power outages; disk failures; and exposure to magnetic fields. The types of human actions that result in these threats fall into five areas: innocent mistakes, inappropriate access by insiders for curiosity reasons, inappropriate access by insiders for spite or for profit, unauthorized intruders who gain access to patient data, and vengeful employees and outsiders (National Academy of Sciences, 1997).

Innocent Mistakes

Innocent mistakes are errors made by people who have legal access to the system and who, in the process of using the system, accidentally disclose data or damage the integrity of data. Examples can be as simple as a healthcare provider recording data in the wrong medical record or a lab sending a fax to the wrong fax number. In school, it may take the form of a teacher entering the wrong grade on the student's academic record. M. Eric Johnson documented several incidences of accidental disclosure of medical data in a paper titled "Data Hemorrhages in a Health Care Sector." Examples given in this paper include: accidentally posting medical data to the Internet such as occurred when the Wuesthoff Medical Center in Florida posted information on more than 500 patients; the Tampa-based WellCare Health Plans posted information on 71,000 Georgia residents; and the University of Pittsburgh Medical Center posted names and medical images of nearly 80 individuals (Johnson, 2009). Additional case examples of HIPAA Resolution Agreements can be viewed at http://www.hhs.gov/ocr/privacy/hipaa/enforcement/examples/index.html.

Inappropriate Access by Insiders for Curiosity Reasons

Sometimes people with legal access to the system make an intentional decision to abuse their access privileges. Browsing is a problem with many electronic record systems—and health records are not immune to this problem. In this type of access, the person looks at medical records for the express purpose of satisfying his or her own curiosity or goals; the access to the medical record provides no benefit to the patient. The auditing functions in many healthcare information systems, however, make it easy to identify these browsers and discipline those individuals. **Table 13-2** includes several current examples of employees who

TABLE 13-2 EXAMPLES OF EMPLOYEES FIRED FOR INAPPROPRIATE ACCESS OF MEDICAL RECORDS

News Source and Date of Publication	Headline	URL
PHIprivacy.net December 21, 2012 2:30 P.M.	CCS Medical employee may have accessed and disclosed Social Security numbers for a tax refund fraud scheme	http://www.phiprivacy.net/?p=11056
MSN News Canada July 25, 2012 16:58:18	5 employees fired after Eastern Health privacy breaches	http://news.ca.msn.com/canada/5-employees-fired-after-eastern-health-privacy-breaches
HeraldNet March 14, 2012, 12:01 A.M.	Everett Clinic fires 13 for snooping	http://heraldnet.com/article/20120314/NEWS01/703149862
New4Jax October 14, 2011 11:59:07 A.M.	20 Hospital Workers Fired for Viewing Collier's Medical Records	http://www.news4jax.com/news/20-Hospital-Workers-Fired-for-Viewing-Collier-s-Medical-Records/-/475880/2062868/-/r6ctbjz/-/index.html
Huffington Post Media Group: NCAAF Sporting News February 3, 2011 at 2:30 P.M.	Iowa hospital employees fired over Hawkeyes' medical records breaches	http://aol.sportingnews.com/ncaa-football/story/2011-02-03/iowa-hospital-employees-fired-over-hawkeyes-medical-records-breaches
Arizona Daily Star January 12, 2011	3 UMC workers fired for records access	http://azstarnet.com/news/local/crime/umc-workers-fired-for-records-access/article_4f789a48-1e8c-11e0-929a-001cc4c002e0.html

were fired for this very reason. In educational institutions, browsing an academic record without an academic purpose is a clear violation of Family Educational Rights and Privacy Act (FERPA) regulations.

Inappropriate Access by Insiders for Spite or for Profit

Healthcare professionals play an important role in protecting patients from exploitation for personal or financial gain. Such violations damage the reputation of an institution and can be expensive. Recently, UCLA paid a fine of $865,500 in a settlement reached between the U.S. Department of Health and Human

Services (HHS) and the University of California at Los Angeles Health System (UCLA Health Center) over a breach of patient records (HHS, 2011). News stories reported that multiple internal employees over many years had improperly accessed the medical records of several high-profile/celebrity patients. Neither HHS nor UCLA confirmed the names of the celebrities but media reports have mentioned many of these celebrities (Jenkins, 2011).

Farrah Fawcett, who was a patient under treatment for cancer at UCLA during this period, set up her own sting to prove to UCLA that someone at their health center was leaking her medical information. After information known only to Fawcett and her doctor was quickly leaked to the *National Enquirer*, UCLA investigated. The Institution found that one employee had accessed her records more often than her own doctors. This woman pleaded guilty to a single count of violating federal medical privacy law for commercial purposes, but died of cancer before she could be sentenced (Ornstein, 2009).

Unauthorized Intruders Who Gain Access to Patient Data

Many hospitals rely on physical security, software, and user education to protect the information stored inside a computer from unauthorized intruders. For example, hospitals may locate the computers where it is difficult for others to access or use them. Hospitals may also use passwords and firewalls to control access. In addition, hospitals may set computers to automatically log off users after a few minutes of inactivity.

Vengeful Employees and Outsiders

Examples of data incursions by vengeful individuals include vindictive patients or intruders who mount attacks to access unauthorized information or damage systems and disrupt operations. For this reason, most hospitals terminate an employee's computer access before informing the employee of the termination and physically escort the terminated employee off the premises.

Examples of additional reported HIPAA violations can be located at:

- https://www.privacyrights.org/data-breach/new
- http://www.phiprivacy.net/
- http://www.hhs.gov/ocr/privacy/hipaa/administrative/breachnotificationrule/breachtool.html

Computer Crime

Computer crimes include a wide range of illegal activities, from computer intrusion into a computer system (i.e., hacking) to child pornography or exploitation. Some of these crimes require a certain level of technical skill, but many are as simple as sending an email with false or misleading information. An individual may perpetrate such crimes; large organized crime groups and even governments may carry out other such crimes. Victims range from vulnerable individuals or organizations to corporations and government institutions that are vital to the infrastructure of the country.

> *Like many tough issues, cybersecurity is a cross-cutting problem, affecting not only all Federal agencies, but also state and local governments, the private sector, non-governmental organizations, academia, and other countries. It is a national security, homeland security, economic security, network defense, and law enforcement issue all rolled into one* (Daniel, 2012).

As a result, several government agencies are involved in investigating these types of crimes. **Table 13-3** lists several of these agencies, their URLs, and their missions.

TABLE 13-3 GOVERNMENT AND GOVERNMENT-RELATED AGENCIES PREVENTING AND PROSECUTING COMPUTER CRIMES

Agency	URL	Mission
Computer Crime & Intellectual Property Section United States Department of Justice (CCIPS)	http://www.justice.gov/criminal/cybercrime/	Responsible for implementing the Department's national strategies in combating computer and intellectual property crimes worldwide including electronic penetrations, data thefts, and cyber-attacks on critical information systems.
FBI: Cyber Crime Division	http://www.fbi.gov/about-us/investigate/cyber/cyber	Investigates high-tech crimes, including cyber-based terrorism, espionage, computer intrusions, and major cyberfraud.
Federal Trade Commission (FTC) Bureau of Consumer Protection	http://www.ftc.gov/bcp/index.shtml	Prevents and investigates business practices that are anticompetitive, deceptive, or unfair to consumers including computer and Internet-related practices.
National Security Council: Cybersecurity	http://www.whitehouse.gov/administration/eop/nsc/cybersecurity	Leads the interagency development of national cybersecurity strategy and policy and oversees the agencies' implementation of those policies.
Internet Crime Complaint Center (IC3)	http://www.ic3.gov/default.aspx	Partnership between the Federal Bureau of Investigation (FBI), the National White Collar Crime Center (NW3C), and the Bureau of Justice Assistance (BJA). IC3's mission is to serve as a vehicle to receive, develop, and refer criminal complaints regarding the rapidly expanding arena of cybercrime.

TABLE 13-3 (CONTINUED)

National White Collar Crime Center (NW3C)	http://www.nw3c.org/	A congressionally funded, nonprofit corporation whose mission is to provide training, investigative support, and research to agencies and entities involved in the prevention, investigation, and prosecution of economic and high-tech crime.
United States Postal Inspection Service (USPIS)	http://postalinspectors.uspis.gov/	Investigates crimes dealing with mail fraud involving both postal mail services and the Internet.
United States Secret Service: Electronic Crimes Task Forces and Working Groups	http://www.secretservice.gov/ectf.shtml	Provides the necessary support and resources to investigate economic crimes that meet one of the following criteria: • Significant economic or community impact • Participation of organized criminal groups involving multiple districts or transnational organizations • Use of schemes involving new technology.

As computer crime has evolved, so have the language and terms used to discuss these crimes. **Table 13-4** defines a number of these terms as well as a few data protection terms.

TABLE 13-4 TERMS RELATED TO COMPUTER CRIME

Term	Definition
Adware	A type of software that downloads or displays unwanted advertisements on a computer.
Cracker	A hacker that illegally breaks into computer systems and creates mischief.
Cybercrime	The use of the Internet or other communication technology to commit a crime of any type.
Data Diddling	Modifying valid data in a computer file.
Denial of Service	Any action or series of actions that prevents any part of an information system from functioning. For example, using several computers attached to the Internet to access a Web site so that the site is overwhelmed and not available.
Encryption	Method of coding sensitive data to protect it when sent over the Internet.
Firewall	A software program used to protect computers from unauthorized access via the linternet.

(continues)

TABLE 13-4 TERMS RELATED TO COMPUTER CRIME (continued)	
Hacker	Originally a compulsive computer programmer, it now has a more negative meaning and is often confused with "cracker."
Identity Theft	When someone uses another person's private information to assume their identity.
Keyboard Loggers	Hardware or software installed on a computer to log the keystrokes of an individual. A keyboard logger can be used to monitor computer activities such as time spent on the Iinternet or collect personal information such as passwords.
Logic Bomb	Piece of program code buried within another program, designed to perform some malicious act in response to a trigger. The trigger can involve entering data or a name, for example.
Malware	General term used to refer to viruses, worms, spyware, Trojan Horses, and adware.
Opt-out	A number of measures to prevent receiving unwanted products or services. For example, if you sign up for a free journal on the Internet you may want to opt-out of receiving emails and product announcements from companies that advertise in this journal. In many cases the default is that you opt-in.
Phishing	(Pronounced *fishing*.) Creating a replica of a legitimate Web page to hook users and trick them into submitting personal or financial information or passwords.
Sabotage	The purposeful destruction of hardware, software, or data.
Salami Method	A method of data stealing that involves taking little bits at a time.
Software Piracy	Unauthorized copying of copyrighted software.
Spamming	The act of sending unsolicited electronic messages in bulk.
Theft of Services	The unauthorized use of services such as a computer system.
Time Bomb	Instructions in a program that perform certain functions on a specific date or time such as printing a message or destroying data.
Trapdoors	Methods installed by programmers that allow unauthorized access to programs.
Trojan Horse	Placing instructions in a program that add additional, illegitimate functions; for example, the program prints out information every time information on a certain patient is entered.
Virus	A program that, once introduced into a system, replicates itself and causes a variety of mischievous outcomes. Viruses are usually introduced from infected USB storage devices, email attachments, and downloaded files.
Worm	A destructive program that can fill various memory locations of a computer system with information, clogging the system so that other operations are compromised.

Prosecution of Computer Crime

It is difficult to detect and persecute many computer crimes. Many times, the person initiating the criminal act does not live in this country and may not be subject to U.S. laws. The U.S. Department of Justice maintains a key resource for understanding computer crime and related issues; this website can be found at http://www.justice.gov/usao/briefing_room/cc/index.html. Although the terms in Table 13-4 are more readily identified with computer crime in areas other than health care, all types of crimes can and do occur within healthcare computer systems.

Some computer crimes are detected but not reported. When data are stolen, the information is not always seen as valuable; thus those responsible for its theft may not be prosecuted. Many times, an institution will be more concerned with the poor publicity that can result from disclosure of this event. However, the breach notification provision of HIPAA required notification of patients using criteria outlined in HIPAA. These criteria were strengthened in January 2013 with the implementation of the Health Information Technology for Economic and Clinical Health (HITECH) breach notification requirements, which clarifies when breaches of unsecured health information must be reported to HHS and to patients. Additional information concerning these requirements can be seen at http://www.hhs.gov/ocr/privacy/hipaa/administrative/omnibus/index.html.

Although methods for tracking entry into computer systems are becoming increasingly sophisticated, discovery of computer crime may be difficult. Laws are catching up, but still lag behind computer technology. In some situations, there are questions about who "owns" data. Therefore, early laws in this area protected individuals from having data about them stored in a computer without their knowledge.

Selected Laws Related to Computing

Freedom of Information Act of 1970: This law allows citizens to have access to data gathered by federal agencies.

Federal Privacy Act of 1974: This law stipulates that there can be no secret personal files; individuals must be allowed to know what is stored in files about them and how it is used. This act applies to government agencies and contractors dealing with government agencies, but not to the private sector.

U.S. Copyright Law of 1976: This law stipulates that it is a federal offense to reproduce copyrighted materials, including computer software, without authorization.

Electronic Communication Privacy Act of 1986: The ECP Act updated the Federal Wiretap Act of 1968 and is sometimes referred to as the Wiretap Act. This law specifies that it is a crime to own any electronic, mechanical, or other device used primarily for the purpose of surreptitious interception of wire, oral, or electronic communication. This law does not apply to communication within an organization, such as email between employees.

Computer Security Act of 1987: This law mandated that the National Institute of Standards and Technology (NIST) and U.S. Office of Personnel Management (OPM) create guidance on computer security awareness and training based on functional organizational roles. In response, the NIST created the Computer Security Resource Center (http://csrc.nist.gov/index.html).

U.S. Copyright Law of 1995, amendment: This amendment protects the transmission of a digital performance over the Internet, making it a crime to transmit something for which you do not have proper authorization.

National Information Infrastructure Protection Act of 1996: This law established penalties for interstate theft of information.

U.S. Copyright Law of 1997 (No Electronic Theft Act): This addition to the copyright act creates criminal penalties for copyright infringement even if the offender does not benefit financially.

Digital Millennium Copyright Act of 1998: This legislation placed the United States in conformance with international treaties that prevail in other countries. It provides changes in three areas: protection of copyrighted digital works, extensions of copyright protection by 20 years, and the addition of criminal penalties and fines for attempting to circumvent copyright protections. In addition, it provides for copy protection for the creative organization and structure of a database, but not the underlying general facts in the database, requires that "Webcasters" pay licensing fees to recording companies, and limits Internet service providers' (ISPs') copyright infringement liability for simply transmitting information over the Internet.

Children's Online Protection Act of 2000: This law requires Web sites targeting children younger than age 14 to obtain parental consent before gathering information on children. Regulations related to this legislation issued by the Federal Trade Commission underwent significant revision in 2012 and are available for review at http://ftc.gov/opa/2012/12/coppa.shtm.

USA Patriot Act of 2001: This act gives federal officials greater authority to track and intercept communications for law enforcement and foreign intelligence purposes. With this act, law enforcement agencies now require fewer checks to collect electronic data.

Homeland Security Act of 2002: This act established the Department of Homeland Security as an executive department of the United States. It also expanded and centralized the data gathering allowed under the Patriot Act.

Cyber Security Enhancement Act (CSEA) of 2002: This act was passed along with the Homeland Security Act and reduced privacy by allowing an ISP to voluntarily hand over personal information from its customers to a government agency. Previously, a warrant was required to access such information (SANS Institute, 2004).

Controlling the Assault of Non-Solicited Pornography and Marketing Act of 2003 (CAN-SPAM Act): This act establishes a framework of administrative, civil, and criminal tools to help U.S. consumers, businesses, and families combat unsolicited commercial email or spam.

Computer Fraud and Abuse Act (CFAA) of 1984, amended in 2008: This law specifies that it is a crime to access a federal computer without authorization and to alter, destroy, or damage information or prevent authorized access. The 2008 amendment clarified a number of the provisions in the original section 1030 and criminalized additional computer-related acts. For example, a provision was added that penalizes the theft of property via computer that occurs as a part of a scheme to defraud. Another provision penalizes those who intentionally alter, damage, or destroy data belonging to others; this part of the act covers such activities as the distribution of malicious code and denial-of-service attacks. Finally, Congress included in the CFAA a provision criminalizing trafficking in passwords and similar items (U.S. Department of Justice, Computer Crime and Intellectual Property Section, 2010).

Identity Theft Enforcement and Restitution Act of 2008: This act lowers the bar for what is considered punishable identity theft crimes, thereby making it easier for prosecutors to bring charges against cybercriminals. It also makes it easier for identity theft victims to be compensated, even for costs that are indirectly associated with the harm incurred from the theft.

Since 2008, with the exception of the HIPAA changes in the Health Information Technology for Economic and Clinical Health (HITECH) Act, the federal government has not enacted significant legislation dealing with cybercrime. A comprehensive bill that failed to obtain a super-majority in the U.S. Senate focused on cybersecurity for the nation's infrastructure (U.S. Senate Committee on Homeland Security & Governmental Affairs, 2012). Since that event, additional bills have been introduced. H.R. 624: Cyber Intelligence Sharing and Protection Act passed the House of Representatives in April 2013 and was sent forward to the Senate. This bill provides for the sharing of certain cyberthreat intelligence and information between the intelligence community and cybersecurity entities (Govtrack.us, 2013). As of June 2013, this bill has not passed the Senate. The House version of the Bill and current status can be seen at http://www.govtrack.us/congress/bills/113/hr624/text#. Current federal legislation does not provide for a comprehensive approach to cybersecurity, however, this is a hot issue and future bills can be anticipated.

Protection of Computer Data and Systems

Healthcare agency procedures can help to protect the privacy and confidentiality of data as well as the safety and security of the entire system. In addition, steps that individual healthcare providers take are also important in maintaining data security. Agency responsibilities include protecting data from unauthorized use, destruction, or disclosure, and controlling data input and output. Individuals are also responsible for protecting the privacy, confidentiality, and integrity of data.

To protect data from unauthorized use, destruction, or disclosure, agencies should take the following steps:

1. Develop and maintain an ongoing risk assessment process for the institution and the specific units within the institution.
2. Develop ongoing educational programs to ensure that users understand their responsibilities.
3. Restrict access to data on a need-to-know basis by requiring passwords, personal identification numbers, and/or callback procedures.
4. Develop and enforce encoding and encrypting procedures for sensitive data.
5. Audit access (viewing) and transactions (modifying) activities. Routinely review these records and follow up on any questionable activity.
6. Develop biometric methods such as electronic signatures, fingerprints, iris scans, or retina prints to identify users.
7. Protect systems from natural disasters by locating them in areas safe from water and other potential physical damage.
8. Develop backup procedures and redundant systems so that data are not lost accidentally. In many cases when a hospital backs up the network file servers or other hospital servers it does not back up an individual local hard drive; instead, the individual is responsible for developing a system to back up these data.
9. Develop and enforce policies for both preventing and dealing with risky behavior and breaches of security.
10. Store only needed data.
11. Dispose of unneeded printouts by shredding.
12. Develop alerts that identify potentially inaccurate data such as a weight of 1200 lbs. or a blood pressure of 80/130 mm Hg.

To manage data responsibly, you should:

1. Avoid distractions and other factors that may result in data entry errors.
2. Develop a consistent process to ensure that you are on the right screen and recording the correct data. For example, always look at the patient's name before entering data on a new screen.

3. Refuse to share a password or sign in with another person's password.
4. Attend implementation/orientation classes and clearly understand institutional policies and procedures.
5. Keep the monitor screen and data out of view of other people.
6. Develop passwords that include numbers and letters that are not easy to identify.
7. Keep your own password and means of access to data secure.
8. Do not use one password or version of a password for several different systems.
9. Report unusual computer activity and potential breaches of security.
10. Encourage patients to understand their rights to privacy and confidentiality.
11. Keep harmful materials such as food, drink, and smoke away from computers.

Tools for Protecting Your PC/Mobile Device

Most healthcare agencies store information on mainframes or servers and have policies for protecting these data. However, portable or mobile devices, such as smartphones and tablets, and smaller computers such as PCs and laptops, in place throughout the institution and are much more difficult to monitor. With the increased connectivity that prevails today, many of these devices are connected to a local area network (LAN), thereby creating an intranet. In addition, many of these institutional devices have access to the Internet.

Personal mobile devices such as smartphones and tablets are rarely produced with the hardware and software security applications necessary to safely receive or transmit patient data. Therefore, it is imperative that healthcare institutions assume responsibility for ensuring that patient data are stored only on secure devices. Institutions do this by providing secure devices in the clinical settings and developing policies and procedures related to the use of personal devices.

In today's connected world there is some inevitable overlap in personal and professional communication. For example, an email requesting a volunteer to work an extra shift may be sent to a personal email account. Many healthcare providers check their work email from home. The following sections focus on ways to protect your personal computer and other devices. Protecting these devices now is not only advantageous to you, but also decreases the risk to healthcare institutions and other healthcare providers.

Antivirus Software

Computer viruses are malicious software programs that replicate themselves as they spread from one computer to another. They carry a code that can destroy files, damage hardware, and/or launch an attack on other computers. Often the user is not aware of the virus and its infection of the computer until the damage is done. Antivirus software scans the computer, email, and downloaded files to identify and disable viruses. Several companies produce and sell this type of software. Students should check whether free versions are available from their university, ISP, or a software company before purchasing any of these programs.

The majority of new computers come with antivirus software. There is wide variation as to when this software expires and will no longer receive automatic updates. Sometimes the coverage is a trial version that remains valid for only a few weeks or months. New viruses, however, are being developed and spread every day. Therefore, when installing new antivirus software, make sure that you configure this software to obtain regular updates and perform scheduled scans of your computer. Updates require that your computer be able to access the Internet and download new files from the vendor for your antivirus software. Most antivirus software programs will alert you when your subscription for updating is running out and new software must be obtained. An increasing number of antivirus software vendors are bundling anti-spyware software with the antivirus software.

Even with regular software updates a new virus can infect a computer. Always watch for alerts from your Internet service provider, employer, university, and/or software vendor concerning virus issues. Also watch for symptoms of an infected computer. **Box 13-1** lists common symptoms that can indicate that a virus has infected your computer.

Box 13-1 Selected Symptoms of a Virus and/or Spyware

- Anti-spyware or virus software is turned off.
- Computer performance slows or freezes.
- Files or folders disappear.
- Frequent firewall alerts about an unknown program or process trying to access the Internet.
- Hard drive quickly becomes filled.
- New or different browser icons appear.
- Programs launch on their own.
- Recurring pop-up ads.
- Emails that were never sent bounce back or other email-related problems.
- The hard drive light is constantly lit.
- The Windows Control Panel Add or Remove Program includes new program(s).
- Inability to access the Web site of antivirus software companies.
- The computer makes unusual sounds, especially at random.
- The Internet home page changes even when reset.

Anti-Spyware Software

By definition, a spyware program is a type of computer software designed to install itself on your computer and then send personal data back to a central service without your permission or knowledge. Spyware secretly obtains the information by logging keystrokes, recording Web browsing history, and scanning documents on the computer's hard drive.

Adware is a specific type of spyware designed to collect data for targeted advertisements directed to your computer. As this type of software is becoming more powerful, there is increasing concern about the amount and type of personal data collected by many well-known companies without the knowledge of Internet users. Given the large number of people who search the Internet for health information, collecting these kinds of data raises important issues.

Cookies are small pieces of data that a Web site puts on your computer. They usually consist of a string of characters that identifies you to the site—something like an account number. Cookies can be useful and make the Internet more efficient by storing your preferences. In most cases, first-party cookies do not send personal information back to a central server, but third-party cookies can track Web sites that you visit and report those visits to other third-party Web sites. Of increasing concern is a specific type of cookie call a Flash cookie. This uses Adobe's Flash player technology to store information about your online browsing activities. When you delete or clear cookies from your browser Flash cookies are not deleted. As a result they are often referred to a "super cookies." Anti-spyware software identifies and deletes spyware but is often not able to delete super cookies.

Firewall

A **firewall** is a piece of hardware or a software program that secures the interactions between an organization's inside network of computers and the external computer environment. It achieves this goal by blocking access to the internal computer network from those outside the network and by blocking internal computers from accessing the Internet or select aspects of the Internet. By blocking external access to internal computers, a firewall can prevent a hacker or malicious software from gaining access to an internal computer. It can also prevent these types of problems from persisting on an internal computer and spreading to others.

If you are accessing a home network, such as a wireless network in your home, be sure that the firewall also protects the home network. To access the firewall in Windows, go to **Start**, **Control Panel**, and **Security**. The Windows operating system will also let you select specific programs that can access your computer or access the Internet from your computer. For example, automatic updates that are part of your antivirus and anti-spyware software, as well as Windows updates, require free passage through the firewall.

Web Browser Security Settings

Because your browser is often your interface to the Internet, it is important that you configure it to ensure your computer's protection as well as your own privacy. For example, you may want to protect your computer from a site downloading malware on your computer by blocking cookies from being stored on the computer and by protecting your credit card information while shopping online.

The first step in keeping your browser secure is keeping it current. If possible, set your browser to check for updates on a regular basis. This includes checking for updates for any add-ons or apps installed with your browser. It is helpful if your selected browser provides a Web page for checking to confirm that your browser is current and that installed add-ons are also up-to-date.

Protecting your computer and your privacy can include a **phishing** filter, a pop-up blocker, notification that a Web site is trying to download files onto your computer, and/or notification if a program's digital signature is current and correct when you are trying to download a program or files. Your browser can also provide you with a 128-bit secure encrypted connection for activities such as interaction with online financial or medical sites. With this protection, when you visit a Web site whose URL starts with "https," a small padlock symbol appears in the browser window. This symbol indicates that the Web site is a secure site and uses a digital certificate to notify you of that fact. A few trusted Certification Authorities (CAs) issue those certificates.

Because each browser has its own procedure for configuration, you must search to find the appropriate settings; use the browser's help section to ensure that you have provided your computer with the highest level of protection possible. Key settings include:

- Pop-up blocker
- Do Not Track
- Third-party cookies
- Saving history and cookies
- Overall level of security

As you select each of these settings there are three points that you should carefully evaluate:

1. What are you opening or blocking? For example, if you select **InPrivate Browsing,** your browser won't retain cookies, your browsing history, search records, or the files you downloaded after you log off; however, when you are connecting to the Internet you are connecting to other computers that can record that information. Your ISP, your employer (if using a work computer), and the sites you have visited can track your Internet activities.

The InPrivate Browsing function can be a useful function for an abused client searching for support services on a home computer and trying to keep that search history from the abuser. It would not protect an employee whose employer is tracking their Internet use.

2. How effective is the setting? For example, if you select **Do Not Track** you are instructing the Web site that you visit to not track your activities. There is no way to ensure that the site will honor your request.
3. How will this setting affect your computer use and functionality? For example, you may decide to block third-party cookies. Remember, the difference between a first-party cookie and a third-party cookie is not in the coding of the cookies, but rather is determined by the context of a particular visit. If a cookie is associated with the page you are viewing, it's a first-party cookie. For example, if you visit CNN.com and the cookie is from CNN it is a first-party cookie. A cookie from a different domain is a third-party cookie. As described above, companies often use third-party cookies to track your activity across sites and then use this information to support targeted advertising. However, you can use these same cookies to support more effective Internet searching. You, the user, must evaluate the advantages and disadvantages of third-party cookies.

NOTE: Some sites that you might access, such as your school's email or course management software for online courses, may require that you turn on certain settings. For example, Blackboard—a type of course management software for delivering online and Web-enhanced courses—requires that cookies and JavaScripts be enabled for that Web site. This means you need to turn that feature on for only that Web site.

Password Protection

You can control who has access to the files on your computer by password-protecting the computer itself. In addition, individual files can be password-protected. However, be sure to use good password design to ensure that others cannot easily decipher it and make sure that you can remember it. Password-protected files are lost if you can't remember the password. They *cannot* be reset by IT like your network password nor can Microsoft reset Office program passwords. **Box 13-2** provides guidelines on creating strong passwords.

If you are using a home wireless network like those that many broadband services provide, make sure the network is password-protected. If it is not, anyone with a wireless card can access the connection when they are in range.

Box 13-2 Do's and Don'ts for Creating Strong Passwords

- Use at least eight characters (more is better).
- Combine letters and symbols.
- Use both lower and uppercase letters.
- Select characters from the whole keyboard.
- Use a different password for each application.
- If you write the passwords down, store them in a safe place, not on your computer or device.
- Change passwords regularly.
- Do not use your password on public computers.
- Do not use your name, Social Security number, birth date, or other data that can be associated with you. This includes names spelled backward.
- Avoid dictionary words or common communication abbreviations such as lol or icu.
- Avoid sequences such as qwer or 8765.
- Do not repeat characters.
- Create a complete sentence and use the first letter from each word with numbers in the middle.

User Guidelines for Protecting Your PC

While some of the same guidelines related to safety and security of mainframes and servers are important for the PC, additional guidelines apply when you want to protect the PC system and its data. Often individuals are concerned about the privacy of information on their computers and about the information that others may access on their PCs when they use the Internet. The following is a summary of action steps to protect the data on your PC.

Protecting Your Email

- Install a virus checker to routinely scan your computer's hard drive(s).
- Configure your virus checker to scan email and downloaded files as they come in.
- Scan email attachments before opening them. Do *not* set your mail to automatically open attachments.
- Do not open email or attachments if you do not know the sender.

- If you use a filter to screen your mail, remember to empty the mailbox where the junk mail goes.
- Use whatever methods your email system provides to protect your mail from snooping, tampering, and forgery.
- Report spam or suspicious email to your ISP.

Downloading Files

- Download data only from reputable systems; those systems regularly check their files for viruses.
- Configure your virus software to scan files before downloading them.
- Scan data storage devices that others have given to you before opening the files.

Using the Internet

- Install and routinely update your firewall.
- Do not stay connected to the Internet for long periods when you are not using it.
- If others have access to your computer, install a password so that they can't sign on to the Internet without your permission.
- Do not tape passwords on the wall or hide them under your keyboard.
- Use only reputable cloud and online backup services.

Protecting Your Computer

- Use an approved surge protector to protect the PC. Remember: A power strip may not provide surge protection.
- Load only sealed software from a reputable vendor.

Protecting Your Data

- Regularly perform system backups and rotate the storage media that you use for the backup procedure.
- If data are lost due to a virus, scan the backups before installing them to ensure you are not reinstalling the virus.
- Do not store backups in the same area as the computer; store them offsite or use a fireproof safe.
- Store sensitive data on a secure external hard drive and store the hard drive in a locked area.
- Connect the secure external hard drive to the computer only as needed. Remember to disconnect the external hard drive when you are finished using it.

- Name sensitive files cryptically.
- Hide important files by using utilities and avoid using the computer hard drive by storing sensitive data on other devices such as external hard drives, memory sticks, and so forth.
- Use a cross cut paper shredder when disposing of paper documentation.
- Label storage media such as CDs and DVDs so that you can easily determine the contents of a disc.
- Eliminate old or unnecessary backup files.
- Remove sensitive data before taking a computer in for repair or, better yet, don't store sensitive data on the hard drive (C).

Protecting Your Personal Identity

- Examine the implications of your email address listings and the use of other information that you provide to your online service provider and other Internet resources.
- Never give out personal information on a chat room or online discussion group and never "click here" to provide personal information to an email saying there is an issue with your account.
- Many online companies ask permission to use your email address to send future information. Check No if you do not want that service and want to request that they do not pass your email address on to others.
- Use the secure server when you are given that option. A secure server provides additional protection when you are sending private information such as a credit card number via the Internet.
- Keep one credit card for Internet use only. Some credit card companies will issue a second card with a different number for just this purpose.
- Look for the padlock icon. When you are sending data to a private Internet site, such as your bank, look for the padlock icon on the screen. This icon signifies that your data are encrypted and you are on a secure site. Alternatively, look for the http to be https, which means you are accessing a secure server.
- Know the policies related to using email. If you transfer messages from your ISP to your own computer, you may have more privacy protection than if you leave those messages on the provider's server.

These guidelines provide a foundation for securing your computer and your privacy. However, Internet-related applications used on a computer change rapidly as the use of the Internet continues to expand. **Table 13-5** provides additional resources for protecting your computer. **Table 13-6** provides resources for protecting children on the Internet. **Box 13-3** provides general guidelines for protecting mobile devices, such as smartphones and tablets. Always remember that there is no such thing as total privacy or security when using the Internet.

TABLE 13-5 RESOURCES FOR PROTECTING YOUR COMPUTER AND YOURSELF ONLINE

Resource	URL
U.S. Department of Homeland Security: United States Computer Emergency Readiness Team	http://www.us-cert.gov/cas/tips/
Federal Trade Commission: OnGuard Online	http://www.onguardonline.gov/ Can be viewed in both English and Spanish.
Microsoft Safety & Security Center	http://www.microsoft.com/security/default.aspx
Stanford School of Medicine Information Security Services*	http://med.stanford.edu/irt/security/

* Many schools in the health professions have Web sites similar to this one. You might want to check with your school to see if they have information posted that deals with this topic.

TABLE 13-6 RESOURCES FOR PROTECTING CHILDREN ONLINE

Resource	URL
Center for Schools and Communities: Protecting Children Online	www.center-school.org/pko/resources.php
Federal Bureau of Investigation	www.fbi.gov/stats-services/publications/parent-guide
Federal Trade Commission	www.onguardonline.gov/topics/protect-kids-online
Goodwill Community Foundation, Inc.	www.gcflearnfree.org/internetsafetyforkids
National Cyber Security Alliance	www.staysafeonline.org/teach-online-safety/
South Carolina Information Sharing & Analysis Center	https://sc-isac.sc.gov/content/protecting-children-online

Box 13-3 Protecting Your Mobil Device and Your Privacy

1. Review the product manual, the manufacturer's Web site, and the Internet service provider's (ISP's) Web site for specific directions and advice related to privacy and security settings.
2. Check for updates on a daily basis and install patches to the operating system when they are available.
3. Install security software that includes antivirus, firewall, and spam blocker functionality.
4. Use your device's auto-lock feature and functionality. For example, set the auto-lock to take effect within minutes of your last activity.
5. Create a strong password and/or pin. Do not use your birthdate, house number, last four digits of your Social Security number, or numbers in sequence such as 1234 or 2468 as a pin number.
6. Use unique passwords for applications with sensitive data.
7. Avoid using sensitive apps on open or public networks.
8. Do not share your device with others, especially if you cannot use separate passwords.
9. Turn off your Wi-Fi and Bluetooth when they are not needed. Do not set Wi-Fi to connect automatically.
10. Do not include sensitive personal information such as your driver's license number, Social Security number, password, or account numbers in text messages.
11. Only download mobile applications from authorized application stores like the Apple App Store or Google Play, formerly known as the Android Market.
12. Notify your ISP immediately if your mobile device is missing.
13. Install software or an app that can wipe out information remotely.
14. Keep your mobile device backed up so you do not hesitate to wipe out information if you cannot locate your mobile device.
15. Install a tracking application to locate your device if it is missing or stolen.

Providing Patient Care via a Computer

While most healthcare providers are well aware of the computer as a tool for documenting care and managing the healthcare record, that application is only part of how providers use computers to deliver care and communicate with patients, clients, and consumers. Three key areas of health care now dealing with major security issues in electronic communication include: (1) the electronic transmission of **personal health information (PHI)**, (2) the use of the Web as a health information and emotional support resource, and (3) the use of email between healthcare providers and clients.

Federal Regulations and Guidelines for the Exchange of Personal Health Information

In their early days, healthcare information systems consisted of individual computer systems designed for specific functions. Over time, however, healthcare providers began networking these islands of information. The early networks were simple. For example, one of the early interfaces involved connecting the lab to the clinical units so that the lab could quickly transmit lab results back to the clinical unit.

Today, a group of federal agencies and private organizations are building a Nationwide Health Information Network (NwHIN) to securely exchange electronic health information on a national level. These organizations are developing and implementing the work standards, services, and policies necessary to establish a comprehensive network of interoperable network systems. The NwHIN is transmitting clinical, public health, and personal health information, with the goal of improving decision making by ensuring that health information is available when and where it is needed (U.S. Department of Health and Human Services, Office of the National Coordinator for Health Information Technology, n.d.).

With the increasing use of technology and interconnectivity, local institutions and others serving a number of healthcare institutions store medical information in a variety of computer databases. Needless to say, the security of personal health data within an electronic health system is a growing concern. The Health Insurance Portability and Accountability Act of 1996, which has as its goal the simplification of the administrative processes used to transmit electronic health information, represented a major step forward in building the needed security standards, policies, and procedures. In passing HIPAA, Congress required the U.S. Department of Health and Human Services to adopt national standards for electronic healthcare transactions, code sets, unique health identifiers, and security. This law established standards for transmitting health data, including standards for transmitting PHI. These standards were the first federal regulations to address privacy and security of PHI. In December 2008, the U.S. Department of Health and Human Services' Office of the National Coordinator for Health Information Technology released *The Nationwide Privacy and Security Framework for Electronic Exchange of Individually Identifiable Health Information*, which reads in part:

> *The principles below establish a single, consistent approach to address the privacy and security challenges related to* **electronic health information exchange** *through a network for all persons, regardless of the legal framework that may apply to a particular organization. The goal of this effort is to establish a policy framework for electronic health information exchange that can help guide the Nation's adoption of health information technologies and help improve the availability of health information and health care quality. The principles have been designed to establish the roles of individuals and the responsibilities of those who hold and exchange electronic individually identifiable health information through a network* (p. 1).

The principles underlying this document are summarized in **Table 13-7**.

The Health Information Technology for Economic and Clinical Health (HITECH) Act was enacted as part of the American Recovery and Reinvestment Act of 2009 and it modified HIPAA through several provisions that strengthened the civil and criminal enforcement of the HIPAA rules. The complete suite of HIPAA Regulations includes:

- Transactions and Code Set Standards
- Identifier Standards
- Privacy Rule
- Security Rule
- Enforcement Rule

Additional details about these standards and rules are located at http://www.hhs.gov/ocr/privacy/hipaa/administrative/combined/index.html.

The Web as a Health Information and Emotional Support Resource

Web sites are fast becoming a major—if not *the* major—source of health information for the general public. Discussion boards and social media sites on the Internet are also emerging as a major source of emotional support for those facing difficult health issues. Chapter 10 discusses the use of Web sites as communication tools and related security issues.

Patient Portals and Electronic Communication with Patients

While many healthcare providers have been hesitant to use electronic communication with patients, increasing numbers of patients are demanding this form of communication. Patients are especially interested in scheduling appointments, renewing prescriptions, obtaining test results, and getting the answers to health questions. Healthcare providers are often reluctant to engage in such

TABLE 13-7 PRINCIPLES OF THE NATIONWIDE PRIVACY AND SECURITY FRAMEWORK FOR ELECTRONIC EXCHANGE OF INDIVIDUALLY IDENTIFIABLE HEALTH INFORMATION

Principle	Definition
Individual Access Principle	Individuals should be provided with a simple and timely means to access and obtain their individually identifiable health information in a readable form and format.
Correction Principle	Individuals should be provided with a timely means to dispute the accuracy or integrity of their individually identifiable health information and to have erroneous information corrected or to have a dispute documented if their requests are denied.
Openness and Transparency Principle	There should be openness and transparency about policies, procedures, and technologies that directly affect individuals and/or their individually identifiable health information.
Individual Choice Principle	Individuals should be provided a reasonable opportunity and capability to make informed decisions about the collection, use, and disclosure of their individually identifiable health information.
Collection, Use, and Disclosure Limitation Principle	Individually identifiable health information should be collected, used, and/or disclosed only to the extent necessary to accomplish a specified purpose(s) and never to discriminate inappropriately.
Data Quality and Integrity Principle	Individuals and entities should take reasonable steps to ensure that individually identifiable health information is complete, accurate, and up-to-date to the extent necessary for the person's or entity's intended purposes and has not been altered or destroyed in an unauthorized manner.
Safeguards Principle	Individually identifiable health information should be protected with reasonable administrative, technical, and physical safeguards to ensure its confidentiality, integrity, and availability and to prevent unauthorized or inappropriate access, use, or disclosure.
Accountability Principle	These principles should be implemented, and adherence assured, through appropriate monitoring, and other means and methods should be in place to report and mitigate nonadherence and breaches.

NOTE: The information in this table was developed for U.S. Department of Health and Human Services, Office of the National Coordinator for Health Information Technology (2008). Nationwide privacy and security framework for electronic exchange of individually identifiable health information. Retrieved from http://www.healthit.gov/sites/default/files/nationwide-ps-framework-5.pdf

communication because of concerns related to security issues, malpractice, and the possibility they will not be able to manage the increased workload.

However, financial incentives within HITECH strongly support electronic communication with patients. As a result, increasing numbers of healthcare providers are now beginning to use electronic communication with patients as part of their electronic health record applications. Safe use of electronic communication, however, requires educating both the healthcare provider and the healthcare recipient.

Summary

Storing data and exchanging these data via the computer system raise several privacy, security, and confidentiality concerns. This chapter focused on issues related to confidentiality and privacy of data, as well as methods to ensure the integrity of data, software, and hardware. Securing computers and the data they store pose a challenge both for large healthcare information systems and for individuals using PCs. The development of the Internet has created a whole new level of opportunity—and a source of concern. Protecting the privacy of patients and the integrity of their health-related data depend on carefully crafted laws and on educating both the provider and the consumer of health care. Fundamental to that security is understanding the applications and activities necessary to secure your personal computer, related devices, and data.

References

American Health Information Management Association (AHIMA) e-HIM Workgroup on Assessing and Improving Healthcare Data Quality in the HER (2007). Assessing and improving EHR data quality. *Journal of AHIMA, 78*(3), 69–72.

American Medical Association (AMA) (2007). *The Patriot Act: Implications for physicians.* Retrieved from http://www.ama-assn.org/ama/pub/physician-resources/legal-topics/patient-physician-relationship-topics/patriot-act.page

Burke, L. & Weill, B. (2005). *Information technology for the health professions.* Upper Saddle River, NJ: Prentice Hall.

Computer Crime and Intellectual Property Section (CCIPS), U. S. Department of Justice (2010). *Prosecuting computer crimes.* Retrieved from http://www.justice.gov/criminal/cybercrime/docs/ccmanual.pdf

Daniel, M. (2012, January 8). Collaborative and Cross-Cutting Approaches to Cybersecurity. [The White House Blog]. Retrieved from http://www.whitehouse.gov/blog/2012/08/01/collaborative-and-cross-cutting-approaches-cybersecurity

Federal Trade Commission (2012a). *Medical identity theft.* Retrieved from http://www.consumer.ftc.gov/articles/0171-medical-identity-theft

Federal Trade Commission (2012b). *Child identity theft*. Retrieved from http://www.consumer.ftc.gov/articles/0040-child-identity-theft

Federal Trade Commission (2012c). *Tax-related identity theft*. Retrieved from http://www.consumer.ftc.gov/articles/0008-tax-related-identity-theft

Govtrack.us (2013) H.R. 624: Cyber Intelligence Sharing and Protection Act. Retrieved from http://www.govtrack.us/congress/bills/113/hr624#

Jenkins, M. K. (2011). Medical records of the rich and famous—A huge risk. [Web log]. Retrieved from http://www.physicianspractice.com/blog/medical-records-rich-and-famous-%E2%80%94-huge-risk

Johnson, M. E. (2009). *Data hemorrhages in the healthcare sector.* Retrieved from http://fc09.ifca.ai/papers/54_Data_Hemorrhages.pdf

Medical Information Board (MIB) (n.d.). *The facts about MIB*. Retrieved from http://www.mib.com/facts_about_mib.html

National Academy of Sciences, Computer Science and Telecommunications Board (1997). Privacy and security concerns regarding electronic health information. In *For the record: Protecting electronic health information* (chapter 3). Retrieved from http://www.nap.edu/openbook/0309056977/html/54.html

Ornstein, C. (2009, May 11). Farrah Fawcett 'under a microscope' and holding onto hope. *Los Angeles Times*. Retrieved from http://www.latimes.com/entertainment/news/la-et-fawcett-interview11-2009may11,0,5790379.story?page=1

Privacy Rights Clearinghouse (2012a). *Privacy Rights Clearinghouse fact sheets*. Retrieved from https://www.privacyrights.org/privacy-rights-fact-sheets

Privacy Rights Clearinghouse (2012b). *Fact sheet 8: Medical records privacy*. Retrieved from http://www.privacyrights.org/fs/fs8-med.htm

Privacy Rights Clearinghouse (2012c). *Children's online privacy: A resource guide for parents*. Retrieved from http://www.privacyrights.org/fs/fs21-children.htm

SANS Institute (2004). *Federal computer crime laws*. Retrieved from http://www.sans.org/reading_room/whitepapers/legal/federal-computer-crime-laws_1446

U.S. Department of Health and Human Services (HHS) (2011, July 7) University of California settles HIPAA privacy and security case involving UCLA Health System facilities. *Press release*. Retrieved from http://www.hhs.gov/news/press/2011pres/07/20110707a.html

U.S. Department of Health and Human Services (HHS), Office of the National Coordinator for Health Information Technology (2008). *Nationwide privacy and security framework for electronic exchange of individually identifiable health information*. Retrieved from http://www.healthit.gov/sites/default/files/nationwide-ps-framework-5.pdf

U.S. Department of Health and Human Services (HHS), Office of the National Coordinator for Health Information Technology (n.d.). The Nationwide Health Information Network, Direct Project, and CONNECT Software. [Software] Available from http://www.healthit.gov/policy-researchers-implementers/nationwide-health-information-network-nwhin40

U.S. Department of Health and Human Services, Office of Civil Rights (2008). *The HIPAA privacy rule's right of access and health information technology* (HIT). Retrieved from http://www.hhs.gov/ocr/privacy/hipaa/understanding/special/healthit/index.html

U.S. Senate Committee on Homeland Security & Governmental Affairs (2012). *Senate rejects second chance to safeguard most critical cyber networks*. Retrieved from http://www.hsgac.senate.gov/media/majority-media/senate-rejects-second-chance-to-safeguard-most-critical-cyber-networks-

Exercises 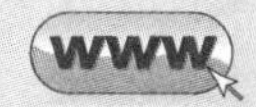

EXERCISE 1 Applying Ethical Principles in Using Computers

■ Objectives

1. Apply ethical concepts in making decisions about the use of computers in commonly encountered situations.
2. Clarify your personal attitude about the ethical use of computer hardware and software.
3. Recognize computer-related criminal behavior.

■ Activity

Your personal ethics are your foundational principles for making decisions about how you will and will not conduct yourself. Health professionals are guided by the ethical code of their specific discipline. In the table below you will see several examples of these codes. As a professional in health care, you will be expected to make ethical decisions about the appropriate use of computers.

1. Start this exercise by first reviewing the codes of ethics posted on the following sites. As you review these documents, pay special attention to the sections on privacy and confidentiality.

Professional Association	URL for the Code of Ethics
American Medical Association (AMA)	http://www.ama-assn.org/ama/pub/physician-resources/medical-ethics/code-medical-ethics.page?
American Nurses Association (ANA)	http://nursingworld.org/MainMenuCategories/EthicsStandards/CodeofEthicsforNurses
Association for Computing Machinery (ACM)	http://www.acm.org/about/code-of-ethics
American Medical Informatics Association (AMIA)	http://www.amia.org/about-amia/ethics/code-ethics
National Association of Social Workers (NASW)	http://www.socialworkers.org/pubs/code/code.asp
International Medical Informatics Association (IMIA)	http://www.imia-medinfo.org/new2/node/39
American Occupational Therapy Association (AOTA)	http://www.aota.org/Practitioners/Ethics/Docs.aspx
American Health Information Management Association (AHIMA)	http://www.ahima.org/about/ethicscode.aspx

In addition to these sites be sure to explore both the Dashboard and Professional Categories located at http://ethics.iit.edu/ecodes/.

2. Beside each situation below, place a check by the term(s) that best reflects your opinion of the behavior of the individual. Provide your reasoning for each of your answers using both the ethical codes of conduct and the information on computer crimes presented in this chapter.
   a. John and Beth are both enrolled in the same section of a computer class. The textbook is expensive so they decide to split the cost and share the required textbook. The book includes access to a Web site; however, it is designed so only one account can be established. They elect to establish one account in Beth's name and share the password.

      John: Ethical___ Unethical___ Computer crime___
      Beth: Ethical___ Unethical___ Computer crime___

   b. At the end of the term John and Beth decide to sell the textbook and the Web access to a student, Robert, who will be taking the course next term. While the password for the Web site can be changed the user name cannot be changed.

      John: Ethical___ Unethical___ Computer crime___
      Beth: Ethical___ Unethical___ Computer crime___
      Robert: Ethical___ Unethical___ Computer crime___

   c. Susan is a senior nursing student recovering from a respiratory infection that required treatment with antibiotics. She was glad to be told by her doctor that by Wednesday she will no longer be contagious. This term Susan is taking Nurs 401. In this course the students are expected to obtain their clinical assignment on Tuesday and prepare for a 6-hour clinical on Wednesday. Susan asks a classmate, Betty, who is assigned to the same clinical unit to check her assignment and to make notes of the information she will need to research, such as the patients diagnosis, significant diagnostic tests, medications, and treatment. The classmate is glad to be of help because they often work together in preparing for clinical and helping each other on the clinical unit.

      Susan: Ethical___ Unethical___ Computer crime___
      Betty: Ethical___ Unethical___ Computer crime___

   d. Betty was surprised to discover that she was not able to help Susan. On Tuesdays nursing students are only able to access the patient(s) on the hospital computer system that are included in their assignments. Betty notifies Susan, who then calls her clinical instructor, Dr. H. Ple to explain her dilemma. Dr. H. Ple comes to the clinical unit and prints off the information. She blacks out the patient's name and gives the printout to Betty who takes it back to Susan.

Susan: Ethical___ Unethical___ Computer crime___
Betty: Ethical___ Unethical___ Computer crime___
Dr. H. Ple: Ethical___ Unethical___ Computer crime___

e. James is assigned to an observational learning experience in a busy emergency department. Five patients from a multiple-car accident have just been admitted and more are expected. James is observing Dr. Smith who is gloved and intubating one of the patients. All of the staff are currently busy caring for the other patients. Dr. Smith's beeper emits a series of beeps. Dr. Smith explains to James that the beeper is hospital issued and requires a password. She tells James that the series of beeps indicates an emergency and she asks James to use her password to sign on and read the text message aloud. James signs in with Dr. Smith's password and reads the message, which includes a patient's name, a brief description of the problem, and requests for a return call STAT.

James: Ethical___ Unethical___ Computer crime___
Dr. Smith: Ethical___ Unethical___ Computer crime___

f. Brian is creating a Web page and finds a terrific background graphic on another page. He copies the background to use on his page. He also includes at the bottom of the page in small print a link acknowledging the source of the background.

Brian: Ethical___ Unethical___ Computer crime___

g. Several healthcare providers are collaborating on an important research study that includes a review of the patient's history, a guided interview, and a computed tomography scan (CT) for each patient participating in the study. The hospital Institutional Board of Review (IRB) has given permission for data collection of the patients' health history via computerized patient records for patients who have signed the informed consent forms. In the past, once the IRB approval was obtained, the principal investigator (PI) sent a list of names of the co-investigators to the IT department to establish their research-related computer accounts. The co-investigators would then review the patient's records and set up the data collection format for each patient. Late Friday afternoon the PI receives a memo explaining that the IT procedures have been changed and the accounts will not be established until the co-investigators have signed the appropriate forms and received training that includes the policies and procedures for using the computerized patient records. Several patients have already been scheduled for interviews and CTs on

Saturday. All of the co-investigators currently have access to the computerized record for these patents via their hospital responsibilities. The PI and co-investigators decide to use their hospital access and deal with the change in procedures on Monday.

PI: Ethical___ Unethical___ Computer crime___
Co-investigators: Ethical___ Unethical___ Computer crime___
IT Department: Ethical___ Unethical___ Computer crime___

h. Terri has taken 21 credits this term and has had a very difficult time keeping up. In 48 hours she must turn in a term paper on the use of computers in health care. She discovers an online term paper titled *The Use of Computers in Rural Hospitals*. The outline is perfect so she uses the paper as a "jumping off point," making significant revisions to the paper. Since she does not cite a specific section of the paper she does not include the paper in her references.

Terry: Ethical___ Unethical___ Computer crime___

i. Dr. Bob is teaching a computer course. The university purchased a site license for 25 copies of the software he is distributing to students. However, 25 students are registered for the course. Dr. Bob gives each of the students an account and sends in a purchase request for additional copies so he will also have access. A week later he receives a call from the purchasing department informing him that the site licenses are only sold in bundles of 25 and cost $500. Dr. Bob decides to wait a week to determine if any students drop the course. If a student does drop the course Dr. Bob plans to use the student's account for his own access.

Dr. Bob: Ethical___ Unethical___ Computer crime___

j. James is completing his senior year as a nursing student in a BSN program. A patient he cared for a few weeks ago obtained his email address from the online university directory and sent him an email. In the email the patient discussed new and potentially serious symptoms and asks that James keep his concerns confidential. James believes the symptoms may indicate a life-threatening situation. He forwards the email to the charge nurse on the unit where the patient was treated and to the senior resident involved in the patient's care.

James: Ethical___ Unethical___ Computer crime___

3. Based on what you've learned during this exercise, create a personal code of ethics to guide your activities in the classroom and the clinical environment. Save the file as **Chap13-Exercise1-LastName** and submit it to your instructor as directed.

EXERCISE 2 Discovering Personal Information on the Internet

Objectives

1. Gain an appreciation of how much personal information is available on the Web.
2. Understand the options you have and do not have to protect your private information.

Activity

1. Select three different Internet search engines. Use each of the them to search for your professor's name on the Internet. Then search for your name. Note what information you find in each case—what did you learn about your professor and yourself. Did you find information that could be misleading or that was not accurate?
2. Professor Emeritus John W. Hill, JD, PhD http://kelley.iu.edu/Accounting/faculty/page12887.cfm?ID=8277 is a recognized legal expert with a distinguished academic record. Review his bio and then use each of the three search engines to see what else you can learn about this man. Now read the post at http://urbanlegends.about.com/od/government/a/Blue-Cross-On-Medicare.htm. This is an example of how a professional's reputation and credentials can be stolen and used on the Internet.
3. Using only your name or phone number, search the Internet to determine if you can locate a street map or picture of your home and/or your parent's home. Note how long it takes you, from the time you start this search until the time you find the information.
4. Using your Word application, write a brief paper explaining what you learned from this exercise and your reaction to this information. Consider whether any of the information you found would be helpful or would hinder you if you were applying for a position in health care.
5. Save this file as **Chap13-Exercise2-LastName**. If you are using a discussion board, respond to the discussion thread on this exercise.

EXERCISE 3 Copyright and Plagiarism

Objectives

1. Describe copyright restrictions and the fair use doctrine.
2. Identify the difference between copyright violations and plagiarism.
3. Identify methods for adhering to copyright law when writing a research paper.

Activity

1. Copyright and plagiarism
   a. Access and review the following Web sites:
      - www.copyright.gov/ Explore the different links, then review the document located at *Copyright Basics (en Español)* and view the video located at *Taking the Mystery Out of Copyright.*
      - http://www.lib.utsystem.edu/copyright/. Complete the tutorial.
      - http://www.libraries.psu.edu/psul/lls/students/using_information.html.

   b. Evaluate the follow scenarios to determine if there is a copyright violation and/or plagiarism. If there is plagiarism or a violation, how should it be handled? Remember that while any one activity may represent both plagiarism and a copyright violation, plagiarism and copyright violation are different issues.
      1. A student is writing a term paper and asks another student to review the paper. The second student makes several revisions from correcting spelling to rewriting sentences. The second student does not add any new citations. In a couple of places she does add examples that clarify some of the concepts included in the original version of the paper. The second student is not paid for the review but does offer to review future papers for pay.
      2. Three students are reading a newly published article written by one of their previous professors. They are surprised and pleased to discover that the professor has acknowledged them at the beginning of the article. The acknowledgement simply states that their insights have been helpful in writing the article. However, in reading the article, each student has discovered a short section (two to three paragraphs) that is almost a direct quote from a term paper previously submitted to the professor.
      3. As a class assignment a student is writing a manual that includes a list of terms with definitions. The student searches the Internet for these terms and uses definitions from a combination of sites when creating each definition.
      4. A student is writing a paper on Meaningful Use and includes a table posted on a government Web site demonstrating how the Centers for Medicare & Medicaid Services are calculating financial incentives. While the Web site for the Centers for Medicare & Medicaid Services is included in the references (http://www.cms.gov/Regulations-and-Guidance/Legislation/EHRIncentivePrograms/index.html) the table does not include a citation.

2. Based on your review of the Web sites and the analysis of the scenarios, answer the following questions:
   a. What is a copyright?
   b. What is fair use?

c. What is the public domain?
d. What are the guidelines for including information in a term paper so as to be in compliance with the copyright law?
e. What is the difference between copyright violation and plagiarism?

3. Type your answers to the questions and save this file as **Chap13-Exercise3-LastName**. Submit it as directed by your professor.

EXERCISE 4 Preventing Computer Crime

Objectives

1. Apply information about computer crimes to prevent these crimes in commonly encountered situations.
2. Understand current laws as they apply to computer crimes.

Situation

During the school year you are living in a dorm with a roommate. Your roommate has an older computer that is having technical problems. There are only a few more weeks left in the term and you know your roommate does not have the money to buy a new computer. Several times he has asked to use your laptop for both school and personal use. How can you configure your computer to protect your privacy? What guidelines or rules should you require your roommate to observe when he is using your laptop?

Activity

1. Review the materials that are available within this chapter and the Web sites listed.
2. Search for Web sites that provide information about protecting your computer, data, and software.
3. Describe the steps you would take to configure your computer and its browser(s) to protect your privacy.
4. Write a set of rules/guidelines that can be used for the next few weeks.
5. Describe how you would ensure that your guidelines are followed.
6. Save this document as **Chap13-Exercise4-LastName**. Submit it as directed by the professor.

Assignments

ASSIGNMENT 1 Copyright—A Student Government Educational Piece

Situation

Several professors at your university are concerned about increasing incidences of copyright infringement. Many of the faculty believe that the ease with which students can cut and paste information from a Web site or an online document has exacerbated this problem. In response to their concerns the faculty senate asked the student government association to create a video that can be posted on YouTube dealing with the many challenges that students face while researching online databases and the Internet. You are on the student government board of directors and a part of a student group assigned the task of developing the video.

Directions

1. Use the following URLs or find other sites to help you develop your video content:
   http://www.templetons.com/brad/copymyths.htm
   http://www.bitlaw.com/copyright/fair_use.html
   http://library.stanford.edu/using/copyright-reminder/copyright-law-overview
   http://vcuhvlibrary.uhv.edu/studyguides/copyright.htm
   http://www.plagiarism.org/
2. Create a script for the video and an announcement of the video. Use an appropriate variety of fonts, bold, italics, underlining, graphics, or other formatting features so that the announcement has an eye-catching format. If directed by your professor, develop the video and upload it to YouTube.
3. Save the file as **Chap13-Assign1-LastName** and submit as directed by your professor.

ASSIGNMENT 2 Tablet Use Guidelines

Situation

The School of Health Professions Learning Lab faculty and staff received a grant to purchase tablets for student use in the clinical area. The tablets include references that can be used to research medications, diagnoses, diagnostic tests, standards of practice, and other clinical materials. These tablets can also be used to access the university network for recording notes and sending emails. Due to their cost, the tablets must be rotated among two groups of students, and therefore, must be checked out the afternoon before clinical and returned the afternoon of clinical.

As the graduate assistant working with the principal investigator (PI) for this grant your charge is twofold: (1) prepare a handout with guidelines on maintaining the safety and security of the tablets and (2) prepare a short presentation to the tablets including these guidelines. This presentation will be shown during the students' orientation.

Directions

1. Prepare a list of potential issues and the guidelines, you can give to the PI for review. Make sure to format the guidelines appropriately, including any graphics that might reinforce them.

2. Save this file as **Chap13-Assign2a-LastName**. Submit your list of safety and security issues and your guidelines to your instructor.
3. Because you know that most of the students are already oriented to PowerPoint, create a short PowerPoint presentation that can be shown during student orientation. This presentation will be loaded on the laptops to provide a quick reference. Make sure to follow the guidelines for quality presentations. Set the program to run automatically.
4. Save this presentation as **Chap13-Assign2b-LastName** and submit it to your professor.

ASSIGNMENT 3 Issue Critique

■ Directions

1. Select one of the following statements to critique:
   a. Information posted on a public discussion board is public domain and can be freely used in total as long as it is properly cited.
   b. The patient owns their data. Therefore, when those data are stored in an electronic health record, each patient has a legal right to know the name of each person who has accessed their record.
   c. Electronic health records are more secure than paper health records, therefore the more sensitive the data (i.e., history of drug and alcohol abuse, AIDS diagnosis, and mental health status) the more important it is that these data be stored electronically.
   d. If the policies and procedures for using the computer system in a healthcare setting create a safety risk for a patient, you should meet the patient's needs and then deal with the policy issues.
2. Write a one- to two-page paper identifying points that support or refute the statement you select. Conclude by stating your position and reasons for that position.
3. Save the file as **Chap13-Assign3-LastName** and submit it to your professor.

NOTE: If this course has an online component, this assignment can be part of a discussion forum requirement, where you will support or refute the statement selected and respond to classmates' posts.

ASSIGNMENT 4 Guidelines for Electronic Communication

■ Situation

You are the school nurse in a local public school with 428 students in grades K to 6. Today the principal asked to meet with you. At that meeting the principal stated that she is concerned about both the tone and content of electronic communication between:

a. Teachers
b. Teachers and Parents
c. Students and Teachers
d. Students

In her judgment some of the emails are aggressive in tone (maybe even bullying) and some seem to divulge confidential information concerning students' health and learning problems. She has asked that you research this problem and provide a set of recommendations to address it.

Directions

1. Develop a list of references and resources you will use in developing the recommendations.
2. Create an outline of the key topics you would address within the recommendations.
3. Using the information you have found create a flyer with a set of guidelines for the children in grades 4 to 6.
4. Run a readability index on the document to be sure that the reading level is appropriate for the students.
5. Save the file as **Chap13-Assign4-LastName**. Submit the references, resources, outline, and the guidelines to your professor.

c h a p t e r

14

Introduction to Healthcare Informatics and Health Information Technology

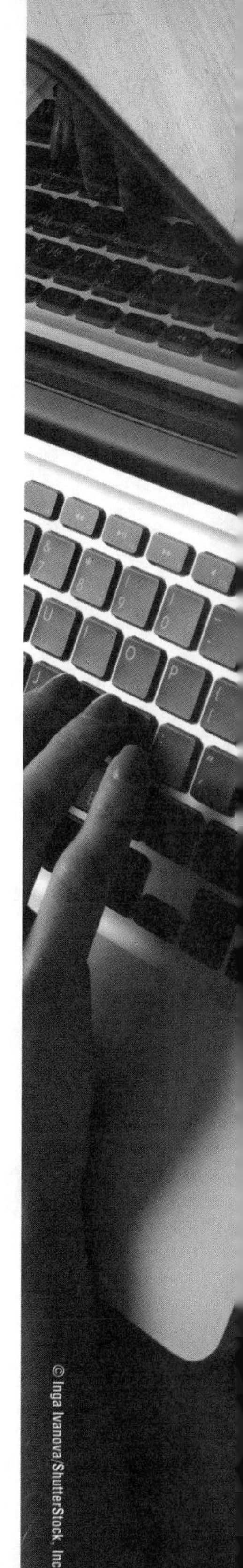

Objectives 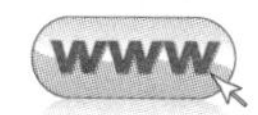

1. Trace the historical development of health informatics.
2. Define health informatics using the concepts of data, information, knowledge, and wisdom.
3. Describe automated healthcare delivery systems.
4. Discuss types of healthcare data and explain how the integration of these data influences the effectiveness of healthcare information systems.
5. Identify selected types and levels of computer-related personnel.

Introduction

This book is designed to support healthcare professionals and students in learning the computer and information literacy skills necessary for safe and effective healthcare delivery in today's increasingly automated healthcare delivery system. **Health informatics** involves the application of these skills to health care. However, the use of computer and information technology in health care does not define the scope of practice in health informatics. Computer fluency and information literacy are foundational skills necessary as a basis for understanding concepts, theories, and tools that you use in the practice of health informatics. Just as a basic understanding of anatomy and physiology is necessary to understand pathology, understanding health informatics requires computer and information literacy. This chapter is an introduction to health informatics.

Historical Perspective of Health Informatics

Over the last several decades, health informatics has evolved as both a discipline (field of study) and as an area of specialization within the health professions. Incorporating processes, procedures, theories, and concepts from computer science, information science, the health sciences, and the social sciences, health informatics is both interprofessional and interdisciplinary in nature. The goal of health informatics is to improve the health of individuals, families, and communities by improving the efficiency and safety of the healthcare delivery system. To achieve this goal health informatics professionals use technology to collect, store, process, and communicate health data, information, knowledge, and wisdom (Nelson, 2014). In tracking the evolution of health informatics as a discipline and as a specialty you must appreciate three key trends. These are:

- The increasing use of computers and automation in healthcare delivery.
- The recognition that all professionals working within health care require health informatics-related knowledge and skills.
- The evolving definition of health informatics as a field of study.

Increasing Use of Computers and Automation in Healthcare Delivery

One can trace the beginning use of computers in health care to the 1950s and 1960s. Experimenting with the use of the technology in medicine and in nursing education characterized this phase. For example, in 1960 the National Institutes of Health (NIH) established a Health Advisory Committee on Computers in Research to review grant requests dealing with problems in biomedical computing (Collen, 1995). In the late 1960s Connie Settlemeyer, in a graduate project at the School of Nursing, University of Pittsburgh, designed a mainframe-based computer-assisted instruction program for teaching nursing students how to chart nurses' notes using the common problem-oriented format called SOAPIE or SOAP.

In the 1970s, after this initial period of experimentation, hospitals began using computers to deal with selected medical data. Beginning in 1971, El Camino Hospital, working in partnership with Lockheed, installed the first computer-aided medical information system, known as MIS (El Camino Hospital, n.d.). Over the next 15 to 20 years a number of hospitals followed by installing information systems to manage the business aspects of health care. Because room changes were key to the business aspect of health care, the backbone of the hospital information system was usually an admission, discharge, and transfer (ADT) system that captured patients' demographic and insurance information data.

Health information system vendors began developing systems for individual departments such as radiology, laboratory, and cardiac cauterization.

Capturing charges from these departments was another important aspect of the business of health care and, as a result, the first attempts at communication between these stand-alone applications consisted of order entry/results reporting systems. A unit clerk or nurse selected a patient from the ADT system and entered new orders that the system communicated to the appropriate department. Upon completion of the order, the results were sent back to the clinical units. Depending on the order and the system configuration, the system could capture a charge either when placing the order or when reporting the results. In these early systems, the unit clerk or staff nurses assumed responsibility for entering orders into the computer system that had been written by physicians on a paper chart. Today these original order entry systems serve as the basis for **computerized provider order entry** (CPOE) systems that enable clinicians (e.g., physicians, nurses, therapists, pharmacists) to enter orders for tests, medications, services, or other clinical processes into the healthcare information system. To ensure increased accuracy and implementation of evidence-based healthcare delivery, decision support systems often supplemented these systems (Agency for Healthcare Research and Quality, 2008).

With the expanded functions of different types of healthcare information systems and the need to integrate data stored in stand-alone systems, larger integrated systems with new and expanded functions emerged. These new and innovative systems often exist alongside older legacy systems. As a result, modern-day healthcare information systems range from small stand-alone systems (i.e., a scheduling system used to make appointments in a private office) to fully integrated healthcare information systems (i.e., electronic health records maintained by large integrated health delivery systems).

By the late 1980s and early 1990s health related agencies and organizations began to propose the concept of automating patient records. In 1991 the Institute of Medicine (IOM) published the *Computer-Based Patient Record: An Essential Technology for Health Care*. This report offered seven recommendations. The first and last recommendations stated:

- Healthcare professionals and organizations should adopt the computer-based patient record (CPR) as the standard for medical and all other records related to patient care.
- Healthcare professional schools and organizations should enhance educational programs for students and practitioners in the use of computers, CPRs, and CPR systems for patient care, education, and research (Dick, Steen, & Detmer, 1991, p. 50).

In 1997 the revised edition of *Computer-Based Patient Record: An Essential Technology for Health Care* included a commentary on the extent of change both in terms of technology and health care during the intervening six years. However, what did not change was the format for patient records. Patient records continue to be almost totally paper based and the commentary notes that "The cost of capitalizing CPR systems remains a significant hurdle for individual institutions, and it is a serious policy issue that must be addressed" (Dick, Steen, & Detmer, 1997, p. ix).

What was becoming increasingly clear is that paper patient records were not only inefficient but they are also unsafe. In 2000 the IOM published *To Err is Human,* which reported that almost 100,000 people die each year from medical error (Kohn, Corrigan, & Donaldson, 2000). It is clear in this report that technology is increasingly seen as the key to improving an inefficient and unsafe healthcare system. In 2004 President George W. Bush declared in his State of the Union Address that "By computerizing health records, we can avoid dangerous medical mistakes, reduce costs, and improve care" (para 1). He followed up this statement with a technology plan, announcing the "ambitious goal of assuring that most Americans have electronic health records within the next 10 years" (The Whitehouse 2004). To achieve this goal he established the Office of the National Coordinator (ONC) by Executive Order. However, with limited funding, progress on this initiative was slow.

The Health Information Technology for Economic and Clinical Health (HITECH) Act of 2009 mandated the creation of the Office of the National Coordinator. During the period between the initial IOM report and the HITECH Act, the terminology moved from computer-based health records to three different types of electronic health records, shown in **Box 14-1**. This new terminology clarified the difference between episodic, longitudinal, and personal health records and became a framework for the activities of the ONC.

Part of the American Recovery and Reinvestment Act (ARRA), the HITECH Act contains incentives designed to accelerate the adoption of health information technology (Health IT) by the healthcare industry, healthcare providers, consumers, and patients. Its goal is to enable improvements in healthcare quality, increase affordability by decreasing cost, and improve healthcare outcomes (Health IT.Gov, 2009).

The programs and activities in the HITECH Act fall into five areas.

1. Support the adoption of electronic health records through financial incentives and technical support to achieve meaningful use.
2. Encourage the development of policies, interoperability requirements, and business practices that increase the electronic health information exchange on a local, state, and national level while ensuring the privacy and security of that data.
3. Establish a Health IT Workforce Development Program to train health IT professionals who are ready to help providers implement electronic health records.

4. Empower citizens to become full partners in their health care with the support of e-health tools that gives them access to their health information in an actionable format.
5. Ensure the development of interoperability standards and policies that make it possible for providers to safely share information with one another and make meaningful use of that information.

With technology's impact on healthcare delivery the need for healthcare professionals who are computer, information, and informatics literate is obvious.

All Professionals Working Within Health Care Require Informatics Knowledge and Skills

In 2002, more than 150 experts from health professions in education, regulation, policy, advocacy, quality, and industry attended a Health Professions Education Summit. Their goal was to assist the Institute of Medicine Committee on Health Professions Education Summit to develop strategies to ensure that educational systems for health professionals are consistent with the principles of the twenty-first

Box 14-1 Types of Electronic Health Records

Electronic medical records (EMRs) are digital versions of the paper charts in clinician offices, clinics, and hospitals. EMRs contain notes and information collected by and for the clinicians in that office, clinic, or hospital.

Electronic health records (EHRs) contain information from all the clinicians involved in a patient's care and all authorized clinicians involved in a patient's care can access the information to provide care to that patient. EHRs also share information with other healthcare providers, such as laboratories and specialists.

Personal health records (PHRs) contain the same types of information as EHRs but are accessed, and managed by patients in a private, secure, and confidential environment. PHRs can include information from a variety of sources including clinicians, home monitoring devices, and patients themselves.

Source:
Office of the National Coordinator for Health Information Technology, U.S. Department of Health and Human Services, Health IT.Gov (n.d.). What are the differences between electronic medical records, electronic health records, and personal health records? Retrieved from http://www.healthit.gov/providers-professionals/faqs/what-are-differences-between-electronic-medical-records-electronic.

century health system. Based on this summit, key position papers, and other resources, the IOM issued a report titled *Health Professions Education: A Bridge to Quality* (Greiner & Knebel, 2003). The report stated that doctors, nurses, pharmacists, and other health professionals are not adequately prepared to provide the highest-quality and safest medical care possible. To meet this challenge, the report called upon educators, as well as accreditation, licensing, and certification organizations, to ensure that students and working professionals develop and maintain proficiency in five core areas: patient-centered care, interdisciplinary teams, evidence-based practice, quality improvement, and informatics.

The IOM publication established the need for all healthcare professionals to be computer, information, and informatics literate and called upon the educational institutions for health professions to make this a reality. Several of the health professional organizations took up this call. For example, the Joint Task Force of the American Health Information Management Association (AHIMA) and the American Medical Informatics Association (AMIA) focused on the education of the healthcare workforce:

> *There are several important cross-cutting issues, including the wide variety of health professionals—from physicians and nurses to therapists and admissions staff—who are or will be using Electronic Health Records (EHRs) as part of their day-to-day activities. This, in turn, has an impact on the broad range of training needed, from basic computer literacy to more sophisticated computer applications and health* (AHIMA and AMIA, 2008, p. 5).

In nursing, the American Nurses Association (ANA), the National League for Nursing (NLN), and the American Association of Colleges of Nursing (AACN) also answered the call. The ANA's report, *Nursing Informatics: Scope and Standards of Nursing Informatics Practice*, identified informatics competencies required of all nurses. "These competencies are categorized in three overall areas: computer literacy, information literacy, and professional development/leadership" (ANA, 2008, p. 36). **Table 14-1** demonstrates the inclusion of informatics in each of the Essentials Documents that the AACN has created since the IOM report. The NLN focused on the need to prepare nursing faculty and administrators who can provide the needed education. The position paper, *Preparing the Next Generation of Nurses to Practice in a Technology-Rich Environment: An Informatics Agenda* (2008), outlines the NLN's recommendations for faculty and administration preparation (NLN, 2008).

In pharmacy, the Accreditation Council for Pharmacy Education (ACPE) answered the call. ACPE includes seven curriculum-related standards that provide the needed education for the accreditation of pharmacy programs leading to the doctor of pharmacy degree. These standards are introduced with the following statement: "As recommended by the Institute of Medicine for all healthcare

TABLE 14-1 INFORMATICS IN THE AMERICAN ASSOCIATION OF COLLEGES OF NURSING'S ESSENTIAL SERIES

The Essentials of Baccalaureate Education for Professional Nursing Practice (2008)	*The Essentials of Master's Education in Nursing (2011)*	*The Essentials of Doctoral Education for Advanced Nursing Practice (2006)*
IV: Information Management and Application of Patient Care Technology	V: Informatics and Healthcare Technologies	IV. Information Systems/ Technology and Patient Care Technology for the Improvement and Transformation of Health Care

professionals, pharmacists must be educated to deliver patient-centered care as members of an interprofessional team, emphasizing evidence-based practice, quality improvement approaches, and informatics" (ACPE, 2011, p. 17).

The impact of the IOM report can also be seen in the accreditation standards for Physical Therapy programs. Note the following Commission on Accreditation of Physical Therapy Education (CAPTE) curriculum content expectations in *Professional Practice Expectations: Evidence-Based Practice:*

> CC-5.21 Consistently use information technology to access sources of information to support clinical decisions.
> CC-5.22 Consistently and critically evaluate sources of information related to physical therapist practice, research, and education and apply knowledge from these sources in a scientific manner and to appropriate populations.
> CC-5.23 Consistently integrate the best evidence for practice from sources of information with clinical judgment and patient/client values to determine the best care for a patient/client.
> CC-5.24 Contribute to the evidence for practice by written systematic reviews of evidence or written descriptions of practice.
> CC-5.25 Participate in the design and implementation of patterns of best clinical practice for various populations (CAPTE, 2013, p. 31).

This last example from the report does not use the term informatics but clearly demonstrates how information literacy concepts are the basis of evidence-based practice, and evidence-based practice is one of the foundational concepts within health informatics. A review of other health professional educational standards will generate similar examples of the recognized need for computer, information, and informatics knowledge and skills in the education programs of all health professionals.

Informatics as a Specialty

While all healthcare professionals require a foundation in health informatics, health informatics is also an area of specialization within healthcare. There are a number of overlapping approaches used to prepare for the specialty role of health informatics. These educational programs range from nondegree certificate programs to postdoctoral programs; however, these programs can be grouped into two basic types.

First are educational programs in which the primary field of study is health informatics. **Table 14-2** provides examples of educational programs offering a degree in health informatics.

TABLE 14-2 EXAMPLES OF EDUCATIONAL PROGRAMS IN HEALTH INFORMATICS

Degree Offered	College or University	URL
Associate of Science in Healthcare Informatics	St. Petersburg College St. Petersburg, FL	http://www.spcollege.edu/Hec/informatics/program_options.html
Bachelor of Science in Health Informatics	Western Governors University	http://www.wgu.edu/online_it_degrees/health_informatics_degree_domains
Post Baccalaureate Certificate in Health Informatics	East Carolina University	http://www.ecu.edu/cs-dhs/hsim/informatics.cfm
Masters in Health Informatics	University of Michigan at Ann Arbor	http://healthinformatics.umich.edu/curriculum
Post Masters or Graduate Certificate in Health Informatics	University of Illinois at Chicago	http://healthinformatics.uic.edu/
Ph.D. in Informatics, with emphasis in Health Informatics	University of Missouri	http://hmi.missouri.edu/prospective/phdhi_description.html
Postdoctoral Program in Biomedical and Health Informatics	University of Washington Seattle, WA	http://www.bhi.washington.edu/postdocprog

In contrast to these degree-based programs are non-degree educational programs such as certificate programs. The HITECH Act introduced the second type of health informatics educational program: a workforce development component with both a community college and a university program. The community college program is offered by a consortium of 82 community colleges. The six month academic programs are designed for professionals with an IT or healthcare background and focus on training students for the following professional roles:

- Practice workflow and information management redesign specialists
- Clinician/practitioner consultants
- Implementation support specialists
- Implementation managers
- Technical/software support
- Trainers

As part of this effort, six Health IT Professional Exams (HIT Pro Exam) were developed to assess the basic competencies in each of six health IT workforce roles. Additional information, including the exam blueprints for each exam, can be found at http://www.healthit.gov/policy-researchers-implementers/competency-examination-program.

The university educational programs are for health professionals, such as physicians, nurses, and dentists, who study informatics as a sub-speciality of their primary discipline. These are usually graduate-level programs offered within the respective schools of each discipline. For example, a master's program in nursing informatics is generally in a school of nursing. These specialists integrate their respective health science specialty with cognitive science, computer science, and information science to manage and communicate data, information, knowledge, and wisdom in the delivery of healthcare services.

In addition to completing formal educational programs, another option for demonstrating competency in health informatics is through certification; however, these options are limited. The ANA offers certification in nursing informatics for nurses with a BSN or higher degree and the required clinical experience in informatics. The American Board of Medical Specialties, working with AMIA, offers a board certification in clinical informatics for physicians. Healthcare Information and Management Systems Society (HIMSS) offers an opportunity to obtain certification as a Certified Professional in Healthcare Information & Management Systems (CPHIMS) for individuals who have completed:

- A baccalaureate degree plus five (5) years of associated information and management systems experience with three of those years in health care, or
- A graduate degree plus three (3) years of associated information and management systems experience with two (2) of those years in health care.

In considering educational preparation for a specialty in health informatics, it is important to note that **health information management** programs should not be confused with health informatics programs. Health information management programs evolved historically from medical records programs. For additional information about the educational programs and certifications related to the profession of health information management please see http://www.ahima.org/certification/credentials.aspx.

The Evolving Definition of Health Informatics

The term **informatics** is the English translation of related terms used in the Russian, French, and German languages starting in the 1960s. Because of differences in translations, it is difficult to determine whether the initial use of the word informatics was referring to the discipline of informatics, information science, computer science, or a combination of these. The term **medical informatics** began to appear in publications in the early 1970s. While the term medical informatics was not defined in these initial publications, it was generally accepted to mean the use of a computer to process medical data and information (Collen, 1995).

Many physicians within the informatics field initially felt that the term medical was inclusive of all the health professions. Evidence of this can be seen, for example, in 1989 when the name American Medical Informatics Association (AMIA) was selected as the title for the professional association. The membership in AMIA was never limited to physicians and has always been open to all health professionals. However, a number of people from other health professions such as nursing, dentistry, and health information management did not agree that the term medicine referenced their disciplines; consequently, discipline names were added to the term informatics, creating the disciplines of nursing informatics, dental informatics, public health informatics, and so forth. Different models were proposed for describing the interrelationships and overlap of the different disciplines (Nelson, 2002). However, none of these gained general acceptance across the various groups.

In 2006 Shortliffe and Blois, key medical informatics leaders, questioned the use of the term medical informatics. "In an effort to be more inclusive and to embrace the biological applications with which many medical informatics groups had already been involved, the name medical informatics has gradually given way to biomedical informatics. Several academic groups have already changed their names, and a major medical informatics journal *Computers and Biomedical Research* was reborn as *The Journal of Biomedical Informatics*." (p. 23). In the same chapter they provided their rationale for eliminating the names health or healthcare informatics. Over the next several years this approach to naming informatics gained momentum within AMIA.

In 2012 the AMIA Board formally approved the white paper titled, *Definition of Biomedical Informatics and Specification of Core Competencies for Graduate Education in the Discipline*. With the acceptance of this paper AMIA now defines **biomedical informatics (BMI)** as "the interdisciplinary field that studies and pursues the effective uses of biomedical data, information, and knowledge for scientific inquiry problem-solving and decision making, motivated by efforts to improve human health" (Kulikowski et al. 2012, p. 3). A figure demonstrating this model can be seen at http://jamia.bmj.com/content/early/2012/06/07/amiajnl-2012-001053.full. As demonstrated in this figure clinical informatics, which is one of three major areas within BMI, includes the practice of informatics in medicine, nursing, dentistry as well as other forms of informatics applied to patients or consumers.

The AMIA approach to naming the discipline has not been accepted by all informatics groups. For example, in response to this issue the faculty at Northwestern University Feinberg School of Medicine, Department of Preventive Medicine, selected the name "Health and Biomedical Informatics" for their educational programs (http://www.preventivemedicine.northwestern.edu/divisions/hbmi/about.html).

In this book we use the term healthcare informatics and health informatics interchangeably and define health or healthcare informatics as an interdisciplinary science and interprofessional area of health-related practice developed from the integration of information science, computer science, cognitive science, and the healthcare sciences. "Health informatics professionals use the tools of information technology to collect, store, process, and communicate health data, information, knowledge, and wisdom. The goals of health informatics are to support healthcare delivery and improve the health status of all" (Nelson, 2014, p. 3).

Analyzing Health Informatics Concepts and Theories

Information science as a discipline evolved from the field of library science and focuses on the study of information generation, transmission, and use. The study of information as a science is usually considered to have originated with Shannon and Weaver's (1949) theory of information. Their work focused on the communication of information and their communication model, which demonstrates the transmission of a message from a sender to a receiver, is the standard used in teaching communication concepts to healthcare providers. Since their work was published, the study of information theory has been approached from several different conceptual frameworks. The primary information model used to explain healthcare informatics was established by Blum (1986). In giving a historical overview of computers in health care, Blum found the model useful in grouping medical applications according to the objects they processed. He identified three groups of applications: data processing, information processing, and knowledge processing. Using Blum's model, Graves and Corcoran (1989), in their classic article, "The Study of Nursing Informatics," proposed that nursing informatics includes nursing data, information, and knowledge. Later that same year, Nelson and Joos (1989) proposed the addition of wisdom to this continuum.

Understanding the definition of healthcare informatics requires an understanding of several key concepts—*data, information, knowledge,* and *wisdom*—as well as an appreciation of the interrelationships between these concepts. In 2008, the ANA *Nursing Informatics: Scope and Standards of Practice* included wisdom in defining the meta-structures of nursing informatics. **Figure 14-1** illustrates the terms and their interrelationships.

Data

Data are raw facts. They exist without meaning or interpretation. Data are the attributes that healthcare professionals collect, organize, and name. The individual elements in a history and physical or a nursing assessment are data elements. For example, the observation that a patient's hair is red, that his weight is 150 pounds, or that his blood sugar is 200 are attributes are raw facts that can be interpreted

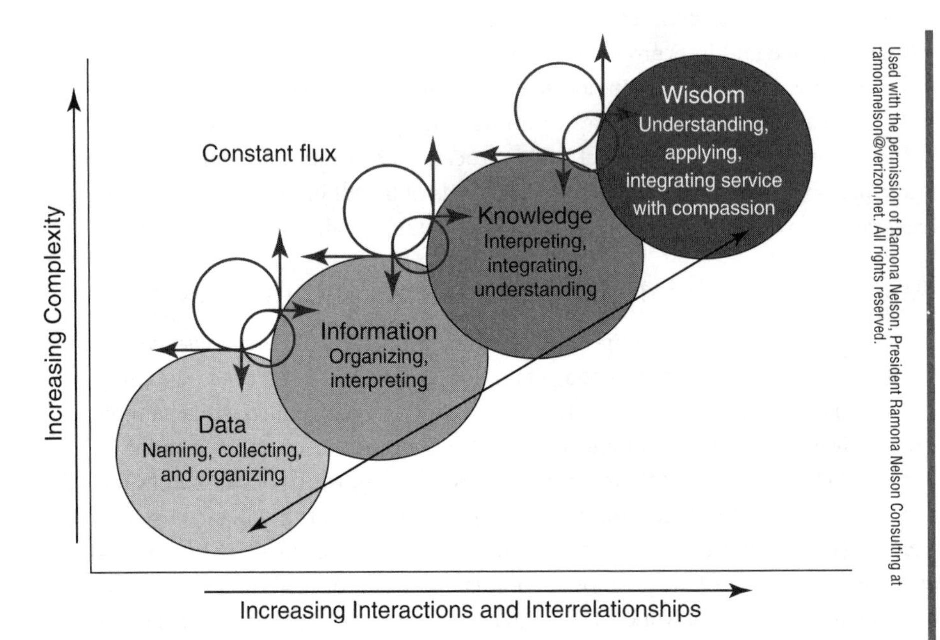

Figure 14-1 Nelson Data-to-Wisdom Continuum

in many different ways. By itself, each piece of these data is meaningless. The red hair may be the result of illness or a hair color product, or just the natural color. The weight may be too high, too low, or the ideal weight for this individual. Depending on the circumstances, this blood sugar could be normal, indicate that the patient is improving, or indicate that the patient is becoming sicker. The process of populating the fields in a database, as described in Chapter 8, involves entering these types of data elements into the database.

Information

Information is a collection of data that has been processed to produce meaning. Classifying, sorting, organizing, summarizing, graphing, and calculating are techniques used to process data. Some of the tools used to process data include paper and pencil, short-term memory, and computers. Many of the exercises in this book demonstrate how computers can be used to process and prepare data so that they can be interpreted. The actual interpretation is a cognitive process whereby data are given meaning and become information. Several factors, including education, attitudes, emotions, and goals, influence how data are interpreted. As a result, each individual gives a unique interpretation to the same collection of data. The various interpretations can be similar, or they can be surprisingly different; however, they are never the same.

For example, suppose a person with newly diagnosed type 2 diabetes has a blood sugar of 350. The client, the physician, and the nurse each place a different significance on this data element; each provides a different interpretation. In other words, this data element is meaningful, but the meaning is different for each individual involved. The physician may interpret this data element as a need for more insulin, the nurse may interpret it as a need for additional patient education, and the client may assume that this blood sugar level is a temporary result attributable to the cake that was eaten the evening before the blood was drawn

An **information system** is a system that processes data, organizing the various elements into meaningful units of information. This definition of an information system does not require that the system be automated. However, in health informatics, the focus is on automated information systems that are used in all aspects of healthcare from basic research to health care delivery. Many different types of automated healthcare information systems exist, several of which are described later in this chapter. The key point to remember is that information from these systems may be interpreted and used differently by different healthcare providers. For example, a chart that tracks the increased independence of a client after a cerebral vascular accident presents vital nursing information. This same chart, when interpreted by the physical therapist, provides key rehabilitation information. Although members of both of these disciplines use the same information to make important decisions about the patient's plan of care, the chart has a different significance for the nurse than for the physical therapist. This is why the development of effective interprofessional documentation systems that are basic to the electronic health record requires the involvement of each of the healthcare disciplines as well as the clients themselves.

It is also important to realize that the same data can produce different types of information. For example, a hospital information system processes order entry data to produce billing information. These same data may be processed by a clinical information system to develop a clinical pathway. Each of these information systems is using the same data, but the information produced is quite different in each case.

Knowledge

While information is built from data, **knowledge** is built from information and data. Knowledge is a collection of interrelated pieces of information and data. In this aggregation, the interrelationships are as important as the individual items of information. An organized collection of interrelated information about a specific topic is usually referred to as a knowledge base. The statement "This student has a good knowledge base in anatomy" would not sound correct if the word "base" was removed from the statement. The information in a knowledge base is organized or structured so that interrelationships can be identified. For instance, the table of contents in any textbook provides an outline of a knowledge base. An effective lecture explains how various facts or pieces of information interrelate. By understanding the information and the interrelationships, you can understand the concepts and theories that are inherent in the specific knowledge base being explained.

Once you develop a knowledge base, you use this knowledge to interpret new data or even reinterpret old data, thereby producing new information. An individual's knowledge base plays a major role in determining how you use data and information in the process of decision making. For example, a diabetic client with an extensive knowledge base about diabetes could be expected to make different decisions than a person with a limited knowledge base in this area. A professional with an extensive knowledge base is a specialist or expert. In this discussion, a knowledge base is more than a large collection of information: It also includes the interrelationships between the pieces of information that produce the knowledge base. An expert builds mental processes that provide quick access to a wide array of interrelationships. As a result, he/she has access to a new level of knowledge. An expert looks at a patient and sees the patient and his or her problems as a whole; in other words, the expert has a gestalt view. In contrast, a novice looks at the same patient and sees only pieces of the information. A novice does not have the quick mental access to all of those interrelationships that the expert has and cannot always see the entire picture of what is happening with a patient. Whereas an expert can look at a client and understand immediately just how sick or anxious that client is, a novice may see the same patient and collect the same data, yet not reach the same conclusion.

This difference is one reason why the teaching–learning process in a clinical setting can be such a challenge. The teacher, who has an expert background, will process the same data and information differently than the student. The student will have no idea how the teacher was able to reach a diagnosis, and the teacher may not understand why the student could not see the "obvious."

The same gap can often be seen between healthcare providers and clients. The client's ability to understand and use health information in making healthcare decisions is referred to as **health literacy**. "Health literacy is defined as the degree to which individuals have the capacity to obtain, process, and understand basic information and services needed to make appropriate decisions regarding their health" (IOM, 2004, p. 2).

A knowledge base can be stored and shared using a variety of media, including oral communication, textbooks, and online databases. As a person gains information, this information is added to his or her internal knowledge base. It is this internal knowledge base that you first use to interpret information and to make decisions. You will not look beyond this internal knowledge base unless you determine that there is an information or knowledge gap. It is very difficult for even an expert to identify what is not known, especially in an area such as health care where the amount of new knowledge and information is exploding. As a result, there is a keen interest in developing the information literacy skills of healthcare professionals as well as the automated decision support systems that can identify information gaps and tap into external knowledge bases.

Automated decision support systems are systems that process information, identifying and demonstrating pertinent interrelationships. These systems may be as simple as the bar chart in **Figure 14-2**, which identifies overtime hours in a healthcare institution, or as complex as a fully automated clinical decision support system within an EHR. Complexity in this situation refers to how much of the knowledge base is stored in the automated system and to the automated rules used to process the data. With a decision support system, the individual's knowledge base interprets the bar chart. Different nurse managers looking at this same bar chart can and do reach different conclusions about staffing on these units.

Although decision support systems can help in the decision-making process, they do not make decisions. For example, you can use an automated scheduling system to generate a work schedule for staff in a clinical setting. The automated system will likely contain an extensive online knowledge base. The system will "know" several facts about the staff as well as the institution's staffing rules.

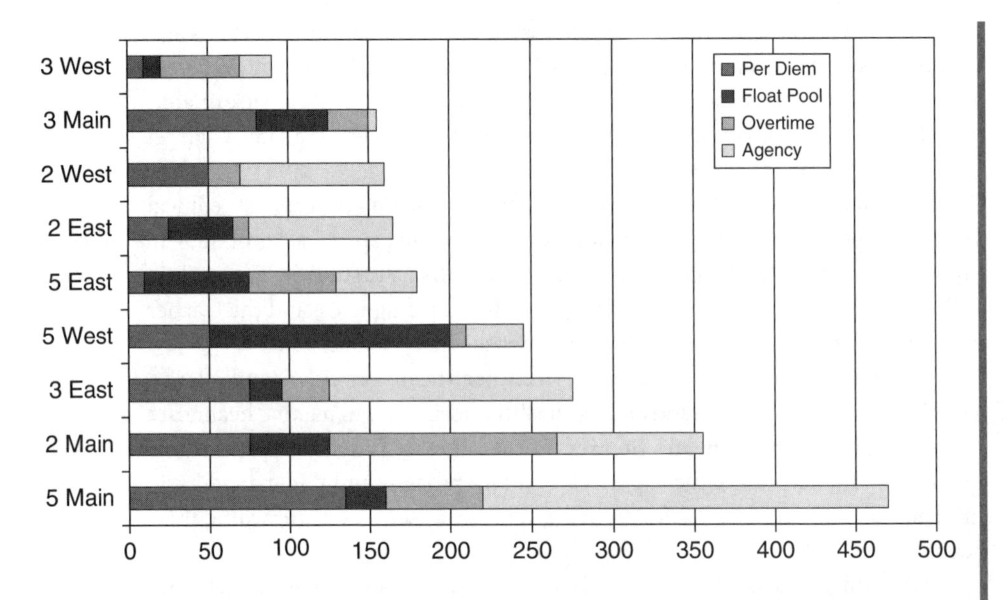

Figure 14-2 Hours of Overtime and Supplemental Staff Used by Clinical Units

However, the scheduling system will not decide who will work when. Instead, the professional in charge is responsible for interpreting the information and approving the schedule.

Decision support systems are an aid to the decision maker. They provide the decision maker with a more complete picture of the interrelations between the information being considered. Ultimately, though, it is the decision maker who interprets the information and decides what action to take. For example, a clinical support system may generate a list of assessment items for a patient with a head injury. This list can be very helpful in ensuring that the healthcare provider does not forget to check a specific assessment item. However, the healthcare provider is still responsible for ensuring that the patient receives a comprehensive and appropriate assessment, including items that are not on the checklist but are nevertheless important because of the patient's overall health status. It cannot be overstated: the key difference between a decision support system and an expert system is that the healthcare provider makes the decision, not the automated system.

Clinical decision support systems are increasingly accepted as a valuable tool for improving safety, decreasing cost, and improving patient outcomes. For these systems to be effective, the knowledge base built into them must reflect best practices based on evidence and be available in a format that allows clinicians to integrate them seamlessly into their workflow. Within current systems examples of clinical decision support systems that can be of aid to clinicians include:

- Immunization, screening, and disease management guidelines for secondary prevention.
- Suggestions for possible diagnoses that match a patient's signs and symptoms.
- Treatment guidelines for specific diagnoses, drug dosage recommendations, and alerts for drug–drug interactions.
- Corollary orders and reminders for drug adverse event monitoring.
- Care plans to minimize length of stay and order sets.
- Duplicate testing alerts and drug formulary guidelines (HIMSS, 2012).

Wisdom

In health care, ethical decision making that ensures cost-effective quality care requires more than an empirical knowledge base. **Wisdom** is knowing when and how to use this knowledge. Knowledge makes it possible for a caregiver to explain the stages of death and dying; wisdom makes it possible for the caregiver to use theories related to death and dying to help terminally ill patients express his or her feelings and plan for the end of life. The development of wisdom requires not only empirical knowledge, but also ethical, personal, and aesthetic knowledge.

Currently, there is no way to automate wisdom, although certain aspects of this concept are being built into automated systems. Expert systems are knowledge-based systems that include built-in procedures for determining when and how to use that knowledge. In the future, the development of decision support systems for experts will require a better understanding of the concept of wisdom and the ways in which wisdom influences the decision-making process of expert practitioners.

Automated Information Systems in Health Care

Computer technology has now been infused into almost every aspect of healthcare delivery. Here, we divide the discussion of automated systems used in health care into two sections. First is an overview of selected types of automated applications. It is followed by a discussion of the types of data that are processed in automated healthcare information systems—including a discussion of levels of integration. Finally, the systems are discussed in terms of healthcare computing roles.

Automated Applications Used in Healthcare Delivery

This section reviews the types of applications commonly used in healthcare delivery. It is becoming increasingly difficult to classify the diverse automated applications used in health care into specific categories. As vendors increase the scope of functions offered within their products, their niches increasingly overlap. In addition, several information systems companies have been purchased or merged so many of their products are also now integrated or merged. For the purposes of our discussion, we group automated information systems used in health care into five types: healthcare information systems (also known as backbone systems), clinical information systems, administrative information systems, consumer information systems, and personnel management systems.

Healthcare Information Systems

While healthcare automation is increasingly more decentralized—a scheme made possible by network connections between systems or interface engines — **healthcare information systems (HISs)** continue to form the backbone of that network within healthcare institutions. Healthcare information systems were originally developed for hospitals. Today you may find them in nursing homes, rehabilitation centers, clinics, private offices, or any other healthcare institution. There are four primary functions of HISs.

First, HISs are often the backbone or primary system used to integrate or interface with the various applications throughout the organization. They communicate information between the point of care or clinical units and the various departments within the institution. This functionality can include sending patient orders to hospital departments and reporting results back to patient health records, as well as requesting supplies and equipment for clinical units or offices. As part of the communication function, HISs may also support the institution's intranet. Second, HISs manage the ADT process. In doing so, they track the location of all patients while maintaining their demographic data. Third, these systems almost always interface with the financial systems used to track the charges and billing process for the institution. Fourth, they are used to produce a number of executive dashboard views (an interface that displays key performance indicators) and administrative reports that support the daily operations of the institution as well as long-term planning. For example, HISs may be used to create a list of patients' dietary orders, which in turn can be used to distribute meal trays or track institutional food costs.

Clinical Information Systems

Clinical information systems process patient data and support patient care. Examples of functions in clinical information systems include collecting patient assessment and health status data, developing plans of care, managing order entry processes and results reporting, tracking treatments including medication administration records, developing work lists, and producing reports such as patient problem lists.

Clinical department systems support the daily work of clinical departments as well as populate the appropriate sections of the EHR. Clinical departmental systems accept patient orders; report results; schedule patients, equipment, and rooms; print labels and work lists; and maintain inventories. The primary benefits of these types of systems include improved efficiency of the department and communication with the clinical units or points of care. The most commonly automated clinical departments interfacing to the EHR include laboratory, radiology, cardiology, and pharmacy. Increasingly, these data are being shared across the total institution, including clinics and private physicians' offices.

In addition to capturing data from clinical department systems, an EHR system can be interfaced to automate monitoring devices, thereby capturing vital signs and other data directly into the clinical record. Additional patient data enters the EHR via direct documentation. One of the primary benefits of an EHR is the improved quality of the data-capture process, thereby increasing access to comprehensive client data. The data are collected and managed by an EHR system much as a database management system manages a database. Data from an individual's EHR can be stored in a clinical data repository, which can be conceptualized as a warehouse or large database where all data elements from all the different systems are stored. This scheme makes it possible to integrate the data and to obtain a different level of information. For example, by integrating the clinical data with the financial data, it becomes possible to evaluate the cost of each problem on the patient problem list. For these systems to be truly effective, a data dictionary that defines each element is required. An example of an actual EHR as it appears to the healthcare provider is depicted in **Figure 14-3** and an example of an Order/Entry screen appears in **Figure 14-4**.

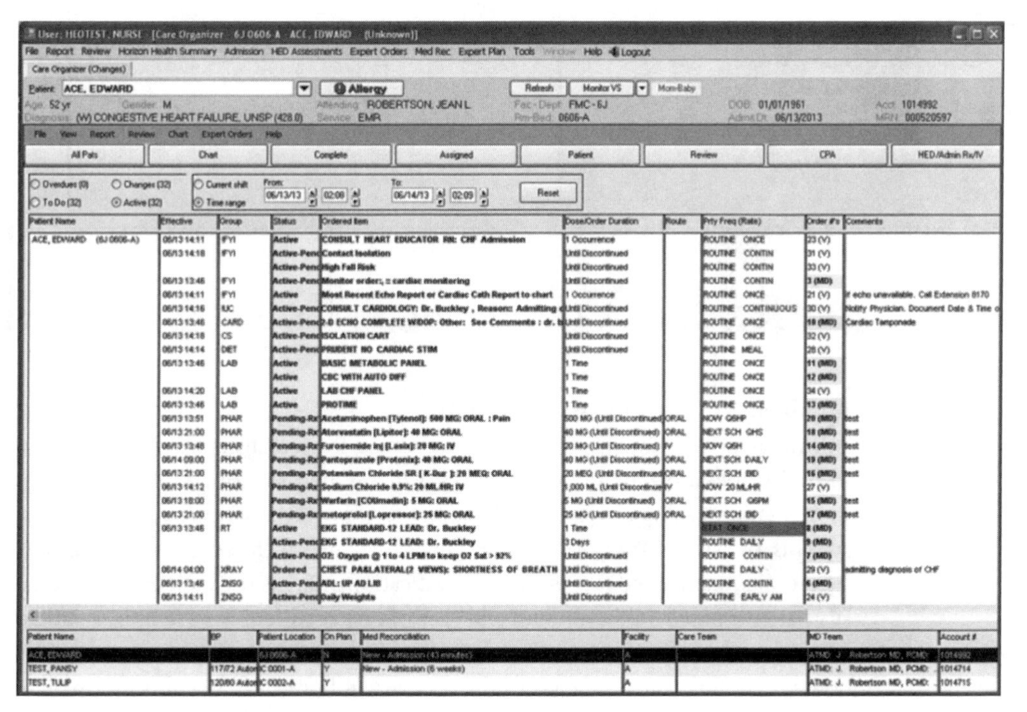

Figure 14-3 Example of EHR Computer Screen

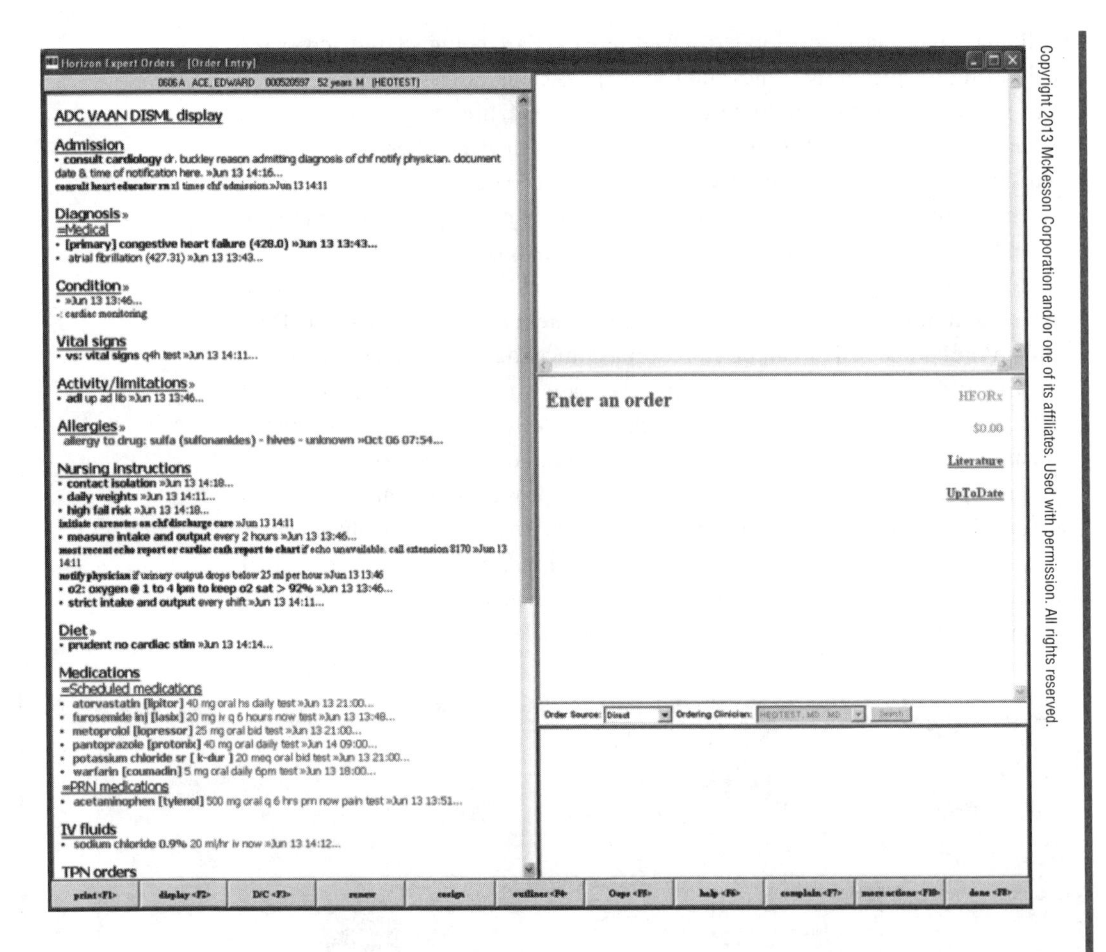

Figure 14-4 Example of an Order/Entry Computer Screen

Administrative Information Systems

Administrative information systems automate the management of data used in the daily operations of an institution as well as data used for strategic and long-range planning. These systems include institution-wide systems, such as financial systems, or systems specific to certain functions, such as the acuity or patient classification systems used for staffing. Classification systems use patient data to classify patients based on the amount and type of care required. For example, a patient with new second- and third-degree burns over 60% of the body may require 6 hours of professional nursing time during every 8-hour shift. In contrast, a patient who is 3 days postoperative from open-heart surgery may require 2 hours of professional nursing time per 8-hour shift. The data from classification systems can be used to decide the amount and type of staff assigned to a clinical unit.

Quality assurance systems attempt to measure and report on cost-effective quality care, resulting in a high level of patient satisfaction. Examples of data processed in quality assurance systems include patient outcomes or variance reports, performance indicators for providers, infection reports, incident reports, patient satisfaction results, and cost data. These data reports can include both individual and aggregate formats.

Material management systems manage the supplies and other inventory of an institution. The goal of these systems is to ensure that the right supplies are at the right site with a minimum of overhead costs. These systems can include an online searchable catalog, an automatic interface to budget systems, automatic reordering of supplies, and alerts issued when there is a significant increase or decrease in inventory orders or costs.

Financial systems include a combination of the information systems used to manage and report the financial aspects of the institution. These include systems that: track income-related data, such as those related to billing and contract monitoring; develop and monitor capital and operating budgets; and track institutional costs, such as payroll and cost accounting. Financial systems usually interface with the ADT and personnel systems. For example, the payroll system typically interfaces with the time-and-attendance or scheduling system to track who has worked and which hours.

Personnel Systems

Personnel systems include a combination of systems that track the characteristics of employees and/or the use of these employees within the institution. Human resources management or personnel records systems maintain individual employee records. For example, healthcare institutions must know the home address, salary, job title and description, professional license number and renewal date, and a number of other details about each employee. Automated systems make it much easier to maintain accurate data and to search for information about individual employees as well as groups of employees. Scheduling systems schedule the actual dates and times that an employee will work and keep a historical record of vacation, holiday, and sick time used.

Some of these systems are now part of the **Enterprise Resource Planning (ERP)** that many organizations use to integrate internal and external management of data and information for the entire organization. ERP systems integrate administrative, financial, personnel, and other systems into one internal system and also manage connections to outside entities.

Consumer Information Systems

Consumer information systems are applications developed for use by the general public, patients, or clients, as opposed to by traditional care providers. A major force supporting the current development of these systems is the Consumer

TABLE 14-3 OFFICE OF THE NATIONAL COORDINATOR: CONSUMER E-HEALTH PROGRAM AIMS

Aim	Definition
Access	Increase access to health information: Consumers and patients are active participants in the secure, easy, and electronic flow of information pertinent to their health and health care.
Action	Enable consumers to take action based on their health information by encouraging the development of tools and services that help make electronic health information useful and meaningful for them.
Attitudes	Shift attitudes thereby empowering consumers to think and act as partners in their care with the support of e-health tools.

Source: Office of the National Coordinator for Health Information Technology, U.S. Department of Health and Human Services, Health IT.Gov (n.d.). Health IT Adoption Programs: Consumer eHealth Program. Retrieved from http://www.healthit.gov/policy-researchers-implementers/consumer-ehealth-program.

eHealth Program (supported by the ONC). The goal of the Consumer eHealth Program is the empowerment of individuals to improve their health and health care through Health IT. The "Three As" (Access, Action, and Attitudes) identify the collective aims of this program (Health IT.Gov, n.d.). See **Table 14-3** for a description of these aims. Additional information about the specific programs supporting each of these aims can be found at http://www.healthit.gov/policy-researchers-implementers/consumer-ehealth-program.

For the purposes of discussion we classify consumer information systems into three basic types of applications:

- Applications that provide information or support services related to health care.
- Applications that assist the general public in maintaining their personal health data.
- Applications such as Blue Button that provide an interface between PHR, EHR, and other health information systems.

Consumer Information and Support

Consumer information and support applications provide information as well as emotional support. These can include Web 1.0-type applications that provide information and Web 2.0 applications based on social media. Both Web 1.0 and 2.0 applications vary greatly in quality and oversight. For example, state and federal government agencies provide a number of excellent information resources, but a number of health-related products of limited value are also marketed as health resources. Examples can readily be found by searching the Internet for products useful in weight loss. In addition to providing information, reputable sites also offer emotional support to consumers. Several voluntary organizations and for-profit businesses maintain virtual groups where patients can exchange information and support for each other. An excellent example of support is the online support groups maintained by the Association of Cancer Online Resources, Inc. (ACOR) at http://www.acor.org/.

Personal Health Records

Personal health records (PHRs) are applications that patients use to maintain copies of their own healthcare information. They may include health information from a variety of sources, including multiple healthcare providers, labs, pharmacies, and the patients themselves. Traditional healthcare institutions, insurance companies, employers, and outside vendors offer a wide range of PHR applications.

Some examples of how patients use PHRs include:

- Emergency care or care while traveling.
- Chronic disease management—collecting data and tracking outcomes is an effective approach to motivating patients to adhere to their treatment plan.
- Care coordination between multiple healthcare providers.
- Family health management for keeping track of appointments, immunizations, and other details for several people.
- Secure communication—some PHRs offer a secure way for patients to communicate with their healthcare providers over the Internet (Office of the National Coordinator for Health Information Technology, 2011).

Additional information on the types of PHRs is located at http://www.hrsa.gov/healthit/toolbox/HealthITAdoptiontoolbox/PersonalHealthRecords/modelsavailable.html.

Blue Button

Blue Button offers a solution for managing one of the major barriers to the use of PHRs. This was the need for patients to collect and enter all their data into their PHR. Tethered systems that are tied to the EHR are maintained by an individual healthcare system can provide a partial solution in that the information from that institution is available to the patient. To be fully effective, PHRs must be able to download healthcare information from *all* providers. Realizing that this was severe limitation with most PHRs, in 2010 the U.S. Department of Veterans Affairs (VA) began the Blue Button program. Blue Button makes it possible for veterans to get easy, secure online access to their health information, which can be downloaded in an understandable format. By August 2012, it had over 1,000,000 users.

In January 2013 the Office of the National Coordinator for Health Information Technology (ONC) announced the implementation of Blue Button Plus, which will make consumers' health data even more accessible through the implementation of interoperable standards that can move EHR data to a third-party consumer health data application. Now both public and private organizations are pledging to also offer Blue Button capabilities to their consumers (Mullin, 2013). With the combination of Meaningful Use requirements for consumer access to their personal health data and the technical support provided by the Blue Button initiative, the implementation and use of PHRs can be expected to grow significantly in the next decade.

Setting-Specific Systems

These systems may include any of the functions already discussed (e.g., clinical, financial, and personnel information management); however, the functions are customized for the specific setting. Examples of setting-specific systems include home health systems, physician office systems, outpatient or ambulatory care clinics, nurse center clinics, and emergency room systems.

Types of Automated Data Used in Healthcare Information Systems

To fully understand the impact of automated systems on health care, it is imperative to consider the types of data being processed. For the purposes of discussion, we classify these data into five major types. This chapter already presented four of these—clinical or client, financial, human resources, and material resources data (Nelson, 2004). New to this chapter is intellectual data. However, it is important to realize that any one piece of data, by itself, is without meaning and can, in fact, fall into any or all of these classifications as explained below.

Clinical or Client Data	These data include all individual client-related data. A comprehensive collection of the client data would be stored in the EHR and/or in the PHR. An example of this type of data would be a patient's blood pressure or a list of the patient's problems.
Financial Data	These types of data include all fiscal data related to the operation of the healthcare institution. Examples include the patient's bill or the budget for an individual unit.
Human Resources Data	These data include all data related to employees as well as individuals who have a contractual relationship with the institution, such as physicians, nurses, students, or volunteers.

Material Resources Data	These data refer to all of the tangible resources used in the operation of the healthcare institution—everything from supplies that are purchased externally to supplies that are created internally.
Intellectual Data	These data comprise the factual data that are stored in the various discipline- or subject-specific databases. Examples include a database with information about medications or a database with published articles and research results.

Levels of Data Sharing

Healthcare applications process the various types of data described previously. The effectiveness of these applications in supporting quality, cost-effective health care is influenced by the level of data sharing made possible by the overall logic and physical design of the total healthcare information system.

Stand-alone systems do not share data or information with any other computer system. Departments tend to develop these systems when they do not trust the institution's systems or when institutional systems do not process data in the format necessary by the department. For example, a department may have frequent changes in its work schedule that are difficult to process in the institutional systems. A PC-based scheduling system developed in that department would be a stand-alone system. Employee schedule changes in the department's system will not be reflected in any other institutional system—the personnel and payroll systems would still show the original schedule. Stand-alone systems result in data redundancy in the system and database discrepancies—and those discrepancies can become a source of conflict between departments and personnel.

Interfaced systems maintain their own database while sharing data across a network. For example, a laboratory system may be interfaced with a HIS; in such a case, the patient orders from the HIS pass directly to the laboratory system, and the laboratory results pass directly back to the HIS. The interfacing of several department systems is called "spaghetti." Because most of these interfaced systems are purchased from different vendors and the computer systems are constantly being updated, maintaining interface-related code becomes a constant battle, and patient data can get lost in this complexity.

Integrated systems use an interface engine and/or share a common database. The clinical data repository or warehouse system discussed earlier is such a system. All of the data related to a client, employee, or financial system are stored in one repository. Although this is a simple concept, the process of building a repository is very complex.

Most healthcare institutions operate with a combination of stand-alone, interfaced, and integrated systems. Data are shared at four different levels:

Level 1 involves integration of a specific institution service or function. For example, an executive information system may pull census, personnel, and financial data together to present an overall picture of the institution's operational status. A product-line system may integrate patient data from several different systems to track how patients in that product line move through the organization.

Level 2 involves sharing data for an individual healthcare institution. Sometimes all patient data are shared in this way; at other times, the sharing involves all institutional data including financial, personnel, and tangible resources.

Level 3 involves the sharing of data across all institutions within the larger organization, a type of system referred to as an enterprise-wide system. This level of sharing is increasingly important with the development of integrated healthcare delivery systems. The best example of this level of integration is the application used by the United States Veterans Health Administration called VistA. A detailed description of VistA can be seen at http://www.ehealth.va.gov/VistA.asp. A key component of VistA is the Computerized Patient Record System (CPRS); CPRS is a longitudinal health record that follows the patient through all VA treatment settings. This application has been installed at all VA medical centers since 1997. VistA data are composed of individual patient records which are the source data for several VA corporate databases, including the National Patient Care Database (NPCD), Decision Support System (DSS), the VA Central Cancer Registry, and the Corporate Data Warehouse (CDW). (U.S. Department of Veterans Affairs, 2012).

Level 4 involves sharing data outside of the institutions owned by the enterprise. These applications serve as regional and national health information networks. Connecting regional and national networks together creates a national "network of networks." Such an effort, known as the Nationwide Health Information Network (NwHIN), has been undertaken by the U.S. federal government. NwHIN is a set of standards, services, and policies that enable the secure exchange of health information over the Internet. It is not a physical network that runs on servers at the U.S. Department of Health and Human Services, nor is it a large network that stores patient records. Rather:

> *These standards, services, and policies will help move health care from a system where patient information is stored in paper medical records and carried from one doctor's office to the next to a process where information is stored and shared securely and electronically. Health information will follow the patient and be available for clinical decision making as well as for uses beyond direct patient care, such as measuring quality of care* (HealthIT.gov, n.d.).

With this level of integration, a patient's record could be accessed from any healthcare institution. If a person living in Pennsylvania is in a car accident in Florida, his or her healthcare record can be accessed from the emergency room in Florida.

In its early stages, healthcare computing relied on stand-alone systems. Today, these systems are becoming increasingly integrated. This sharing of data across disciplines within health care is one of the factors advancing the overall move toward integration of services. As this trend continues, healthcare information systems are becoming more generic—they are becoming patient-focused systems rather than medical or nursing systems. Although this trend is improving the comprehensiveness of the data, no one approach to managing patient data will not meet the information needs for all disciplines. How to develop an integrated, patient-focused healthcare information system that meets the information needs of different disciplines is an important applied research question in healthcare computing. The other side of the coin begs this question: How do we prepare healthcare providers with interprofessional skills to effectively work together to provide patient-centered care?

Healthcare Computing Personnel

There are several levels and types of personnel who work in healthcare computing. Some personnel have a primary background in computer and information science, whereas others have a primary background in health care. A few are prepared in healthcare informatics. The educational preparation of people in healthcare computing varies from on-the-job training to postdoctoral study.

Chief Information Officer or Director of Information Services

The **chief information officer** (CIO) is administratively responsible for the operation of the information services department. Increasingly this individual is part of the executive team responsible for strategic and long-range institutional planning as well as the day-to-day operation of the department. Closely related to this role is the chief medical or nursing informatics officer.

Systems Analysts

Systems analysts work with users to define their information needs and design systems to meet those needs. Their education is usually in information or computer science with knowledge of health care acquired from on-the-job experience. However, with the increased use of computers systems in the clinical setting, a significant number of system analysts now have formal healthcare training, such as in nursing.

Programmers

Programmers design, code, and test new software programs as well as maintain and enhance current applications. These individuals usually receive their educational preparation in computer science or as on-the-job training.

Systems or Network Administrators

Systems administrators are responsible for planning and maintaining multiuser computer systems on a local or wide area network. These individuals may have an associate or baccalaureate degree in computer or information science. They are often certified in the use of the software application used to manage the network.

Microcomputer Specialists

Microcomputer specialists support personal computer users throughout the institution. They may install new software, troubleshoot or repair personal computers, answer user questions, and train users on new software.

Mobile Device Specialists

Mobile device specialists provide support for all mobile devices used in the process of delivering health care, such as smartphones and tablets. They may provide user support desk assistance, create test scenarios, and develop test scripts for a facility's mobile environment.

Healthcare Information Security Officer

The **healthcare information security officer** is responsible for the design, oversight, and ongoing management of the information security program for the facility. This may include writing policies, procedures, conducting security risk assessments, testing the technical systems, or employee training. The purpose of this job is to maintain the confidentiality, integrity, and availability of data within all healthcare organization information systems.

Computer Operators

There are several types of computer operators. The title "**computer operator**" usually refers to an individual who actually runs a mainframe or minicomputer; these individuals generally have minimal interaction with healthcare providers. Microcomputer (PC) operators, by comparison, work closely with users. They troubleshoot, upgrade, and repair computers as well as install software. Network administrators provide this same type of service for local area networks.

Summary

Literacy is the ability to read, write, and use numbers skillfully enough to meet the demands of society. Computer literacy is the ability to use a computer skillfully enough to meet the demands of society. The depth and scope of computer literacy needed by any one person can vary extensively. One person can be very literate when it comes to word processing, but unable to use any other program. Another person may have a general knowledge of several different programs. In today's automated world, all people need to have at least a basic understanding of computers. Healthcare professionals, like all other educated people, need a basic level of computer literacy.

Information literacy refers to the ability to access, evaluate, and use information. With the advent of computers, information literacy requires the ability to access databases, especially literature databases, and the largest database of all—the Internet. Once information has been accessed, the information-literate individual must be able to evaluate the information effectively and to recognize inaccurate and incomplete information. This task is especially difficult if the reader has a limited knowledge base related to the information being accessed. Finally, information literacy requires the ability to use the information.

Healthcare informatics is a field specific to health care. It uses tools from information science, computer science, cognitive science, and the healthcare sciences to help manage healthcare institutions and deliver quality health care. This book provides the reader with a foundation in computer and information literacy. It concludes by introducing the reader to the discipline of healthcare informatics.

References

Accreditation Council for Pharmacy Education (ACPE) (2011). Accreditation standards and guidelines: Professional program in pharmacy leading to the doctor of pharmacy degree. Retrieved from https://www.acpe-accredit.org/standards/default.asp

Agency for Healthcare Research and Quality (AHRQ) (2008). Computerized provider order entry. Retrieved from http://healthit.ahrq.gov/portal/server.pt/community/ahrq_national_resource_center_for_health_it/650

American Association of Colleges of Nursing (AACN) (2006). The essentials of doctoral education for advanced nursing practice. Retrieved from http://www.aacn.nche.edu/education-resources/essential-series

American Association of Colleges of Nursing (AACN) (2008) The essentials of baccalaureate education for professional nursing practice. Retrieved from http://www.aacn.nche.edu/education-resources/essential-series

American Association of Colleges of Nursing (AACN) (2011). The essentials of master's education in nursing. Retrieved from http://www.aacn.nche.edu/education-resources/essential-series

American Health Information Management Association (AHIMA) and American Medical Informatics Association (AMIA) Joint Work Force Task Force (2008). Core competencies for health information management and informatics. Retrieved from http://www.amia.org/reports/core-competencies-health-information-management-and-informatics

American Nurses Association. (2008). *Nursing informatics: Scope and standards of practice.* Silver Spring, MD: NurseBooks.org.

Blum, B. I. (1986). *Clinical information systems.* New York: Springer-Verlag.

Collen, M. F. (1995) *A history of medical informatics in the United States*. Washington, DC: American Medical Informatics Association.

Commission on Accreditation of Physical Therapy Education (CAPTE) (2013). Evaluative criteria for accreditation of PT programs. Retrieved from http://www.capteonline.org/AccreditationHandbook/

Dick, R. S, Steen, E. B, & Detmer, D. E. (eds.) (1997). *The computer-based patient record: An essential technology for health care*, revised edition. Washington, DC: National Academies Press.

Dick, R. S, Steen, E. B, & Detmer, D. E. (eds.) (1991). *The computer-based patient record: An essential technology for health care.* Washington, DC: National Academies Press.

El Camino Hospital (n.d.). *About El Camino hospital: History & milestones.* Retrieved from http://www.elcaminohospital.org/About_El_Camino_Hospital/History_Milestones

Englebardt, E. & Nelson, R. (2002). *health care informatics: An interdisciplinary approach.* St. Louis: Mosby.

Graves, J. & Corcoran, S. (1989). The study of nursing informatics. *Image: Journal of Nursing Scholarship, 21*(4): 227–231.

Greiner, A. & Knebel, E. (eds.). (2003). Institute of Medicine: Committee on the Health Professions Education Summit. Health professions education: A bridge to quality. Retrieved from http://www.nap.edu/catalog.php?record_id=10681

Healthcare Information and Management Systems Society (HIMSS) (2012). Best practices of clinical decision support. Retrieved from http://www.himss.org/ResourceLibrary/ResourceDetail.aspx?ItemNumber=11719

HealthIt.gov (n.d.) Nationwide Health Information Network (NwHIN). Retrieved from http://www.healthit.gov/policy-researchers-implementers/nationwide-health-information-network-

Institute of Medicine, Committee on Health Literacy (2004). *Health literacy: A prescription to end confusion.* Retrieved from http://search.nap.edu/napsearch.php?term=10883

Kohn, L. T, Corrigan, J. M. & M. S. Donaldson (eds.) (2000). *To err is human: Building a safer healthcare system.* Retrieved from http://www.nap.edu/catalog.php?record_id=9728

Kulikowski, C. A., Shortliffe, E. H., Currie, L. M., Elkin, P. L., Hunter, L. E., Johnson, T. R., et al. (2012), Definition of biomedical informatics and specification of core competencies for graduate education in the discipline. *J Am Med Inform Assoc., 19.* Retrieved from http://jamia.bmj.com/content/early/2012/06/07/amiajnl-2012-001053.full

Mullin, R. (2013). ONC introduces blue button plus. Retrieved from http://www.4medapproved.com/hitanswers/blue-button-plus/

National League for Nursing (NLN) (2008). Preparing the next generation of nurses to practice in a technology-rich environment: An informatics agenda. Retrieved from http://www.nln.org/aboutnln/PositionStatements/informatics_052808.pdf

Nelson, R. (2014). Introduction: The evolution of health informatics. In R. Nelson & N, Staggers (Eds,), *Health informatics: An interprofessional approach* (pp. 2–17). St. Louis: Elsevier/Mosby.

Nelson, R. (2004). Incorporating new technology: Nursing informatics. In L. Caputi & L. Englemann (Eds.), *Teaching nursing: The art and the science* (pp. 555–588). Glen Ellyn, IL: College of Dupage Press.

Nelson, R. (2002). Major theories supporting health care informatics. In S. Englebardt & R. Nelson (Eds.), *Health Care Informatics; An Interdisciplinary Approach.* St. Louis: Mosby-Year Book, Inc.

Nelson, R. & Joos, I. (1989). On language in nursing: From data to wisdom. *PLN Visions,* 6(Fall).

Office of the National Coordinator for Health Information Technology, U.S. Department of Health and Human Services, Health IT.Gov (2011). What is a personal health record: What healthcare providers need to know. Retrieved from http://www.healthit.gov/providers-professionals/faqs/what-personal-health-record

Office of the National Coordinator for Health Information Technology, U.S. Department of Health and Human Services, Health IT.Gov (2009). HITECH programs & advisory committees. Retrieved from http://www.healthit.gov/policy-researchers-implementers/hitech-programs-advisory-committees

Office of the National Coordinator for Health Information Technology, U.S. Department of Health and Human Services, Health IT.Gov (n.d.). *Consumer eHealth program.* Retrieved from http://www.healthit.gov/policy-researchers-implementers/consumer-ehealth-program

Shannon, C. E. & Weaver, W. (1949). *The mathematical theory of communication.* Urbana: University of Illinois Press.

Shortliffe, E. H. & Blois, M. S. (2006). The Computer Meets Medicine and Biology: Emergence of a Discipline. In E. H. Shortliffe & J. J. Cimino (Eds.), *Biomedical informatics: Computer applications in health care and biomedicine* (pp. 3–47). New York: Springer-Verlag.

The White House (2004). *Promoting innovation and competitiveness: President Bush's technology agenda.* Retrieved from http://georgewbush-whitehouse.archives.gov/infocus/technology/economic_policy200404/chap3.html

U.S. Department of Veteran Affairs (2012). VA Information Resource Center (VIReC) VistA Overview. Retrieved from http://www.virec.research.va.gov/VistA/Overview.htm

Exercises

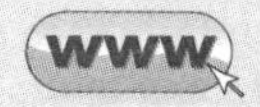

EXERCISE 1 Defining the Scope of Practice for Health Informatics

Objectives

1. Identify the different subspecialties within health informatics.
2. Describe the interrelationships between the subspecialties in health informatics.
3. Describe the informatics positions in a local clinical facility.

Directions

1. Review the following Web sites:
   a. http://mastersinhealthinformatics.com/wp-content/uploads/2010/04/Health-Informatics-Job-Map1.jpg
   b. http://cctsi.ucdenver.edu/RIIC/Pages/WhatisTranslationalInformatics.aspx
   c. http://www.preventivemedicine.northwestern.edu/divisions/hbmi/about.html
   d. http://www.mc.vanderbilt.edu/dbmi/informatics.html
2. List and briefly define at least 10 subspecialties you were able to find in your research.
3. Use PowerPoint or another graphics program to create your own diagram showing the relationships as you see them.
4. Interview the director of information technology in a clinical facility. Find out what informatics positions exist in this facility and what the job descriptions are for those positions.
5. Write a short paper discussing how those positions relate or do not relate to the subspecialties listed for item 2 above.
6. Import the diagram created in step 3 into this paper. Save the paper as **Chap14-Exercise1-LastName** and submit following the directions of the professor.

EXERCISE 2 Selecting a Health Informatics-related Professional Organization

Objectives

1. Assess the advantages and disadvantages of professional associations related to health informatics.
2. Select a professional organization based on your career goals.

■ **Directions**

1. Review each of the professional organization's Web sites below and determine:
   a. Their focus or mission and how this relates to your career goals.
   b. The activities where you could become activity involved. For example, are there committees where you might participate in the organization?
   c. Benefits you can access such as online or print journals, toolkits, conferences, webinars, and opportunities to network with leaders in the field.
   d. Cost to belong including decreased rates for students.
2. Review these Web sites:
   a. Health-related informatics associations with special interest groups
      - American Medical Informatics Association (AMIA)—http://www.amia.org. Review special interest groups; for example, AMIA includes a special interest group in nursing located at http://www.amia.org/programs/working-groups/nursing-informatics. This group is responsible for appointing the nursing representative to the IMIA—Nursing Informatics Special Interest Group.
      - Healthcare Information and Management Systems (HIMSS)— http://www.himss.org/Index.aspx. Be sure to review both the interest groups and the professional community groups.
   b. Health-related informatics associations with specific areas of interest
      - American Telemedicine Association (ATA)—http://www.americantelemed.org/. Check the special interest groups. For example there is a telehealth nursing special interest group located at http://www.americantelemed.org/i4a/pages/index.cfm?pageid=3327
      - American Health Information Management Association (AHIMA)—www.ahima.org. Members are employed mainly in medical records management.
      - College of Healthcare Information Management Executives (CHIME)—http://www.cio-chime.org/
   c. Nursing informatics associations
      - Alliance for Nursing Informatics (ANI)—http://www.allianceni.org/
      - American Nursing Informatics Association(ANIA)—http://www.ania.org/
   d. Other
      - Select one other group not listed here. This can be a local or online group.
3. Based on your analysis, select the one group you would like to join and explain your rationale.

4. Create a presentation explaining the advantages of your selected group.
5. Save the file as **Chap14-Exercise2-LastName** and submit following the directions of the professor.

EXERCISE 3 Selecting a Personal Health Record Application

Objectives

1. Discuss the difficulty of tracking one's personal health history.
2. Analyze the advantages and disadvantages of selected personal health record applications.
3. Explore the challenges involved in integrating personal health data across applications.

Directions

1. Collect your personal health information, including your personal physicians and their contact information, immunizations, medications (including over-the-counter drugs), list of current and previous diagnoses, surgeries, hospitalizations, screening tests and their results, dental and vision history, etc. If you are missing data that you know exists, create a written record from your memory. Old medical bills may help you recreate some of these data.
2. Review the following sites and develop five criteria you would use to select a personal health record application for maintaining your personal health information.
   a. http://www.myphr.com/HealthLiteracy/understanding.aspx
   b. http://patientprivacyrights.org/detailed-phr-privacy-report-cards/#CapMed
   c. http://www.myphr.com/
   d. https://oag.ca.gov/privacy/facts/medical-privacy/health-record
3. Review the following options. Feel free to select additional options. Select one for your personal use.
   a. https://www.healthvault.com/us/en
   b. https://healthmanager.webmd.com/manager/default.aspx?secure=1
   c. https://www.mymediconnect.net/
   d. www.lhncbc.nlm.nih.gov/project/nlm-personal-health-record-phr
4. Record your personal health data and make a list of the challenges you encounter.
5. Write a short blog about your experiences addressing what you experienced, any advice you have for others, and what you found to be the positives and negatives of a PHR.

Assignments

ASSIGNMENT 1 Positions in Health IT and Informatics

Directions

1. Review the following sites for current positions in health IT and/or health informatics.
   a. https://my.usajobs.gov/
   b. http://www.monster.com/
   c. Any local or regional academic medical center
   d. Any local or regional community hospital.
2. Identify five health IT or informatics-related positions. With a brief job description of each one.
3. Write a short paper comparing and contrasting the positions you found with the healthcare computing personnel positions presented in this chapter.
4. Save the file as **Chap14-Assign1-LastName** and follow the professor's direction for submitting the assignment.

ASSIGNMENT 2 Understanding the Data, Information, Knowledge, and Wisdom Continuum

Directions

1. Carry out an Internet search for several diagrams illustrating the data-to-wisdom continuum. Do not limit your search to health care.
2. Do the same search using the literature databases available through your library. The reference librarian can help you with this search.
3. After analyzing the diagrams, create your own figure illustrating these concepts as you understand them.
4. Create a presentation explaining your figure, the concepts illustrated in your figure, and the interrelationship between these figures.
5. Save the file as **Chap14-Assign2-LastName** and follow the professor's direction for submitting the assignment.

ASSIGNMENT 3 Introduction to the ePatient

Directions

1. Answer the following two questions:
   a. Who is ePatient Dave and what implications do his efforts have for health care? This video can be used to start your research http://video.wned.org/video/2305112748.
   b. List and explain the 5 Es of the ePatient. This web site will help you start your research http://blog.himss.org/2013/01/25/part-1-value-of-social-media-in-healthcare-is-already-outlined-just-not-realized/
2. Write a short paper describing five implications your research has for your practice in health care.
3. Save your work as **Chap14-Assign3-LastName** and submit as directed by the professor.

Glossary

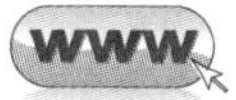

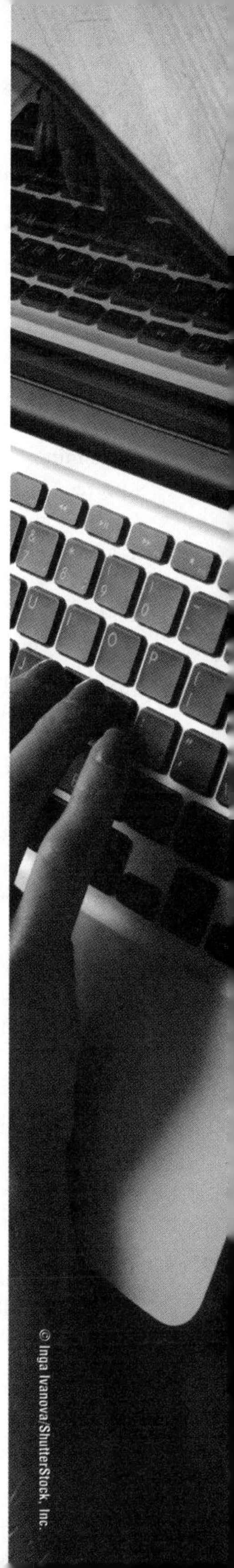

absolute cell addresses: Cell addresses in formulas that remain the same despite other changes in the worksheet; they are indicated by a dollar sign ($) preceding the part of the address that is to remain absolute in Excel.

accelerated graphics port (AGP): The default internal bus between the graphics controller and the main memory, dedicated to, and designed specifically for, video systems.

Access database: A proprietary database that contains tables, forms, reports, queries, macros, and modules.

accessibility: Refers to how easy it is to obtain information. For example, information is accessible when you enter a search term in a Web browser and it produces the desired results.

access providers: Companies that provide access to an Internet host computer. They often supply the software and hardware needed to connect to the Internet.

account: Set up by the school or university, an account allows a student to use the computer laboratory, the university's resources, the school's network, and have access to course materials that reside on course management software servers.

active cell: The cell currently being used; it is outlined or highlighted so that it can be located quickly on the spreadsheet.

add record function: Permits placement of additional records into the database.

ADJACENT: This search terminology is used when searching for terms that are located next to each other.

administrative information systems: Systems that automate the management of data used in the daily operations of the institution as well as data used for strategic and long-range planning.

adware: A specific type of spyware designed to collect data on your Internet-related activities for the purpose of targeting advertisements directly to your computer.

Aero peek: A GUI that shows a thumbnail preview of open objects on the taskbar when hovering over an application.

aggregator: A software application that collects information from various online sources, such as blogs, podcasts, and Web sites, so that this information can be shown together in a single view.

Alt, Ctrl, F4, and **Shift keys:** Special keys that modify normal operations; in combination with other keys, they initiate commands or complete tasks.

analytic graphics: Data presented in graph form for analysis, understanding, and decision making. Presentation graphics, spreadsheet, or statistic programs can be used to create these graphs.

AND: This searching terminology is used when searching for records that include both terms on either side of the AND.

animated files: Files that are streamed together to produce the effect of motion or animation; they generally carry a .gif file extension.

Animations tab: This tab contains commands for previewing a slide show, adding animations, and adding the transitions between slides.

answer table: A temporary table in which the program stores search results.

antivirus software: A program that scans the computer, email, and downloaded files to identify and disable virus software.

application or **apps:** Software that meets specific task needs of the user, such as Word, Excel, and PowerPoint.

application key: This key displays the shortcut menu for the selected item.

area charts: Charts that present or emphasize the total quantity (volume) of several items over time.

ASCII: American Standard Code for Information Interchange.

asynchronous: A communication exchange in which the people can communicate with each other at different times, such as email and discussion boards.

attachments: Files sent along with an email; they can be of any type, such as a Word document to PDF to PowerPoint presentation.

AutoFill: Built-in, time-saving feature in which an application such as Excel automatically inserts data by following a pattern you have begun in a worksheet.

automated decision support systems: Systems that process information, identifying and demonstrating pertinent interrelationships that can be used to support the decision-making process of a care provider.

AutoRecover: A feature in Office that will automatically save your files in case of an unplanned disruption.

AutoReport: A feature that creates a simple report showing all the fields in the table.

AutoSum: The most commonly used function in Excel; it automatically adds a series of numbers in rows, columns, or both.

axis: The horizontal and vertical planes or lines on which data are plotted.

Backspace key: This key deletes characters to the left of the cursor.

Backstage view: The screen default when you click the File tab; this view helps you work with your document.

bandwidth: The amount of data that can travel over a communications channel at one time.

bar graphs: Graphs that compare data against some value at a specific point in time. This type of chart emphasizes comparison, not time.

basic literacy: The ability to locate and use printed and written information to make decisions and to function in society, both personally and professionally.

bibliographic database management system: A specific type of database designed to store data about articles, books, and other informational materials, such as videos.

Big Data: An emerging concept that describes the use of analytics to analyze very large sets of aggregated data.

biomedical informatics (BMI): The interdisciplinary field that studies and pursues the effective use of biomedical data, information, and knowledge for scientific inquiry, problem solving, and decision making, motivated by efforts to improve human health.

bit: The smallest unit of data, the lowest level; the term "bit" is an abbreviation for "binary digit."

bitmapped graphics: Graphics represented as pixels (tiny dots), commonly used for clip art images. Examples include the GIF, PCX, and TIF formats.

blank presentation: The default template used when PowerPoint opens. Slides that use this template have minimal design and no color applied to them.

blank slide: A slide with no placeholders.

blended course or learning (or *hybrid course*): The combination of traditional classroom and online distance learning activities within a single course or group of learning activities.

block: A selected (highlighted) section of text that is treated as a unit.

blog: A self-published Web site containing dated material, usually written in a journal format. Mini-blogs, called *tweets,* have grown in popularity using a social networking service called *Twitter.* They are restricted to 140 characters.

Blue Button: This is a symbol representing a set of applications and standards that makes it possible for patients to get secure online access to their health information in an understandable format.

Bluetooth: A special wireless port that uses radio waves to communicate between the devices. It uses the wireless protocol for exchanging data over short distances.

bookmarks (or *favorites*)**:** These are URLs that have been saved within a browser for future use.

Boolean search: One of the most commonly used search strategies for searching any database; it provides the ability to narrow or expand a search as well as to eliminate some records.

boot: To start a computer so that it can execute the necessary start-up routines. A cold boot means starting a computer when it has been powered off. A warm boot is the process of restarting a computer that is already on.

border: Borders can be inserted into a document to frame a section, page, or other parts of a document.

bounce: The failure of an email message to be delivered. Emails can bounce for numerous reasons, such as an incorrect email address or the recipient's mailbox is full.

brightness: The visible light intensity of the screen; it is measured in nits. The more nits, the brighter the picture.

Broadband: A type of data connection, such as DSL or cable, that provides an ongoing connection to the Internet.

Broadband over Powerline (BPL): An Internet connection that goes through the existing electric power distribution network.

browser: *See* Web browser.

bubble chart: A type of chart that shows the relationship among three values by using bubbles. You can use it instead of a scatter chart but only if you have 3 values or variables.

bulletin board: An online area for posting public messages; it is similar to its counterpart that hangs on a wall. Bulletin boards are typically organized around specific topics and may be part of an online service and accessed through Internet search engines.

bullets (in lists): Small dots, squares, dashes, checks, or other graphics inserted before a phrase or key points.

byte: A string of bits used to represent a character, digit, or symbol. It usually contains 8 bits.

cable: A communications channel option used in many homes and many businesses. Cable is faster than either dial-up or DSL, but degrades in speed as more people access the cable lines at the same time.

cable modem: A device that connects to the network using television cable services.

cache memory: This is a type of computer memory where frequently used instructions and data are stored.

calculated fields: Fields that are generated when mathematical operations are performed on selected fields.

Caps Lock key: This key switches or toggles between all uppercase and all lowercase letters.

cascade windows: All open windows can be arranged from the top of the screen down, with the title bar of each open window visible to the user; works well if it is necessary to see content in all the open windows at same time.

categories: Labels given to the x-axis and y-axis.

cell: A placeholder for data in a spreadsheet. Labeled by column letter and row number, each cell occurs at a specific intersection of a row and a column.

cell address (or *cell reference*)**:** The label for each cell in a spreadsheet. It is used to reference the cell when creating formulas or using functions.

change function: A function that permits the user to alter the contents of a record.

chart style: The range of predefined combinations of formatting elements that control the appearance of a chart.

chart type: The actual graphical display of the data in a particular format. Examples include pie and bar charts.

chat: An application providing real-time communication between two or more users via a computer. Most Internet service providers have built-in chat features.

chatiquette: Similar to netiquette; the words and behavior acceptable while participating in a chat room.

chat room: A designated area or virtual "room" where individuals gather simultaneously and "talk" to one another by typing messages. Everyone who is online in the chat room usually sees the messages.

Chief Information Officer (CIO) or **Director of Information Services:** Administrator responsible for the operation of the information services department.

chip: A tiny piece of semiconducting material (usually silicon) that packs many millions of electronic elements onto an area the size of a fingernail. The circuit boards found in computers consist of many chips.

CINAHL: (Cumulative Index to Nursing and Allied Health Literature) is a group of commercially available literature databases provided by EBSCO that is designed for nurses at all levels including student nurses and allied health professionals.

click: To press and hold the mouse button down, as on a menu item to see the commands, or to scroll through a window until the desired command is selected.

client–server: Computing architecture that is the de facto model for network-oriented computing. Generally the clients are personal computers and servers hold the data accessed by client computers.

clinical or **client data:** All data that are related to an individual client. A comprehensive collection of the client data is stored in the EHR.

clinical information systems: Systems used to process patient data and support patient care.

clip art: A library of symbols (images) prepared by others for use with specific graphics programs.

clipboard: A holding area or buffer for copied or cut data intended to be pasted into another document, another application, or another location within the original document.

clock speed: The rate at which a computer completes a processing cycle. It is a function of the quartz crystal circuit.

cloud computing: The delivery of hosted services over the Internet or a proprietary network.

column graphs: Graphs that show data changes over time or that illustrate comparisons. The data or values are presented vertically (*y*-axis), whereas the categories appear horizontally (*x*-axis).

columns: Columns are vertical groups of cells in a spreadsheet that are labeled with letters that run vertically across the top of the spreadsheet from A to Z.

commerce service providers (CSP): Companies that provide other businesses with tools and services needed to sell their services and products. Many times this includes online services.

communication (or *connectivity*)**:** Refers to the electronic transfer of data from one place to another. It also refers to how people use the technology to enhance their communications with each other and with healthcare consumers.

communication device: Any type of hardware capable of transmitting data and information from one computer to another.

communications channel: The transmission pathway that data take to arrive at the other end of a connection.

comparison layout slide: A presentation layout that includes a title placeholder, two text placeholders below it, and two content placeholders below them.

compression file: A file whose data has been reduced by using a compression utility, generally to allow you to send or receive large or multiple files or to reduce storage requirements.

computer: A programmable machine capable of performing a series of logical and arithmetic operations. Its function is to accept data and instructions from a user, process the data to produce information, store the data for later retrieval, and display the information.

computer-assisted communication: When a computer enhances the communication process by either structuring the message or providing a channel through which to send and receive messages.

computer-assisted instruction software: Programs that help users learn concepts or specific content related to their discipline or area of study.

computer crime: Includes a wide range of illegal activities, from computer intrusion into a computer system (i.e., hacking) to child pornography or exploitation.

computer information system: Hardware (computers) and software plus people, data, communications (connectivity), and policies and procedures.

computerized provided order entry (CPOE): Systems that enable clinicians to enter orders for tests, medications, services, or clinical processes into the healthcare information system.

computer literacy: The ability to use the computer to do practical tasks.

computer operator: An individual who actually runs a mainframe or minicomputer and who generally has minimal interaction with users. Microcomputer operators, by comparison, work closely with users to troubleshoot, upgrade, and repair computers and to install software.

confidentiality: Refers to the healthcare provider's responsibility to limit access to information so that it is shared in a controlled manner for the benefit of the patient.

consumer information systems: Applications that have been developed for the general public, patients, or clients, as opposed to the traditional care providers.

content with caption slide: A presentation layout that features two text placeholders, one for a title and one for explanatory text. The third placeholder is intended to hold content.

contextual tab: A tab that appears in a window which is available only in a certain context or situation.

contrast ratio: The proportion of the brightest color (white) to the darkest color (black) on the screen.

controlled vocabulary: An agreed set of terms with standard definitions that are used to communicate information and to index information for later retrieval.

convertible: A laptop that turns into a tablet when the keyboard is removed or swiveled.

cookies: Small pieces of data designed to enhance the online experience by recording what a visitor does on a Web site to be used in subsequent visits.

copy command: Copies one, several, or all of the files from one place to another.

course management software or **system (CMS):** A software application that facilitates distance learning by centralizing the development, management, and distribution of instructional-related information and materials. Two commonly used CMS programs are Blackboard and Moodle.

cracker: Hacker who illegally breaks into computer systems and creates mischief.

cradle or **docking station:** A device primarily used with PDAs, laptops, iPods, and cameras to upload or download data from the mobile device to the desktop computer and vice versa.

current cell address: Indicates the *active cell* and is displayed on the left side of the formula toolbar.

cursor keys (or *arrow keys*)**:** A cluster of four keys that have directional arrows on them used for moving around a screen.

custom animations: Animations that apply a special visual effect or sound to text or other objects on the slide, such as diagrams, clip art, and charts, on a presentation slide.

cut (delete or **move) command:** A command that removes the selection from the document and moves it to the clipboard; it is the default option for the drag-and-drop method.

cybercafe: A local business, such as a coffee shop or deli, that offers Internet access.

cybercrime: A crime committed by using the Internet or other communication technology.

data: Raw facts, which exist without meaning or interpretation. Data are the attributes that healthcare professionals collect, organize, and name.

database: A collection of data that are organized in files. The files can be analogous to a file cabinet that holds related drawers of records.

database function: A function that allows users to create table structures, edit data or records, search tables, sort records, and generate reports.

database management system (DBMS): A program that enables users to work with electronic databases to store, modify, and retrieve data from the database.

database model (or *schema*)**:** The structure of a database, which includes how that database is organized and used. These structures are generally stored in a data dictionary and are often depicted graphically.

database software: A program that helps organize, store, retrieve, and manipulate data for the purpose of later retrieval and report generation.

data buses: A collection of wires that connect the internal parts of the computer and its peripherals that are used to carry data.

document camera: A camera mounted on a stand and connected to a project that permits the projection of documents and objects onto a larger screen.

data dictionary: A file that defines the basic organization of a database.

data diddling: Refers to modifying valid data within a computer file.

data integrity: Refers to data that are accurate and complete.

data mart: A subset or smaller-focus database designed to help managers make strategic decisions. Sometimes it comprises a subset of a data warehouse.

data mining: Refers to database applications that look for patterns in already-created databases.

data projectors: Devices used to display graphic presentations to an audience by projecting the image onto a larger screen.

data protection: Ensuring that data is not accessed for unauthorized use or storage.

data relationships: How the data in a database are related.

data series: A group of related data points on a chart that originate from rows and columns in the worksheet. These values are used to plot the chart.

Data tab: A tab on the Excel ribbon that allows you to import external data, view linked spreadsheets, sort and filter data, outline data, and use data tools.

data type: Refers to the description of which data should be expected to appear in a field.

data validation: A tool that restricts the entering of data not permitted by the validation rule.

data warehouse: A collection of data designed to support decision making. Its purpose is to present a picture of the general conditions of the entity both at a particular time and historically.

default: The setting a computer uses unless told otherwise.

defragmentation utility: A program that consolidates files and folders on the storage device so that each one is stored in a contiguous space.

Delete command: A command that removes files from the storage device; also used to remove text, rows, columns, or slides from a document.

Delete key: This key deletes text to the right of the cursor.

denial-of-service attack: Any action or series of actions that prevents any part of an information system from functioning—for example, using several computers attached to the Internet to access a Web site so that the site is overwhelmed and not available.

density per inch (DPI): Indicates the pixel density—that is, the number of dots (pixels) per inch. Resolution quality increases with larger DPI.

Design tab: A tab on the PowerPoint ribbon that contains options for changing the page setup, themes, and background in the graphics presentation.

desktop: The main window or screen that is seen after logging on to the computer.

desktop publishing software: Programs that permit users to create high-quality specialty publications such as newspapers, bulletins, and brochures.

dialog box: A special window that requires the user to make selections to implement a command.

Dialog Box launcher: A small icon that appears in the lower-right corner of a group in Office programs. When the user clicks this icon, a custom dialog box opens.

dial-up modem: A device that prepares data for transmission over a telephone line by converting digital data into its analog (wave) form and then reverses the process at the other end of the connection.

dial-up service: Also referred to as plain old telephone service (POTS). This is a method of accessing a network by using telephone wires.

digital camera: A camera that can upload photographs to a computer or to a special picture printer, eliminating the need for both film and film development.

digital literacy: The ability to effectively and critically use digital technology to navigate, evaluate, and create information.

directory: Within a computer-based information system, a directory is an approach to organizing folders, subfolders, and files in a hierarchical format.

directory site: A hierarchical grouping of World Wide Web links on the Internet, arranged by subject and related concepts; it is generally manually created and the links are prescreened.

disk cleanup: The process of removing unwanted files usually accomplished through a utility available on a computer.

distance education: The delivery of education when the student and the instructor are in physically different locations, often over the Internet.

distributed database: Data that are stored in more than one physical place instead of in a single, central location.

distribution list (or *alias* or *mailing list*)**:** An email application that can be used to send a message to a group of people.

distributive education: A comprehensive term that includes both distance and hybrid learning.

documentation: Handout(s) or documents available online to read and/or print that provide helpful information for using computers and learning specific software programs.

documentation management and exchange software: A stand-alone or add-in application that allows individuals and teams to share ideas and information in a common format.

documentation systems: Healthcare information systems that collect assessment and patient status data from a variety of healthcare providers and which are increasingly used as interdisciplinary communication tools.

domain name: An address, similar to that used by the postal service, that points to a computer with a specific IP address. It is a description of a computer's location on the Internet.

dot pitch: The measurement (in millimeters) of the distance between the red, green, and blue phosphors that make up the colors of the monitor.

double-click: To press and release the left mouse button twice in quick succession.

doughnut: A type of pie chart. It compares parts to the whole but can combine more than one data series.

download: To move a file from one computer (generally a server) to another (generally a local PC).

drag: To left-click an icon, menu option, or window border, then, without lifting the finger off the mouse button, moving the object to another place on the screen.

drag and drop: An alternate to cut/copy and paste, where you select the text to be moved and drag it to the new spot.

DSL (digital subscriber line) connection: A communications channel option, usually delivered through the phone system. A faster connection than dial-up service.

DSL (digital subscriber line) modem: A device that connects to the network over a DSL connection.

DVD: A high-capacity optical disk used to store computer data or a video recording—hence the name "digital video disc." As use of these discs increased for data storage, DVD has come to mean "digital versatile disc."

editing features: Inserting, deleting, and replacing items within a document.

eLearning: All the types of education and instruction that various entities deliver to learners via a digital medium.

electronic discussion group: An email service in which individual members post messages for all group members to read.

electronic health information exchange: The exchange of health-related information, including protected health information between health institutions and other covered entities via an interoperable health information technology infrastructure.

electronic health record (EHR): A collection of records that contain information from all the clinicians involved in a patient's care; all authorized clinicians involved in a patient's care can access the information to provide care to that patient. EHRs also share information with other health care providers, such as laboratories and specialists.

electronic mail (email): Programs that permit the sending and receiving of electronic messages from one person to one or many other people.

electronic pen: A pen that permits the construction of electronic signatures and requires the user to hold the pen and write on a special pad.

email: A message that is composed and sent over a computer network to a person or group of people who have an electronic mail address. Email can be sent over a local area network or over the Internet.

emoticon: The use of icons to show an emotion via text on the computer. These symbols or combinations of symbols substitute for facial expressions, body language, and voice inflections.

encryption: A method of coding sensitive data to protect those data from access when they are sent over the Internet.

end users: Healthcare providers who use computers as tools to assist them in delivering care and consumers who access healthcare information on the Internet and/ or store their personal health records (PHR) on Internet-accessible servers.

Enter: Refers to the Enter or Return key and sends text to the next line.

entertainment software: A class of software that the industry has designed for fun, including games.

Esc key: Generally backs out of a program or menu one screen or one menu at a time.

Ethernet: A communications standard typically used by LANs.

Ethernet card: A card that fits into a computer slot and provides connectivity to an internal network.

exact match: A search that finds only entries that are an exact match for a specified word. Any minor difference results in exclusion of that entry from the results.

expansion bus: The internal collection of wires connected to the expansion slot, which vary in speed and communication protocol.

expansion slot: The place on the system board where you can add cards, adapters, or other computer boards.

Fiber-optic connections (such as those used in Verizon's FiOS service)**:** A broadband option for connecting to a network using the fiber-optic cable run to the home and businesses by some companies.

field (or *attribute*)**:** The space within a file that has a predefined location and length. Only one data item is placed in each field, a concept referred to as the use of atomic data.

file: A collection of related records that contain data and which is created by an application program; the place where the work or task is done.

file formats: How a program stores data, such as in text, graphic, or image form, which is an important consideration for importing or transferring files. Users must have an application program that can "read" the file format before they can view it.

file nomenclature: The file name, a delimiter, and a file extension.

File Transfer Protocol (FTP): A communications protocol and program that transfers files from one computer to another over the Internet.

filter: A tool that automatically moves incoming emails into separate folders according to criteria that either you or your Internet provider have specified. Filters can also be included in a virus checker or a software program used to manage your email.

filtering: A tool that allows you to select specific records for review. It does not rearrange data, but rather hides rows you do not want displayed.

financial data: All of the fiscal data related to the operation of a healthcare institution.

financial systems: A combination of information systems that manage and report the financial aspects of an institution.

find and replace: To locate, or locate and substitute, specific files or words within a folder or document.

firewall: A piece of hardware or a software program used to protect computers from unauthorized access via the Internet as well as to secure the interactions between an organization's inside network of computers and the external computer environment.

FireWire: A special-purpose port that is similar to a USB port in that the user can attach multiple devices to it.

flash memory: A type of nonvolatile memory that the user can erase and rewrite on, making it easier to update the memory contents.

folder: A storage place for files and other folders.

font: The visual appearance (font face or typeface), size, style, and weight of a group of characters or symbols that make up text in a document.

footer: An information area that appears consistently at the bottom of each page of a document. It can hold the name of the document, page number, date, or other identifying information.

footprint: Refers to the amount of physical space occupied by any piece of computer-related equipment.

format painter: A tool used to copy formatting from one selection of text and apply it to another.

formatting: The process of setting the appearance of a document by using indentations, margins, tabs, justification, pagination, and so forth.

formula: Helps you analyze the data on a worksheet. With a formula, it is possible to perform operations such as addition, multiplication, and comparison and to enter the calculated value on the worksheet.

formula bar: The location where data or an entered formula appears on the screen in Excel.

function: A prewritten formula in Excel that simplifies the process of entering calculations; examples include SUM and AVERAGE.

function key: A special key that application programs use to complete tasks.

gadgets: Special applications that customize your desktop. For example, to show you the current weather or a stock report.

gaming input device: Devices created specifically to interact with games; examples include light guns, joysticks, dance pads, and motion sensing controllers.

Get Started tab: This group, which is found in the Home and Student versions of Microsoft Office, helps the new user get started with Word.

global positioning system (GPS): A device that uses satellite beacons to determine your location.

Goal Seek: A spreadsheet feature that permits you to identify a target or goals and then manipulate current arguments or values to achieve those goals.

grammar checker: A tool that provides feedback to the user about errors in grammar.

graphical user interface (GUI): An interface that takes advantage of the computer's graphic and mouse capabilities and makes it easier to use the commands and applications.

graphics software: Programs that facilitate the creation of a variety of graphics. There are three types: *Presentation* graphics permit the user to create or alter symbols, display a variety of chart styles, make transparencies and slides, and produce slide shows. *Paint* programs permit users to create symbols or images from scratch. *Computer-aided drafting* programs meet the drawing needs of architects and engineers.

gray literature (or *grey literature*)**:** Works that are not formally reviewed and have not appeared in standard, recognized publications.

groups: Commands organized in logical groups that are collected together under tabs in each ribbon.

hacker: Originally this referred to a compulsive computer programmer; now this term has a more negative connotation of someone who intends to cause harm to a computer; it is often confused with cracker.

handheld computers: Computers small enough to fit in your hand. They have full functionality but include much smaller screens and keyboards (and sometimes specialized keyboards).

handles: Squares that surround a selected image or block of text when it is viewed on screen.

handout: Documentation provided to an audience that outlines the graphics presentation, defines selected terms, or presents complex information.

hard disk (or *hard drive*)**:** A fixed data storage device in a sealed case that reads stored data on platters in the drive. This magnetic storage device stores data in sizes ranging from gigabytes to the terabytes.

hard return: A code inserted in a document by pressing the Enter key. It is usually placed at the end of a paragraph to force a new line or paragraph to start.

hardware (for a computer system)**:** Consists of input devices, the system unit (processing unit, memory, boards, and power supply), output devices, and secondary storage devices.

header: An information area that appears consistently at the top of each page of a document. It can hold the name of the document, page number, date, or other identifying information.

healthcare informatics: Study of how healthcare data, information, knowledge, and wisdom are collected, stored, processed, communicated, and used to support the process of healthcare delivery to clients, providers, administrators, and involved organizations.

healthcare information security officer: The individual responsibility for the design, oversight, and ongoing management of the information security program for the facility.

healthcare information systems (HISs): Previously referred to as hospital information systems, this term is now used to refer to the backbone or primary system used to integrate or interface with the various applications throughout any healthcare delivery organization. They communicate information between the point of care or clinical units and the various departments within the institution or throughout the enterprise.

Health Insurance Portability and Accountability Act of 1996 (HIPAA): Legislation intended to simplify the administrative processes used to transmit electronic health information.

health literacy: The degree to which individuals have the capacity to obtain, process, and understand basic information and services needed to make appropriate decisions regarding their health.

Help feature: Accessed through the blue question mark on the ribbon or the Help option on a menu bar, this is how to access help on the program you are using both offline or online.

history list: A list of Internet sites that have been visited over the past several days, offering a convenient means of redisplaying those pages.

hits: A list of links or records that are returned as search results when a search engine is used.

Home tab: The groups on this tab allow you to format the document.

human resources data: Includes all data related to employees as well as individuals who have a contractual relationship with the institution, such as physicians, nurses, students, or volunteers.

hyperlinks: Text that is formatted in such a way that clicking on it takes the user someplace else or provides additional information about a topic.

hypertext database model: A growing database concept for use with large amounts of disparate information such as text, pictures, film, and sounds, where any object can be linked to any other object.

Hypertext Markup Language (HTML): Provides a mechanism for displaying text- and graphics-based documents in Web browsers. HTML files are static Web pages in which the content is created at the time the page is created.

Hypertext Transfer Protocol (HTTP): A communications protocol that is used for accessing and working with the World Wide Web. Do not confuse it with HTML, which is a tagging language.

icon: A pictogram on a computer screen that represents applications, such as Internet Explorer and special programs, such as the Recycle Bin.

identity theft: A crime in which someone assumes another person's identity to access that person's private information.

impact printer: Any printing device in which the printing mechanism touches the surface of the paper; that is, a mechanism that strikes against a ribbon. Common examples include dot matrix and line printers or plotters.

indent: To establish, by adjusting document paragraph settings, how far text should be spaced from the margin.

informatics: The use of a computer to process data, information, and knowledge within any discipline or field of study.

informatics specialists: Professionals who bridge the gap between the healthcare provider as end user and the technical expert. Their education and professional experience includes both health care and computer/information science.

information: A collection of data that has been processed to produce meaning. Techniques that are used to process data include classifying, sorting, organizing, summarizing, graphing, and calculating.

information attributes: Attributes used to develop criteria for evaluating the quality of information from any source.

information literacy: The knowledge and set of skills needed to find, retrieve, analyze, and use information.

information science: The study of information generation, transmission, and use.

information system: A system that produces information by using an input/process/output cycle. A basic information system consists of four elements: people, policies and procedures, communication, and data.

inkjet printer: A type of printer that produces higher-quality output than a dot matrix printer, and is an excellent middle ground alternative between the laser and dot matrix printer.

input device: A hardware component that converts data from an external source into electronic signals that are understood by the computer.

insert: To add characters in the text at the point of the cursor.

Insert key: This key is a toggle switch that moves between typeover and insert modes; to add new text, slides, rows, columns, and so forth. In word processing programs, insert mode is the default.

Insert tab: The groups on this tab allow you to add a cover page or insert a blank page, page break, table, chart, SmartArt, or clip art using this tab.

instant messaging (IM): A communication service that permits you to send real-time messages via a private chat room to other individuals who are also online.

integrated software: Multiple capabilities included in one program, such as word processing, database, spreadsheet, graphics, and communication programs.

integrated systems: Systems that share a common database.

integrity: The accuracy and comprehensiveness of data.

intellectual data: Comprises the factual data that are stored in the various discipline- or subject-specific databases.

interactive video conferencing: Connecting two or more traditional classrooms with room-based video equipment and a sound system that transmits voice communication between the rooms.

interactive whiteboard: A large interactive display device that connects to and allows a user to interact with the computer. This interaction can take place through remote controls, special pens, a writing tablet, or a finger.

interfaced system: A system that maintains its own database while sharing data across a network.

Internet: Sometimes referred to as the information or global superhighway, a loose association of millions of networks and billions of computers around the world, all of which work together to share information.

Internet/application buttons: Buttons used to control selected application functions such as email, documents, photos, gadgets, and Web access.

Internet backbone: The collective name for the high-speed lines that carry the bulk of Internet traffic.

Internet front-end software: Software with which the user interacts (the browser). It might be a comprehensive program, such as Firefox or Internet Explorer, or a program provided by the service provider.

Internet or Web conferencing: A type of communication in which two or more individuals interact over the Internet in real time, receiving more or less immediate replies. This communication can involve interaction via text, audio, or video.

Internet Protocol (IP): An address with a unique identification number that distinguishes each computer on the Internet.

Internet service providers (ISPs) (or *commerce service providers,* or *CSPs*)**:** Through their interconnection, these networks create high-speed communication lines for access to email and the Internet.

Invisible Web: The part of the Web, such as nonindexed pages or databases, that is not searched when using a search engine and that often requires a password to enter.

IrDA port: An infrared light beam port that connects wireless devices to the computer using light waves. Abbreviated form for Infrared Data Association.

jump lists: Shortcuts to files and commands that are frequently used.

justified: Text that is aligned relative to both the left and right margins.

kernel: The central module of the operating system that loads first and remains in memory as long as the computer is turned on.

keyboard: The input device for typing data into the computer.

keyboard logger: Either hardware or software installed on a computer to log the keystrokes of an individual, either to monitor computer activities, such as time spent on the Internet, or to collect personal information, such as passwords.

KeyTip badges: Letters and numbers that appear on the ribbon when you press the Alt key and that make it easier to carry out tasks.

key field: In Excel, this is constituted by one or more fields within a computer record that contains a unique identifier. Using unique identifiers within key fields ensures that no duplicate records will occur.

keywords: Terms that may have been selected by the author, the publisher, or the developer of the literature database management system to identify the topic of an article.

keyword search: Using terms or tags that have been selected by the author, the publisher, or the developer of the database management system to search for a file or document.

keyword search site: An Internet site that permits the user to type in "keywords" to retrieve links to sites that contain needed information; it comprises a server or a collection of servers dedicated to indexing Internet pages, storing the results, and returning lists of links that match particular queries.

knowledge: A collection of interrelated pieces of information and data. In this aggregation, the interrelationships are as important as the individual items of information.

labels: The group that represents the content of graph slides. They help the user to understand the graph (e.g., the names given to each pie wedge or bar).

landscape orientation: Presents a document, spreadsheet, or slide in a wide or horizontal view.

language: Consists of a vocabulary and an accompanying set of rules that tell the computer how to work.

laptop (or *notebook*)**:** A portable computer; generally more expensive than a personal computer, but with the same power and capabilities.

laser printer: A type of printer that produces high-quality print, is fast, and generates little noise.

LCD (liquid crystal display): The technology used for flat panel monitors.

learning management system (LMS): An application that supports learning.

legend: Information that identifies the pattern or color of a specific data series or category.

level 1 data sharing: Involves integration of a specific institution service or function.

level 2 data sharing: Involves sharing data for an individual healthcare institution.

level 3 data sharing: Involves the sharing of data across all institutions within the larger organization, a type of system referred to as an enterprise-wide system.

level 4 data sharing: Involves sharing data outside of the institutions owned by the enterprise. These applications serve as regional or community health information networks.

light pen: A light-sensitive pen-like device often used in hospital or clinical information systems.

line graph: A graph that presents a large amount of data to show trends over time.

line spacing: The space between lines or the space before and after paragraphs in a document.

link: The logical association between tables based on the values in corresponding fields; it is a connection between two tables in a relational database program. This term may also be used to refer to a hyperlink.

lists: Bulleted and numbered lists are used in Word documents to format, arrange, and/or emphasize a sequence of points or steps.

ListServ: The trade name of a software program that manages automated discussion lists. This term is commonly used to refer to all automated discussion lists.

local area network (LAN): A type of network with distance limitations. A building or small campus environment might use a LAN. A LAN typically uses a communications standard called *Ethernet.*

lock key: A key used to lock part of a keyboard.

log in: The procedure used to access the system or network.

logic bomb: A piece of program code buried within another program, designed to perform some malicious act in response to a trigger. For example, the trigger can involve entering data or a name.

macro: An automated sequence of operations that can perform repetitive tasks.

Mailings tab: The groups on this tab help you prepare envelopes, labels, mail merge letters, and recipient lists.

mainframe: A large computer that accommodates hundreds of users simultaneously. It has a large data storage capacity, a large amount of memory, multiple input/output (I/O) devices, and speedy processor(s).

massive open online course (MOOC): A model for delivering free, usually noncredit courses, via the Internet to anyone who has an interest in learning.

material management systems: Systems that manage the supplies and other inventory of an institution.

material resources data: Refers to all of the tangible resources used in the operation of the healthcare institution—everything from supplies that are purchased externally to supplies that are created internally.

maximize button: This button expands the window to fill the computer screen.

media control buttons: Buttons that control the media player, access the DVD drive, and control the speakers.

medical identity theft: When someone uses another individual's personal information without their knowledge or consent to obtain medical care.

medical informatics: The use of a computer to process medical data, information and knowledge.

MEDLINE: The primary U.S. National Library of Medicine's (NLM) bibliographic database. It contains over 19 million references to journal articles in life sciences, with a concentration on biomedicine, and is indexed using MESH.

memory: A form of semiconductor storage that resides inside the computer, generally on a motherboard, and that takes the form of one or more chips. It stores operating system commands, programs, and data.

menu: A list of commands or tasks that are available to the user.

menu bar: An area in the window that contains the names of available commands.

MeSH (Medical Subject Headings): The U.S. National Library of Medicine (NLM) comprehensive controlled vocabulary of predefined terms and concepts in a hierarchical structure that permits searching at various levels of specificity. MeSH is used for indexing articles for PubMed, MEDLINE, and Cochrane library, among others.

message area: In Excel, this area shows which actions will occur when a function or button is activated. It may also show error messages. It is usually located in the left corner of the status bar.

metadirectory: A directory of links to other directories; sometimes called a directory of directories or directories of directories.

meta search engine: Not really a search engine, but rather a Web site that works by taking the user's query and searching the Web using several search engines at one time.

metropolitan area network (MAN) (also *Wide Area Network* or *WAN*)**:** A high-speed network that covers a large geographic distance. A MAN may include a city or Internet service provider (ISP) that provides the connection for city agencies or individual users with access to the Internet.

microcomputer: A small, one-user computer system with its own central processing unit (CPU), memory, and storage devices. Also referred to as a personal computer or desktop, these models are growing in processing power, speed, and storage capacity.

microcomputer specialist: An individual who supports personal computer users throughout an institution. He or she may install new software, troubleshoot or repair personal computers, answer user questions, and train users on how to use new software.

microphone: A voice input device that permits the user to speak into the computer to enter data or give instructions.

microprocessor: A processor that fits on one integrated circuit chip.

Microsoft Office OneNote: A program that provides an electronic tool for organizing and storing information such as notes from class, reference materials, or Internet sources.

MIDI port: A port that permits the connection of musical instruments to the computer.

midrange computer (formerly called a *minicomputer*)**:** A medium-sized computer that is faster and stores more data than a personal computer (PC).

minimize button: When an application is minimized using this button, an icon representing the program appears on the taskbar; the program remains open but is running in the background.

mobile device: A small handheld computing device. Examples are laptops, PC tablets, handheld computers (also called ultra-mobile PCs), PDAs, and smartphones like the iPhone and BlackBerry.

mobile device specialists: Individuals who provide support for all mobile devices.

modem: Devices that provide an interface between a computer and a transmission channel and that convert the data into a form that the ISP can transmit via a transmission line.

monitor: A device that displays graphic images from the video output of a computer. Other terms used for this device include display screen and flat panel.

motherboard (or *system board*)**:** The main circuit board of the system unit. It contains slots for the processor chip, memory slots, and slots for adapter cards for video, sound, and connection to peripheral devices.

mouse: An input device for a computer.

move command: This command takes a file or folder from one place and puts it in another, but does not duplicate the file in the process; this can also refer to placing data in another location in a document.

movie: A video file that has an extension such as .avi, .mov, or .mpeg.

multifunction device: An all-in-one input/output device. It typically incorporates a printer, scanner, copier, and fax machine into a single unit.

nanotechnology: The design and manufacture of circuits and devices at the molecular level of 100 nanometers or less.

National Health Information Infrastructure (NHII): A comprehensive network of interoperable network systems transmitting clinical, public health, and personal health information, created to improve decision making by making health information available when and where it is needed.

NEAR: A term used when searching for information, which limits the terms of interest to within a few words of each other.

netbook: An ultraportable laptop that is smaller and cheaper than a traditional laptop, but also less powerful.

netiquette: The name given to electronic communication behavior conventions.

network: A collection of computers and other hardware devices, such as a printer, scanner, or file server, that are connected using communication devices and transmission media.

network administrator: The individual responsible for planning and maintaining multiuser computer systems on a local area network.

network card: A card installed into a computer to enable a direct connection to a network.

newsgroup: Informational material and articles organized around a particular topic, such as Alzheimer's disease or child abuse. Newsreaders can post a message to the newsgroup for all to read and respond.

nonimpact printer: Any printing device in which the printing mechanism does not touch the surface of the paper. Examples include laser, thermal, and ink jet printers.

Normal view: The default view in a presentation. It contains three parts: the slide, the notes pane at the bottom, and the left pane for seeing all of the slides or outline view.

NOT: A term used when searching for information, which deliberately excludes specific words to avoid hits that are not of interest.

notebook (or *laptop*)**:** A portable computer; generally more expensive than a personal computer, but with the same power and capabilities.

notification area: The area on the screen that contains icons for programs that run in the background.

Num Lock key: A toggle key that turns the numeric keypad on and off.

object: A small picture or graphic representation of icon, file, folder, or shortcut found on the desktop.

online document sharing: When groups work together on a common document even when the group members are separated in space Document sharing applications let you upload files to a collaborative Web site.

operating system (OS): The most important program that runs on a computer: It tells the computer how to use its own components or hardware. The most common operating system for PCs is the Windows family (e.g., Windows Vista, Windows 7 and Windows 8). Apple computers use the Macintosh operating system (e.g., OS 10).

opt out: A number of measures designed to prevent online users from receiving unwanted products or services.

optical drive: An alternative to magnetic storage. It holds large amounts of data, which are usually written (pressed) once and accessed many times. The most common example is the CD-ROM (compact disc read-only memory).

OR: This term is used when searching for documents or information that includes all of the terms of interest. For example, any document that contains either the term cardiac OR the term heart.

outliner: A feature of many word processing programs that enables the user to plan and rearrange large documents in an outline form.

overtype: To replace the character under the cursor with the character typed.

page break: The place where one document page ends and the next page begins.

Page Layout tab: The groups on this tab help you select the font style and color, margins, paragraph indents, and spacing, and allow you to add watermarks, add a page border, or change the page color or arrangement.

page orientation: The vertical or horizontal layout of a page.

page tabs (or *tabbed browsing*)**:** Tabs that permit you to open a new Web site in a separate tab for quick access when you are working in multiple Web sites.

Page Up/Down, Home, and **End keys:** Used to move quickly from one place in the document or on the screen to other locations.

pagination: The numbers or marks that are used to indicate the sequence of the pages.

parallel ports: Unidirectional ports that send data in parallel—that is, as groups of eight bits (one byte) of information in a row much like a parade. Parallel ports are rarely used today, having been replaced by UBS ports.

Paste command: The method for placing files that have been copied or cut.

password: A combination of symbols such as letters and numbers used to gain access to a restricted resource on a computer or network.

patches: Generally, fixes for software problems discovered after its original release. Many of these patches focus on fixing security problems inherent in the software that might make the user's computer vulnerable to hackers and viruses.

pattern searching: This approach to searching permits the use of wild cards in place of a character. This is different from truncation, which deals with shortening a word.

PC card bus: This bus moves data from a digital camera through a PC card slot into the computer.

PCI/PCI-E bus: The Peripheral Component Interconnect (PCI) bus and the PCI-Express (PCI-E) bus are relatively new standards for connecting high-speed devices, such as the local hard drive, network cards, sound cards, and video cards. PCI-E is intended to replace the PCI and AGP buses.

PC video camera: An input device that the operator uses to capture video. It may be used to send video images as email attachments, to make video telephone calls (video conferencing), and to post live, real-time images to a Web server.

personal digital assistants (PDAs) (or *palmtop computers*)**:** A mobile device with applications for organizing personal and professional data and communication.

personal health information (PHI): Health data and/or information that can be connected to an identified individual. This concept is closely related to Protected Health Information (PHI), which is defined in HIPAA as individually identifiable health information transmitted by electronic media, maintained in electronic media, or transmitted or maintained in any other form or medium.

personal health records (PHRs): These applications contain the same types of information as EHRs but are accessed and managed by patients in a private, secure, and confidential environment. PHRs can include information from a variety of sources including clinicians, home monitoring devices, and patients themselves.

personal software: Programs that help people manage their personal lives. Examples include appointment calendars, checkbook balancing applications, money management applications, and calculators.

personnel systems: Systems that track the characteristics of employees and/or the use of these employees within the institution.

phishing: Pronounced *fishing*; the creation of a replica of a legitimate Web page to trick users into submitting personal information, such as financial data or passwords. It also refers to fraudulent email that solicits private information, such as passwords or credit card numbers. It can result in identify theft.

pictures: Digital photographs that can be imported and used in a graphic presentation. They are generally in .jpg file format.

picture with caption slide: This layout includes two text placeholders and one content placeholder that will accept only pictures.

pie chart: A type of chart that compares parts to a whole or several values at one point in time. These charts also help to emphasize a particular part or to show relationships between sets of items.

pitch: The number of characters printed in 1 inch (cpi).

PivotTable: A table that provides a summary report that allows you to quickly compare long lists of values and look at data in ways not normally apparent from a regular worksheet or table.

pixels: More formally, picture elements. Tiny dots that make up the screen image. The more pixels used, the sharper the image (resolution).

plagiarism: The act of stealing another person's ideas or work and presenting it as your own.

plotters: An output device that draws images by moving a pen over the paper.

plug-ins: An application that adds specific functions or services to a larger application. For example, the plug-in Adobe Reader makes it possible to read PDF files.

podcast: An audio and/or video file that can be uploaded to a Web site, YouTube, or a podcast hosting service.

point: To move the mouse so that the cursor is on or over a particular command or icon on the screen.

pointer: A symbol used to represent the mouse location on the screen.

pointer shapes: The actual appearance of the pointer.

point size: The height of the font given in printing language, measured as 72 points per inch of height.

pointing stick: A pointing or navigation device that looks like a pencil eraser and uses pressure to detect mouse movement.

policies and procedures: An outline of the guiding principles related to using information and technology, providing and step-by-step directions to accomplish the end results.

portrait orientation: Presents a document, spreadsheet, or slide in an upright or vertical view.

ports: Highways that lead into, out of, and around the computer. They take the form of plugs, sockets, or hot spots that are found on the back, front, and sides of most system units.

posters: A graphic presentation used to present the results of a research study or to communicate ideas.

power management keys: Keys that provide the ability to place the computer in sleep mode and to power up the computer when it has been in sleep mode.

power-on self-test (POST): A test that analyzes the buses, clock, memory, drives, and ports to make sure that all of the hardware is working properly.

PowerPoint: A graphic presentation program provided as part of the Microsoft Office suite.

power supply box: A device that converts the power available at the wall socket (120-volt, 60-MHz, AC current) to the power necessary to run the computer (+5 and +12 volt, DC current).

presentation: A group of slides that makes up the actual material to be presented (generally in PowerPoint). It can vary from an unlimited number of slides to only a few.

presentation graphics program: A software program that is used to create presentations.

Press Wheel button: To click the wheel once and move the mouse on the desktop. This action causes the mouse pointer to scroll along the document automatically until the user presses the wheel button again.

pretty good privacy (PGP): Software that is used to encrypt and protect email as it moves from one computer to another. PGP can be used to verify a sender's identity.

primary source: The original source of information.

Print Preview: A view of how the document will look when it is printed.

Print Screen key: Used either in combination with the Alt key or alone, this key places a snapshot of the screen or active window onto the clipboard.

privacy: Refers to a person's desire to limit the disclosure of personal information.

processor: The central unit in a computer, which contains the circuitry for performing the instructions that computer programs provide. An older term for the processor is central processing unit (CPU).

programmer: An individual who designs, codes, and tests new software programs as well as maintains and enhances current applications.

quality assurance systems: Systems that measure and report on cost-effective quality care.

query: Refers to the combination of terms that you enter into a search engine to conduct a search.

Quick Access Toolbar: Located on the left of the title bar, this is a customizable toolbar that contains a set of commands that are independent of the tab that is currently displayed. Commands can be added to the toolbar.

Quick Print: A way to print a document directly, without having to use the print dialog box.

radar charts: Charts that compare the aggregate values of multiple data series.

radio frequency identification (RFID): The use of radio signals to communicate information found on a tag attached to an object or person, first to an RFID reader and then to the computer.

random-access memory (RAM): Temporary data storage for computer processes. This type of memory is volatile—the data disappears from RAM when the power is off. The most common unit of measurement for RAM is the byte, which is the amount of storage space it takes to hold a character.

range(database): This operation selects records based on the operators such as greater than, less than, equal to, or some combination of them, which are called logical operators.

range (spreadsheet): A group of cells in a rectangular pattern defined by the upper-left and lower-right corners is called a range or block of cells. For example, the range of cells from A1 to E6 would include all of the cells in columns A, B, C, D, and E in rows 1, 2, 3, 4, 5, and 6.

ranking: The process of indicating how relevant a search hit may be. Many times a search engine will organize the search results by their ranking.

readability statistics: The reading level of a Word document. Readability level can be measured using the Flesch Reading Ease or the Flesch-Kincaid Grade Level tests. These scores are based on the number of syllables per word and the number of words per sentence.

read-only memory (ROM): Memory that has been burned on the chip at the factory; the computer can read instructions from it but cannot alter them. This memory is permanent.

record: A collection of fields related or associated with a focal point.

References tab: The groups on this tab include Table of Contents, Footnotes, Citations and Bibliography, Captions, Index, and Table of Authorities (cases, statutes).

registers: Temporary, high-speed storage spaces that the processor uses when it processes data. They are part of the processing unit, not the memory.

relative addresses: Cell addresses in Excel formulas that are designed to change when the formula is copied to other cells in Excel.

rename command: Gives a file or folder a new name.

replace: To substitute one thing for another; highlighting or selecting the text puts the application into the replace mode.

resolution: Describes the number of horizontal and vertical pixels (dots) found on the screen.

response time: The time (in milliseconds) that it takes to turn a dot on or off. Response times vary with monitors and can range from 3 to 16 milliseconds.

restart option: With this option the computer will turn off and then restart itself.

restore button: The button that restores a window to the size it was before it was maximized or minimized.

Review tab: The groups on this tab enable users to proof documents; for example, check spelling and grammar, do a word count, track changes, insert comments, enable ScreenTips for showing a word in another language, or protect a document from changes by someone else.

ribbon: Microsoft Office uses a "fluent user interface" that is presented as a "ribbon." The tab names resemble menu names, and the ribbon resembles a toolbar, as in previous versions of Word.

right-click: To press and release the right mouse button once. This operation is used to activate the shortcut menu.

right-drag: To hold down the right mouse button, move the mouse to a different location, and then release the mouse button. This operation generally results in the appearance of a shortcut menu from which to select a command.

robots (or *spiders* and *crawlers*)**:** Used to create a database of links that are accessed when you conduct a search. These computer programs search the Web, locate links, and then index the links to create the results database.

root level: The top level on which folders reside. This level stores files the computer needs to access at start-up.

rotate wheel: To move the mouse wheel forward and backward. Use this action to scroll up and down in a document or at a Web site.

rows: Cells that run horizontally across the spreadsheet. Beginning with 1, they are numbered down the left side of the spreadsheet.

RSS (Really Simple Syndication): A scheme that makes it possible for users to subscribe to and receive information about a specific topic that has been published on blogs, podcasts, and other social networking applications.

rules (policies): All users of computer-networked computer systems are subjected to acceptable use policies and procedures.

sabotage: The purposeful destruction of hardware, software, and data.

salami method: Method of data stealing that involves taking little bits at a time.

satellite Internet connection: Uses a satellite dish antenna and a transceiver (transmitter/receiver) that operates in the microwave portion of the radio spectrum.

Save: The process by which you save a file for the first time.

Save As: To save a file to a file name, format, and location that you specify. It permits saving files in another format, such as a previous version of an application, a PDF file, or a Web page.

Scan Disk: An error-checking tool that checks the file system for errors and bad sectors.

scanner: An input device that converts character or graphic patterns into digital data (discrete coded units of data).

scatter graphs: Graphs that show trends or statistics, such as averages, frequency, regression, or distribution.

scenario: A type of what-if analysis tool and a set of values that Excel saves and can substitute automatically in the worksheet. They are used to forecast the outcome of a worksheet model.

screen savers: Moving or static pictures displayed on the desktop when no activity takes place for a specified period of time.

ScreenTip: When the mouse arrow is held over an option in the ribbon, a tip appears that describes its function; a small window that displays descriptive text when you rest the pointer on a command or control.

scroll bars: The bars located along the right and bottom of the window that can be used to move through a document.

scrolling: The process of moving around in a document to view a specific portion of a page of text within a document.

SCSI (Small Computer System Interface; pronounced *scuzzy*)**:** A parallel port that supports faster data transfers than are possible with traditional parallel ports. SCSI ports permit attachment of as many as seven peripheral devices in a linked chain fashion.

search engines: Software programs that are used to find and index information.

search sites: Places on the Internet where you go to find information.

secondary source: A source that summarizes, describes, analyzes, or interprets a primary source.

section break: Creates layout or formatting changes within or between pages in a document.

section header: Use this layout when you have to break a presentation into separate parts. It has two text placeholders.

secure digital (SD): Nonvolatile cards used in portable devices such as smartphones, PDAs, digital cameras, and tablet computers.

security: The measures an organization implements to protect information and systems.

selecting text (or *object*)**:** To highlight the text or object, such as a word or a cell in a spreadsheet.

select fields: A type of search that uses some mark to select the fields to be displayed in the search results. All of the fields or only selected ones may be chosen.

serial ports (or *com ports*)**:** To arrange data in serial form, sending it to the destination one bit at a time.

series: A collection of related numbers located in a column or row under a common heading.

server: A computer that controls access to the software, hardware (like printers on the network), and data located on a network.

setting-specific systems: Functions such as clinical, financial, and personnel information management; they are customized for the specific setting.

shading: To set text in color.

shapes: Predesigned forms used to enhance the look of the slide and include rectangles, circles, arrows, callouts, and so forth.

shortcut: A pointer to an object; it tells the computer where to find the object but is not the actual object.

Shut down command: Powers down the computer. Most computers today will turn off their system units automatically, but the monitor may need to be turned off separately.

sidebar: A vertical bar on the right side of the window in a Window computer.

single-click: To press and release the left mouse button once to activate a command or to select an icon or menu option.

size: Refers to the diagonal measurement from corner to corner of the display unit (monitor).

slides: Individual screens that make up a presentation.

slide layout: Refers to the way in which the placeholders for the text and images are arranged on the slide.

slide show: An automated presentation of slides.

Slide Show tab: The groups on this tab include options for starting a presentation, setting it up, and determining how it will be displayed.

Slide Show view: Transitions from one slide to another and any special effects or sounds can easily be seen in this view. This is the best way to view a slide show.

Slide Sorter view: In this view, the entire presentation is displayed so that slides can be easily rearranged.

Slide transitions: Animation-like effects that appear when moving from one slide to the next during an onscreen presentation.

SmartArt: A feature in Office that permits you to easily create a visual representation of your information. Use SmartArt to create graphic lists, show a process, or demonstrate hierarchies.

smart cards: A credit card-sized card that contains a microprocessor, input and output functions, and storage.

smart phones: Communication devices such as the BlackBerry and the iPhone that provide access to the Internet, email, phone, references, GPS, books, games, and so forth.

smart tag: A pop-up that appears when you place the insertion point over certain text.

SmartTV: Televisions that integrate Internet and Web 2.0 tools.

social media: Web-based and mobile technologies that support social networking and allow users to share information.

social networking: The use of a Web-based service to construct a profile and to identify and communicate with a list of other users with whom you share a personal connection.

soft return: Code inserted in the document automatically when a typed line reaches the right margin.

software piracy: Unauthorized copying of copyrighted software.

software program: The step-by-step instructions that direct the computer hardware to perform specific tasks such as multiplying, dividing, fetching, or delivering data. The three major categories of software are operating systems (OS), languages, and applications.

solid-state storage media: A type of computer storage made from silicon microchips and that consist of electronic components (instead of mechanical) and so have no moving parts. Examples include flash memory cards and USB storage devices.

sorting: The process of placing data in a specific order like numeric or alphabetic.

source: Refers to both the author information and the location where information is found on the Internet.

space bar: The keyboard bar that enters a space between words.

spacing: There are two types of spacing. *Proportional* spacing means that a variable amount of space is allotted for each character depending on the character width. *Fixed space* or *monospace* means a set space is provided for each character regardless of the character width.

spam: Electronic junk mail. This type of email is unsolicited and/or not from an identifiable source.

spamming: The act of sending unsolicited electronic messages in bulk. The most common form of spam is that delivered in email as a form of commercial advertising.

speakers and headphones: Listening accessories that come with most computers and reproduce high-quality sound.

spell checker: A program that checks text for spelling errors.

spim: Part spam and part instant message, spim is being used by an increasing number of advertisers.

spreadsheet software: A program that permits the manipulation of numbers in a format of rows and columns. Spreadsheet programs contain special functions for adding and computing statistical and financial formulas.

spyware: A type of computer software designed to install itself on your computer and then send personal data back to a central service without your permission or knowledge.

stacked and side-by-side: An arrangement of windows that partition the screen into quadrants depending on the number of windows that are open.

stand-alone systems: A system that does not share data or information with any other computer system.

standard language: Set of terms that may have been accepted for indexing concepts or content. This is another term used to refer to a controlled vocabulary.

Stand By option: Thus puts the computer into a low-power state, but lets the user quickly resume working. The computer looks like it is turned off, but the power lights remain on.

Start button: The button used to open the Start menu. The Start button has now been replaced by the Windows Logo Key; however, when you hover over the Windows Logo key you will see the word *start*.

statistics software: A program that permits statistical analysis of numeric data.

status bar: A part of the document window that shows the page number, number of words in the document, some view buttons, and the Zoom slider.

stock charts: Charts that show the high, low, opening, and closing prices for individual stocks over time.

stop word: A word that is ignored in a query because the word is so commonly used that it makes no contribution to relevancy. Examples include *and, get, the,* and *you.*

storage: A place or space for holding data and application programs.

Structured Reference: A tool used in formulas and functions that uses a table element as a reference in a formula.

style: The appearance of a character—normal (upright), condensed, or italic (oblique).

stylus (or *digital pen*)**:** A tool used with a tablet to create an image on the tablet surface. The tablet then converts the marks or images to digital data that the computer can use.

subfolders: Storage places contained within other folders. They provide further division or structure to the organization of files.

subject terms: Standardized sets of subject terms; often referred to as a *controlled vocabulary.*

suite: A value package of software that includes a word processor, a spreadsheet, a database, a presentation graphics program, and sometimes a personal information manager.

supercomputers: The fastest, most expensive, and most powerful type of computers available. They tend to focus on running a few programs that require a lot of computations; uses of supercomputers include animation graphics, weather forecasting, and research applications.

surface charts: Charts that indicate the optimum combinations between two sets of values.

surfing (or *browsing*)**:** The process of clicking hyperlinks to go to another part of a document, to a different document, or to another site.

surge protector: A device that sits between the electrical outlet and the computer supply source, which protects the computer from low-voltage surges in electrical power by directing the extra power to the outlet's grounding wire.

Switch User option: Lets another user log on to a computer while keeping the previous user's programs and files open.

symbols: The clip art or images that are available within, or can be imported into, a presentation program.

symbol set: The characters and symbols that make up a font.

synchronous communication: A situation in which people communicate with one another at the same time via their computers. Chat rooms and Internet meetings are examples of synchronous communication, because all of the individuals involved are on their computers at the same time.

system: A set of interrelated parts.

system administrators: Individuals who plan and maintain multiuser computer systems on a local or wide area network.

systems analyst: An individual who works with users to define their information needs and design systems to meet those needs.

system unit: The control center or "brains" of the computer; it is not visible to the eye on most computers unless someone removes the cover of the computer.

T1 and **T3:** Communication connections used by large businesses. A telecommunications company generally provides these services.

tab: A setting that places the subsequent text on that line a certain number of spaces or inches in from the left margin.

Tab key: This key moves the cursor along the screen at defined intervals or to the next field in a dialog box.

table: A structure that consists of columns and rows for holding and displaying data. Table structures are used in Word, Excel, Access, and PowerPoint.

tablet: A computer that is smaller than a laptop, but bigger than a smartphone.

tagging: The process of indicating the appearance of Web page contents by specifying fonts and font-related attributes as well as the location or layout of the text and graphics.

tags: Terms that function as keywords associated with online content, such as blog postings, bookmarks, and Web sites. Tags make it possible for an aggregator to effectively search the Internet and group together related information.

tape drive: A secondary storage device that allows the back up or duplication of stored data on a hard disk.

taskbar: A long horizontal bar that is used to launch and monitor running applications. It contains the Start button, Quick Launch toolbar, open applications, and notification area. Its default position is at the bottom of the desktop but it can be moved to the top, right, or left of the screen.

task pane: A small window that displays additional options and commands for certain features.

technical professionals: Individuals who develop, maintain, and evaluate the technical aspects of information systems. They are generally responsible for the network, databases, software and hardware updates, security, communications, and respond to end-user problems and questions.

technology-assisted communication and collaboration: When people use computer/information systems for both the communication and the collaboration processes by which they share information and create new information.

templates: Predesigned (formatted) documents or files used as a starting point for creating output; they are used in Word, Excel, and PowerPoint to save the user from having to redesign the document or file each time it is used.

temporary Internet file: A file sent to the computer for the purpose of speeding the loading of graphics files when a Web site has been visited multiple times.

tertiary source: A source, such as a textbook, that cites secondary sources.

theft of services: Unauthorized use of services such as those provided by a computer system.

themes (or *presentation styles* in some programs)**:** Professionally designed format and color schemes for a presentation.

thermal printer: A printing device that presses heated pins against special paper to produce the printed image; the quality of this output is low.

thesaurus: A built-in feature that helps you search for alternative words.

threaded discussion: An online information exchange that is similar to a bulletin board, except that topics within each interest area are identified and organized together so that users can access and read only the discussions pertaining to a particular interest area.

time bomb: Instructions hidden in a program that perform certain functions on a specific date or time, such as printing a message or destroying data.

title and content slides: A layout that includes one text placeholder, usually for the title, and one content placeholder.

title bar: A horizontal bar at the top of a window.

title slide: A slide that introduces the presentation or is used to separate sections within a presentation.

toggle: To switch from one mode of operation to another.

touchpad: A stationary pointing device upon which the user moves the cursor by moving a finger around on a pad.

touchscreen: A screen that allows commands or actions to be entered by pressing specific places on a special screen with a finger.

trackball: A stationary mouse with a ball on top of it.

Transitions tab: The tab where a developer can add transitions to each slide of a presentation.

Transmission Control Protocol/Internet Protocol (TCP/IP): The base protocol (set of rules) that every computer on the Internet must use and understand for sending and receiving data.

transmission media: Materials or substances capable of transmitting a signal. They are of two types: physical media and wireless media.

transparencies: Thin sheets of transparent flexible material, onto which documents or slides can be printed and then displayed using an overhead projector. This system is still used in schools, but is being largely replaced by LCD projectors.

trapdoors: Methods installed by programmers that allow unauthorized access into programs.

triple-click: To press and release the left mouse button three times. In word processing programs, this operation selects an entire paragraph.

trojan horse: Instructions placed in a program that add illegitimate functions; for example, a Trojan horse may cause information to be printed every time information on a certain patient is entered.

truncation: Use of a symbol to indicate that you are searching for any citation that includes a term beginning with certain letters. For example, "Inter*" will bring all results beginning with the letters Inter.

two content slide: A layout that includes one text placeholder for the title and two side-by-side content placeholders.

typeface: The specific design of a character or symbol; commonly referred to as the font face.

uninterruptible power supply (UPS): A device that provides electrical power generated by a battery in the event of a power outage. The battery keeps the computer going for several minutes after the outage occurs. During this time, the user can save data and properly shut down the computer.

updates: Generally, these are enhancements to software that provide additional features or functions.

upgrade: To enhance a piece of equipment or buy the newest release of a software program. Many computers are "upgradeable," meaning that the user may add more memory, additional storage devices, and so forth.

upload: The act of transferring a file from a local computer to a remote server (the opposite of downloading); this process is used when moving local HTML files to a Web server for publishing on the Internet.

URLs: An address that helps a computer find a Web page's exact location on the Web server.

USB cellular modem: A wireless adapter that connects a laptop to a cellular telephone for data access and transfer.

USB port (universal serial bus port): A port standard that supports fast data transfer rates (12 million bits per second).

Usenet: A type of online bulletin board. With this service, users read and post messages or articles in categories called newsgroups.

user domain: The location address for everyone who uses that mail system. This part of the address functions like the home address of a person in postal service mail delivery.

UserID (or *user name*)**:** The public name you use to access a restricted resource such as an email system or network. No one else on that system will have the same UserID.

utilities: A group of software programs that help with the management or maintenance of the computer and protection of the computer from unwanted intrusion.

vector graphic: An image created with lines, arcs, circles, and squares. This file format stores images as vector points. Examples include CGM and PGL.

version: Unique numbers (sometimes names) assigned to software programs as they are revised; the interface, commands, and functions can change with each version.

video camera: An input device that an operator uses to capture video.

video conferencing: Conference involving a computer, video camera, microphone, and speakers. Along with broadcasting audio, whatever images appear in front of the video camera are delivered to the participant's monitor. A "virtual" conference can involve two participants or many.

View tab: The groups included in this tab allow you to view the document in print layout, full screen reading, Web layout, outline, or draft form.

virtual classroom: A digital learning environment that exists solely online. The content is stored, accessed, and exchanged through networked computer and information systems.

virtual keyboard: A software component that permits the user to type on an optical-detectable surface instead of pressing physical keys.

virus: Small malicious programs or scripts that can negatively affect the health of your computer by creating, moving or erasing files; consuming memory; and causing the computer to function incorrectly.

virus definition: The signature file used to ensure that your computer can detect the newest viruses.

voice over Internet Protocol (VoIP): Technology that makes it possible to transmit voice or sound via the Internet.

Using this protocol, your voice is converted into a digital signal that travels over the Internet.

Web 1.0: The first generation of Web utilization, which refers to static information.

Web 2.0: The second generation of Web utilization. This term does not refer to a change in technology, but rather a change in how Web technology and applications are being creatively used to enhance and expand information sharing, communication, and collaboration.

webcam: A digital camera used to transmit the images over the Internet.

webinar: An interactive presentation, lecture, workshop, or seminar delivered over the Internet.

Web browser: A software program that is used to display Web pages on the World Wide Web.

Web browser security settings: Protection that can include a phishing filter, a pop-up blocker, notification that a Web site is trying to download files or software onto your computer, and notification if a program's digital signature is current and correct when you are trying to download a program or files.

Web servers: Computers that hold information that users request, then process the request, and then make them available to the end user.

What-if Analysis: A set of tools that permits you to predict or test future results by manipulating some variables.

wide area network (WAN) (see also *Metropolitan Area Network* or *MAN*)**:** A high-speed network that covers a large geographic distance. The best example of a WAN is the Internet, which uses the Transmission Control Protocol/Internet Protocol (TCP/IP) communications standard.

Wi-Fi (wireless fidelity): A communications protocol used by wireless devices.

wiki: A Web page or a collection of Web pages that can be viewed and modified by anyone who has access to a browser and the Internet. One of the most commonly used wikis is Wikipedia, an online editable encyclopedia.

window: A place on the desktop where the contents of an application, files, or folders, are displayed.

Windows Logo key: Displays or hides the Start menu.

Wireless Application Protocol (WAP): A standard used by mobile devices, such as smartphones, when they are communicating with Internet services.

wireless card: A card that fits into a computer slot, which permits the computer to access a wireless network via radio-based connection.

wireless connection: A connection that employs a microwave dish, generally located outside the house.

wireless home network: Part of the broadband services that many telecommunications companies offer. Each computer or device that connects to the wireless network must have a wireless network card or built-in wireless networking capabilities.

wireless local area network (WLAN): A network that does not use wires for communication between the "server" and the client computer or mobile device. Most WLANs physically connect to a LAN for the purpose of accessing resources on the LAN.

wireless modem: A device with an external or built-in antenna for use with mobile devices such as laptops and cell phones. Some mobile phones, smartphones, and PDAs can function as data modems.

wireless router: A fiber-optic connection that relies on a wireless router to provide the connectivity between the computer, phone wire, and fiber-optic panel.

wisdom: In health care, ethical decision making that ensures cost-effective quality care requires more than an empirical knowledge base. Knowing when and how to use this knowledge is referred to as wisdom.

wizard: A step-by-step process that guides you through the creation of a document or file.

word processing software: A program that permits the creating, editing, formatting, storing, and printing of text. Most include spelling and grammar checkers.

word wrap: A setting that automatically carries words over to the next line if they extend beyond the margin.

workbook (or *notebook*)**:** A collection of spreadsheet pages. Workbook pages are called worksheets in most programs.

worksheet (or *spreadsheet*)**:** A file made up of labels (letters), values (numbers), lines or borders, and formulas. It can also contain charts, illustrations, tables, links, and special text like WordArt and text boxes.

workstation: A desktop computer, but with more power, memory, and enhanced capabilities for performing specialized tasks.

World Wide Web (WWW) (or *the Web*)**:** The part of the Internet that stores graphical electronic files, called Web pages, on servers that are accessed from the user's computer.

Worldwide Interoperable Microwave Access (WiMAX): A network that includes use of wireless towers.

worm: A destructive program that can fill various memory locations of a computer system with information, clogging the system so that other operations are compromised.

***x*-axis:** Horizontal reference lines or coordinates of a graph.

***y*-axis:** Vertical reference lines or coordinates of a graph.

zoom: A view setting that allows you to examine part of a document more closely or to see a complete page of the document at once.

Index

Note: Page numbers followed by *b*, *f*, or *t* indicate material in boxes, figures, or tables, respectively.

E

F

O

P

Q

R

U

V

W